W9-DDP-659

The Practice of Nursing Research: Conduct,
Critique, and Utilization

Burns, N. & Grove, S.

THE PRACTICE OF NURSING RESEARCH

CONDUCT, CRITIQUE AND UTILIZATION

Nancy Burns, R.N., Ph.D.

Professor of Nursing
University of Texas
  at Arlington
School of Nursing
Arlington, Texas

Susan K. Grove, R.N., Ph.D.

Associate Professor of Nursing
University of Texas
  at Arlington
School of Nursing
Arlington, Texas

1987
W.B. SAUNDERS COMPANY
Philadelphia, London, Toronto, Sydney, Tokyo, Hong Kong

W. B. Saunders Company: West Washington Square
                          Philadelphia, PA 19105

Library of Congress Cataloging-in-Publication Data

Burns, Nancy, Ph. D.

The practice of nursing research: conduct, critique
and utilization.

1. Nursing—Research—Methodology.   I. Grove, Susan K.
   II. Title.   [DNLM: 1. Nursing.   2. Research.
   WY 20.5 B967p]

RT81.5.B86   1987   610.73′072   86–26136

ISBN 0–7216–1095–1

Editor: Dudley Kay
Developmental Editor: Alan Sorkowitz
Designer: W. B. Saunders Staff
Production Manager: Carolyn Naylor
Manuscript Editor: Ann Blum
Illustrator: Richard Burke
Illustration Coordinator: Walt Verbitski

The Practice of Nursing Research: Conduct, Critique and Utilization   ISBN   0–7216–1095–1

Last digit is the print number: 9   8   7   6   5   4   3   2   1

To my family:

To Jerry, my husband, whose love and support have made it possible for me to reach out for achievements beyond the expected.

To daughters Robin Bell and Melody Davidson, sons-in-law Ronnie Bell and Sam Davidson, and grandsons Brady Bell and Layton Davidson, who have endured my absence from our close family unit many times when they would have preferred my nearness.

Nancy

To my husband Jay Suggs for helping me make my dream a reality.

To Monece and Samantha, may your futures be full of dreams you desire to accomplish.

Susan

Preface

Our aim in developing this book is to create an excitement about research and a desire to search for knowledge through the performing of research. We recognize the increasing emphasis being placed on research and the development of a unique research tradition in nursing. Nursing research has become an integral part of baccalaureate education, graduate education and clinical practice. There is a growing interest in critiquing and utilizing research findings as well as in conducting research. Nurse researchers are conducting both quantitative and qualitative studies that reflect an increasing sophistication.

We believe that our text, a comprehensive book written by nurse researchers, can facilitate the movement of research into the mainstream of nursing. It incorporates a variety of unique strategies that (1) clarify the similarities and unique aspects of nursing research and emphasize the importance of a nursing practice background in conducting nursing research; (2) include a strong conceptual framework that links nursing research with theory, knowledge and nursing practice; (3) illustrate the development of the steps of the research process for quantitative and qualitative research strategies; and (4) provide numerous examples taken from actual clinical nursing research. The examples clearly illustrate points under discussion and demonstrate the direct connection between research and clinical practice.

Our text provides a comprehensive introduction to nursing research for undergraduate, graduate and practicing nurses. At the master's level, the text provides not only substantive content related to research but also practical applications based on the authors' experiences in conducting various types of nursing research, familiarity with the research literature and experience in teaching nursing research at various educational levels. In a baccalaureate program, in which research is a separate course at the upper division or senior level or in which the research content is integrated throughout the curriculum, this text can be used to direct the student's study of the entire field of nursing research (critique, utilization and conduct), or it can be used in a course that focuses primarily on critique and utilization. We also believe that the book will be a valuable resource for practicing nurses in critiquing and utilizing research findings and in conducting studies in clinical settings.

Our text is organized into four units, which contain 22 chapters. Unit I introduces the reader to the world of nursing research. The content and presentation of this unit has been designed to assist the reader in overcoming the barriers frequently experienced in understanding the language used in nursing research. This unit also includes a classification system of types of quantitative and qualitative research and introduces the reader to these two types of research. Unit II provides an in-depth discussion of the steps of the research process, including implications for both quantitative and qualitative strategies. The pragmatics for implementing the research process are presented in Unit III. Some of the information, such as suggestions for seeking funding and data collection strategies, has traditionally been communicated orally from experienced researchers to the neophyte researcher. Unit IV addresses the implications of research for nursing, including the critique process, utilization of research and future directions for research in nursing.

NANCY BURNS
SUSAN GROVE

Acknowledgments

Developing this book was a three-year project and there are many people that we would like to thank. We would like to express our appreciation to the Dean and faculty of the School of Nursing at the University of Texas at Arlington for their support during the long and sometimes tedious times that are inevitable in developing a book of this magnitude. We would also like to express gratitude to our students for the questions they have raised regarding the content of this text. The book was pilot tested over a two-year period as the basic text for an undergraduate nursing research course. Our students' interest and encouragement during this period were essential.

We would like to recognize the invaluable input from the many colleagues who provided blind reviews of the content:

Elsie Simms, R.N., Ph.D.
Northeast Missouri State University

Emily S. Tompkins, Ph.D., R.N., C.
Fairleigh Dickinson University

Jackie King, R.N., Ph.D.
Southeast Missouri State University

Barbara L. MacDermott, R.N., M.S.
Syracuse University

Patricia Bailey, R.N, Ed.D.
University of Scranton

Joan K. Austin, R.N., D.N.S.
Indiana University

Margaret T. Beard, R.N., Ph.D.
Texas Woman's University

Margaret Dimond, R.N., M.A., Ph.D.
University of Utah

Theresa M. Valiga, R.N., Ed.D.
Villanova University

Sally Decker, R.N., M.S.N.
Saginaw Valley State College

Sylvia Squires Britt, R.N., D.S.N.
Formerly University of Alabama School of Nursing

Patricia J. Morin, R.N., Ph.D.
Nebraska Wesleyan University

Frances M. Hicks, R.N., M.S., Ph.D.
University of Portland

Joan Thiele, R.N., Ph.D.
Intercollegiate Center for Nursing Education

Judith A. Floyd, R.N., Ph.D.
Wayne State University

Patricia Brugge-Wiger, R.N., Ph.D.
Minneapolis VA Medical Center

Brenda P. Haughey, R.N., Ph.D.
State University of New York at Buffalo

Lorna M. Facteau, R.N., D.N.Sc.
The Catholic University of America

Pat Mahon, R.N., Ph.D.
Texas Woman's University

Alene Harrison, R.N., M.S.
Wilkes College

We would also like to thank our editor, Dudley Kay, Publisher of Nursing and Allied Health; our developmental editor, Alan Sorkowitz; our copy editor, Ann Blum; and Al Beringer of the typesetting department at W. B. Saunders, who worked with us in a pilot project to typeset the text from computer disks. The support and guidance we received from these individuals throughout the development of this book was invaluable. A special thanks to Jay Suggs for the time and energy he spent in critiquing and editing the entire text and for his endless support.

Table of Contents

Chapter 3
Introduction to Quantitative Research 45

Chapter 4
Introduction to Qualitative Research 75

UNIT III
THE PRAGMATICS OF IMPLEMENTATION

Chapter 13
Proposal Writing for Research Approval

Chapter 14
Seeking Funding for Research

I

NURSING RESEARCH—
WHAT IS IT?

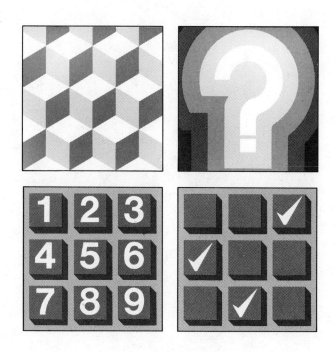

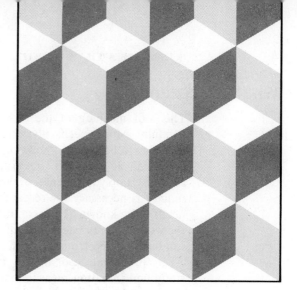

1

Introduction to the World of Nursing Research

Welcome to the world of nursing research. It may seem strange to consider research a "world," but it is truly a new way of experiencing reality. When entering a new world, a person must learn a unique language, incorporate new rules and use new experiences to learn how to effectively interact within that world. As one becomes a part of a new world, perceptions change and methods of reasoning are modified. To many nurses, nursing research is a relatively new world. To facilitate entry into this world, one needs a guide. We believe a guidebook such as this text can facilitate entry into the world of nursing research.

Initially, in any guidebook, it is necessary to broadly explain the world to be explored. That is the function of this chapter. A general definition of research is included, and the value of research to nursing is examined. The chapter concludes with the presentation of a framework that connects nursing research to the rest of nursing. This framework introduces concepts and relationships that are further developed throughout the text.

3

What Is Research?

The root meaning of the word *research* is to search again or to examine carefully. More specifically, research is diligent, systematic inquiry or investigation to validate old knowledge and generate new knowledge. The concepts *systematic* and *diligent* are critical to the meaning of research. These two concepts imply planning, organization and persistence. Systematic, diligent inquiry is necessary for researchers to address the following questions: What needs to be known? How can it best be measured? How can other elements of the world be prevented from interfering with this measurement? What meaning can be extracted from these measurements?

Investigation or inquiry in research involves systematically designing a study and initiating measurement. The data obtained from measurement are then analyzed to produce findings. Interpreting the findings and linking the findings from many studies help to explain nursing phenomena. These activities—questioning, planning, observing, analyzing and explaining—are the elements of the research process. This process facilitates the discovery of knowledge or the verification of present world views. Nursing research and the research process are discussed further in Chapter 2.

Why Is Research Necessary?

Research is essential to the development of any profession. Through research, a scientific body of knowledge is generated and theories are developed and tested. The knowledge and theories generated through nursing research are necessary to provide a scientific basis for planning, predicting and controlling the outcomes of nursing practice. The development of a scientific basis for practice through research can lead to professional accountability.

GENERATING A KNOWLEDGE BASE

The primary goal of nursing research is to develop a scientific knowledge base for nursing practice. At the present time, our knowledge base has evolved primarily from beliefs, common sense, intuition and past experiences that have developed into rules (Gortner, 1980a). In very few cases can a particular nursing action be justified by referring to nursing research findings. Seldom has nursing research been used to demonstrate that a particular nursing intervention is the most effective means of treating a person with a particular nursing diagnosis.

Dependence on research conducted by other disciplines is no solution to our problems. For example, in the past, nurses have tended to learn primarily the medical knowledge base in order to assist the physician in medical practice. Some nurses have considered nursing practice to be secondary to medical practice, and even have trouble distinguishing between nursing practice and medical practice. One way to determine whether a particular segment of care is actually a component of nursing practice (and thus of interest to nursing research) is to evaluate the extent to which the nurse can make decisions and take actions related to that care. One of the consequences of using another discipline's orientation is that the focus shifts away from the nursing orientation. Nursing involves ways of seeing people and the world that are different from those of other sciences. Other scientists who study the same phenomena or situations may not look at them in the same way that nurses would. They may not see in them what nurses see because nursing has a different philosophy and different conceptual models than do other scientific disciplines.

Nursing has adopted a holistic view of humans and their environments. Holism is a philosophical perspective in which all characteristics of people and their environments are interrelated and to some degree inseparable. People are considered to be greater than the sum of their parts. This is an important idea from a researcher's point of view. From a holistic frame of reference, measurement and research can never give us the total picture. The whole is always greater than the part being studied and that part can never completely explain the whole. Therefore, we can expect great complexity and multidimensionality in the areas we study. Multiple variables will often have to be studied simultaneously, requiring complex statistical analyses. Interpreting findings in the light of our holistic perspective is not a simple task.

In nursing, we must identify our particular areas of concern, conduct our own research and use our own research strategies. As previously indicated, nursing, viewed from the nursing body of knowledge, sees the health situation from a different perspective than do other health professions. As our body of knowledge is strengthened through nursing research and theory development, this different perspective will become more evident (Newman, 1982).

DEVELOPING AND TESTING NURSING THEORIES

In order to be useful, information acquired through nursing research must be developed into nursing theories that describe, explain or predict nursing phenomena. Stray facts from a study are not useful alone. These facts must be linked together within the nursing knowledge base to form theories. The theories explain the meaning of the research findings. The theories must then be tested through further nursing research and then refined to enhance their usefulness in nursing practice. Of course, not all nursing theory will be originally developed from research findings. Sometimes the theory originates as an idea, and then research is conducted to test its accuracy. Either way, research has a role in further developing our theories (Bohny, 1980; Johnson, 1974).

BECOMING MORE ACCOUNTABLE

Generating a body of scientific knowledge and developing and testing theory through research is necessary to enhance accountability (Gortner, 1974). Broadly, nursing is accountable to society for providing quality care and for seeking ways to improve that care. More specifically, we are accountable to our clients. This accountability is reflected in our relationships with other health professionals and with the health institutions within which we practice.

A solid research base will provide evidence of the nursing actions necessary to provide effective nursing care. If we have little scientific predictability of the effect of our nursing actions, we cannot be held accountable for taking or not taking a specific action in a specific situation. Although nursing practice will always involve a degree of uncertainty, research can greatly reduce it.

The utilization of research will render the nurse more credible as an expert in nursing care and more powerful as a decision maker. As this occurs, control over nursing interventions and outcomes will increase, as will accountability. Credibility, power, control and accountability are all interrelated and are essential to the attainment of true professional status.

How Does Nursing Research Relate to the Rest of Nursing?

In exploring the world of nursing research, it is helpful to have a framework by which to establish connections between research and the various elements of nursing. A framework of the world of nursing is presented in the following pages, and this framework is used as an organizing model for the textbook. The framework demonstrates the idea that nursing research is not an entity disconnected from the rest of nursing but rather is influenced by and influences all other nursing activities. All elements and their relationships are illustrated in the model in Figure 1–1. The model is explained in the following sections, beginning with the most concrete elements and then moving to the more abstract components of nursing thought.

CONCRETE AND ABSTRACT THINKING

The model demonstrates that nursing thought flows along a continuum of concrete and abstract thinking. *Concrete thinking* is oriented toward and limited

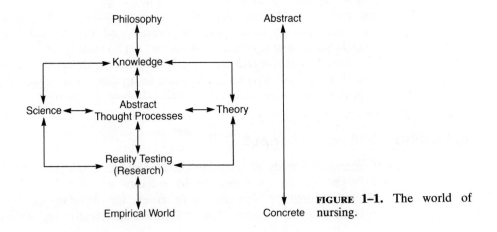

FIGURE 1–1. The world of nursing.

by tangible things or events that are observed and/or experienced in reality. The focus of concrete thinking is immediate events that are limited by time and space.

In the past, nursing was seen as a doing profession rather than as a thinking profession. The nurse was expected to do the work, not to ask why. Therefore, nurses tended to be very concrete, "practical" thinkers. This type of thinking and behavior was valued and rewarded. Problem solving was considered important only if the effect was immediate. The rudiments of this set of values are still present in nursing. Our basic nursing education is designed primarily using concrete thinking. Therefore, nurses tend to be unskilled in abstract thinking and even slightly fearful of it.

Abstract thinking is oriented toward the development of an idea without application to, or association with, a particular instance. Abstract thinkers tend to look for meaning, patterns, relationships and philosophical implications. This type of thinking is independent of time and space. In the past, the nurse who was able to think in abstract ways was often considered a "dreamer," with her head in the clouds. Such a nurse was not considered a "good nurse," and great effort was expended to try to suppress this type of thinking. In other words, nurses were often punished for thinking abstractly; this still happens occasionally today.

Nursing research requires skills in both concrete and abstract thinking. Abstract thought is required to identify researchable problems, to design studies and to interpret findings. Concrete thought is necessary in both planning and conducting studies. This back-and-forth flow between abstract and concrete thought may be one reason why nursing research seems so "foreign." In more recent years, activities involving abstract thinking, such as theory development and research, have been achieving a greater prominence in nursing and are becoming more accepted.

The Empirical World

The empirical world is experienced through our senses and is the concrete portion of our existence. It is what is often called reality. "Doing" kinds of activities are part of the empirical world. There is a sense of certainty about the real world; it seems predictable, controllable, understandable. It appears to have more substance to it than do ideas, and it feels safe and secure.

Concrete thinking is focused on the empirical world. Words associated with concrete thinking in the empirical world include practical, down to earth, solid and factual. The concrete thinker wants facts. Whatever he or she knows must be immediately applicable to the current situation.

The practice of nursing takes place in the empirical world, as demonstrated in the model. Some components of the research process also take place in the empirical world. For example, research ideas, which are developed into research problems, are primarily derived from the empirical world. Data collection involves the actual measuring of some aspect of the empirical world (measurement of reality). For example, a yardstick and a weight scale are among the truest means of measuring reality. Research findings are utilized in clinical practice, which is also within the empirical world.

Reality Testing

We tend to validate or test the reality of our existence through our senses. In everyday activities, we constantly check out the messages received from our senses. For example, "Am I really seeing what I think I am seeing?" Sometimes our senses can play tricks on us. This is why we have developed instruments to more accurately record our sensory experiences. For example, does the patient just feel hot or does he have a fever? We have thermometers to test this sensory perception more accurately.

Research is a way of validating reality. This measurement of reality is done in terms of the researcher's perception. For example, the researcher might ask: "Do patients consume more oxygen when they use a bedside commode than when they use a bedpan?" Our senses would tell us that getting up on a bedside commode would use more oxygen. Nursing research indicates that this may not be true (Winslow, Lane & Gaffney, 1984). Thus, nursing research is a way of testing reality—a way of getting a better "handle" on what really goes on in the empirical world.

Abstract Thought Processes

Abstract thinking is particularly important in research. In research, we must consider not only what we see but also the meaning behind what we see. Examining meaning requires abstract thought. For example, we make clinical observations (requiring concrete thinking) to which we attach meaning, and that provides us with an idea (abstract thinking) for a research study. After we have collected research data (using concrete thought), our next question is "What does it mean?" Answering this question moves us again into abstract thought.

Abstract thinking is a key process in every element of the nursing world. In a sense, it links all the elements together. Without skills in abstract thought, a person is trapped in a flat existence in the empirical world, an existence in which that world can be experienced but not understood (Abbott, 1952). It is through abstract thinking that theories (which explain our nursing world) can be tested and moved into the body of science. Abstract thinking allows scientific findings to be developed into theories. It allows both science and theories to be blended into a cohesive body of knowledge, guided by a philosophic framework, and applied in clinical practice. Abstract thinking is actually more useful in clinical practice than one might think. For example, it is the abstract thinker who will recognize patterns in the incidence of infection in patients receiving a specific treatment and who will contemplate ideas about the relationships between the infection and other elements of the patient's care.

There are three major abstract thought processes: introspection, intuition and reasoning (Silva, 1977). These thought processes are important in practicing nursing, developing and evaluating theory, understanding and using scientific findings, planning and implementing research and adding to nursing's body of knowledge.

INTROSPECTION

Introspection is a process of turning your attention inward toward your own thoughts. It occurs at two levels. At the more surface level, you are aware of the thoughts you are experiencing. You have an increased awareness of the flow and interplay of feelings and ideas that occur in constantly changing patterns. These thoughts or ideas can rapidly fade from view and disappear if they are not quickly written down. Sometimes they surface and then slip away so fast and in such rapid succession that it is impossible to write them down. One trick that sometimes works to avoid losing these important thoughts is to jot down key words for each idea.

When introspection is allowed to occur in more depth, thoughts are examined more critically and in detail. Patterns or links between thoughts and ideas emerge, and you may recognize fallacies or weaknesses in your thinking. You may question what brought you to this point in your thinking and find yourself really enjoying the experience.

Imagine the following clinical situation. You have just left John Brown's home. John has a colostomy and has been receiving home health care for several weeks. Although John is caring for his colostomy, he is still reluctant to leave home for any length of time. You experience feelings of irritation and frustration with this situation. You begin thinking back over your nursing actions and recalling other clients who have reacted in similar ways. What were the patterns of their behavior?

You have an idea—perhaps the patient's behavior is linked to the level of family support. You feel unsure about your ability to help the patient and family deal with this situation effectively. You recall other nurses describing similar reactions of patients and wonder just how many of the patients with colostomies have this problem. Your thoughts jump to reviewing the charts of other patients with colostomies and reading relevant ideas discussed in the literature. Some research has been conducted on this topic recently, and you could critique the findings for use in practice. If the findings are inadequate, perhaps other nurses would be interested in studying this situation with you.

INTUITION

Intuition is an awareness or knowing that seems to come unbidden. It is a feeling or sense that usually cannot be logically explained. It may be described as a "gut feeling" or a "hunch." Because intuition cannot be "scientifically" explained with ease, many people are uncomfortable with it. Some even say that it does not exist. So, sometimes, the feeling or sense is pushed down, ignored or dismissed as "silly." But intuition is not the lack of knowing. It is rather a result of "deep" knowledge—tacit knowing or personal knowledge

(Polanyi, 1962, 1966; Silva, 1977). The knowledge is incorporated so deeply within that it is difficult to consciously bring it to the surface. Thus, intuitive knowledge cannot easily be expressed in a logical manner (Benner, 1984; Beveridge, 1950; Kaplan, 1963).

Intuition is generally considered unscientific and unacceptable for use in research. And, in some instances, that concern is valid. For example, a "hunch" that there is a significant difference between one set of scores and another set of scores is not particularly useful as a final measure. But, however unexplainable that intuition is, it has some important scientific uses. One does not always need to be able to explain something in order to be able to use it. A burst of intuition may identify a problem for study, indicate important variables to measure or link two ideas together in the interpretation of findings. The trick is to recognize the feeling, value it and hang on to the idea long enough to consider it.

Imagine the following situation. You have been working in an outpatient cardiac rehabilitation unit for the last 3 years. You and two other nurses working on the unit have been meeting with the clinical nurse specialist to plan a study to determine the factors important in patients' responses to the rehabilitation program. The group has met several times with a nursing professor at the university who is working with the group to develop the study. At present, the group is concerned with identifying the factors that need to be measured and how to measure them.

You have had a busy morning. Mr. Green, a patient, stops by to chat on his way out of the clinic. He chats and you listen, but not attentively. Then you become more acutely aware of what he is saying. While listening, you begin to have a feeling about one variable that should be studied. You cannot really explain the origin of this feeling. You cannot identify any specific thing that Mr. Green said that triggered the idea, but somehow the flow of words stimulated a burst of intuition. The variable you have in mind has not been previously studied. You feel both excited and uncertain. What will the other nurses think? If it has not been studied, is it really significant? But somehow you feel that it is important to consider.

REASONING

Reasoning is thinking that links ideas together in order to reach conclusions. It is through reasoning that we "make sense" of both our thoughts and our experiences. This thinking is often evident in the verbal presentation of a logical argument in which each part is linked together to reach a logical conclusion. Reasoning is used to develop theories, solve problems and interpret research findings. Specific patterns of reasoning are described in Chapter 2.

Reasoning is used in the following example. You are working in a nursing home and are presently meeting with two nurses from the local home health care agency. The three of you are discussing the findings from a study that examined the satisfaction of caregivers providing home care for the elderly (Worcester & Quayhagen, 1983). The group's intent is to prevent premature admission of the elderly to the nursing home. To prevent premature admissions, the study recommended that the family caregiver of the elderly be provided with support in three areas: handling psychological and behavioral problems, communicating with physicians and seeking temporary caregivers.

You reason that if a community support group could be developed, family caregivers would be able to meet regularly with nurses to consider ways to manage problems. The nursing home would be a good site for the meeting. You propose that families who had help from a home health nurse or the support group would be less likely to seek early admission of their elder family member to the nursing home. The home health care nurse argues that the most important action is to gather a list of available home health aides, because a support group will not help if the caregiver is getting inadequate help at home. You agree. The group concludes that both activities would tend to decrease early nursing home admission.

Science

Science is a coherent organization of research findings and tested theories related to a specific field of knowledge. Science is both a product and a process. For example, within physics is Newton's Law of Gravity, which was developed through extensive research. The knowledge of gravity (product) is a part of the science of physics that evolved through formulating and testing theoretical ideas (process). The science of a field determines the accepted process for obtaining knowledge within that field. Research is an accepted process for obtaining scientific knowledge.

Some sciences will rigidly limit the types of research that can be used to obtain knowledge. The acceptable method for developing a science is the traditional research process (quantitative research). According to this process, the information gained from one study is not sufficient for its inclusion in the body of science. The study must be repeated several times and must show the same results each time before that information can be considered a "fact." Consider the research on the relationship between smoking and lung cancer. Numerous studies of animals and humans have been done, and the findings all indicate a relationship between smoking and lung cancer, although certainly not everyone who smokes develops lung cancer. Enough research has been done so that it is now considered a "fact" that smoking is a major factor in the development of lung cancer.

"Facts" from research are systematically related to each other in a way that seems to best explain our empirical world. Abstract thought processes are used to make these linkages. The linkages are called *laws*, *principles* or *axioms*, depending on the certainty of the facts and relationships within the linkage. The certainty is dependent on the amount of research conducted to test it and to some extent on skills in abstract thought processes. The "truths" or explanations of the empirical world reflected by these laws, principles and axioms are never absolutely certain and may be disproved by further research.

The ultimate goal of science is to be able to explain the empirical world and, thus, to have increased control over it. In order to accomplish this, the aims of science are to discover new knowledge, expand existing knowledge and reaffirm previously held knowledge (Andreoli & Thompson, 1977).

Science has been developed using predominantly quantitative research methods. However, in the last 20 years, there has been an increasing interest in developing a qualitative research tradition. Qualitative research is based on a different philosophical orientation toward reality than quantitative research. Within the qualitative research tradition, many of the long held tenets about science and ways of obtaining knowledge are being questioned. The philosophical orientation of qualitative research is holistic, and the purpose of this research is examining the whole rather than the parts. Qualitative researchers are more interested in obtaining understanding of complex phenomena than in determining cause-and-effect relationships among specific variables.

Nursing is in only the beginning stages of developing a science (Greene, 1979). Little research and very little replication of studies have been conducted. Major studies with findings significant to nursing practice must be replicated. If researchers repeatedly find the same results each time they replicate a study, they become increasingly certain that they are accurately describing the empirical world. The cluster of findings from replicated research then becomes a part of science. Nursing science must be developed on a broad base with the utilization of a variety of research methods, both qualitative and quantitative. These research methods are described in Chapter 2. Nursing research must search for meaning as well as facts to support the holistic perspective (Munhall, 1982).

Theory

A theory is a way of explaining some segment of the empirical world. It is an expression of a perception of a part of the empirical world (Dubin, 1978). For example, Selye developed a theory about stress; Freud, a theory of human personality; and Maslow, a theory about needs. A theorist develops a theory from a combination of personal experiences, research findings and abstract thought processes.

Nursing theories provide a framework for practicing nursing. Roy's (1984) theory proposes that the nursing role is to help the patient adapt. Orem's (1985) theory indicates that the nurse's role is to help the client achieve self-care. Rogers' (1970) theory suggests that the nurse's role is to help man reach his fullest potential. Theories are as important as science and become a part of science when they have been adequately tested. Because theories are so important to research, their use in research is discussed further in Chapter 7.

A theory may be developed in one of two ways. Findings from research may be used as a starting point, with the theory emerging as the theorist organizes the findings to best explain the empirical world. Or the theorist may use abstract thought processes and personal knowledge or intuition to explain some phenomenon. The theory is then tested by research to validate the theorist's ideas. In nursing, more progress has been made in developing nursing theories than in developing a scientific body of knowledge.

All research has the effect of either developing theory or testing theory, with or without the conscious intent of the researcher. However, most nursing research currently being conducted is designed to test theories other than nursing theories. Nursing is reaching a point of theory development that will allow testing. Since nursing research is examining phenomena of interest to practice, conceptual ideas from the non-nursing theories may eventually be incorporated into nursing theories.

The Relationship Between Science and Theory

Science and theory are different and yet very dependent on one another. They both require the use of abstract thought processes. The purpose of each is to promote understanding or "knowing" of the empirical world. Science is seen as being closer to "truth," whereas theory is associated with conjectures or possibilities. Science is thought of as being more certain than theory. People who favor a strong science tend to discount the value of theories, whereas those who stress the greater importance of theories tend to discount the wisdom of using scientific knowledge alone for adequate explanations of the empirical world (Benoliel, 1977).

Knowledge

Knowledge is a very complex concept and there are many facets of this concept. For example, we may say that we "know" our friend John, "know" how to give an injection, "know" that the earth rotates around the sun and "know" algebra. These are examples of knowing—being familiar with a person, acquiring a psychomotor skill, comprehending facts and mastering a subject. Knowing presupposes order or imposes order on thoughts and ideas (Engelhardt, 1980). Carper (1975, 1978) identifies four fundamental patterns of knowing in nursing: (1) empirical, (2) esthetic, (3) ethical and (4) personal. These patterns of knowing are discussed in Chapter 2.

There are differences in types of knowing, yet there are also similarities. People have a desire to know what to expect (Russell, 1948). There is a need in our world for certainty, and we seek it by trying to decrease uncertainty through knowledge (Ayer, 1966). Think of the questions you ask of a person related to some bit of knowledge. "Is it true?" "Are you sure?" "How do you know?" We have some expectations of what we consider knowledge. We expect knowledge to be an accurate reflection of reality that is more than opinion or belief. Experience, perception and memory play a role in knowledge but are not knowledge themselves. We seek to be "sure" by verifying our information, and one such way is research. Research is a means of validating our experiences, perceptions and memory. It is also a means of gaining proof for our beliefs and opinions.

Two additional expectations of knowledge are that it be acquired through acceptable means and that the person has a right to know (White, 1982). Acceptable routes include experience, education, abstract reasoning and access to authorities. The right to know involves recognition of the credibility of the person as an expert in a given area of knowledge. This recognition often comes from formal education in a particular field of knowledge that has been carefully generated through experience, theory development and scientific studies. For example, we would feel certain that we were getting accurate knowledge about the law of gravity from a physicist.

In nursing, a body of knowledge must be obtained (learned), incorporated and assimilated by each member of the profession and collectively by the profession as a whole. This body of knowledge guides the thinking and behavior of the profession and individual practitioners. It will guide the directions of further development and interpretation of science and theory in the field of nursing. Nursing's development of a body of knowledge will initially give us the confidence that we "know" what we are doing. This is the basis for recognition of nursing as a science by health professionals, consumers and society.

Philosophy

Philosophy provides a broad, global explanation of our world. It is the most abstract and all-encompassing concept in the model (see Fig. 1–1). Philosophy gives unity and meaning to our world and provides a framework within which our thinking, knowing and doing occur. Our philosophical position influences our knowledge. The way we use science and theories to explain the empirical world will depend on our philosophy. Ideas about truth and reality as well as beliefs, values and attitudes are part of philosophy. Philosophy asks such questions as "Is there an absolute truth or is truth relative?" "Is there one reality or is reality different for each individual?" "What is Man?" "What is Man's purpose in life?"

Our world is modified by our philosophy as a pair of glasses would modify our vision. Our perceptions are influenced first by our philosophy and then by our knowledge. If what we see or think is not within our ideas of truth or reality, if it does not "fit" our belief system, we may not "see" it. Our minds may reject it altogether or modify it to fit within our philosophy (Scheffler, 1967; Tucker, 1979).

Philosophical positions commonly held by the nursing profession include our view of human beings as holistic, rational and responsible. We believe that people desire health. Health is considered to be better than illness, life better than death. We consider quality of life to be important. Good nursing care is that care which facilitates improved patterns of health. In nursing, truth is seen as relative and reality tends to vary with perception (Silva, 1977).

Nursing's philosophical positions have a strong influence on our research (Baer, 1979; Ludemann, 1979). The research problems identified in nursing are a reflection of our philosophy. For example, our desire to find ways to measure quality of life reflects our philosophical concern with that idea. The designs of our studies are also influenced by our philosophy. For example, our holistic orientation requires study designs that measure multiple interacting variables such as coping abilities, social supports, attitudes and ego strength in the same study. Our need to understand holistic responses prompts us to use qualitative designs to explore meaning. The data collected and the way that data are collected are affected by our philosophy. Our philosophy will guide the interpretation of findings and the use of these findings in nursing practice.

Philosophy influences how we see the empirical world and how we interact with it. For example, because we believe that reality varies with perception and that truth is relative, we would not try to impose our views of truth and reality on clients. Rather, we would accept their view of the world and help them seek health from within their world view. The way the nurse relates to clients to produce health will be influenced by philosophy. For example, our view of people as rational, responsible individuals who desire health means that we assist clients to achieve their goals. We have no need to force unwilling persons to meet our goals rather than their own (Curtin, 1979). The care we provide is influenced by our philosophy. For example, we will provide care that is mutually agreeable and is oriented toward improving health.

In conclusion, the most abstract of our concepts (philosophy) links in a very direct and meaningful way with the most concrete concept, the empirical world. Within the model (see Fig. 1–1), all the elements interact; research is not off to the side, disconnected from the rest of nursing. In order to utilize nursing's body of knowledge in practice, one must incorporate all the elements of the nursing world. If one element is missing, the rest of the elements lose meaning. One cannot be only concrete, only abstract, only theoretical or only scientific. One cannot attend to only clinical practice and disregard the rest of the nursing world—not if one is a nurse in the whole sense of the word.

Summary

The intent of this chapter is to introduce the reader to the world of research. Research is defined as diligent, systematic inquiry to validate old knowledge and generate new knowledge. Research is essential to the development of any profession because it generates a scientific body of knowledge and develops and tests theories. Generating a body of knowledge for nursing through research is necessary to enhance accountability.

This chapter presents a framework for exploring the world of nursing research (see Fig. 1–1). This framework establishes connections between research and the various elements of nursing. The major elements of this framework, described from the most concrete to the most abstract, include concrete and abstract thinking, empirical world, reality testing, research, abstract thought processes, science, theory, knowledge and philosophy.

Nursing research requires skills in both concrete and abstract thinking. Concrete thinking is oriented toward tangible things or events. Abstract thinking is oriented toward the development of an idea without application to, or association with, a particular instance. The empirical world is the concrete portion of our existence experienced through our senses and is validated through reality testing. Research is a form of reality testing.

Abstract thought processes are particularly important in research because they involve examining meaning. Three types of abstract thought are described: introspection, intuition and reasoning. Abstract thought processes are necessary for the development of science. Science is a coherent organization of research findings and tested theories related to a specific field of knowledge. Theory is a way of explaining some segment of the empirical world. Theories are developed and tested through research, and when the theories are adequately tested, they become part of science.

Knowledge is generated through experience, theory development and scientific studies. In nursing, a body of knowledge must be obtained, incorporated and assimilated by each member of the profession and collectively by the profession as a whole. The most abstract element of the framework is philosophy. Philosophy gives unity and meaning to our world and provides a structure within which our thinking, knowing and doing occur. Nursing's philosophical positions, such as the holistic perspective, have a strong influence on our research. The framework demonstrates the idea that nursing research is not an entity disconnected from the rest of nursing but rather is influenced by and influences all other nursing activities. This framework provides an organizing model for this textbook.

REFERENCES

Abbott, E. A. (1952). *Flatland*. New York: Dover Publications, Inc.

Andreoli, K. G. & Thompson, C. E. (1977). The nature of science in nursing. *Image*, 9(2), 32–37.

Ayer, A. J. (1966). *The Problem of Knowledge*. Maryland: Penguin Books.

Baer, E. D. (1979). Philosophy provides the rationale for nursing's multiple research directions. *Image*, 11(3), 72–74.

Barnard, K. E. (1980). Knowledge for practice: directions for the future. *Nursing Research*, 29(4), 208–212.

Benner, P. (1984). *From novice to expert: excellence and power in clinical practice*. Menlo Park, California: Addison-Wesley Publishing Company.

Benoliel, J. Q. (1977). The interaction between theory and research. *Nursing Outlook*, 25(2), 108–113.

Beveridge, W. I. B. (1950). *The art of scientific investigation*. New York: Vintage Books.

Bohny, B. J. (1980). Theory development for a nursing science. *Nursing Forum*, 19(1), 50–67.

Carnegie, M. E. (1974). The shifting of research emphasis and investigators. *Nursing Research*, 23(3), 195.

Carper, B. A. (1975). *Fundamental patterns of knowing in nursing*. Unpublished doctoral dissertation, Teachers College, Columbia University, New York.

Carper, B. A. (1978). Fundamental patterns of knowing in nursing. *Advances in Nursing Science*, 1(1), 13–24.

Curtin, L. L. (1979). The nurse as advocate: a philosophical foundation for nursing. *Advances in Nursing Science*, 1(3), 1–10.

Donley, Sr. R. (1980). Why has nursing been slow in developing a theoretical base? *Image*, 12(1), 2.

Downs, F. S. & Fleming, W. J. (1979). *Issues in nursing research*. New York: Appleton-Century-Crofts.

Dubin, R. (1978). *Theory building* (rev. ed.). New York: The Free Press.

Engelhardt, H. T., Jr. (1980). Knowing and valuing: looking for common roots. In H. T. Engelhardt

& D. Callahan (Eds.), *Knowing and valuing: the search for common roots* (Vol. 4, pp. 1–17). New York: The Hastings Center.

Gortner, S. R. (1974). Scientific accountability in nursing. *Nursing Outlook*, 22(12), 764–768.

Gortner, S. R. (1975). Research for a practice profession. *Nursing Research*, 24(3), 193–197.

Gortner, S. R. (1980a). Nursing research: out of the past and into the future. *Nursing Research*, 29(4), 204–207.

Gortner, S. R. (1980b). Nursing science in transition. *Nursing Research*, 29(3), 180–183.

Greene, J. A. (1979). Science, nursing and nursing science: a conceptual analysis. *Advances in Nursing Science*, 2(1), 57–64.

Henderson, V. (1977). We've "come a long way," but what of the direction? *Nursing Research*, 26(3), 163–164.

Jacox, A. (1980). Strategies to promote nursing research. *Nursing Research*, 29(4), 213–218.

Johnson, D. E. (1974). Development of theory: a requisite for nursing as a primary health profession. *Nursing Research*, 23(5), 372–377.

Kaplan, A. (1963). *The conduct of inquiry*. New York: Harper & Row, Publishers.

Ludemann, R. (1979). The paradoxical nature of nursing research. *Image*, 11(1), 2–8.

Munhall, P. L. (1982). Nursing philosophy and nursing research: in apposition or opposition? *Nursing Research*, 31(3), 176–181.

Newman, M. A. (1982). What differentiates clinical research? *Image*, 14(3), 86–88.

Notter, L. E. (1975). The case for nursing research. *Nursing Outlook*, 23(12), 760–763.

O'Connell, K. A. & Duffey, M. (1976). Research in nursing practice: its nature and direction. *Image*, 8(1), 6–12.

Orem, D. E. (1985). *Nursing: concepts of practice* (3rd ed.). New York: McGraw-Hill Book Company.

Polanyi, M. (1962). *Personal knowledge*. Chicago: The University of Chicago Press.

Polanyi, M. (1966). *The tacit dimension*. New York: Doubleday & Company.

Rogers, M. E. (1970). *The theoretical basis of nursing*. Philadelphia: F. A. Davis Company.

Roy, Sr. C. (1984). *Introduction to nursing: an adaptation model* (2nd ed.). Englewood Cliffs, New Jersey: Prentice-Hall, Inc.

Russell, B. (1948). *Human knowledge, its scope and limits*. Brooklyn, New York: Simon and Schuster.

Scheffler, I. (1967). *Science and subjectivity*. Indianapolis: The Bobbs-Merrill Company, Inc.

Schlotfeldt, R. M. (1960). Reflections on nursing research. *American Journal of Nursing*, 60(4), 492–494.

Schlotfeldt, R. M. (1973). Planning for progress. *Nursing Outlook*, 21(12), 766–769.

Silva, M. C. (1977). Philosophy, science, theory: interrelationships and implications for nursing research. *Image*, 9(3), 59–63.

Stanford, E. D. (1980). Directions for research in nursing. *Nursing Research*, 29(4), 203.

Stevens, B. J. (1984). *Nursing theory: analysis, application, evaluation* (2nd ed.). Boston: Little, Brown and Company.

Swanson, J. M. & Chentiz, W. C. (1982). Why qualitative research in nursing? *Nursing Outlook*, 30(4), 241–245.

Toulmin, S. (1960). *The philosophy of science*. New York: Harper & Row, Publishers.

Tucker, R. W. (1979). The value decisions we know as science. *Advances in Nursing Science*, 1(2), 1–12.

Verhonick, P. J. (1971). Clinical investigations in nursing. *Nursing Forum*, 10(1), 80–88.

Walker, L. O. (1971). Toward a clearer understanding of the concept of nursing theory. *Nursing Research*, 20(5), 428–435.

White, A. R. (1982). *The nature of knowledge*. Totowa, New Jersey: Rowman and Littlefield.

Winslow, W. H., Lane, L. D. & Gaffney, F. A. (1984). Oxygen consumption and cardiovascular response in patients and normal adults during in-bed and out-of-bed toileting. *Journal of Cardiac Rehabilitation*, 4(8), 348–354.

Worcester, M. I. & Quayhagen, M. P. (1983). Correlates of caregiving satisfaction: prerequisites to elder home care. *Research in Nursing and Health*, 6(2), 61–67.

2

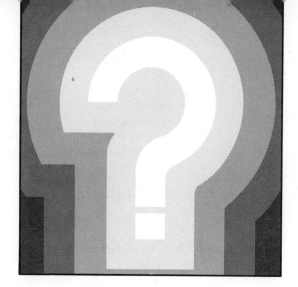

What is Nursing Research?

"What distinguishes nursing research from research in other disciplines?" This is a question that is often debated in nursing circles. In some ways, there is no difference, because the knowledge and skills required for research do not vary from one discipline to another. However, looking at a different dimension of research, there are distinctions. The research within any discipline must be consistent with the philosophical orientation and theories of that discipline. Therefore, nursing research must be consistent with nursing's philosophy and theories. Since the philosophical orientation and theories are gained through nursing education, the conduct of nursing research requires the involvement of a nurse.

The theoretical orientations and body of knowledge of a discipline define the variables for study, and the gaps in a discipline's body of knowledge determine what needs to be known. The gaps in nursing's body of knowledge determine what needs to be known for the practice of nursing. The congruence between what needs to be known, the philosophical orientation and theories define what is "nursing research."

In order to gain a true sense of nursing research, one must understand how nursing has historically acquired knowledge and how research has developed within the discipline. Knowledge of the scope of nursing research and the methods of scientific inquiry used to develop an empirical knowledge base for nursing are essential to explore "what is nursing research." This chapter describes the ways of obtaining knowledge in nursing; compares the research process, problem solving process and nursing process; describes the development of research in nursing; and identifies nursing research methods.

Ways of Obtaining Knowledge

If nursing is to be considered a science, a unique body of knowledge is required (Schlotfeldt, 1971; Gortner, 1974; Donaldson & Crowley, 1978; Feldman, 1981). A discipline's body of knowledge includes information, facts, principles and theories that are organized according to the beliefs accepted by the discipline at a given time. A body of knowledge is dynamic and constantly changes as new information is discovered. This body of knowledge is derived from the focus or unique perspective of the discipline and provides an organizing framework for the discipline's practice (McMurrey, 1982). For example, the unique body of knowledge that directs medical practice includes the information, facts, principles and theories of pathophysiology that are used in the diagnosis and treatment of disease.

The focus of nursing's unique body of knowledge includes the responses of the holistic person to health and illness as the person interacts with an everchanging environment. Nursing acts are implemented to promote the holistic person's health and to facilitate the person's growth toward his or her potential within the environment (Keller, 1981). Nursing has historically acquired knowledge through traditions, authority, borrowing, trial and error, intuition, personal experience, role-modeling, reasoning and research. These ways of obtaining knowledge are not separate and distinct; one way of obtaining knowledge influences and expands upon the other ways of obtaining knowledge.

TRADITIONS

Traditions include "truths" or beliefs that are based on customs and past trends. Traditions that were accepted from the past continue to influence the present practice of nursing; they have been transferred to the present by either written or oral communication. For example, many of the policy and procedure manuals in hospitals and other health care facilities contain traditional ideas; and nursing interventions are commonly transmitted orally from one nurse to another over the years. Traditions can positively influence nursing practice, because they were developed from effective past experiences of nurses. For example, the principle of hygiene currently used in practice is a product of Florence Nightingale's emphasis on a clean, safe environment.

However, traditions can also narrow and limit the knowledge sought for nursing practice. For example, nursing units are frequently organized and run according to set rules or traditions. Tradition has established the time and pattern for giving bed baths, taking vital signs, giving q.i.d. medications and selecting needle length for giving injections. The nurses on patient care units quickly inform new staff members about the accepted or "traditional" behaviors for the unit.

Traditions are very difficult to change because they have existed for long periods of time and are frequently supported by people with power and authority. Many traditions have not been evaluated or tested for accuracy or efficiency. However, even those traditions that have been disproved through research tend to persist. Nursing's body of knowledge must be more empirically than traditionally based.

AUTHORITY

An authority is a person with expertise and power who is able to influence opinion and behavior. A person is given authority because it is thought that she or he knows more in a given area than do others. Knowledge gained from authority is illustrated when one person credits another person as the source of information. Nurses who write books or develop theories are frequently considered authorities. Students view their instructors as authorities, and clinical nursing experts are considered authorities within clinical settings. To be considered a source of knowledge, authorities in nursing must have both expertise and power. The use of only power and control does not make someone an authority.

Many customs or traditional ways of knowing are maintained by authorities, but the knowledge obtained from authorities, like traditions, can be inaccurate. Like tradition, much of the knowledge gained from authorities has never been validated, and, although it may be useful, it must be verified through research.

BORROWING

Some nursing leaders have described part of nursing's knowledge as information borrowed from other disciplines such as medicine, sociology, psychology, education and business administration (Andreoli & Thompson, 1977; Paletta, 1980; Feldman, 1981; McMurrey, 1982). Borrowing in nursing involves the appropriation and use of knowledge from other fields or disciplines to guide nursing practice. Nursing has borrowed in two ways. For years, some nurses have taken information from other disciplines and applied it "directly" to nursing practice. This information was not integrated within the unique focus of nursing. For example, nurses have used the medical model as their primary knowledge base to guide their nursing practice, thus focusing on the diagnosis and treatment of disease.

Another way of borrowing, which is more acceptable in nursing, is the integration of information from other disciplines within the focus of nursing. Since disciplines share knowledge, it is sometimes difficult to know where the boundaries exist between nursing's knowledge base and those of other disciplines. There is a blurring of boundaries as the knowledge bases of disciplines evolve (McMurrey, 1982). For example, the knowledge of self-esteem is associated with the discipline of psychology but is important in providing nursing care to clients. Nurses use content on self-esteem in assessing the psychological needs of clients. However, borrowed knowledge has not been adequate for answering many questions that are generated in practice.

TRIAL AND ERROR

Trial and error is an approach with unknown outcomes used in a situation of uncertainty, where other sources of knowledge are unavailable. Since each client responds uniquely to a situation, there is uncertainty in nursing practice. Because of this uncertainty, nurses must use some trial and error in providing nursing care. However, with trial and error, there is frequently no formal documentation of effective and ineffective nursing actions. Using this strategy, knowledge is gained only from experience, and the knowledge gained is often not shared with other nurses. In addition, the trial and error way of obtaining knowledge can be time consuming, because nurses might have to try many interventions before they find one that is effective. The use of trial and error may even lead to the implementation of unsafe nursing actions.

INTUITION

Intuition, which was described in Chapter 1, is helpful to the individual nurse in providing nursing care but is difficult to communicate to other nurses. It has been the basis for many effective nursing actions in the past and continues to be so. However, some nurses claim that their actions are intuitive to avoid having to think or justify these actions. In nursing, there is a need to clarify the knowledge that has been obtained intuitively.

PERSONAL EXPERIENCE

Personal experience involves gaining knowledge by being personally involved in an event, situation or circumstance. In nursing, personal experience enables one to gain skills and expertise by providing care to patients and families in clinical settings. Nonverbal learning occurs during personal experience and enables the nurse to cluster (or chunk) ideas into a meaningful whole. For example, you may be told how to give an injection in a classroom setting, but you do not "know" how to give an injection until you observe other nurses giving injections to patients and you actually give several yourself.

The extent of personal experience has an effect on the complexity of a nurses's knowledge base. Benner (1982, 1983, 1984) identified five levels of experience to describe the development of clinical knowledge and expertise: (1) novice, (2) advanced beginner, (3) competent, (4) proficient and (5) expert.

Novice nurses have no personal experience in the work that they are to perform, but they have preconceived notions and expectations about clinical practice that are challenged, refined, confirmed or disconfirmed by personal experience in a clinical setting. The advanced beginner has just enough experience to recognize and intervene in recurrent situations. For example, the advanced beginning nurse is able to recognize and intervene to meet the hygiene and elimination needs of patients.

Competent nurses frequently have been on the job for 2 or 3 years, and their personal experiences enable them to generate and achieve long-range goals and plans. Through experience, the competent nurse is able to use personal knowledge to take conscious, deliberate actions that are more efficient and organized. From a more complex knowledge base, the proficient nurse views the patient as a whole and as a member of a family and community. The proficient nurse recognizes that each patient and each family respond differently to illness and health. The expert nurse in clinical practice has an extensive background of experience and is able to accurately identify and skillfully intervene in a situation. Personal experience increases an expert nurse's ability to intuitively grasp a situation with accuracy and speed.

With an adequate knowledge base developed through research, an increasing number of nurses can attain the expert level in clinical practice. The dynamics of expert nursing practice need to be clarified through nursing research. In addition, the transmission of expertise from one nurse to another needs to be described and utilized in developing effective methods for nursing education.

ROLE-MODELING

Role-modeling is learning by imitating the role and behaviors of an exemplar. The role model is viewed as knowing the appropriate and rewarded roles for a profession; these roles include the standards and norms of behavior (Erickson, Tomlin & Swain, 1983). In nursing, role-modeling enables the novice nurse to learn through interaction with or examples set by highly competent nurses. Examples of role models are "admired teachers, practitioners, researchers or illustrious individuals who inspire students through their examples" (Werley & Newcomb, 1983, p. 206).

An intense form of role-modeling is mentorship. In mentorship, the expert nurse serves as a teacher, sponsor, guide, exemplar and counselor for the novice nurse (Vance, 1982). In a mentor–mentee relationship, there is an investment of time and a mutual exchange of ideas and aspirations relative to the mentee's career plans. The mentee assumes the values, attitudes and behaviors of the mentor while gaining intuitive knowledge and personal experience.

REASONING

Reasoning is processing and organizing knowledge for application to selected situations in order to reach conclusions. These conclusions are then integrated into one's knowledge base. Different patterns of reasoning provide the organization for the development of theory and research. Stevens (1984) identified four patterns of reasoning as being essential to nursing: (1) problematic, (2) operational, (3) dialectic and (4) logistic. One uses all four types of reasoning, but frequently one type of reasoning is more dominant than the others. Reasoning is also classified by the discipline of logic into inductive and deductive modes.

Problematic Reasoning

Problematic reasoning involves problem identification, identification of all factors influencing the problem and resolution of the problem situation. For example, the nurse uses problematic reasoning in the nursing process to identify actual and potential nursing diagnoses and to implement nursing interventions to resolve these problems. Problematic reasoning is evident in the identification of a researchable problem.

Operational Reasoning

Operational reasoning involves the identification and discrimination between many alternatives or viewpoints. The focus is on the process (debating alternatives) rather than on the resolution (Stevens, 1984). The nurse uses operational reasoning in developing realistic, measurable goals to be achieved by clients and families. Debating which data analysis techniques to use in research requires operational thought.

Dialectic Reasoning

Dialectic reasoning involves looking at situations in a holistic way. A dialectic thinker believes that the whole is greater than the sum of the parts and that the whole organizes the parts (Stevens, 1984). For example, a nurse using dialectic reasoning would view a client as more than and different from the sum of his or her biological, psychological and social behaviors. Dialectic reasoning also includes examining factors that are opposites and making sense of them by merging them into a single unit or idea which is greater than either alone. Analyzing the research literature and determining the current knowledge regarding a potential research problem requires dialectic reasoning.

Logistic Reasoning

Logistic reasoning is in some ways the opposite of dialectic reasoning. Logistic reasoning breaks the whole into parts that can be carefully examined, as can the relationships among the parts. A logical reasoner assumes that the whole is the sum of the parts and that the parts organize the whole (Stevens, 1984). For example, a patient states that he is cold, and the nurse logically examines the following parts and their relationships: (1) room temperature, (2) patient's temperature, (3) patient's clothing and (4) patient's activity. The room temperature is 65°F, the patient's temperature is 98.6°F and the patient is wearing lightweight pajamas and is drinking ice water. The patient is obviously cold because of external environmental factors. One way that logistic reasoning is used in research is to determine the subproblems.

Inductive and Deductive Reasoning

Logic is a science that involves valid ways of relating ideas to promote understanding. The aim of logic is to determine "truth" or to explain, predict and control (Kaplan, 1964). The science of logic deals with thought processes, such as concrete and abstract thinking, and methods of reasoning, such as logistic, inductive and deductive. Inductive and deductive reasoning are constantly used by everyone, although the choice of types of reasoning may not always be conscious (Kaplan, 1964). *Inductive reasoning* is reasoning from particular instances to a general premise or conclusion (Chinn & Jacobs, 1983). A premise or hypothesis is a statement of the proposed relationship between two or more variables. The following is an example of inductive reasoning:

Particular Instances

A headache is an altered level of health that is stressful.
A fractured bone is an altered level of health that is stressful.
A terminal illness is an altered level of health that is stressful.

General Premise

Therefore, all altered levels of health are stressful.

In this example, inductive reasoning is used to move from the specific instances of altered levels of health that are stressful to the general premise that all altered levels of health are stressful. Research is necessary to test whether each of these specific instances is valid or accurate. The testing of many different altered levels of health to determine whether they are stressful is necessary to confirm the premise that all types of altered health are stressful.

Deductive reasoning is reasoning from a general premise to a particular situation or conclusion (Chinn & Jacobs, 1983). The following is an example of deductive reasoning:

General Premise

All persons experiencing the loss of a close family member grieve.

Particular Situation

Mary Jones' husband died, therefore she grieves.

In this example, deductive reasoning is used to move from the general premise that all persons experiencing the loss of a close family member grieve to the particular situation in which one specific individual grieves over the loss of a specific close family member.

In logistic reasoning, premises are linked together to form conclusions. The conclusions generated are valid only if they are based on valid premises. For example:

General Premises

All health professionals are caring.
All nurses are health professionals.

Conclusion

All nurses are caring.

In this example, the premise that all health professionals are caring is not valid or an accurate reflection of reality. Research is a means to test and confirm a premise, so valid premises can be used as the basis of nurses' reasoning in practice.

Deduction is the common method of reasoning used in conducting traditional (quantitative) research. The aim of quantitative researchers is to reduce things to their parts and to study the parts, not the whole. Researchers are now conducting more qualitative studies that require inductive reasoning to understand the whole rather than to explain the parts. Nurse researchers must be skilled in both inductive and deductive reasoning.

RESEARCH

Nursing has obtained knowledge in different ways, which have positively influenced nursing practice. However, if nursing is to be accepted as a scientific discipline with a unique body of knowledge, much of our knowledge must be generated through research (Schlotfeldt, 1971; Silva, 1977; Notter, 1978; Barnard, 1980; Gortner, 1983). Researchers generate empirical knowledge by testing the real world. The knowledge developed from research can be used for description, explanation, prediction and control within the practice of nursing.

Description

Description involves identifying the nature and attributes of nursing phenomena but does not focus on the relationships of phenomena (Chinn & Jacobs, 1983). Through research, nurses are able to describe what already exists in nursing practice, discover new information or classify information for use in nursing. Studies identifying criteria for nursing diagnoses are a form of descriptive research (Kim & Moritz, 1982). Since nursing's knowledge base is relatively undeveloped, description is essential groundwork for studies that will focus on explanation, prediction and control.

Explanation

In explanation, the relationships among phenomena are clarified and the reasons "why" certain events happen are identified. For example, the etiologies and criteria of nursing diagnoses identified through descriptive research require further study. Theorists have developed tentative explanations of the relationships among the various criteria of a specific nursing diagnosis. The next step is to conduct explanatory research to test these proposed relationships and the relationships between etiologies and criteria. In addition, the relationships among nursing interventions and patient outcomes require examination through explanatory research.

Prediction

Through prediction, one can estimate the probability of a specific outcome in a given situation (Chinn & Jacobs, 1983). However, predicting an outcome does not necessarily enable one to modify the outcome. With predictive knowledge, nurses could anticipate the effects nursing interventions would have on patients and families. For example, predictive research on immobility might provide nurses with the knowledge to estimate the effects of prolonged bedrest but would not enable them to alter the outcome of bedrest.

Control

If one can predict the outcome of a given situation, the next step is to control or manipulate the situation to produce the desired outcome. Dickoff, James and Wiedenbach (1968) described control as the ability to write a prescription (prescriptive theory) to produce the desired results. Nurses could prescribe certain interventions to help clients achieve their goals. Nurses might prescribe exercise interventions to increase a patient's activity tolerance or prescribe therapeutic communication and empathy to help a patient and family cope with their fears of death. Few studies have developed knowledge that is useful for prediction and control in the practice of nursing. Expanding research activities will provide the empirical knowledge needed for description, explanation, prediction and control of phenomena within the practice of nursing.

Problem-Solving Process Background—
Relevance for Research

Research is a process and is similar in some ways to other processes. Therefore, the background in the problem-solving process and nursing process, acquired early in nursing education, is useful in research. Relating the research process to these processes can be helpful in assisting the beginning researcher to use familiar ways of thinking to facilitate the incorporation of new skills and knowledges.

A process includes a purpose, a series of actions and a goal. The purpose provides direction to the process, and the series of actions are organized into steps to achieve an identified goal. A *process* is continuous and can be revised and/or reimplemented in order to reach an endpoint or goal. There are three processes of particular interest to nursing: (1) problem-solving process, (2) nursing process and (3) research process (Table 2–1).

Comparison of the Problem-Solving Process
and the Nursing Process

The problem-solving process is the systematic identification of a problem, determination of goals related to the problem, identification of possible solutions to achieve those goals, implementation of selected solutions and evaluation of goal achievement. Problem-solving is frequently used in daily activities and in nursing practice. For example, you use problem solving when selecting clothing, deciding where to live and communicating with a patient.

TABLE 2–1
Comparison of the Problem-Solving Process, Nursing Process
and Research Process

Problem-Solving Process	Nursing Process	Research Process

Data collection	Assessment
	    Data collection
	    Data interpretation
		Knowledge of the world of
		    nursing

Problem definition	Nursing diagnosis	Problem identification

Plan
    Goal setting
    Identify solutions
	Plan
	    Goal identification
	    Planned interventions
		Design—methodology

Implementation	Implementation	Data collection and analy- sis
Evaluate and revise process	Evaluation and modification	Outcomes

The nursing process is a subset of the problem-solving process (Table 2–1). The steps of the nursing process are assessment, nursing diagnosis, plan, implementation, evaluation and modification. Assessment involves the collection and interpretation of data for the development of nursing diagnoses. Nursing diagnoses are developed through reasoning from data provided by assessment. These diagnoses provide direction to the remaining steps of the nursing process, just as the step of defining the problem directs the remaining steps of the problem-solving process. The planning step in the nursing process is the same as the problem-solving process. Both processes involve implementation, or putting the plan into action. The final step in both processes is evaluation, which involves determining the effectiveness of the process. The problem-solving process and the nursing process are cyclic. If the process is not effective, all steps are reviewed and revised (modified), and the process is reimplemented.

COMPARISON OF THE NURSING PROCESS AND THE RESEARCH PROCESS

There are important similarities and differences between the nursing process and the research process. The similarities between these two processes are that both involve abstract, critical thinking and complex reasoning. Thus, these processes are not an automatic or rote application of steps. Through the nursing process and research process, one is able to make connections or discover relationships among phenomena. In these two processes, information is gathered, observations are made, problems are identified, plans are developed (design) and actions are taken (data collection and analysis) (Blumer, 1969). Both processes are reviewed for effectiveness and efficiency—the nursing process is evaluated, and outcomes are determined in the research process (Table 2–1). These processes are iterative and spiraling, which means that implementing them expands the user's knowledge. In addition, process utilization leads to change in the user, resulting in greater complexity in future use.

The research process and the nursing process also have definite differences. Knowledge of the nursing process is not sufficient to enable one to conduct the research process. The research process is more complex and requires the understanding of a unique language and the rigorous application of a variety of research methods.

The research process has a broader focus. In the nursing process, assessment focuses on a specific client and family and the nurse's perceptions of them. In the research process, there is a need to be aware of and knowledgeable about the world of nursing in order to identify the phenomena requiring investigation. This knowledge of the world of nursing helps to clarify what area one desires and is qualified to study.

The nursing process and the research process differ in purpose. The nursing process organizes and directs the provision of care to specific clients. The purpose of the research process is more general. The conduct of the research process requires greater precision, rigor and control than the implementation of the nursing process. The outcomes from research are frequently shared with a larger number of nurses, and they have the potential to create a lasting impact on nursing practice.

Nursing Research—Past and Present

Reviewing the history of nursing research enables one to better understand the present status of research in nursing. Some people think that research is new to nursing, but Florence Nightingale initiated nursing research more than 100 years ago. Following the work of Nightingale (1850–1910), research received minimal attention until the 1950s. Since then, the value placed on research has gradually increased. However, few nurses had the educational background to conduct studies until the 1970s. Table 2–2 identifies the key historic events influencing nursing research.

FLORENCE NIGHTINGALE

Florence Nightingale was described as a reformer, reactionary and researcher. Her research has influenced health care in general, and nursing more specifically. Nightingale's (1859) initial research activities are found in her notes on nursing. She discussed the importance of a healthy environment in promoting the physical and mental well-being of a patient. She identified the need to gather data on the environment (ventilation, cleanliness, temperature, purity of water and diet) to determine the influence on patients' health (Herbert, 1981).

Nightingale is most noted for her data collection and statistical analyses during the Crimean War. She gathered data on soldier morbidity and mortality and the factors influencing them. Her statistical data were clearly presented in tables and pie diagrams, a very sophisticated type of data presentation for this time period (Palmer, 1977).

Nightingale's research enabled her to instigate attitude, organization and social change. She changed the attitudes of the military and society toward the

TABLE 2–2
Historical Events Influencing Nursing Research

1850	Nightingale, First Nurse Researcher
1897	Nurses' Associated Alumnae
	(Renamed American Nurses' Association in 1911)
1900	American Journal of Nursing (first published)
1952	Nursing Research (first published)
1953	Institute of Research and Service in Nursing Education
1955	American Nurses' Foundation
1956	ANA Committee on Research and Studies
1956	Hughes Study, Nursing Functions and Activities
1957	Southern Regional Educational Board (SREB)
	Western Interstate Commission on Higher Education in Nursing (WICHEN)
	New England Board of Higher Education (NEBHE)
1963	International Journal of Nursing Studies (first published)
1965	ANA Sponsored Nursing Research Conferences
1967	Image (Sigma Theta Tau Publication) (first published)
1970	ANA Commission on Nursing Research
1971	ANA Council of Nurse Researchers
1978	Research in Nursing and Health (first published)
	Advances in Nursing Science (first published)
1979	Western Journal of Nursing Research (first published)

care of the sick. The military began to view the sick as having the right to adequate food, suitable quarters and appropriate medical treatment. She improved the organization of army administration, hospital management and hospital construction. Because of Nightingale's influence, society began to accept the responsibility for testing public water, improving sanitation, preventing starvation and decreasing morbidity and mortality (Cook, 1913; Palmer, 1977).

EARLY 1900s

From 1900 to 1950, research activities were limited, but there were a few studies that advanced nursing education. Some of these studies were the Nutting Report, 1912; Goldmark Report, 1923; and Burgess Report, 1926 (Abdellah, 1972; Johnson, 1977). In 1900, the *American Journal of Nursing* was first published, and late in the 1920s and 1930s, case studies began appearing in this journal. Case studies involve an in-depth analysis and/or systematic evaluation of an individual patient or a group of similar patients to promote understanding of nursing interventions. These case studies were the beginning of practice-related research and are a valuable means of identifying nursing research problems and selecting methods to investigate them.

A research trend that started in the 1940s and continued in the 1950s focused on the organization and delivery of nursing services. Studies were conducted on the numbers and kinds of nursing personnel, staffing, patient classification according to nursing needs, patient and personnel satisfaction and unit arrangement. Types of care such as comprehensive care, home care and progressive patient care were evaluated. These evaluations of care laid the foundation for the development of self-study manuals, which are similar to the quality assurance manuals of today (Gortner & Nahm, 1977).

NURSING RESEARCH IN THE 1950s AND 1960s

Major advances were made in nursing research during the 1950s for several reasons. Research became a higher priority with the strong support of such nursing leaders as Henderson and Abdellah. There was an increased number of masters-prepared nurses who had taken courses in research; some had completed theses, which provided them with a background for conducting research. In the 1950s and 1960s, schools of nursing began introducing research and the steps of the research process at the baccalaureate level. In addition, funding for research became more available. In 1955, $500,000 was awarded for federal research grants in nursing (de Tornyay, 1977). The increase in research activities promoted the initial publication of the journal *Nursing Research* in 1952. This journal provided nurses with a means of communicating their findings.

In 1950, American Nurses' Association (ANA) made plans to conduct a 5-year study of nursing functions and activities. The findings of this study were reported in *Twenty Thousand Nurses Tell Their Story*. As a result of this study, ANA developed statements on functions, standards and qualifications for professional nurses in 1959. Also during this time period, clinical research began expanding as the specialty groups (community health, psychiatric, medical–surgical, pediatrics and obstetrics) developed standards of care. The research conducted by ANA and the specialty groups provided the basis for the nursing practice standards that currently guide professional nursing practice (Gortner & Nahm, 1977).

Educational studies were conducted in the 1950s and 1960s in an attempt to determine the most effective educational preparation for the registered nurse. Montag developed and evaluated the 2-year nursing preparation (associate degree) in the junior colleges. Student characteristics, such as admission and retention patterns and the elements that promoted success in nursing education, were also studied at this time (Downs & Fleming, 1979).

There were several other developments that took place in the 1950s and 1960s that influenced nursing research. In 1953, an Institute for Research and Service in Nursing Education was established at Teacher's College, Columbia University, which provided learning experiences in research for doctoral students (Werley, 1977). The American Nurse's Foundation was chartered in 1955. The functions of this foundation have included receiving and administering research funds, conducting research programs, consulting with nursing students and engaging in research. In 1956, a Committee on Research and Studies was established to guide ANA research (See, 1977).

A Department of Nursing Research in the Walter Reed Army Institute of Research was established in 1957. This was the first nursing unit in a research institution that emphasized conducting clinical nursing research (Werley, 1977). Also in 1957, the Southern Regional Educational Board (SREB), Western

Interstate Commission on Higher Education (WICHE), and the New England Board of Higher Education (NEBHE) were developed. These organizations are actively involved in promoting research and disseminating the findings of studies. In 1965, ANA sponsored the first of a series of nursing research conferences. These conferences continue to be an essential means of disseminating research findings. The criteria of these conferences required that the studies presented be relevant to nursing and be conducted by a nurse researcher, thus promoting research in nursing (See, 1977).

In the 1960s, there was an increasing number of clinical studies that focused on quality care and the development of criteria to measure patient outcomes. Intensive care units were being developed, which promoted investigations of nursing interventions, staffing and cost-effectiveness (Gortner & Nahm, 1977).

RESEARCH IN THE 1970s

In the 1970s, the groundwork for clinical research was laid. Clinical research remains a priority today. O'Connell and Duffey (1976) reviewed the studies published in *Nursing Research* from 1970 to 1974 and noted that of the 275 studies published, 71 (26 per cent) involved nursing practice. Forty-six per cent of these nursing practice studies focused on monitoring techniques, such as temperature, pulse and blood pressure; 25 per cent dealt with physical treatment procedures; and 29 per cent with psychological treatment procedures. Subjects in these studies were mainly adults (65 per cent) and inpatients (77 per cent). Since this review, other authors have reviewed more recently published studies and described the focus of research during the 1970s (Lindsey, 1982, 1983).

The nursing process became the focus of many nursing studies, such as attempts to determine the best methods to assess a client and family. In 1973, the first Nursing Diagnosis Conference was held, and these conferences continue to be held every 2 years. Studies have been conducted to identify appropriate nursing diagnoses and to determine an effective diagnostic process.

The educational studies of the 1970s were concerned with the evaluation of teaching methods and student learning experiences. Some studies focused on the use of computers in nursing education. For example, Newman and O'Brien (1978) developed a computer program to provide nursing students with an opportunity to experience the research process through computer simulation. A number of studies have been conducted to differentiate the practice of the baccalaureate-prepared nurse and the associate degree nurse. These studies, which primarily measured abilities to perform technical skills, were unable to differentiate the two levels of education.

In the service setting, primary patient care was the trend of the 1970s, and studies were conducted related to its implementation and evaluation. Researchers continued to study quality assurance methods in the service setting. Nurse practitioners and clinical nurse specialists (both master's-prepared clinicians) began to modify the perception of the nursing role in the 1970s. Limited research has been conducted on the clinical nurse specialist role; however, the nurse practitioner role has been researched to determine its impact on productivity, quality and cost of health care. The studies have consistently indicated that the nurse practitioner provided quality care for a minimal price (Downs & Fleming, 1979).

In the late 1960s and 1970s, nurses were involved in the development of models, conceptual frameworks and theories to guide nursing practice. The nursing theorists' works provided direction for future research in nursing. In 1978, Chinn began publishing the journal *Advances in Nursing Science*, which includes the works of the nursing theorists and the research conducted on theories relevant to nursing.

The number of doctoral programs in nursing and the number of nurses (approximately 2,500) prepared at the doctoral level increased in the 1970s (Jacox, 1980). This has facilitated more sophisticated studies; however, many nurses with doctoral preparation have not become actively involved in nursing research.

Another event influencing research in the 1970s was the establishment of the ANA Commission on Nursing Research. In 1972, the commission established the Council of Nurse Researchers to advance research activities, provide an exchange of ideas and recognize excellence in research. The commission also prepared position papers on subjects' rights in research and on the federal guidelines concerning research and human subjects and sponsored research programs nationally and internationally (See, 1977).

Federal funds for nursing research have increased significantly, with a total of just over $39 million awarded for research in nursing from 1955 to 1976. Even though this is a large increase, in 1974 alone, the schools of medicine received $493 million in federal research funds (de Tornyay, 1977).

The dissemination of research findings was a major issue in the 1970s (Barnard, 1980). Sigma Theta Tau, the national honor society for nursing, sponsored national and international research conferences, and the chapters of this organization sponsored many local conferences. *Image*, initially published in 1967 by Sigma Theta Tau, includes many articles concerning the research process and relevant studies conducted in nursing. Two journals of research began publication in the 1970s: *Research in Nursing and Health* in 1978, and the *Western Journal of Nursing Research* in 1979. Progress has been made in nursing in conducting studies and in disseminating findings. However, the research endeavors of the 1980s are moving the profession forward at a much more rapid pace. These activities are described in Chapter 22.

PRESENT SCOPE OF NURSING RESEARCH

The historical events discussed provide a basis for the current scope of nursing research. Scope defines the range or dimensions of operation. In nursing research, scope addresses what needs to be studied and how the studies should be conducted. In addition to scope, an important consideration is that the research of a discipline should be derived from and consistent with the philosophy of that discipline (Silva, 1977). Thus, the scope of nursing research must "fit" or be congruent with the philosophy and theories of the profession. Donaldson and Crowley (1978) hold the position that the unique perspective of nursing includes (1) the life processes of human beings in sickness and wellness, (2) the patterning of human behavior in interaction with the environment in critical life situations and (3) the processes whereby positive changes in health are effected. There are different philosophical orientations among nurse researchers; therefore, there are differing views regarding the scope of nursing research.

One view is that nursing research should be limited to only those studies that generate knowledge that is directly useful in clinical practice. This view has received increasing support during the last 10 years (Newman, 1982). For example, the ANA (1981) defined nursing research as "the development of knowledge about health and the promotion of health over the full lifespan, care of persons with health problems and disabilities, and nursing actions to enhance the ability of individuals to respond effectively to actual or potential health problems" (p. 2).

Another view is that the scope of nursing research includes studies of nursing education, nursing administration, health services and characteristics of nurses and the nursing role as well as clinical situations. The argument is that findings from these studies indirectly influence nursing practice and thus add to nursing's body of knowledge. Educational research is necessary to provide an efficient, effective educational background. Nursing administration and health services research studies are necessary to determine and promote quality in the health care system. Management studies influence the organization and provision of nursing care.

In the broadest scope, some nurses believe that any research conducted by a nurse is nursing research. This means that a nurse participating in research designed by a physician to answer medical questions would be conducting nursing research. Therefore, the nurse who works with a physician to gather data concerning the effects of different chemotherapy agents in the treatment of cancer would be conducting nursing research. The fact is that these studies add to medicine's body of knowledge, not nursing's. The nurse functions as an assistant to a medical researcher in the above example, not as a nurse researcher (Hodgman, 1979).

There are nurses with advanced degrees in fields such as psychology, biology or sociology who are involved in research in these areas. Nurses who are doctorally prepared in another discipline do provide different perspectives in research methodology. However, nurses who investigate problems in other related disciplines do not necessarily generate findings that will be meaningful or useful in nursing (Donaldson & Crowley, 1978). Only if the research focus of these nurse scientists is within the perspective of nursing can their studies make a significant contribution to nursing.

The scope of nursing research requires clarification and direction. This is currently a concern of the nursing profession. In this text, *nursing research* is defined as a scientific process that validates old knowledge and generates new knowledge that directly and indirectly influences clinical nursing practice.

Nursing Research Methods

Scientific method incorporates all procedures that scientists currently use or may use in the future to pursue knowledge (Kaplan, 1964). This eliminates the idea that there is "the" scientific method or that there is only one way to conduct research (Kaplan, 1964; Silva, 1977; Munhall, 1982a, 1982b, 1983; Tinkle & Beaton, 1983). This broad definition of scientific method includes quantitative and qualitative research.

Since 1930, many researchers have narrowly defined scientific method to include only quantitative research. *Quantitative research* is a formal, objective, systematic process in which numerical data are utilized to obtain information about the world. This research method is used to describe, test relationships and examine cause-and-effect relationships. The predominantly used method of scientific investigation in nursing is quantitative research. Many researchers believe that quantitative research provides a more sound knowledge base to guide nursing practice and is better accepted by other scientific disciplines than is qualitative research.

Qualitative research is a systematic, subjective approach used to describe life experiences and give them meaning. Qualitative research is not a new idea in the social or behavioral sciences (Kaplan, 1964; Glaser & Strauss, 1967; Scheffler, 1967; Blumer, 1969; Baumrind, 1980). However, nursing's interest in qualitative research is more recent, having begun in the 1970s. This type of research is a means of understanding such human experiences as rejection, pain, caring, powerlessness, anger and comfort. Since human emotions are difficult to quantify (assign a numerical value), qualitative research seems to be a more effective method of investigating these emotional responses than is quantitative research. In addition, qualitative research focuses on understanding the whole, which is consistent with the holistic philosophy of nursing (Ludemann, 1979; Baer, 1979; Munhall, 1982b).

COMPARISON OF QUANTITATIVE AND QUALITATIVE RESEARCH

Quantitative and qualitative research complement each other, because they generate different kinds of knowledge that are useful in nursing practice. In some studies, the two approaches are combined. The problem area to be studied will determine which type of research needs to be conducted, and the researcher's knowledge of both types of research will promote accurate selection of the research process for the problem selected. A comparison of the two methods is presented in Table 2–3.

Quantitative research is considered a "hard" science that is based on rigor, objectivity and control. The quantitative approach toward scientific inquiry emerged from a branch of philosophy called *logical positivism*, which operates on strict rules of logic, truth, laws, axioms and predictions (Watson, 1981). Quantitative researchers hold the position that "truth" is absolute and that there is a single reality that one could define by careful measurement. In

TABLE 2-3
Quantitative and Qualitative Research Characteristics

Quantitative Research	Qualitative Research
Hard science	Soft science
Focus: concise and narrow	Focus: complex and broad
Reductionistic	Holistic
Objective	Subjective
Reasoning: logistic, deductive	Reasoning: dialectic, inductive
Basis of knowing: cause-and-effect relationships	Basis of knowing: meaning, discovery
Tests theory	Develops theory
Control	Shared interpretation
Instruments	Communication and observation
Basic element of analysis: numbers	Basic element of analysis: words
Statistical analysis	Individual interpretation
Generalization	Uniqueness

order to find truth, one must be completely objective, which means that values, feelings and personal perceptions cannot enter into the measurement of reality. Quantitative researchers believe that all human behavior is objective, purposeful and measurable. The researcher needs only to find or develop the "right" instrument or tool to measure the behavior.

Qualitative research is considered a "soft" science, or an artistic, philosophical approach. The primary concern with qualitative research is that it lacks the objectivity and control that are essential to "hard" scientific research. Qualitative research evolved from the behavioral and social sciences as a method of understanding the unique, dynamic, holistic nature of humans. Qualitative researchers believe that "truth" is dynamic and can be found only by studying persons as they interact with and in their sociohistorical settings (Tinkle & Beaton, 1983).

In Table 2–3, the focus of quantitative research is identified as concise, narrow and reductionistic. Reductionism involves breaking the whole into parts so that the parts can be examined. Quantitative researchers remain detached from the study and try not to influence the study with their values (objectivity). Researcher involvement in the study is thought to bias or sway the study toward the perceptions and values of the researcher, and biasing a study is considered poor scientific technique.

The focus of qualitative research is complex and broad, and the intent of the research is to give meaning to the whole (holistic). The qualitative researcher has an active part in the study, and the findings from the study are influenced by the researcher's values and perceptions. Thus, this research approach is very subjective, but the approach assumes that subjectivity is essential for the understanding of human experiences.

Quantitative research is conducted to describe variables, identify relationships among variables, and examine cause-and-effect relationships. Thus, this method is very useful in testing theory, by testing the validity of relationships that compose the theory. Quantitative research incorporates logistic and deductive reasoning as the researcher examines particulars in order to make generalizations about the universe.

Qualitative research is conducted to generate knowledge concerned with meaning and discovery. Inductive and dialectic reasoning are predominant in these studies. For example, the qualitative researcher studies the whole person's response to pain; this is accomplished by examining premises about human pain and by determining the meaning that pain has for a particular person. Since qualitative research is concerned with meaning, the findings from these studies can be used to identify the relationships among the variables, and these relational statements are used in theory development.

Quantitative research requires control. The investigator uses control to identify and limit the problem to be researched and attempts to limit the effects of extraneous or outside variables that are not being studied. For example, in studying the relationship between decubitus ulcer healing and the treatment of heat, the researcher controls the use of heat on the ulcer (by manipulating the amount and the way heat is applied) and attempts to control all other variables (such as the use of massage and ointment) that might influence the ulcer's healing. The intent of this control is to facilitate a more precise examination of the effect of heat on ulcer healing.

Quantitative research also requires the use of instruments or tools that will generate numerical data. Statistical analysis is used to reduce and organize the data and to determine significant relationships. Control, instruments and statistical analysis are used in the attempt to render the research findings an accurate reflection of reality. Thus, the researcher will be able to generalize the study findings. Generalization involves the application of trends or general tendencies (which are identified by studying a sample) to the population from which the research sample was drawn. For example, a controlled, experimental study indicated that heat was effective in healing decubitus ulcers of a selected sample of a population; therefore, the researcher generalizes that heat is an effective treatment for healing "similar" decubitus ulcers of patients. Researchers must be cautious in making generalizations; a sound generalization requires the support of many studies.

Qualitative researchers use structured and unstructured observation and communication as means of gathering data. The data include the shared interpretations of the researcher and the subjects, and no attempts are made to control the interaction. For example, the researcher and subjects might share their experiences of powerlessness in the health care delivery system. The data are subjective and incorporate the perceptions and beliefs of the researcher and the subjects (Eisner, 1981; Leininger, 1985).

Qualitative data are in the form of words and are analyzed in terms of individual responses or in terms of descriptive summaries or both. The researcher identifies categories for sorting and organizing the data (Wooldridge, Leonard & Skipper, 1978). The intent of the analysis is to organize the data into a meaningful, individualized interpretation or framework that describes the phenomenon studied. The findings from a qualitative study are unique to that study, and it is not the intent of the researcher to generalize the findings to a larger population. However, understanding the meaning of a phenomenon in a particular situation is useful for understanding similar phenomena in similar situations.

TYPES OF QUANTITATIVE RESEARCH

The quantitative method includes different types of research. This text classifies quantitative research methods into five types, which are listed in Table 2–4, described briefly below and further discussed in Chapter 3.

Exploratory Research

Exploratory or formative research is conducted to gain new insights, discover new ideas and/or increase knowledge of a phenomenon. These studies are usually conducted when little is known about a research topic. The major purpose of exploratory research is to formulate problems or hypotheses for further, more precise study (Selltiz, Wrightsman & Cook, 1976).

Descriptive Research

Descriptive research provides an accurate portrayal or account of characteristics of a particular individual, situation or group (Selltiz, Wrightsman & Cook, 1976). These studies are a means of discovering new meaning, describing what exists, determining the frequency with which something occurs and/or categorizing information (Marriner, 1981). In descriptive research, the researcher uses structured observations (observations guided by a checklist) or questionnaires or both to describe the phenomenon studied. Descriptive studies provide the knowledge base needed to conduct correlational, quasi-experimental and experimental studies.

Correlational Research

Correlational research involves the systematic investigation of relationships between (among) two or more variables. If the relationships exist, the researcher determines the type (positive or negative) and the degree or strength of the relationships. The primary intent of correlational studies is to explain the nature of relationships in the real world, not to determine cause-and-effect. However, correlational studies are the means for generating hypotheses to guide quasi-experimental and experimental studies that do focus on examining cause-and-effect relationships.

TABLE 2–4
Types of Quantitative Research

Exploratory Research
Descriptive Research
Correlational Research
Quasi-Experimental Research
Experimental Research

Quasi-Experimental Research

The purpose of quasi-experimental research is to explain relationships or clarify why certain events happened or both (Cook & Campbell, 1979). These studies are also a means of examining causal relationships; thus, they are a basis for prediction of phenomena. Quasi-experimental studies are not as powerful as experimental studies, because they do not have the same degree of control. Quasi-experimental studies lack sufficient control in at least one of three areas: (1) manipulation of the treatment variable, (2) manipulation of the setting or (3) random selection of subjects. When studying human behavior, frequently there are variables that researchers are unable to manipulate or control.

Experimental Research

Experimental research is an objective, systematic, controlled investigation for the purpose of predicting and controlling phenomena. The purpose of this type of research is to examine causality. Experimental research is considered the most powerful quantitative method because of the rigorous control of variables. Experimental studies have three main characteristics: (1) there is a manipulation of some sort (such as manipulation of a treatment variable), (2) some of the subjects in the study receive the treatment (experimental group) and some do not (control group) and (3) there is a means of randomly selecting subjects so that they have an equal chance of being included in the study.

TYPES OF QUALITATIVE RESEARCH

Qualitative research can be viewed as a type of exploratory research. However, this type of exploratory research is different from the exploratory quantitative research previously discussed. Quantitative exploratory research is conducted to obtain sufficient information to conduct more controlled quantitative studies. Qualitative studies, exploratory in nature, are conducted to increase insights and generate meaning for whole situations and abstract concepts. The outcome of qualitative research is the development or expansion of theory. Because of the uniqueness of qualitative approaches, they are being considered separately. This text includes four types of these studies, which are presented in Table 2–5, described briefly below and further discussed in Chapter 4.

Phenomenological Research

Phenomenological research is an inductive, descriptive approach, developed from phenomenological philosophy. The focus of phenomenological philosophy

---

TABLE 2–5
Types of Qualitative Research

Phenomenological Research
Grounded Theory Research
Ethnographic Research
Historical Research

is understanding the response of the whole human being, not just understanding specific parts or behaviors (Omery, 1983). The aim of phenomenological research is to describe an experience as it is lived by the person, such as describing a person's experience of pain as it is lived by the person (Oiler, 1982).

Grounded Theory Research

Grounded theory research, developed by Glaser and Strauss, was initially described in a 1967 publication. This research approach is useful in discovering what problems exist in a social scene and how the persons involved handle them. Grounded theory methodology emphasizes observation and the development of practice-based intuitive relationships between variables. The research process involves formulation, testing and redevelopment of propositions until a theory evolves. The theory developed through grounded theory research is empirically based (Simms, 1981).

Ethnographic Research

Ethnographic research is the investigation of cultures through an in-depth study of the members of the culture. This type of research attempts to tell the story of people's daily lives and to describe the culture of which they are a part. The ethnographic research process is the systematic collection, description and analysis of data to develop a theory of cultural behavior. The researcher (ethnographer) actually lives in or becomes a part of the cultural setting in order to gather the data. Ethnographers describe specific cultures and also compare cultures to determine similarities and differences (Aamodt, 1982).

Historical Research

Historical research is a narrative description or analysis of events that occurred in the remote or recent past. Data are obtained from records, artifacts or verbal reports (Krampitz, 1981). Historical research is useful so that past mistakes are not repeated and it helps in our understanding of present situations. In addition, this type of research has the potential to provide a foundation for and direct the future movement of the profession. Only a minimal amount of historical research has been conducted in nursing, with the majority of the studies focusing on past and current nursing leaders (Newton, 1965).

Summary

This chapter addresses the question "What distinguishes nursing research from research in other disciplines?" In some ways, there are no differences. However, nursing research must be consistent with nursing's philosophy and theories. Research is an essential means of obtaining knowledge. Historically, however, nursing has obtained knowledge through tradition, authority, borrowing, trial and error, intuition, personal experience, role-modeling and reasoning. Six types of reasoning were described: problematic, operational, dialectic, logistic, inductive and deductive. Deduction is the common method of reasoning used in conducting quantitative research. The predominant method of reasoning in qualitative research is induction. All methods of obtaining knowledge are important to nursing. However, more of nursing's knowledge must be generated through research in the future. The purpose of research is to describe, explain, predict and control phenomena in nursing practice. Currently, most of the research in nursing is descriptive and explanatory, and ultimately needs to be at the level of prediction and control.

Research is a process, and, in some ways, is similar to other processes such as the problem-solving process and the nursing process. A background in the problem-solving process and the nursing process, acquired early in nursing education, provides a foundation for understanding the research process. A comparison of the problem-solving process, nursing process and research process is included in this chapter.

Key historical events have facilitated the development of nursing research. Florence Nightingale is considered the first nurse researcher. However, following her work, little research was conducted in nursing until the 1950s. Nursing research has moved from an educational focus to a clinical practice focus. The increasing value placed on nursing research is demonstrated by the number of research conferences, journals and organizational support systems that have emerged. These historical events provide a basis for understanding the current scope of nursing research. In this text, nursing research is defined as a scientific process that validates old knowledge and generates new knowledge that directly and indirectly influences clinical nursing practice.

Nursing research incorporates both quantitative and qualitative research methods. Quantitative research is a formal, objective, systematic process of using numerical data to obtain information about the world. This research method is used to describe, test relationships and examine cause-and-effect relationships. In this text, quantitative research is classified into five types: exploratory, descriptive, correlational, quasi-experimental and experimental. Qualitative research is a systematic, subjective approach used to describe life experiences and give them meaning. Four types of qualitative research are included in this text: phenomenological, grounded theory, ethnographic and historical.

There seem to be essentially two sides to the nature of humans: one rational, logical, mathematical and rule oriented; and the other intuitive, feeling and holistic. The ability to use both of these aspects of self and to achieve a balance between the two are important to one's health. In nursing research, a balance is needed, because the focus of research is the client's response to the health situation. There is a need in nursing practice to predict and control; to have knowledge of the average, or normals; and to categorize and generalize. Quantitative research will provide this knowledge. Knowledge generated from qualitative research will provide meaning and understanding of the specific, not the general; of values; and of life experiences. Both quantitative and qualitative research are necessary to generate nursing's unique body of knowledge.

References

Aamodt, A. M. (1982). Examining ethnography for nurse researchers. *Western Journal of Nursing Research*, 4(2), 209–221.

Abdellah, F. G. (1972). Evolution of nursing as a profession. *International Nursing Review*, 19(3), 219–235.

American Nurses' Association (1981). Research priorities for the 1980s: Generating a scientific basis for nursing practice. Commission on Nursing Research.

Andreoli, K. G. & Thompson, C. E. (1977). The nature of science in nursing. *Image*, 9(2), 32–37.

Baer, E. D. (1979). Philosophy provides the rationale for nursing's multiple research directions. *Image*, 11(3), 72–74.

Barnard, K. E. (1980). Knowledge for practice: directions for the future. *Nursing Research*, 29(4), 208–212.

Baumrind, D. (1980). New directions in socialization research. *American Psychologist*, 35(7), 639–652.

Benner, P. (1982). From novice to expert. *American Journal of Nursing*, 82(3), 402–407.

Benner, P. (1983). Uncovering the knowledge embedded in clinical practice. *Image*, 15(2), 36–41.

Benner, P. (1984). *From novice to expert: excellence and power in clinical nursing practice*. Menlo Park, California: Addison-Wesley Publishing Company.

Blumer, H. (1969). *Symbolic interactionism: perspective and method*. Englewood Cliffs, New Jersey: Prentice-Hall, Inc.

Chinn, P. L. & Jacobs, M. K. (1983). *Theory and nursing: a systematic approach*. St. Louis: The C. V. Mosby Company.

Conway, M. E. (1978). Clinical research: instrument for change. *Journal of Nursing Administration*, 8(12), 27–32.

Cook, Sir E. (1913). *The life of Florence Nightingale* (Vol. 1). London: Macmillan Publishing Co., Inc.

Cook, T. D. & Campbell, D. T. (1979). *Quasi-experimentation: design & analysis issues for field settings*. Chicago: Rand McNally College Publishing Company.

de Tornyay, R. (1977). Nursing research—the road ahead. *Nursing Research*, 26(6), 404–407.

Dickoff, J., James, P. & Wiedenbach, E. (1968). Theory in a practice discipline: practice oriented theory (Part 1). *Nursing Research*, 17(5), 415–435.

Donaldson, S. K. & Crowley, D. M. (1978). The discipline of nursing. *Nursing Outlook*, 26(2), 113–120.

Downs, F. S. & Fleming, W. J. (1979). *Issues in Nursing Research*. New York: Appleton-Century-Crofts.

Eisner, E. W. (1981). On the differences between scientific and artistic approaches to qualitative research. *Educational Researcher*, 10(4), 5–9.

Erickson, H. C., Tomlin, E. M. & Swain, M. A. (1983). *Modeling and role-modeling: a theory and paradigm for nursing*. Englewood Cliffs, New Jersey: Prentice-Hall, Inc.

Fawcett, J. (1984). *Analysis and evaluation of conceptual models of nursing*. Philadelphia: F. A. Davis Company.

Fawcett, J. (1986). A typology of nursing research activities according to educational preparation. *Journal of Professional Nursing*, 1(2), 75–78.

Feldman, H. R. (1980). Nursing research in the 1980s: issues and implications. *Advances in Nursing Science*, 3(1), 85–92.

Feldman, H. R. (1981). A science of nursing—to be or not to be? *Image*, 13(3), 63–66.

Glaser, B. G. & Strauss, A. L. (1967). *The discovery of grounded theory: strategies for qualitative research*. Chicago: Aldine.

Gortner, S. R. (1974). Scientific accountability in nursing. *Nursing Outlook*, 22(12), 764–768.

Gortner, S. R. (1975). Research for a practice profession. *Nursing Research*, 24(3), 193–197.

Gortner, S. R. (1983). The history and philosophy of nursing science and research. *Advances in Nursing Science*, 5(2), 1–8.

Gortner, S. R. & Nahm, H. (1977). An overview of nursing research in the United States. *Nursing Research*, 26(1), 10–33.

Herbert, R. G. (1981). *Florence Nightingale: saint, reformer or rebel?* Malabar, Florida: Robert E. Krieger Publishing Company.

Hodgman, E. C. (1979). Closing the gap between research and practice: changing the answers to the 'who', the 'where' and the 'how' of nursing research. *International Journal of Nursing Studies*, 16(1), 105–110.

Hodson, K. E. (1986). Research in nursing education and practice: the ecological methods perspective. *Western Journal of Nursing Research*, 8(1),33–48.

Jacox, A. (1980). Strategies to promote nursing research. *Nursing Research*, 29(4), 213–218.

Johnson, W. L. (1977). Research programs of the National League for Nursing. *Nursing Research*, 26(3), 172–176.

Kaplan, A. (1964). *The conduct of inquiry: methodology for behavioral science.* New York: Chandler Publishing Company.

Keller, M. J. (1981). Toward a definition of health. *Advances in Nursing Science*, 4(1), 43–64.

Kerlinger, F. N. (1973). *Foundations of behavioral research.* New York: Holt, Rinehart and Winston, Inc.

Kim, M. J. & Moritz, D. A. (1982). *Classification of nursing diagnoses: proceedings of the third and fourth national conferences.* New York: McGraw-Hill Book Company.

Krampitz, S. D. (1981). Research design: historical. In S. D. Krampitz & N. Pavlovich (Eds.), *Readings for nursing research* (pp. 54–58). St. Louis: The C. V. Mosby Company.

Lawson, L. (1981). Research design: experimental. In S. D. Krampitz & N. Pavlovich (Eds.), *Readings for nursing research* (pp. 67–74). St. Louis: The C. V. Mosby Company.

Leininger, M. M. (1985). *Qualitative research methods in nursing.* Orlando: Grune & Stratton, Inc.

Lindsey, A. M. (1982). Phenomena and physiological variables of relevance to nursing, review of a decade of work: part I. *Western Journal of Nursing Research*, 4(4), 343–364.

Lindsey, A. M. (1983). Phenomena and physiological variables of relevance to nursing, review of a decade of work: part 2. *Western Journal of Nursing Research*, 5(1), 41–63.

Ludemann, R. (1979). The paradoxical nature of nursing research. *Image*, 11(1), 2–8.

McMurrey, P. H. (1982). Toward a unique knowledge base in nursing. *Image*, 14(1), 12–15.

Marriner, A. (1981). Research design: survey/descriptive. In S. D. Krampitz & N. Pavlovich (Eds.), *Readings for nursing research* (pp. 59–66). St. Louis: The C. V. Mosby Company.

Munhall, P. L. (1982a). Ethical juxtapositions in nursing research. *Topics in Clinical Nursing*, 4(1), 66–73.

Munhall, P. L. (1982b). Nursing philosophy and nursing research: in apposition or opposition? *Nursing Research*, 31(3), 176–177, 181.

Munhall, P. L. (1983). Methodologic fallacies: a critical self-appraisal. *Advances in Nursing Science*, 5(4), 41–49.

Newman, M. A. (1982). What differentiates clinical research? *Image*, 14(3), 86–88.

Newman, M. A. & O'Brien, R. A. (1978). Experiencing the research process via computer simulation. *Image*, 10(1), 5–9.

Newton, M. E. (1965). The case for historical research. *Nursing Research*, 14(1), 20–26.

Nightingale, F. (1859). *Notes on Nursing: what it is, and what it is not.* Philadelphia: J. B. Lippincott Company.

Notter, L. E. (1978). *Essentials of nursing research.* New York: Springer Publishing Company.

O'Connell, K. A. & Duffey, M. (1976). Research in nursing practice: its nature and direction. *Image*, 8(1), 6–12.

Oiler, C. (1982). The phenomenological approach in nursing research. *Nursing Research*, 31(3), 178–181.

Omery, A. (1983). Phenomenology: a method for nursing research. *Advances in Nursing Science*, 5(2), 49–63.

Paletta, J. L. (1980). Nursing research: an integral part of professional nursing. *Image*, 12(1), 3–6.

Palmer, I. S. (1977). Florence Nightingale: reformer, reactionary, researcher. *Nursing Research*, 26(2), 84–89.

Scheffler, I. (1967). *Science and subjectivity.* Indianapolis: The Bobbs-Merrill Company, Inc.

Schlotfeldt, R. M. (1971). The significance of empirical research for nursing. *Nursing Research*, 20(2), 140–142.

See, E. M. (1977). The ANA and research in nursing. *Nursing Research*, 26(3), 165–171.

Selltiz, C., Wrightsman, L. S. & Cook, S. W. (1976). *Research methods in social relations* (3rd ed.). New York: Holt, Rinehart and Winston.

Silva, M. C. (1977). Philosophy, science, theory: interrelationships and implications for nursing research. *Image*, 9(3), 59–63.

Simms, L. M. (1981). The grounded theory approach in nursing research. *Nursing Research*, 30(6), 356–359.

Stevens, B. J. (1984). *Nursing theory: analysis, application, evaluation* (2nd ed.). Boston: Little, Brown and Company.

Swanson, J. M. & Chentiz, W. C. (1982). Why qualitative research in nursing? *Nursing Outlook*, 30(4), 241–245.

Tinkle, M. B. & Beaton, J. L. (1983). Toward a new view of science: implications for nursing research. *Advances in Nursing Science*, 5(2), 27–36.

Trussell, P., Brandt, A. & Knapp, S. (1981). *Using nursing research: discovery, analysis, and interpretation*. Wakefield, Massachusetts: Nursing Resources.

Vance, C. (1982). The mentor connection. *Journal of Nursing Administration*, 12(4), 7–13.

Visintainer, M. A. (1986). The nature of knowledge and theory in nursing. *Image: Journal of Nursing Scholarship*, 18(2),32–38.

Watson, J. (1981). Nursing's scientific quest. *Nursing Outlook*, 29(7), 413–416.

Werley, H. H. (1977). Nursing research in perspective. *International Nursing Review*, 24(3), 75–83.

Werley, H. H. & Newcomb, B. J. (1983). The research mentor: a missing element in nursing? In N. L. Chaska (Ed.), *The nursing profession: a time to speak* (pp. 202–215). New York: McGraw-Hill Book Company.

Wooldridge, P. J., Leonard, R. C. & Skipper, J. K. (1978). *Methods of clinical experimentation to improve patient care*. St. Louis: The C. V. Mosby Company.

3

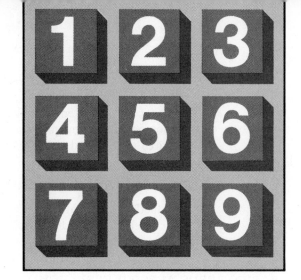

Introduction to Quantitative Research

What do you think of when you hear the word *research?* Frequently the term *experiment* comes to mind. One might equate experiments with randomizing subjects into groups, collecting data and conducting statistical analyses. Frequently, one thinks that an experiment is conducted to prove something, such as proving that one mouthwash is more effective than another. These common notions are associated with the classic experimental design originated by Sir Ronald Fisher (1935). Fisher is noted for adding structure to the steps of the research process with such ideas as the null hypothesis, research design and statistical analysis.

Fisher's experimentation provided the ground work for what is now known as experimental research. Throughout the years, a number of other quantitative approaches have been developed. Campbell and Stanley (1963) developed the quasi-experimental approaches. Karl Pearson developed statistical approaches for examining relationships between variables and expanded correlational research techniques. The fields of sociology, education and psychology are noted for their development and expansion of strategies for conducting exploratory and descriptive research. The steps of the research process used in these different quantitative approaches are the same, but the philosophy and strategies for implementing these steps vary with the approaches.

Nurses use a broad range of quantitative approaches in developing nursing knowledge. Therefore, it is important that they understand the concepts and process associated with quantitative research. This chapter provides information on conducting quantitative research, an introduction to the quantitative research process and examples of quantitative nursing studies.

Conducting Quantitative Research

Conducting quantitative research requires familiarity with such concepts as basic research, applied research, rigor and control. The following section defines these concepts and includes examples from quantitative studies.

BASIC VERSUS APPLIED RESEARCH

Basic, or *pure, research* is a scientific investigation that involves the generation of "knowledge for knowledge sake" or for the pleasure of learning and finding truth. The findings of basic research are frequently not directly useful in practice (Nagel, 1961; Wysocki, 1983). An example of basic research is the study conducted by Martinson and Anderson (1983) examining the effects of thermal applications on the abdominal temperature of dogs. The findings from this study indicated "that a wide range of thermal applications to the abdominal skin of the dog do not alter deep abdominal temperatures" (p. 89). These findings of selected dogs' responses to thermal application cannot be directly applied in nursing practice. Additional applied research is needed to provide sufficient knowledge related to the application of heat to the abdomen of a patient. Basic research usually precedes or is the basis for applied research.

Applied research is a scientific investigation conducted to answer a clinical question or solve a practice-related problem. If researchers want to solve problems, make decisions or predict or control outcomes related to nursing actions in real-life practice situations, they conduct applied research (Abdellah & Levine, 1979). Applied research is conducted to refine and utilize the knowledge generated from basic research; therefore, these approaches are complementary. Many of the studies that have been conducted in nursing are applied because researchers have chosen to focus on answering immediate clinical questions, such as validating conventional nursing actions or documenting cost-effectiveness of these actions. In addition, most federal funding has been granted for applied research (Wysocki, 1983).

Perry (1981) conducted an applied study to examine the effectiveness of the educational aspect of a rehabilitation program. This study was conducted to solve a practice-related problem of examining the effectiveness of a specific teaching process in the rehabilitation of patients experiencing chronic bronchitis and emphysema. The findings from this study indicated "that a rehabilitation program that maximized patient involvement in learning fostered the patients' ability to make decisions and take actions that increased their ability to cope with their illness" (p. 222). The findings from this study have the potential, with replication, for impacting nursing practice by validating the effectiveness of a specific teaching process in rehabilitation. More research is needed before the information from this study can be generalized to other types of teaching processes, patients and rehabilitation programs.

RIGOR IN QUANTITATIVE RESEARCH

Rigor is the striving for excellence in research. The concept *rigor* is associated with discipline, scrupulous adherence and strict accuracy. A rigorous quantitative researcher constantly strives for more precise measurement tools and tightly controlled study designs. Characteristics valued in these researchers include critical examination of reasoning and attention to precision.

The types of reasoning considered essential to the development of the quantitative research process are logistic and deductive. During the development of the research process, the researchers constantly examine their reasoning processes. Their critical examination of these processes is done to decrease errors in such areas as measurement, design, statistical analysis and generalization. Reducing these errors is considered necessary for research findings to be an accurate reflection of reality. The nature of these errors within the research process is further explained in later chapters of this text.

Another aspect of rigor is precision, which encompasses accuracy, detail and order. Precision is evident in the concise statement of the research purpose and detailed development of the study design. But the most explicit use of precision is evident in the measurement or quantification of the study variables. Measurement involves objectively experiencing the real world through the senses: sight, hearing, touch, taste and smell. The researcher continually searches for new and more precise ways to measure the real world.

RESEARCHER CONTROL IN QUANTITATIVE RESEARCH

Control involves the imposing of "rules" by the researcher to decrease the possibility of error and thus increase the probability that the study's findings are an accurate reflection of reality. These rules used to achieve control are referred to as *design*. Through control, the researcher reduces the influence of extraneous variables (variables that are not being studied) on the research variables. Controlling extraneous variables enables the researcher to clarify the "true" relationships among the study variables and to examine the "true" effect(s) of one variable on another.

There are different mechanisms for control within a quantitative study: (1) subject selection (sampling), (2) subject's knowledge of the study (Hawthorne effect) and (3) the research setting (Cook & Campbell, 1979). Varying degrees of control, ranging from uncontrolled to highly controlled, are implemented in quantitative approaches (Table 3–1).

Sampling

Sampling is a process of selecting subjects that are representative of the population being studied. Random sampling provides a sample that is most

TABLE 3–1
Control in Quantitative Research

Type of Quantitative Research	Researcher Control	Sampling	Research Setting
Exploratory research	Uncontrolled	Nonrandom	Natural setting
Descriptive research	Uncontrolled	Nonrandom	Natural setting
Correlational research	Uncontrolled/ partially controlled	Nonrandom/ random	Natural setting/ partially controlled
Quasi-experimental research	Partially controlled	Nonrandom/ random	Partially controlled
Experimental research	Highly controlled	Random	Highly controlled/ laboratory

representative of a population, because each member of the population has an equal chance or probability of being included in the study. In quantitative research, both random and nonrandom samples are used (Table 3–1). A more in-depth discussion of population and sampling is presented in Chapter 9.

Hawthorne Effect

The Hawthorne effect describes a particular response that sometimes occurs when individuals are involved as research subjects. It is a psychological response in which the research subjects change their behavior simply because they are subjects in a study, not because of the research treatment. The concept *Hawthorne effect* was developed from the classical experiments at the Hawthorne plant of the Western Electric Company during the late 1920s and early 1930s.

In these studies, the researcher manipulated the working conditions (altered the lighting, decreased work hours, changed payment and increased rest periods) to examine the effect on worker productivity (Homans, 1965). The subjects in both the treatment group (work conditions were changed) and control groups (no change in work conditions) increased their productivity. Even those groups in which lighting was decreased showed an increase in productivity. It appeared that the subjects were influenced by their knowledge that they were part of a study. Based on the findings from these studies, the researchers proposed that if the subjects know the research hypothesis, they might not respond to the treatment in the study but instead respond in such a way as to support the hypothesis of the study.

An example of the Hawthorne effect in a nursing study is demonstrated with the following hypothesis: Patients experiencing a specific type of preoperative teaching on coughing and deep breathing (treatment group) have clearer breath sounds on the first postoperative day than patients not receiving this planned instruction (control group). If the patients in both the treatment and control groups know the study hypothesis, they might alter their coughing and deep breathing patterns just because they are in a study, not because of the preoperative instruction. In addition, the subjects might alter their coughing and deep breathing patterns just to support the study hypothesis.

In any quantitative study, the researcher should make every attempt not to influence the subjects' responses. For example, the researcher could give a simple explanation of the study without indicating the relationship between this specific preoperative instruction on coughing and deep breathing and the patients' performance of these activities postoperatively. Another strategy is to not inform the subjects as to whether they are in the treatment or the control group, provided that this can be done without infringing upon the subjects' rights. Informed consent is discussed in Chapter 12.

Research Settings

There are three common settings for conducting research: natural, partially controlled and highly controlled (Table 3–1). *Natural settings*, or field settings, are uncontrolled, real-life situations (Abdellah & Levine, 1979). Conducting a study in a natural setting means that the researcher does not manipulate or change the environment for the study. For example, Robb (1985) conducted a descriptive study to verify "the amount and frequency of incontinent urine loss in an outpatient population" (p. 278). The setting for this study was the patient's home.

A *partially controlled setting* is an environment that is manipulated or modified in some way by the researcher. Many nursing studies are conducted in partially controlled settings. Wells (1982) examined the "effect of relaxation on postoperative muscle tension and pain" (p. 236). Within the hospital, Wells could control the implementation of the treatment, such as who would or would not receive the relaxation training and the timing and quality of the training. However, the researcher did not control other aspects of the environment, such as family support and different types of nursing care on the hospital units, that might have influenced the patients' postoperative muscle tension and pain.

Highly controlled settings are artificially constructed environments that are developed for the sole purpose of conducting research. Laboratories, research centers, experimental centers and test units are highly controlled settings where experimental studies are conducted. This type of setting reduces the influence of extraneous, environmental variables. Therefore, the researcher is able to accurately examine the cause-and-effect relationship of the variables studied. Until recently, very few settings existed in which nurses could conduct highly controlled studies, but this is changing. Experimental studies require a highly controlled setting; however, other quantitative studies may be conducted in this setting. For example, the following study is an exploratory study using a highly controlled setting.

Updike, Accurso and Jones (1985) studied the "physiologic circadian rhythmicity in preterm infants" (p. 160). The setting for this study was a neonatal intensive care unit–clinical research center that was "staffed by five registered nurses hired on a full-time basis for the sole purpose of operating the clinical research center. Their primary responsibilities center on clinical research and involve direct clinical patient care only when necessary for a specific study'' (p. 160). The lighting of the unit, temperature of the isolettes, scheduling of feeding, repositioning and other nursing measures were controlled.

Steps of the Quantitative Research Process

The quantitative research process includes planning and implementing a study and communicating the study's findings. The steps of the process are outlined in Figure 3–1. This figure demonstrates the logical flow and flexibility of this process. In conducting the research process, there is a flow back and forth among the steps as the researcher strives to clarify points and strengthen the development of the study. The research process is cyclic in this diagram because each study provides a basis for generating further research.

FORMULATING A RESEARCH PROBLEM

A research problem is a question or statement that clarifies the focus of a study. Formulating a research problem involves moving from a general research

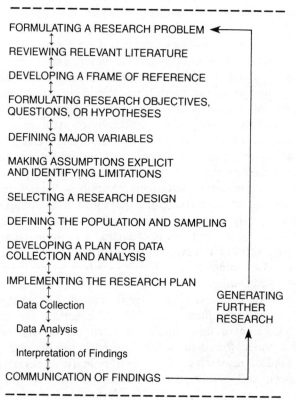

FIGURE 3–1. Steps of the quantitative research process.

topic to a specific researchable problem. A research topic is a general area of personal interest that is relevant to nursing. In the final phase of formulating the problem, the researcher struggles to refine the problem statement, frequently rewriting it several times to achieve clarity and narrowness of scope.

Using deductive reasoning, the research problem is generated from the research topic, and the purpose is generated from the problem. The population, setting and major variables to be studied are identified in the research purpose. Based on the study purpose, the researcher formulates specific subproblems that direct the design of the study. Formulating a research problem and purpose is described in Chapter 5, and developing research subproblems is described in Chapter 8. These steps of the research process are illustrated by Killeen's (1985) study that examined taking risks with health.

PROBLEM

Is the extent to which an individual approaches risk related to participation in behaviors that threaten health? (p. 117)

PURPOSE

... to determine whether a relationship exists between individuals' general propensity to take risks and the extent of their participation in selected behaviors that put their health at risk. (p. 117)

RESEARCH QUESTIONS

1. "Does a relationship exist between an individual's general propensity to take risk and his or her participation in the health-threatening behaviors of smoking, consuming alcohol, using mood-altering drugs, being overweight, failing to use seat belts, and exposing oneself to dangerous situations?
2. If so, is this relationship influenced by the demographic characteristics of age, gender, and education?" (pp. 117–118)

REVIEWING RELEVANT LITERATURE

A review of relevant literature is conducted to determine the knowledge that currently exists concerning a selected research problem. The concepts and interrelationships of the concepts in the problem guide the researcher in reviewing the literature. The investigator reviews relevant theories and studies. Theories are reviewed to clarify the definitions of concepts and to refine the frame of reference for the problem to be investigated. Reviewing relevant studies enables the researcher to clarify which problems have been investigated, which require further investigation and which have not been investigated. In addition, the literature review directs the researcher in designing the study and interpreting the outcomes. The process of reviewing relevant literature is described in Chapter 6.

DEVELOPING A FRAME OF REFERENCE

A frame of reference is an abstract conceptualization that places the study within a context of meaning. It is the structure within which a study is developed and links all components of a study together. One important purpose of a framework is to provide a context for the interpretation of study findings. A frame of reference can be either theoretical or conceptual. The terms *conceptual framework* and *theoretical framework* have been used interchangeably by nurse researchers. In this textbook, a distinction is made between the two terms.

A conceptual framework is an organization or matrix of concepts that provides a focus for inquiry (Newman, 1979). The conceptual framework of a study focuses the researcher's attention on the concepts that are to be clarified or described (Table 3–2). Conceptual frameworks are developed by linking concepts selected from theories, experience or studies.

A theoretical framework is a general, abstract explanation of the interrelationships of the concepts to be investigated in a study (Silva, 1981). A theoretical framework is an expression of an existing theory, and only one theory can be used in a theoretical framework. When a theoretical framework is used, the purpose of the study is to test a proposition from a theory (Table 3–2). The proposition selected from a theory serves as a basis for formulating the hypotheses, as illustrated below.

$$\text{Theory} \longrightarrow \text{Proposition} \longrightarrow \text{Hypotheses}$$

The works of nursing theorists have greatly increased during the 1970s and 1980s. These works (King, 1981; Orem, 1985; Rogers, 1970; Roy & Roberts, 1981) are excellent sources for the development of theoretical frameworks to guide nursing research. The focus of Chapter 7 is the development of a frame of reference.

TABLE 3–2
Developing a Frame of Reference

Type of Quantitative Research	Frame of Reference
Exploratory studies	Conceptual framework
Descriptive studies	Conceptual framework
Correlational studies	Conceptual/theoretical framework
Quasi-experimental studies	Theoretical framework
Experimental studies	Theoretical framework

FORMULATING RESEARCH SUBPROBLEMS

The problem and purpose identified in a study contain several research subproblems (Leedy, 1980). These subproblems can be stated as objectives, questions or hypotheses. Exploratory and descriptive studies include objectives or questions. Correlational studies include questions or hypotheses. Quasi-experimental and experimental studies include hypotheses. The development of research objectives, questions and hypotheses is discussed in Chapter 8. Examples of objectives, questions and an hypothesis from nursing studies follow:

RESEARCH OBJECTIVES

1. To identify a list of nursing diagnoses;
2. To examine the usefulness and completeness of this list; and
3. To identify types, frequency and distribution of nursing problems encountered by nurses in selected settings. (Jones, 1982, p. 141)

RESEARCH QUESTIONS

1. Is there a relationship between nurses' levels of anxiety and their levels of self-disclosure? and
2. Is there a relationship between patients' levels of anxiety and their levels of self-disclosure to nurses? (Johnson, 1979, p. 9)

RESEARCH HYPOTHESIS

The effectiveness of oral hygiene nursing care of the acutely ill surgical patient (dependent variable) is influenced by the agent used (independent variable) provided that the frequency and technique of application are standardized. (Passos & Brand, 1966, p. 197)

DEFINING RESEARCH VARIABLES

The research purpose and the objectives, questions or hypotheses of a study contain concepts to be investigated. These concepts are research variables. Research variables are characteristics, properties or attributes of persons, events or objects that are examined in a study (Abdellah & Levine, 1979). The conceptual definitions, from the framework of the study, direct the way variables are defined operationally. Variables are operationally defined to make them measurable in the real world. A more extensive discussion of research variables is provided in Chapter 8. Examples of conceptual and operational definitions are presented from Newman and Gaudiano's (1984) study of the relationship between depression and subjective time in the elderly.

DEPRESSION

Conceptual Definition—An affective state characterized by a negative self-concept associated with self-reproach and self-blame. (p. 138)
Operational Definition—Measured by the Beck Depression Inventory (BDI). (p. 138)

SUBJECTIVE TIME

Conceptual Definition—Newman defined perceived duration, referred to as subjective time, as a ratio of awareness to the content of events in one's life (p. 137):

$$\text{Subjective time} = \frac{\text{Awareness}}{\text{Content}}$$

Operational Definition—An individual's perceived duration of a short interval as determined by having the subjects produce their subjective estimate of an interval of 40 seconds. (p. 138)

MAKING ASSUMPTIONS EXPLICIT AND IDENTIFYING LIMITATIONS

Assumptions are statements that are taken for granted or are considered true, even though these statements have not been scientifically tested (Silva, 1981). Assumptions are embedded (unrecognized) in thinking and behavior, and uncovering these assumptions requires introspection. Sources of assumptions are universally accepted truths (all humans are rational beings), theories, previous research and nursing practice (Myers, 1982).

In studies, assumptions are embedded in the philosophical base of the frame of reference, study design and interpretation of findings. Theories and instruments are developed based on assumptions that may or may not be known by the researcher. In addition, the researcher has personalized assumptions. All these assumptions influence the development of the research process. The recognition of assumptions by the researcher is a strength, not a weakness. Assumptions influence the logic of the study, and their recognition leads to more rigorous study development.

Williams (1980) reviewed published nursing studies and other health care literature to identify 13 commonly embedded assumptions:

1. People want to assume control of their own health problems.
2. Stress should be avoided.
3. People are aware of the experiences that most affect their life choices.
4. Health is a priority for most people.
5. People in underserved areas feel underserved.
6. Most measurable attitudes are held strongly enough to direct behavior.
7. Health professionals view health care in a different manner than do lay persons.
8. Human biological and chemical factors show less variation than do cultural and social factors.
9. The nursing process is the best way of conceptualizing nursing practice.
10. Statistically significant differences relate to the variable or variables under consideration.
11. People operate on the basis of cognitive information.

12. Increased knowledge about an event lowers anxiety about the event.
13. Receipt of health care at home is preferable to receipt of care in an institution. (p. 48)

Williams (1972) stated the following assumptions in her study of factors contributing to skin breakdown:

ASSUMPTIONS

1. Nonambulatory patients are more likely to develop decubitus ulcers than are ambulatory persons;
2. Assessable variables other than pressure are associated with decubitus ulcer formation; and
3. Most patients in the health care facilities utilized for data collection in this study would develop breakdown within four weeks of admission if they developed skin breakdown at all. (p. 238)

Limitations are restrictions in the study that may decrease the generalizability of the findings. There are two types of limitations: conceptual and methodological. *Conceptual limitations* restrict the abstract generalization of the findings. The conceptual limitations are reflected in the frame of reference and conceptual and operational definitions. The *methodological limitations* restrict the population to which the findings can be generalized. Methodological limitations result from such factors as nonrandom sample, weak designs, single setting, uncontrolled data collection and inaccurate use of statistical analyses. Limitations are discussed from the point of view of threats to validity in Chapter 10. Johnson (1979) cited the following limitation in her study on anxiety/stress and the effects on disclosure between nurses and patients.

LIMITATIONS

The generalizability of this study is limited by the fact that all data were collected in one hospital; therefore, any conclusions and generalizations that are reached may be applicable only to this particular population and sample. (p. 11)

SELECTING A RESEARCH DESIGN

Research designs provide guidelines for investigating specific research objectives, questions or hypotheses. This step of the research process directs the selection of a population, a sampling procedure and a plan for data collection and analysis. The choice of research design depends on the researcher's knowledge, the research problem investigated, the purpose of the study and the desire to generalize the findings (Brophy, 1981).

Designs are specific to the research approach. In exploratory, descriptive and correlational studies, no treatment is administered. These designs focus on improving the precision of measurement. Quasi-experimental and experimental designs usually involve treatments and control groups. These designs focus on achieving higher levels of control as well as precision in measurement. Specific research designs are presented in Chapter 10.

Defining the Population and Sampling

The population is all elements (individuals, objects or substances) that meet certain criteria for inclusion in a given universe (Kerlinger, 1973). The researcher needs to carefully define the criteria for inclusion in the population. A study might be conducted to describe the responses of patients to their first hospitalization, and the study might be conducted in Hospital X on Unit Y. The population could be defined in different ways and include all patients hospitalized for the first time in: (1) Hospital X on Unit Y, (2) all units in Hospital X, (3) all hospitals in City Z or (4) all hospitals in the United States. The definition of population will depend on the criteria established and the similarity of subjects in these various systems. The question that the researcher needs to answer in defining the population is "Which population is best represented by the research sample?"

A sample is a subset of the population that is selected for a particular investigation. The members of a sample are subjects who participate in a study. The sample must be representative of the population and can be selected by a variety of strategies. In Williams' 1972 study of skin breakdown, she described a convenience sample consisting of "26 nonambulatory, i.e., bedfast or chair-fast, patients admitted to specific nursing care units in a county general hospital and in a private extended care facility in a southwestern urban community" (p. 239). Chapter 9 describes sampling and population theory and specific sampling techniques.

Developing a Plan for Data Collection and Analysis

Data collection is the precise, systematic gathering of information relevant to the research subproblems. The data collected in quantitative studies are numerical. There are numerous methods of data collection, such as interviews, questionnaires and research tools or instruments (Eells, 1981a). Precise tools to measure the variables of interest in nursing need to be developed. For example, Yonkman (1982) studied the effect of cool and heated aerosol on the oral temperature; a thermometer was the precise data collection instrument for measuring the oral temperature. Measurement theory and data collection tools are discussed in Chapter 11.

Planning data collection enables the researcher to anticipate problems that are likely to occur and to explore possible solutions. Researchers usually develop detailed procedures for the data collection process. A schedule is often developed that identifies the initiation and termination of data collection and when data will be collected. Planning and implementing data collection are the focus of Chapter 16.

Planning data analysis is an essential step in developing a study. The data analysis techniques used in a study depend on the research subproblems, data collected, research design, researcher expertise and availability of computer resources. A variety of statistical analyses exist that can describe the sample, examine a relationship or determine significant differences.

IMPLEMENTING THE RESEARCH PLAN

Implementing the research plan involves data collection, data analysis and interpretation of research findings. In this step of the research process, some researchers conduct a pilot study.

Pilot Study

A *pilot study* is a smaller version of a proposed study conducted to refine the methodology. It should be as similar to the proposed study as possible, using similar subjects, the same setting and the same data collection and analysis techniques. A pilot study is conducted for one or more of the following reasons:

1. To determine whether the proposed study is feasible (*e.g.*, are the subjects available, does the researcher have the time and money to do the study)
2. To identify problems with the design
3. To determine whether the sample is representative of the population or whether the sampling technique is effective
4. To refine the data collection instrument
5. To refine the data collection and analysis plan
6. To give the researcher experience with the subjects, methodology and research instruments (Ort, 1981).

Data Collection

Data collection is the generation of numerical data to answer the research subproblems. In order to collect data, the researcher must obtain the consent from the setting or agency where the study is to be conducted. Getting approval to conduct a study is described in Chapter 13. Consent must also be obtained from the research subjects to indicate their willingness to participate in the study. Frequently, the subjects are asked to sign a consent form, which describes the study, promises the subjects confidentiality and indicates that the subject can stop participation at any time. In data collection, the investigator measures variables using such activities as observing behaviors, conducting an interview, administering a questionnaire and using precise measurement tools. The data collection process is described in Chapter 16.

Data Analysis

Data analysis is conducted to reduce and organize the data to produce findings that must then be interpreted by the researcher. Data analysis may involve simple descriptive procedures or sophisticated mathematical computations. Most analyses are now performed by computer. Entering data in the computer and interpreting the analysis obtained require extensive knowledge and skills. The use of computers in research is discussed in Chapter 15 and analysis techniques are described in Chapter 17.

Interpretation of Findings

Findings are not meaningful until they are interpreted. They are interpreted in terms of the research subproblems, research design and the study framework. Interpretation of findings involves the researcher drawing conclusions from the findings and making recommendations for further study. The conclusions drawn from the findings can be significant and predictive, nonsignificant, significant and not predictive, unexpected or mixed. Having drawn conclusions about the study findings, the researcher is able to make recommendations for further research. Interpretation of findings is discussed in Chapter 18.

COMMUNICATION OF RESEARCH FINDINGS

The research is not complete until the findings are communicated. Communication of findings involves the dissemination of study findings to appropriate populations. These populations include nurses, other health professionals and health care consumers. Research conferences and journals are frequently used to communicate findings. The communication of findings is the focus of Chapter 19.

Types of Quantitative Research

Five types of quantitative research are included in this text: exploratory, descriptive, correlational, quasi-experimental and experimental. The type of research selected is determined by the level of existing knowledge for the research problem. When little knowledge is available, exploratory and descriptive studies are conducted, and, as the knowledge level increases, correlational, quasi-experimental and experimental studies are carried out. The purpose of each approach is described and is further illustrated with an example that includes the steps and results of a specific study.

EXPLORATORY RESEARCH

Purpose

The purpose of exploratory research is the exploration and description of phenomena. This approach is used to generate new knowledge about concepts or topics about which little is known. The exploratory study by Triplett (1970) entitled "Characteristics and perceptions of low-income women and use of preventive health services" is used as an example.

STEPS OF THE RESEARCH PROCESS

1. *Research Problem* □ "Do poor users of health services perceive interactions with health workers differently than good users, do they react differently in similar situations, and are there personal or demographic characteristics which differentiate the two groups?" (p. 141)
2. *Research Purpose* □ The purpose of this study was to describe the demographic and personal characteristics of low-income women who are either good or poor users of preventive health services.
3. *Review of Relevant Literature* □ The review of literature identified certain social-psychological characteristics of the poor that interfered with their health care–seeking behavior. The two characteristics focused on were social isolation and low self-esteem. The author also identified perceived threat as a factor in the patient–health worker relationship, and threat may be present when there is a high degree of disparity between the health worker's expectations of patients and their desire to meet these expectations.
4. *Frame of Reference* □ The conceptual framework included the following concepts: perception of self (self-esteem and ability to cope), utilization of services, interaction with health workers, perception of disparity of expectations, perception of threat and social isolation. The authors identified relationships among these concepts. The model developed for this text to illustrate these relationships (Fig. 3–2) indicates the direction of the relationships and whether the suggested relationships are positive or negative. In a positive relationship, both variables vary or change in the same direction. Thus, as one concept increases, the other concept increases; or both concepts decrease together. A negative relationship proposes that as one concept increases, the other concept decreases. The authors suggested that as the perception of self decreases, the utilization of services decreases (positive relationship). As

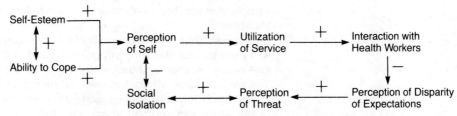

FIGURE 3–2. Conceptual model derived from Triplett's framework.

utilization of services decreases, the interaction with health workers decreases (positive relationship). As interactions with health workers decrease, there is an increase in the perception of disparity of expectations (negative relationship). As perception of disparity of expectations increases, the perception of threat increases. An increased perception of threat leads to an increase in social isolation. This relationship is bidirectional, which means that increased social isolation also leads to an increased perception of threat. As social isolation increases, perception of self decreases (which is also bidirectional). The relationships in the model reflect a circular phenomenon.

5. *Research Objectives* □ "To explore whether: (a) medically indigent women perceived disparity or threat in interactions with health workers, (b) perceptions of threat and disparity were related to each other and to the degree of utilization, (c) the women's perceptions of themselves influenced use or perceptions of threat and disparity and (d) these variables and certain demographic characteristics were related." (p. 141)

6. *Research Variables* □ The three research variables—disparity, threat and perception of self—were conceptually and operationally defined as follows:
Disparity—"the degree to which a patient perceives the expectations of the health worker to be unrealistic in respect of the patient's resources (or her ability and desire to mobilize her resources) as measured by a series of questions to the respondent." (p. 141)
Threat—"the degree to which the patient demonstrates or expresses feelings that indicate reluctance to continue with, or engage in, new activities for fear of exposing her ignorance, encountering disrespect, or feeling at a disadvantage as measured by a series of questions to the patient." (p. 141)
Perception of Self—"the feelings expressed by the patient as to (a) her self-esteem (as measured by Rosenberg's scale) and (b) her ability to cope with ordinary demands and responsibilities related to family health care as reflected by the respondent's perceptions of how the health workers feel about her and as measured by a series of questions." (p. 141)

7. *Assumptions and Limitations* □ The researcher assumed that the responses of the subjects were reflective of their true feelings. The study was limited by the sample, which was drawn from a population that was referred by staff, who might have been biased in their selection. The researcher indicated that the sample size was too small to permit controlling for several variables.

8. *Implementation of the Research Plan* □ An exploratory design was used to describe the characteristics and perceptions of the low-income women and their use of preventive health services. The subjects were 40 women selected by public health nurses in an Iowa public health agency, and half were identified as good health care users and half were poor health care users. The

data were gathered only by the researcher through interviews conducted in the subjects' homes. The data were analyzed to determine percentages and areas of significance.

9. *Results* ☐ A disparity was found between the subjects (low-income women) and the health care workers, with the greatest disparity being between the physician and subjects, and the least disparity being between the nurse and subjects. Poor users of health care perceived a greater threat in interacting with health care workers than the good users of health care. There was a significant relationship between disparity of expectations and threat, for those women who perceived a high disparity also perceive a high threat. These findings were supportive of the study framework. The good users of health care tended to have lower self-esteem than the poor users, and the good users admitted more feelings of isolation and loneliness (which is not supportive of the study framework). There was no relationship found between the subjects' use of health care and their education, age or social class.

DESCRIPTIVE RESEARCH

The purpose of descriptive research is the description of phenomena. This approach is used to clarify concepts and generate relationships for use in further research or theory development. Common types of descriptive research include the case study and descriptive survey. An example of a case study and a survey follows.

Case Study Purpose

The purpose of a *case study* is to describe in-depth many characteristics or attributes of a single subject or a specific group. The case study presented is "Assessment and treatment of psychosocial problems of the cancer patient: a case study" by Freidenbergs, Gordon, Hibbard and Diller (1980).

STEPS OF THE RESEARCH PROCESS

1. *Research Problem* ☐ The multitude of problems and complexity of issues that exist for cancer patients often interfere with the effort of health care providers to reduce the distress from the frequent sequela to cancer.
2. *Research Purpose* ☐ The purpose of this study was to more clearly define the assessed elements of psychosocial distress and to begin examining the effectiveness of health care workers' treatments on this distress.
3. *Review of the Literature* ☐ The literature reviewed included studies and sources on the potential and actual psychosocial

problems of cancer patients and the methods used to intervene with these problems.

4. **Conceptual Framework** □ The framework addressed the relationship between the diagnosis of cancer and the increased levels of psychosocial distress. Through psychosocial assessment, the specific problems associated with psychosocial distress from the diagnosis of cancer can be identified and can direct the treatment of health care workers. The effect of the health care worker's treatment on psychosocial distress is unclear in the framework. A possible approach to modeling of these relationships is presented in Figure 3–3.

5. **Research Objectives** □ The objectives were to assess the psychosocial problems of one cancer patient and to treat the psychosocial problems of the selected patient.

6. **Research Variables** □ The variables were psychosocial assessment and psychosocial intervention.
   Psychosocial Assessment—"was a problem-oriented interview that assessed 122 potential cancer-related problems that were grouped into 13 areas of life-functioning: physical discomfort, medical treatment, hospital service, mobility, housework, vocational, financial, family, social, worries, affect, body image and communication." (p. 113)
   Psychosocial Intervention—"was psychosocial services in the program that were developed and provided by a multidisciplinary group of professionals who functioned as oncology counselors. The interventions were divided into three groups: educational, counseling and environmental." (p. 114)

7. **Assumptions and Limitations** □ No assumptions were identified in the study. The researchers did identify the limitation of using one subject.

8. **Implementation of the Research Plan** □ The subject was a 70-year-old female with the diagnosis of malignant melanoma of the thigh. The data were gathered using structured clinical interviews. The subject's psychosocial problems were assessed four times: (1) when the subject was admitted to the hospital for surgery to remove the tumor, (2) at hospital discharge, (3) 3 months after discharge and (4) 6 months after discharge. Psychosocial interventions were provided during hospitalization and for 6 months following discharge. The data were analyzed to identify what the psychosocial problems of the cancer patient

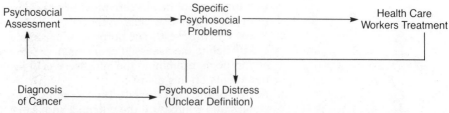

FIGURE 3–3. Conceptual model derived from Freidenbergs *et al* framework.

were and whether these problems changed with the psychosocial intervention.

9. *Results* □ The final assessment of the patient showed that her problems were in the areas of physical discomfort, mobility, worry and body image. The reported psychosocial problems had decreased in number from the first assessment to the last; the subject had reported 90 psychosocial problems in the first assessment and 44 in the last. The researchers noted that the decrease in problems might have been due to the psychosocial intervention but could have resulted from the passing of the crisis. These findings have implications for nursing because the assessment tool could be useful to increase the identification of psychosocial problems in cancer patients.

Descriptive Survey Purpose

A descriptive survey is conducted to identify or describe a concept in a real-life situation. Generally, questionnaires or interviews are used to collect data from large samples. The descriptive survey presented is "Health needs of the elderly" by Hain and Chen (1976).

STEPS OF THE RESEARCH PROCESS

1. *Research Problem* □ "Although increasing numbers of elderly persons are moving into high-rise apartments, health needs of these residents have not been documented to any extent." (p. 433)
2. *Research Purpose* □ "This study attempted to identify health needs of the elderly in two high-rise apartments for senior citizens in Erie, Pennsylvania." (p. 433)
3. *Review of the Literature* □ The literature reviewed focused on studies and sources that identified the health needs of the elderly.
4. *Conceptual Framework* □ The conceptual framework of this study is limited, since it is based only on the empirical findings of previous studies. The concepts examined include health condition, physical functioning and access to medical care. The researchers indicated that the elderly have chronic health problems of one kind or another that can result in physical and emotional disability. Health problems are perceived by the elderly as being normal and inevitable; therefore, help is frequently not sought. Access to care is limited by lack of knowledge and decreased energy to reach available services.
5. *Research Questions* □ What are the health conditions of the elderly? What is the physical functioning of the elderly? What is the access of the elderly to medical care?
6. *Research Variables* □ The research variables were health

condition, physical functioning and access to medical care and were operationally defined as follows:

Health Condition—"included the number of days of illness, status of ambulation and difficulty with symptoms during the month prior to the interview.

Physical Functioning—indicated the capacity during the month prior to the interview in five activities of daily living adapted to the apartment setting: getting about in the apartment; doing own laundry; washing, bathing, dressing, putting on shoes (self-care factors); getting around outside the apartment complex; and cutting toenails.

Access to Medical Care—included situations of emergency, nonemergency and routine health care." (p. 433)

7. *Assumptions and Limitations* □ The researchers made two assumptions about the sample: (1) that the elder member of the pairs of adults living together would be males, and (2) the health needs of older adults living alone or in pairs might differ. The limitations were that the subjects were suspicious of the survey and were reluctant to respond. In addition, they were hard to locate because of their involvement in numerous activities. The subjects were also difficult to communicate with because of their hearing impairments. The final limitation was a sample loss of nine elderly subjects, which might have influenced the results.

8. *Implementation of the Research Plan* □ The sample consisted of 128 subjects: 20 males living alone, 71 females living alone, and 37 pairs. The subjects were residents of two high-rise apartment buildings in Pennsylvania. The data were gathered during an interview by one researcher in order to reduce the interviewer bias. The subjects were asked to complete a 20-item questionnaire that was developed for this study. The questionnaire was developed to cover health condition, physical functioning and access to medical care. A pilot study had been conducted on this questionnaire, in which five elderly persons had been asked to respond to the items on the questionnaire. They indicated no difficulty in responding to the items, so the questionnaire was finalized for the study based on their responses. The data were analyzed using means and percentages (descriptive statistics) to identify the health condition, physical functioning and access to medical care of the elderly.

9. *Results* □ The findings indicated that 24.3 per cent of the elderly surveyed were not in good health and that the common health conditions of the elderly were hypertension, heart conditions, diabetes and arthritis. Thirty-two per cent of the elderly surveyed needed assistance in physical functioning. The predominant difficulty was with ambulatory activities, especially for the females living alone. The findings also indicated that 11.7 per cent of the elderly surveyed did not have access to medical care or that the access to medical care was uncertain.

The researchers made three recommendations: (1) A nurse practitioner could assess the health status of the elderly at a specified health center or in their own apartments, (2) community groups or a home health aide could provide the assistance for the elderly who indicated difficulty with physical functioning and (3) a counseling or referral service could be provided for those persons without access to medical care.

CORRELATIONAL RESEARCH

Purpose

Correlational research is conducted to examine whether relationships occur between or among two or more variables. If a relationship exists, a correlational study also clarifies the type (positive or negative) and degree of the relationship. The correlational study in this example is "The relationship among health beliefs, health values, and health promotion activity" by Brown, Muhlenkamp, Fox and Osborn (1983).

STEPS OF THE RESEARCH PROCESS

1. **Research Problem** □ "What is the relationship among individuals' health locus of control, health values, and their health-promotion activities?" (p. 158)
2. **Review of Relevant Literature** □ The review of literature included the concepts of health beliefs, health values, locus of control and health-related behaviors. Previous studies that examined locus of control, health values and health behaviors were summarized.
3. **Theoretical Framework** □ "The framework for this study was the health belief model of Hochbaum and Rosenstock, which focuses specifically on the influence of social, psychological and cognitive variables on health behavior. According to this model, one's behavior in a particular situation is determined by the way one perceives the surrounding world." (p. 155)
4. **Research Questions** □ "What is the relationship between the Multidimensional Health Locus of Control (MHLC) subscales, health value, and health-promotion activities? Is there a relationship between health locus of control and health information–seeking activities?" (p. 158)
5. **Research Variables** □ The research variables were locus of control, health values and health promotion activities. The conceptual definitions were not provided, but the operational definitions are as follows: (a) *Locus of control* was measured by the Multidimensional Health Locus of Control Scale; (b) *Health values* were measured by the Rokeach's Value Survey; (c) *Health*

promotional activities were measured by a Personal Lifestyle Activities Questionnaire developed by the researchers.

6. ***Assumptions and Limitations*** □ No assumptions were stated within the study. The limitations identified were that the sample was not random, which limits the generalizability of the findings, and the sample was small for the type of statistical analysis conducted.

7. ***Implementation of the Research Plan*** □ The sample was one of convenience and consisted of 67 subjects obtained from a church social group and secretaries from a university and a law office. The subjects were provided with the questionnaires (MHLC Scale, Value Survey, Personal Lifestyle Activities Questionnaire and demographic data) to complete and return by mail. The data were analyzed to determine the type and degree of correlation among the variables, which included health locus of control, health values and health promotion activities.

8. ***Results*** □ There was a significant negative relationship (correlation of −0.325) found between health promotion activities and chance health locus of control (person believes health is a product of chance), which means that the subjects who identified more health promotion activities identified less chance health locus of control. There was also a significant negative relationship (correlation of −0.395) between health promotion activities and powerful other health locus of control (person believes health is influenced by powerful others). There was not a significant relationship (correlation of 0.023) between health promotion activities and internal health locus of control (person believes he or she controls own health). There were no significant relationships found between the variable health values and the other two variables, health locus of control and health promotion activities.

QUASI-EXPERIMENTAL STUDY

Purpose

The purpose of quasi-experimental research is to examine cause-and-effect relationships. The quasi-experimental study presented is "The effect of teaching on medication knowledge" by Osguthorpe, Roper and Saunders (1983).

STEPS OF THE RESEARCH PROCESS

1. ***Research Problem*** □ The problem was that the effect of teaching methods on patient's knowledge level is unknown.

2. ***Research Purpose*** □ The purpose of this study was to examine "the most effective method of teaching psychiatric inpatients

about their medication. The secondary purpose was to evaluate the three instruments developed for the study: the drug information sheet, the videotaped nurse explanation and the multiple choice pre/post-test to measure medication knowledge." (p. 206)

3. *Review of the Literature* □ The literature review included studies and sources on health education and teaching-learning methods. The researchers' major focus was on the findings from studies concerning patient teaching.

4. *Theoretical Framework* □ "The framework for this study was based on Orem's work and the following proposition: Health education should bring the patient to an understanding of illness and treatments so that adequate comprehension occurs to allow the patient to follow actively through on the recommended regimen after discharge." (p. 205)

5. *Research Hypotheses* □ (a) "Psychiatric inpatients taught about their medications through the drug information sheet and/or the videotaped nurse explanation will score higher on the post-test than those who were taught through the usual ward practices (the control group)... (b) Subjects taught about their medications through the usual ward practices will have no change in their test scores from pretest to post-test. (c) Test scores will not be influenced by either age or level of schooling of the subjects." (pp. 207–208)

6. *Research Variables* □ The independent (treatment) variable was teaching method. The teaching methods used were a drug information sheet and a videotaped nurse explanation. The dependent variable was knowledge. The psychiatric patients' knowledge of their medications was measured with a multiple-choice examination that was developed by the researchers.

7. *Assumptions and Limitations* □ One assumption of the authors was "that patients have a right to learn about their health care needs and that nurses are appropriate teachers" (p. 205). They further "believed that patient education could be achieved with a variety of techniques" (p. 207). Although it was not stated, the authors also had to assume that the subjects would respond to the best of their ability on the multiple-choice test. Limitations recognized by the authors were that the measurement tools used in the study had limited reliability and validity, which limits generalizability.

8. *Implementation of the Research Plan* □ The researchers ran a pilot study to test the instruments used in this study. The study was conducted using a quasi-experimental, four-group pretest-post-test design. The sample was 202 patients in nine general psychiatric wards in a large urban Veterans Administration psychiatric hospital. The nine wards and not the subjects were randomly assigned to the treatment groups and the control group. The four groups received the following treatments: Group A received the drug information sheet; Group B received the drug information sheet and the videotaped nurse

explanation; Group C received the videotaped nurse explanation; and Group D (control group) received no experimental treatment. The number of subjects per group was not identified. Each subject was pretested by a researcher within the first 2 weeks of being on medication, and 1 week following the pretest, the subject received the specified treatment. One week after receiving the treatment, the post-test was given to the subject. The data were analyzed, using analysis of variance, to examine the effect of the treatments (drug information sheet and videotaped nurse explanation) on the psychiatric inpatients' knowledge of their medication.

9. *Results* □ The findings indicated that there was no significant difference in the four groups of subjects regarding their knowledge of their medications as measured by the multiple choice test. This means that the drug information sheet and the videotaped nurse explanation (treatments) did not significantly change the knowledge of the subjects as compared with that of the control group when measured by the multiple-choice test. The researchers, in an attempt to explain these findings, indicated that the multiple-choice test might have been oversimplified and was not effective in examining the effect of the teaching methods. It was also possible that the teaching methods did not impart new information. The researchers recommended further study in this area using less simplified teaching methods and testing measures.

EXPERIMENTAL RESEARCH

Purpose

The purpose of an experimental study is to examine cause-and-effect relationships between variables in highly controlled settings. Very few nursing studies are "purely" experimental. The experimental study presented is "The effect of oxygen inhalation on oral temperature" by Lim-Levy (1982). In this example, the subjects were randomly assigned to groups but were not randomly selected. However, the study is a good example of the process of conducting experimental research.

STEPS OF THE RESEARCH PROCESS

1. *Research Problem* □ The effect of oxygen inhalation on oral temperatures has not been clearly determined.
2. *Research Purpose* □ The purpose was "to determine the effect of oxygen inhalation by nasal cannula on oral temperatures" (p. 150).
3. *Review of the Literature* □ The literature review included other studies that had been conducted on the effect of oxygen on the

oral temperature. The researcher made references to the difficulties in taking rectal and axillary temperatures versus the oral temperature.

4. ***Theoretical Framework*** □ The framework, not specifically identified, is derived from physics and physiology. The researcher stated that "It has been thought that the increased air current directed to the nasal cavity lowers the oral temperature" (p. 150). This idea could have been supported with a proposition from physics or physiology theory.

5. ***Research Hypothesis*** □ "Oxygen inhalation by nasal cannula of up to 6 liters per minute (LPM) does not affect oral temperature measurement taken with an electronic thermometer." (p. 150)

6. ***Research Variables*** □ The independent (treatment) variable was the administration of oxygen. The oxygen was administered by nasal cannula at 2 LPM, 4 LPM and 6 LPM. The dependent variable was temperature. The subject's temperature was measured with an electric thermometer, which registered a temperature in approximately 30 seconds and covered a range of temperatures from 94° to 108° F. There were several extraneous variables that the researcher controlled because of their possible effects on the oral temperature. These variables were recent ingestion of food and beverages, smoking, gum chewing and local inflammatory process.

7. ***Assumptions and Limitations*** □ The researcher assumed that the subjects would refrain from vigorous activity, eating, drinking and smoking 1 hour before the experiment, which had been requested. No limitations were identified.

8. ***Implementation of the Research Plan*** □ The sample consisted of 100 healthy adults (59 females and 41 males), ranging in age from 18 to 56 years. The subjects were employees of a general hospital and students of a school of nursing. They were randomly assigned to the control group and the three treatment groups. Twenty-five subjects were in the control group, 24 subjects received 2 LPM of oxygen by nasal cannula, 26 subjects received 4 LPM and 25 subjects received 6 LPM. All subjects initially had their temperature taken, and their temperatures were taken again 30 minutes later after the treatment groups had been on oxygen 30 minutes. An analysis of variance was conducted on the data to determine whether there were significant differences between the control group and the treatment groups.

9. ***Results*** □ This study showed no significant effect of oxygen inhalation by nasal cannula on oral temperature. These findings have implications for nursing because the oral temperature will cause less patient embarrassment and anxiety and decrease nursing time. The researcher recommended further research "using higher oxygen flow, longer treatment and including febrile patients" (p. 152).

Summary

Quantitative research is the traditional approach in nursing research. Nurses use a broad range of quantitative approaches—exploratory, descriptive, correlational, quasi-experimental and experimental—for developing nursing knowledge. Conducting quantitative research requires familiarity with such concepts as basic research, applied research, rigor and control. Basic, or pure, research is a scientific investigation that involves the generation of "knowledge for knowledge sake" or for the pleasure of learning and finding truth. Applied research is a scientific investigation conducted to answer a clinical question or solve a practice-related problem. Many of the studies that have been conducted in nursing are applied because researchers have chosen to focus on answering immediate clinical questions.

Conducting quantitative research involves rigor, which is associated with discipline, scrupulous adherence and strict accuracy. A rigorous quantitative researcher constantly strives for more precise measurement tools and tightly controlled study designs. Control involves the imposing of "rules" by the researcher to decrease the possibility of error and thus increase the probability that the study's findings are an accurate reflection of reality. Some mechanisms for control within a quantitative study include subject selection (sampling), subject's knowledge of the study (Hawthorne effect) and the research setting.

The quantitative research process includes planning and implementing a study and communicating the study's findings. The different steps of this research process have been introduced in this chapter and are described in depth later in the text. The steps of the process follow:

1. *Formulating a research problem*—the identification of a question or statement that clarifies the focus of a study.
2. *Reviewing relevant literature*—an organized search of the literature to determine the knowledge that currently exists concerning a selected research problem.
3. *Developing a frame of reference*—the formulation of an abstract conceptualization that places a study within a context of meaning. It is the structure within which a study is developed and links all components of a study together.
4. *Formulating subproblems*—the identification of objectives, questions or hypotheses for a specific study.
5. *Defining research variables*—the development of conceptual definitions and operational definitions for the variables to be investigated.
6. *Making assumptions explicit and identifying limitations*—the identification of assumptions and limitations for a specific study. Assumptions are the statements that are taken for granted or are considered true, even though these statements have not been scientifically tested. Limitations are restrictions in the study that may decrease the generalizability of the findings.

7. *Selecting a research design*—a structure that provides a blueprint for the development of a study.
8. *Defining the population and sampling*—Population is all elements that meet certain criteria for inclusion in a given universe. A sample is a subset of the population that is selected for a particular investigation.
9. *Developing a plan for data collection and analysis*—the identification of a particular strategy for collecting and analyzing data for a study.
10. *Implementing the research plan*—involves data collection, data analysis and interpretation of research findings.
11. *Communicating findings*—the dissemination of study results to the appropriate populations.

Five types of quantitative research are included in this text: exploratory, descriptive, correlational, quasi-experimental and experimental. The purpose of each quantitative approach is described and further illustrated with an example that includes the steps and results of a specific study.

References

Abdellah, F. G. & Levine, E. (1979). *Better patient care through nursing research* (2nd ed.). New York: The Macmillan Publishing Company, Inc.

Armstrong, R. L. (1981). Hypothesis formulation. In S. D. Krampitz & N. Pavlovich (Eds.), *Readings for nursing research* (pp. 29–39). St. Louis: The C. V. Mosby Company.

Brophy, E. B. (1981). Research design: general introduction. In S. D. Krampitz & N. Pavlovich (Eds.), *Readings for nursing research* (pp. 40–48). St. Louis: The C. V. Mosby Company.

Brown, N., Muhlenkamp, A. Fox, L. & Osborn, M. (1983). The relationship among health beliefs, health values, and health promotion activity. *Western Journal of Nursing Research*, 5(2), 155–163.

Butts, P. A. (1982). Dissemination of nursing research findings. *Image*, 14(2), 62–64.

Campbell, D. T. & Stanley, J. C. (1963). *Experimental and quasi-experimental designs for research*. Chicago: Rand McNally College Publishing Company.

Cook, T. D. & Campbell, D. T. (1979). *Quasi-experimentation: design & analysis issues for field settings*. Chicago: Rand McNally College Publishing Company.

Downs, F. S. (1984). *A source book of nursing research* (3rd ed.). Philadelphia: F. A. Davis Company.

Downs, F. S. & Fleming, J. W. (1979). *Issues in nursing research*. Norwalk, Connecticut: Appleton-Century-Crofts.

Downs, F. S. & Newman, M. A. (1977). *A source book of nursing research* (2nd ed.). Philadelphia: F. A. Davis Company.

Dubin, R. (1978). *Theory building*. New York: The Free Press, A Division of Macmillan Publishing Company, Inc.

Eells, M. A. W. (1981a). Data collection: philosophical and theoretical perspectives. In S. D. Krampitz & N. Pavlovich (Eds.), *Readings for nursing research* (pp. 80–92). St. Louis: The C. V. Mosby Company.

Eells, M. A. W. (1981b). The research problem. In S. D. Krampitz & N. Pavlovich (Eds.), *Readings for nursing research* (pp. 3–10). St. Louis: The C. V. Mosby Company.

Fisher, Sir R. A. (1935). *The designs of experiments*. New York: Hafner Publishing Company.

Freidenbergs, I., Gordon, W., Hibbard, R. M. & Diller, L. (1980). Assessment and treatment of psychosocial problems of the cancer patient: a case study. *Cancer Nursing*, 3(2), 111–119.

Gunter, L. (1981). Literature review. In S. D. Krampitz & N. Pavlovich (Eds.), *Readings for nursing research* (pp. 11–16). St. Louis: The C. V. Mosby Company.

Hain, Sr. M. J. & Chen, S. C. (1976). Health needs of the elderly. *Nursing Research*, 25(6), 433-439.

Homans, G. (1965). Group factors in worker productivity. In H. Proshansky & B. Seidenberg

(Eds.), *Basic studies in social psychology* (pp. 592–604). New York: Holt, Rinehart and Winston.

Johnson, M. N. (1979). Anxiety/stress and the effects on disclosure between nurses and patients. *Advances in Nursing Science*, 1(4), 1–20.

Jones, P. E. (1982). Developing terminology: a university of Toronto experience (1978). In M. J. Kim & D. A. Moritz (Eds.), *Classification of nursing diagnoses: proceedings of the third and fourth national conferences* (pp. 138–145). New York: McGraw-Hill Book Company.

Kaplan, A. (1964). *The conduct of inquiry: methodology for behavioral science*. New York: Chandler Publishing Company.

Kerlinger, F. N. (1973). *Foundations of behavioral research*. New York: Holt, Rinehart and Winston.

Killeen, M. L. (1985). Taking risks with health. *Western Journal of Nursing research*, 7(1), 116–124.

King, I. M. (1971). *Toward a theory for nursing*. New York: John Wiley & Sons.

King, I. M. (1981). *A theory for nursing: systems, concepts, process*. New York: John Wiley & Sons.

Leedy, P. D. (1980). *Practical research: planning and design*. New York: Macmillan Publishing Company, Inc.

Lim-Levy, F. (1982). The effect of oxygen inhalation on oral temperature. *Nursing Research*, 31(3), 151–152.

Martinson, I. M. & Anderson, S. E. (1983). Effects of thermal applications on the abdominal temperature of dogs. *Research in Nursing and Health*, 6(2), 89–93.

Mason, D. Data analysis: introduction. In S. D. Krampitz & N. Pavlovich (Eds.), *Readings for nursing research* (pp. 108–113). St. Louis: The C. V. Mosby Company.

Myers, S. T. (1982). The search for assumptions. *Western Journal of Nursing Research*, 4(1), 91–98.

Nagel, E. (1961). *The structure of science: problems in the logic of scientific explanation*. New York: Harcourt, Brace & World, Inc.

Neale, J. M. & Liebert, R. M. (1980). *Science and behavior: an introduction to methods of research*. Englewood Cliffs, New Jersey: Prentice-Hall, Inc.

Newman, M. A. (1979). *Theory development in nursing*. Philadelphia: F. A. Davis Company.

Newman, M. A. & Gaudiano, J. K. (1984). Depression as an explanation for decreased subjective time in the elderly. *Nursing Research*, 33(3), 137–139.

Orem, D. E. (1985). *Nursing: concepts of practice* (3rd ed.). New York: The McGraw-Hill Book Company.

Ort, S. V. (1981). Research design: pilot study. In S. D. Krampitz & N. Pavlovich (Eds.), *Readings for nursing research* (pp. 49–53). St. Louis: The C. V. Mosby Company.

Osguthorpe, N., Roper, J. & Saunders, J. (1983). The effect of teaching on medication knowledge. *Western Journal of Nursing Research*, 5(3), 205–216.

Passos, J. Y. & Brand, L. M. (1966). Effects of agents used for oral hygiene. *Nursing Research*, 15(3), 196–202.

Perry, J. A. (1981). Effectiveness of teaching in the rehabilitation of patients with chronic bronchitis and emphysema. *Nursing Research*, 30(4), 219–222.

Robb, S. S. (1985). Urinary incontinence verification in elderly men. *Nursing Research*, 34(5), 278–282.

Rogers, M. E. (1970). *An introduction to the theoretical basis of nursing*. Philadelphia: F. A. Davis Company.

Roy, Sr. C. (1984). *Introduction to nursing: an adaptation model* (2nd ed.). Englewood Cliffs, New Jersey: Prentice-Hall, Inc.

Roy, Sr. C. & Roberts, S. (1981). *Theory construction in nursing: an adaptation model*. Englewood Cliffs, New Jersey: Prentice-Hall, Inc.

Ruth, M. V. & White, C. M. (1981). Data collection: sample. In S. D. Krampitz & N. Pavlovich (Eds.), *Readings for nursing research* (pp. 93–97). St. Louis: The C. V. Mosby Company.

Selltiz, C. Wrightsman, L. S. & Cook, S. W. (1976). *Research methods in social relations* (3rd ed.). New York: Holt, Rinehart and Winston.

Silva, M. C. (1981). Selection of a theoretical framework. In S. D. Krampitz & N. Pavlovich (Eds.), *Readings for nursing research* (pp. 17–28). St. Louis: The C. V. Mosby Company.

Triplett, J. L. (1970). Characteristics and perceptions of low-income women and use of preventive health services: an exploratory study. *Nursing Research*, 19(2), 140–146.

Updike, P. A., Accurso, F. J. & Jones, R. H. (1985). Physiologic circadian rhythmicity in preterm infants. *Nursing Research*, 34(3), 160–163.

Waltz, C. F. & Bausell, R. B. (1981). *Nursing research: design, statistics and computer analysis*. Philadelphia: F. A. Davis Company.

Wells, N. (1982). The effect of relaxation on postoperative muscle tension and pain. *Nursing Research*, 31(4), 236–238.

Williams, A. (1972). A study of factors contributing to skin breakdown. *Nursing Research*, 21(3), 238–243.

Williams, M. A. (1980). Editorial: assumptions in research. *Research in Nursing and Health*, 3(2), 47–48.

Wysocki, A. B. (1983). Basic versus applied research: intrinsic and extrinsic considerations. *Western Journal of Nursing Research*, 5(3), 217–224.

Yonkman, C. A. (1982). Cool and heated aerosol and the measurement of oral temperature. *Nursing Research*, 31(6), 354–357.

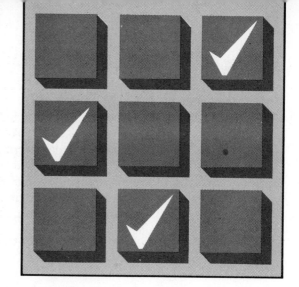

4

Introduction to Qualitative Research

Qualitative research is a relatively new approach to research in nursing, and being new, it is not as well understood as quantitative research. Qualitative research seeks to gain insight through discovering the meanings attached to a given phenomenon. These insights can then be used to improve nursing practice. As with quantitative research, the goals are to describe, explain, predict and control. However, this is accomplished not through establishing causality but through improving our comprehension of the phenomenon as a whole. Within a holistic framework, qualitative research seeks to explore the depth, richness and complexity inherent in the phenomenon.

The terminology used in qualitative research and the methods of reasoning are very different from those of more traditional methods. The concepts and reasoning are reflections of the philosophical orientations within the qualitative research approaches. These philosophical orientations, which differ with each approach, direct the methodology. Even though the various qualitative research approaches have many ideas in common, each approach uses different terminology to explain those ideas. Although the terminology is different, there are some commonalities in the "mind set" of qualitative researchers as they implement the research process. Ideas important to most qualitative approaches will be explained in this chapter using the terminology of phenomenology. These ideas are gestalt, bracketing, intuiting and sedimented views.

Published findings from qualitative studies are beginning to appear more frequently in journals and books. Comprehension of these research methodologies is necessary in order to critique the studies in publications and utilize the findings in practice. To provide this background, gestalts, the conduct of qualitative research and four of the most prominent approaches to qualitative research (phenomenological, grounded theory, ethnographic and historical) are described in this chapter. The methodology used in each of the four approaches is explained.

Gestalts

The concept of *gestalts* is closely related to holism. This view proposes that knowledge about a particular phenomenon is organized into a cluster of linked ideas, a gestalt. This clustering, or interrelatedness, enhances the meaning of the ideas. A theory is in some ways like a gestalt. A theory is a cluster of linked ideas that explains a phenomenon. If we are trying to understand something new and are offered a theory that explains it, our reaction may be "Now that makes sense" or "Oh, I see." It has "come together" for us. However, once we understand a phenomenon by using a particular theory, it is difficult for us to "see" the phenomenon outside of the meaning given it by the theory. Therefore, in addition to giving meaning, a theory can limit meaning. "Seeing" the phenomenon from the perspective of one point of view may limit our ability to see it from another point of view. For example, because we are so familiar with it, it is difficult to examine the phenomenon of stress without using Selye's theory of stress.

The purpose of a qualitative research approach is to form new gestalts in order to generate new theories. To accomplish this, the researcher has to "get outside of" the theories or gestalts that currently explain a phenomenon. The qualitative researcher cannot be limited by existing theories; rather, the mind must be open to new gestalts emerging through the abstract thinking processes of the researcher. Since personal experiences of the researcher are an important part of conducting the study, it is crucial that the researcher be open and receptive to new perceptions (new gestalts) being formed from information received during the research process.

EXPERIENCING GESTALT CHANGE

One qualitative researcher, Ihde (1977), has explained the process of forming a gestalt, "getting outside" of that gestalt and developing a new gestalt in such a way that you can experience the process. According to qualitative points of view, experiencing the process is the best way to understand it.

Ihde's extensive research has been in the area of vision or seeing, which is a very empirical sense. He has studied how our eyes and brain actually perceive an image, for example, how our eyes sometimes see one line as shorter or longer than another when the lines are equal in length. Ihde has related the vision of the eye with the way we "see" mentally. Consider the concrete thinking behind sayings such as "Seeing makes it real," "Seeing is believing," or "I saw it with my own eyes." It is easy to generalize from seeing to the other senses (hearing, touching, smelling, tasting), or empirical ways of knowing, and from there to perception. In fact, we often use phrases such as "I see" or "I hear" to mean "I understand."

Ihde proposes that we have an initial way of perceiving (or seeing) a phenomenon that is naive and inflexible. It is based on the assumption that the way the phenomenon is being seen at the time is the one and only way of seeing that is real. This is generally the way we think about "facts." If it is a fact, we see it as true or real. One cannot argue with a fact, since that information is fixed and will not change. But "seeing" occurs within a specific context of beliefs, which Ihde calls natural, or *sedimented*. In other words, we see things within a specific frame of reference, world view or theory. This gives us a sense of reality, certainty, security and, seemingly, control. Ihde uses line drawings to demonstrate this sedimented view. Examine the following line drawing:

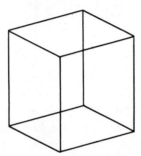

Most people who passively view this figure will see a cube. If you continue to gaze at it, you will find that the cube reverses itself. The figure actually seems to move. It jumps and then becomes fixed again in your view. With practice, you can see first one view and then the other, and then reverse it again. Ihde (1977) developed five alternative ways to view the drawing and suggests that there are more. See the figure on page 78.

Suppose, now, that the cube drawing is not a cube at all, but is an insect in a hexagonal opening... Suppose I tell you that the cube is not a cube at all, but is a very oddly cut gem. The central facet (the shaded area of the guide picture) is nearest you, and all the other facets are sloping downwards and away from it... Now, suppose I tell you that the gem is also reversible. Suppose you are now inside the gem, looking upwards, so that the central facet (the shaded area of the guide picture) is the one farthest away from you, and the oddly cut side facets are sloping down towards you. (pp. 96–98)

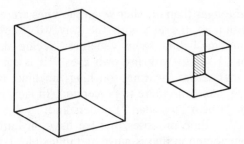

Ihde proposes that in order to see an alternate view of the drawing, you must first deconstruct your original sedimented view. Then you must reconstruct another view. This activity involves the use of intuition. He sees this as jumping from one gestalt to another. Try examining a second line drawing. What is your sedimented view? Can you reconstruct another gestalt or view?

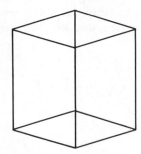

Ihde found that one of the important strategies in switching from one view of a drawing to another was to change your focus. Try focusing on a different point of the drawing or looking at it as two-dimensional rather than as three-dimensional. If you concentrate and gaze for a long enough period of time, you can experience the change in gestalt. Ihde cautions that a new reconstruction tends to be considered odd at first and unnatural, but attains stability and naturalness after a while.

Once you have accomplished this jump, you are no longer naive; you cannot go back to the idea that the phenomenon you have observed can be seen only in one way. You have become more open and receptive to examining more variations in the phenomenon; you can explore deeper layers of the phenomenon. Viewing these deeper layers requires a second-order deconstruction and an increase in openness. Ihde refers to this as *ascendence to the open context*. It allows you to see the depth and complexity within the phenomenon you examine; you have increased your insight. Ihde suggests that ascendence to the open context gives you "multi-stability" and far greater control than the sedimented view.

CHANGING GESTALTS IN NURSING

Nursing has a strong traditional base. With tradition comes a sedimented view of such phenomena as patients, illness situations, health and the effects of nursing care. We are introduced to these sedimented views very early in our nursing experiences. When we ask questions, the sedimented view is often explained. These explanations are gestalts that have been held for many years. Now, we are beginning to question many of these long-held ideas, and the insights gained are changing nursing practice. For example, for many years, nurses perceived the patient as being passive, dependent and unable to take responsibility for his or her care. Now, patients are more often perceived as participating in their care and being responsible for their health. Ascendence to the open context requires more than just switching from one sedimented view to another. The nurse functioning within an open context would be able to view the patient from a variety of perspectives, passive and dependent in some ways, participating with health care givers in other ways and directing his or her care in some cases.

Qualitative research is a tool by which we can examine a phenomenon outside the context of existing gestalts or sedimented views. The earliest and perhaps most dramatic demonstration of the influence qualitative research can have on nursing practice was the 4-year study conducted by Glaser and Strauss (1965). This study was reported in a book entitled *Awareness of dying,* which described the environment of dying patients in hospitals. At that time, the "gestalt" commonly held was that people could not cope with knowing that they were dying and must be protected from that knowledge. The environment of care was designed to protect the patient from that knowledge. Glaser and Strauss examined the meaning that environment had to the patient. The study changed our gestalt. Instead of protecting, we saw the traditional care of the dying as creating loneliness and isolation. We began to "see" the patient in a new light, and our care began to change. Kubler-Ross, perhaps influenced by the work of Glaser and Strauss, then began her studies of the dying. From this new orientation to care for the dying, hospice care began to develop, and now, 20 years later, the environment of care for the dying is changing.

Conducting Qualitative Research

Qualitative research is not easy to conduct. A long period of time (often years) is required to complete a study. The techniques used differ from those of quantitative studies, and the researcher must be rigorous in utilizing qualitative techniques. Data collection usually involves large amounts of handwritten notes, which must be sorted and organized. Qualitative researchers tend to use words as the basis for analysis rather than numeric data. To generate the findings, the researcher examines all the notes and tabulations and begins to organize them in some way that "makes sense." This organizing, or clustering, of data is a critical part of qualitative research. Abstract thinking processes are used to develop research findings from which meanings and theoretical implications emerge. In order to be useful, the theory that emerges from qualitative research must clearly reflect the phenomenon. In addition, others should be able to verify the findings intuitively and through their own personal experiences.

RIGOR IN QUALITATIVE RESEARCH

The concept *rigor* is associated with discipline, scrupulous adherence and strict accuracy. In quantitative research, rigor is associated with problem identification, research design and statistical analysis. The rigor in quantitative research leads to narrowness, conciseness and objectivity. Qualitative research does not have this type of rigor but demands its own type. The difference in type of rigor is due to the differences in focus and outcomes of the two types of research. The qualitative researcher uses his or her own personality in the research process. In order to be effective in conducting qualitative research, the researcher must have ascended to an open context and be willing to continue to let go of sedimented views (deconstructing). This openness requires discipline. The researcher will be examining many dimensions of the area being studied and forming new ideas (reconstructing) while continuing to recognize that the present reconstructing is only one of many possible ways of organizing data. Lack of rigor in qualitative research is associated with the failure to "get away from" older ideas, inadequate time spent collecting data, poor observations and failure to give careful consideration to all the data obtained. Evaluation of the rigor of a qualitative study is often based on the logic of the emerging theory and the clarity with which it sheds light on the studied phenomenon.

Use of Researcher's Personality

The use of the researcher's personality is a key factor in qualitative research. Empathy and intuition are deliberately used, and skills in these areas are cultivated by these researchers. The researcher must become closely involved in the subject's experience in order to interpret it. In addition, the researcher must remain open to the perceptions of the subject rather than attach his or her own meaning to the experience. In order to accomplish this, researchers have developed specific strategies, such as bracketing and intuiting, to facilitate openness during data collection and analysis.

Bracketing

One of the methodological strategies used during qualitative research is bracketing. To *bracket*, the researcher suspends or lays aside what is known about the experience being studied (Oiler, 1982). This is similar to the idea of achieving an open context. The researcher gets rid of sedimented views and deconstructs. This procedure facilitates "seeing" all the facets of the phenomenon and the formation of new gestalts.

Intuiting

Bracketing must have taken place before intuiting can occur. *Intuiting* is the process of actually "looking at" the phenomenon. During intuiting, the researcher focuses all awareness and energy on the subject of interest. This is thought to allow an increase in insight. Intuiting requires absolute concentration and complete absorption with the experience being studied (Oiler, 1982).

Intuiting is a strange idea to those of us in the Western world. It is a more common practice in Eastern thought and is related to meditation practices and the directing of personal energy forces.

APPROACHES TO QUALITATIVE RESEARCH

There are several approaches to conducting qualitative research that have emerged from very different fields of study. Since qualitative research is relatively new and still actively evolving, different approaches are still emerging. Four common types of qualitative research are examined here: phenomenological, grounded theory, ethnographic and historical. These four approaches are commonly used in nursing research and together provide an overview of the characteristics of qualitative research. Each section will describe the purpose of the type of research, the terminology used, the process of conducting the study and the expected outcome. An example of a nursing study is included in each section. Many direct quotes from the researchers are used to demonstrate the involvement of the researcher's personality in the study and the approach to interpreting and reporting findings.

Phenomenological Research

PURPOSE

Very little phenomenological research in nursing has been published in the literature. This particular approach to nursing research is the most recent and probably the least accepted or understood of the qualitative methods discussed in this text. The goal of phenomenological research is to describe experiences as they are lived, in phenomenological terms, the "lived experience." The philosophers and theorists from which phenomenology emerged include Husserl, Kierkegaard, Heidegger, Marcel, Sartre and Merleau-Ponty. The discussion of phenomenological research in this text is based on the explanations of nurse researchers who use the approach (Lynch-Sauer, 1985; Munhall & Oiler, 1986; Oiler, 1982; Parse, Coyne & Smith, 1985).

Phenomenological research examines the particular experiences of unique individuals in a given situation. It is based on a philosophy that espouses the idea that there is not a single reality; each individual has his or her own reality. Reality is considered subjective; thus, an experience is considered unique to the individual. This is considered true even of the researcher's experiences. This research approach attempts to explore meaning within the personal knowledge realm. The studies explore—not what is (reality)—but what is perceived to be (Oiler, 1982). Nurse researchers who have used this method include Paterson and Zderad (1976), Watson (1979) and Parse, Coyne & Smith (1985). Parse, Coyne & Smith (1985) stated that the method should not be used until the researcher has received guidance from a mentor experienced in phenomenological research.

The first detailed explanation of phenomenological research was presented by Parse, Coyne and Smith (1985) in *Nursing research: qualitative methods*. The book also describes Parse's theory, Man-Living-Health, which was developed from a philosophical base of existential phenomenology. In the book, the authors described a phenomenological study of the lived experience of health. The purpose of the study was to develop a definition of health "as it is experienced in everyday life" (p. 27). This study is used throughout the following discussion to illustrate the process of conducting phenomenological research.

DEVELOPING RESEARCH QUESTIONS

The first step in conducting a phenomenological study is to identify the phenomenon to be explored. In the case of Parse's study, the phenomenon to be explored is the lived experience of health. Next, the researcher will develop a research question. Two factors must be considered in developing the research question: "(1) What are the necessary and sufficient constituents of this feeling or experience? (2) What does the existence of this feeling or experience indicate concerning the nature of the human being?" (Omery, 1983, p. 55). Parse, Coyne and Smith's (1985) research question asked: "What are the common elements in experiencing a feeling of health among several different age groups?" (p. 27).

METHODOLOGY

Methodology in quantitative research is usually defined in precise steps, and identification of these steps requires recognition of a process that occurs over time. However, the methodology of phenomenological research is difficult to explain because it has no clearly defined steps. This is due, in part, to the reluctance of phenomenologists to place a major importance on time or sequencing of events. Phenomenologists also believe that the clear definition of a methodology tends to limit the creativity of the researcher. The phenomenological researcher prefers to be free to find unique ways to explore phenomena (Paterson & Zderad, 1976; Omery, 1983).

Sampling and Data Collection

After developing the research question, the researcher identifies sources of the phenomenon being studied. The researcher seeks individuals who are willing to describe their experience(s) with the phenomenon in question. These individuals must understand and be willing to express inner feelings and describe the physiologic experiences that occur with the feelings.

Several strategies can be used for data collection, and it is possible to use combinations of strategies. In one strategy, the subjects are asked to describe their experiences of a phenomenon. This verbal data should be collected in a relaxed atmosphere with sufficient time allowed to facilitate a complete description by the subject. Another strategy is to ask the subjects to write down their experiences. Parse, Coyne and Smith used this strategy for their study. In order to answer the research question, they obtained 50 volunteers who were willing to participate in the study. The subjects were asked to write a description of an occasion when they felt healthy and to describe their feelings, thoughts and perceptions of the experience.

Another strategy requires that the researcher be more directly involved in the experience. The researcher actually observes the subject during the experience. The researcher simultaneously observes verbal and/or nonverbal behavior, the environment and his or her own responses to the situation. Written notes may be used, or the experience may be tape-recorded or videotaped. When observed behavior is being recorded, the researcher must describe rather than evaluate observations. In order to conduct these data collection strategies, the researcher involves his or her personality and uses bracketing and intuiting.

Data Analysis

Data collection and data analysis take place simultaneously; both use the researcher's personality, bracketing and intuiting. Omery (1983) describes three approaches to data analysis, with the techniques developed by van Kaam, Giorgi and Colaizzi. Van Kaam's (1966) method, frequently used in nursing, suggests classifying data and ranking the classifications according to the frequency of occurrence. This ranking is verified by a panel of judges. The number of categories is then reduced to eliminate overlapping, vague or intricate categories. For the second time, agreement of the panel of judges is sought. Hypotheses are developed to theoretically explain the categories, and these hypotheses are tested on a new sample. This process is continued until no new categories emerge (Omery, 1983).

Giorgi (1970) uses a similar process but prefers to maintain more of the sense of wholeness. Although individual elements of the phenomenon are identified, their importance to the phenomenon is not established by the frequency of their occurrence but rather by the intuitive judgment of the researcher. Giorgi considers it important to identify the relationships of the units to each other and to the whole (Omery, 1983).

A third method of data analysis is described by Colaizzi (1978). This method involves examining experiences that are "beyond human experiential awareness or to examine those experiences that cannot be communicated" (Omery, 1983, p. 58). This strategy is useful in studying many subjects or situations that frequently occur in nursing, such as behaviors of preverbal children, subjects with Alzheimer's disease, combative behavior of the unconscious patient and body motion of subjects with new amputations.

OUTCOMES

Findings are often described from the orientation of the subjects studied, rather than being translated into scientific or theoretical language. For example, the actual words used by the subjects to describe an experience will often be used

TABLE 4–1
Group 2. Common Elements with Descriptive Expressions

Spirited Intensity	Fulfilling Inventiveness	Symphonic Integrity
1. Being enthusiastic	1. Finishing a project that takes up time	1. Being at ease
2. Catching a second wind	2. Accomplishment	2. Feeling of worth
3. Exercising and walking	3. Winning the game of life	3. Enjoying own space at that moment
4. Feel in peak condition	4. Trying some new endeavor	4. Peaceful feeling inside while bicycling
5. Positive outlook on life	5. Feeling something enriching my life	5. A "just right" feeling about everything
6. Feeling of refreshment	6. Doing what I struggled for	6. Drinking in the beauty of the day
7. Feeling full of energy	7. Pushing a little extra	7. Peaceful attitude
8. A glowing light of energy burning brightly in my eyes	8. Feel successful as a person	8. Rhythmical, easy, warm
9. A whip the world feeling	9. Ability to extend to limits of endurance	9. Glowing and good inside
10. A surge of energy	10. Accomplishing something	10. Feeling loved

From Parse, Coyne and Smith. *Nursing research: qualitative methods.* Bowie, Maryland: Brady Communications Company, p. 32.

when reporting the findings. The researcher identifies "themes" found in the data. From these themes, a structural explanation of the findings is developed. From a sample of 100 subjects between 20 and 45 years of age, Parse, Coyne and Smith (1985) identified 30 descriptive expressions (Table 4–1) and three themes that they considered central to the experience of health. The three themes emerging from the descriptive expressions were "spirited intensity, fulfilling inventiveness and symphonic integrity" (p. 31).

From these elements Parse, Coyne and Smith (1985) developed a statement that defines health for this particular sample. "Health is symphonic integrity manifested in the spirited intensity of fulfilling inventiveness" (p. 31). The interaction between the researcher and the analysis process in phenomenological research is illustrated by the compatibility of this definition with Parse's (1981) theory.

Published Phenomenological Studies

Anderson, J. M. (1985). Perspectives on the health of immigrant women: a feminist analysis. *Advances in Nursing Science*, 8(1), 61–76.
Drew, N. (1986). Exclusion and confirmation: a phenomenology of patients' experiences with caregivers. *Image*, 18(2), 39–43.
Lynch-Sauer, J. (1985). Using a phenomenological research method to study nursing phenomena. In M. M. Leininger (Ed.), *Qualitative research methods in nursing* (pp. 93–107). Orlando: Grune & Stratton, Inc.
Norris, C. M. (1975). Restlessness: a nursing phenomenon in search of meaning. *Nursing Outlook*, 23(2), 103–107.
Parse, R. R., Coyne, A. B. & Smith, M. J. (1985). *Nursing research: qualitative methods*. Bowie, Maryland: Brady Communications Company, 1985.
Chapter IV: The lived experience of health: a phenomenological study (pp. 27–38).

Chapter V: The lived experience of persisting in change: a phenomenological study (pp. 39–68).

Chapter XII: The lived experience of reaching out: a phenomenological investigation (By Nancy J. Andre) (pp. 119–132).

Rieman, D. J. (1986). The essential structure of a caring interaction: doing phenomenology. In P. A. Munhall & C. J. Oiler (Eds.), *Nursing research: a qualitative perspective* (pp. 85–108). Norwalk, Connecticut: Appleton-Century-Crofts.

Grounded Theory Research

PURPOSE

Grounded theory is an inductive research technique presented by Glaser and Strauss (1967). It is most useful in studying areas in which little previous research has been conducted and in gaining a new viewpoint in familiar areas of research. This approach to theory development requires that the researcher collect data without using a pre-existing theory as an organizing framework. The researcher is to remain open-minded about what will be found and how it will be organized. The intuitive process plays an important role in this approach.

One significant study using a grounded theory approach that is relevant to clinical nursing practice is Fagerhaugh and Strauss's (1977) study of the politics of pain management. This study emerged from the previous work of Glaser and Strauss in the care of the dying (Glaser & Strauss, 1965, 1968; Strauss & Glaser, 1970) and chronic illness care (Strauss, 1975; Strauss, Corbin, Fagerhaugh, Glaser, Maines, Suczek & Wiener, 1984)). The study of pain involved five researchers, 2 years of systematic observations in 20 wards, two clinics and nine hospitals. The purposes of the study were twofold: to develop an approach to pain management that was radically different from established approaches, and to develop a substantive theory about "what happens in hospitals when people are confronted with pain and attempt to deal with it" (Fagerhaugh & Strauss, 1977, p. 13). The research questions were "Under what conditions is pain encountered by staff?" and "How will it be handled?"

METHODOLOGY

Contrary to the logically prearranged steps of traditional research, the steps of grounded theory research occur simultaneously. The researcher will be observing, collecting data, organizing the data and forming theory from the data at the same time. An important methodological technique in grounded theory research is the constant comparative process in which every piece of data is compared with every other piece. The methodological techniques used in grounded theory research are explained in depth in a book by Glaser (1978) entitled *Theoretical sensitivity*.

Data Collection and Analysis Techniques

Data may be collected by interview, observation, records or a combination of these. Data collection usually results in large amounts of handwritten notes that must be sorted and analysed. This process is initiated by coding and categorizing the data. These procedures are further described in Chapter 17. Handwritten notes and tape recordings are the most common means of recording data. If tape recordings are used, they must be transcribed. Techniques used during the process of data collection and analysis can be described in three major steps: concept formation, concept development and concept modification and integration.

Concept Formation □ A beginning conceptual framework is developed from the data. The categories created during data collection become concepts that can then be examined theoretically.

Concept Development □ During this phase, the emerging theory is further developed and thinking moves from inductive to deductive. Concept development includes four processes:

1. *Reduction.* Categories, which at this point in the research have become numerous, are clustered by linking them into higher-order categories.
2. *Selective Sampling of the Literature.* Unlike that in traditional research, the literature in grounded theory research is not extensively searched at the beginning of the study in order to avoid development of a sedimented view. At this point in the research, the literature is examined to merge findings from earlier studies with present findings.
3. *Selective Sampling.* Data collection becomes more specific. The concepts that have been developed into an emerging theory are compared with data to determine conditions under which they occur and whether they are central to the theory. Hypotheses are developed from the theory and tested on the data. Further data collection may be conducted, with the goal of exploring specific hypotheses. Through these activities, the conceptual framework may be modified or expanded.
4. *Emergence of the Core Variable.* Through the aforementioned activities, the concept most important to the theory emerges. This concept or core variable becomes the central theme or focus of the theory.

Concept Modification and Integration □ This step is a wrapping-up process in which the theory is finalized and is again compared with the data (Stern, 1980).

OUTCOMES

The research report presents the theory supported by examples from the data. The literature review and numerical reports of data are not used in the report. Thus, these reports will not contain tables showing frequency of occurrence of a particular variable or statistical analysis of the findings. The reports tend to be narrative discussions of the study process and findings.

In the pain study, the researchers wished to observe a variety of situations in which pain was a common phenomenon. The areas studied included an intensive care unit for severe burns, a cardiac care unit, an obstetrics ward, a physical rehabilitation unit, a neurology and neurosurgery unit, a routine surgery unit, a medical ward, an x-ray department, an emergency department, a kidney transplant unit and a cancer ward. The following excerpt is from the report on the grounded theory study on pain. It focuses on a description of the sampling process and demonstrates the care and detailed thought that must go into the development of sampling categories.

> On all these wards we made "internal comparisons" along the theoretical dimensions. That is, we continued our theory-directed sampling: for instance, high-pain regimens versus low-pain regimens; experienced inflicters of regimen pain versus new inflicters; delivering mothers who had the fathers supporting their efforts to endure pain versus those who had no such supporting or controlling agents. Meanwhile, we were also looking at an activity that spanned separate wards and which would maximize variables as they related to pain infliction. We followed a number of personnel who drew blood from patients. We observed some who were very experienced, some who were not; some who were able to work in a leisurely fashion, some who were not; some who met "first-time" patients, others who met patients very experienced at this particular procedure; some who encountered patients with much ongoing pain and some who did not; some who had recently had experiences with accusations of incompetence and some who had not. (Fagerhaugh & Strauss, 1977, p. 308)

In the pain study, the core categories that evolved were pain work, pain trajectories, legitimation, balancing and accountability. Pain work was further classified into relief of pain, the handling of pain expression, diagnosing the meaning of pain, inflicting pain, minimizing or preventing pain, patients enduring pain and the staff members' controlling their own reactions to the patient's response to pain. The patient's cooperation in the pain work and negotiation between the staff and the patient were identified as important factors. An example of negotiation is described by Glaser (1973):

> "This won't take long," I said to her... "It's not going to hurt... I think I can inject it right into the IV tubing and not have to stick you."
> She looked unconvinced.
> "Honestly I won"t stick you unless I have to." (1973, p. 130.)

Pain trajectories were divided into expected and unexpected trajectories. For example, an expectant mother would have a very different pain trajectory than a person with intractable back pain.

> An unexpected trajectory—unexpected for a given ward, that is—carries a potential for staff and patient disturbance and ward upset. Both the sentimental order and the work order of the ward are threatened...

> Patients with an unexpected or atypical trajectory tend to be labeled as "uncooperative" or "difficult," and relations between them and the staff are likely to grow progressively worse. (Fagerhaugh & Strauss, 1977, p. 22–23)

The researchers also concluded that the pain trajectory was influenced by the patients' illnesses, their previous experience with pain, the medical care they were receiving and their social history. They observed that the nursing and medical staff seldom know anything about the patient's pain trajectory other than what was currently occurring.

Assessing and legitimating pain was also an important factor. Staff often suspected patients of claiming more pain than they had or of claiming pain when they had none. This left the patient in the position of attempting to convince the staff that they were actually having the pain they claimed to have (legitimating). The staff and patient were often involved in the process of balancing priorities during pain work. Decisions were based on what was considered to be the most important by staff.

> The staff members may not always agree among themselves, and the balancing done by the patient may not agree with the staff's. Patient and staff may even opt for opposite choices, disagreeing over the value of living a bit longer versus enduring terrible pain. They may be balancing quite different considerations. The staff may be balancing more work versus quicker pain relief, while the patient may be balancing pride in not complaining about pain versus difficulty of enduring it without more medication. (Fagerhaugh & Strauss, 1977, p. 25)

In terms of accountability, the researchers found that pain work was not a major priority of staff. Staff tended to be more responsible for controlling the patient's expression of pain than for controlling the experience of pain.

As can be seen from the study described, grounded theory research examines a much broader scope of dimensions than is usually possible with quantitative research. The findings can be intuitively verified by the experiences of the reader. The clear, cohesive description of the phenomenon can allow greater understanding and, thus, more control of our nursing practice. Fagerhaugh and Strauss (1977) concluded the following from their study:

> Genuine accountability concerning pain work could only be instituted if the major authorities on given wards or clinics understood the importance of that accountability and its implications for patient care. They would then need to convert that understanding into a commitment that would bring about necessary changes in written and verbal communication systems. This kind of understanding and commitment can probably come about only after considerable nationwide discussion, such as now is taking place about terminal care, but that kind of discussion seems to lie far in the future. (p. 27)

Published Grounded Theory Studies

Forsyth, G. L., Delaney, K. D. & Gresham, M. L. (1984). Vying for a winning position: management style of the chronically ill. *Research in Nursing and Health, 7*(3), 181–188.

May, K. A. (1982). Three phases of father involvement in pregnancy. *Nursing Research, 31*(6), 337–342.

O'Brien, M. E. (1982). Pragmatic survivalism: behavior patterns affecting low-level wellness among minority group members. *Advances in Nursing Science, 4*(3), 13–26.

Pyles, S. H. & Stern, P. N. (1983). Discovery of nursing gestalt in critical care nursing: the importance of the gray gorilla syndrome. *Image, 15(2), 51–57.*

Saunders, J. M. (1981). A process of bereavement resolution: uncoupled identity. *Western Journal of Nursing Research, 3*(4), 319–336.

Simms, L. M. (1981). The grounded theory approach in nursing research. *Nursing Research, 30*(6), 356–359.

Stern, P. N. (1982). Affiliating in stepfather families: teachable strategies leading to stepfather–child friendship. *Western Journal of Nursing Research, 4*(1), 75–89.

Wilson, H. S. (1986). Presencing—social control of schizophrenics in an antipsychiatric community: doing grounded theory. In P. L. Munhall & C. J. Oiler (Eds.). *Nursing research: a qualitative perspective* (pp. 131–144). Norwalk, Connecticut: Appleton-Century-Crofts.

Ethnographic Research

Ethnographic research was developed by the discipline of anthropology as a mechanism for studying cultures. There are two basic research approaches in anthropology—ethnography and ethnoscience—which differ somewhat in research strategies and the elements of the culture that are studied. *Ethnography* "can be defined as the systematic process of observing, detailing, describing, documenting, and analyzing the lifeways or particular patterns of a culture (or subculture) in order to grasp the lifeways or patterns of the people in their familiar environment" (Leininger, 1985, p. 35). *Ethnoscience* research "permits the nurse researcher to obtain insights into the meaning of particular things and events as understood by participants of a culture" (Evaneshko & Kay, 1982, p. 49). Most nurses involved in these types of research obtained their doctoral preparation in anthropology and have used the techniques to examine issues related to culture that are of interest to nursing.

A group of nurse scientists, led by Madeleine Leininger, have developed a strategy for nursing research, referred to as *ethnonursing* research, emerging from Leininger's theory of transcultural nursing. Ethnonursing "focuses mainly on observing and documenting interactions with people of how these daily life conditions and patterns are influencing human care, health, and nursing care practices" (Leininger, 1985, p. 238). Nurse researchers conduct studies using all three approaches: ethnography, ethnoscience and ethnonursing. Although "mini" ethnographic studies can be conducted by novice researchers, Leininger suggests that well-designed studies in ethnography and ethnonursing require formal coursework and mentorship with a nurse researcher experienced in this type of research.

PURPOSE

The purpose of ethnographic research is to describe cultures. Leininger (1985) suggests the following eight purposes for using ethnography and ethnonursing research:

1. When there is virtually no knowledge or very limited knowledge about a phenomenon.
2. When the researcher wants to grasp the totality of a human lifestyle or of a broad world view about individuals, families, and cultures from their viewpoints and their modes of knowing and understanding life.
3. When the researcher wants data relating to some quite new or different types of questions that have not been asked by scientists or humanists.
4. To obtain meanings-in-context data, and meanings-in-familiar or recurrent environmental contexts.
5. To generate concepts, theories, and hypotheses or to identify salient variables that have not been identified or that merit study.
6. To conduct cross-cultural comparative studies of human and nursing care phenomena.
7. To identify recurrent and patterned lifeways of people.
8. To provide detailed accounts of events, situations, and circumstances that are usually difficult to discover by other research methods. (p. 39–41)

For an ethnographic study, culture is defined very broadly; for example, an ethnographic study could range from examining a specific tribe in Africa to studying the culture of an intensive care unit or an oncology unit. Germain's (1979) book entitled *The cancer unit: an ethnography* is an example of ethnographic research.

STEPS OF ETHNOGRAPHIC RESEARCH

The steps of ethnographic research are more sequential than those of phenomenology or grounded theory and include the following:
1. Identification of the culture to be studied
2. Identifying the significant variables within the culture
3. Literature review
4. Gaining entrance
5. Cultural immersion
6. Acquiring informants
7. Gathering data (elicitation procedures)
8. Analysis of data
9. Description of the culture
10. Theory development

In her study, Germain (1979) describes her research experience in such a graphic way that the reader can experience some of the process of conducting this type of research. This style of writing is typical of qualitative researchers and although lengthy, gives the reader a clear picture of the whole phenomenon being explained. Germain viewed the oncology unit as a subculture whose members were affected by many variables. Variables that Germain identified included the following:

1. Societal factors
   (a) Attitudes toward cancer and its treatment
   (b) Greater openness toward those who are dying
   (c) Changing patterns of higher education
   (d) The women's liberation movement
   (e) Increased consumer demands for participation
2. Institutional factors
   (a) Bureaucratic control patterns in hospitals
   (b) Professional-bureaucratic role conflicts
   (c) Traditional pattern of role dominance
   (d) Grouping of persons with varying stages of cancer in a confined area
3. Ideology-reality conflict within the profession of nursing
4. Complexities of cancer care
5. The individual psychological variables of all those involved in the subculture (patients, nurses, doctors, families and other hospital department members)

Germain believed that these variables could not be examined separately but must be studied holistically because of each variable's impact on the other variables. The ethnographic approach allowed her to examine the total context of the oncology unit rather than individual variables. Germain's discussion of the purpose of the study gives some insight into the scope of the study.

The principal goal of the study was an ethnographic description of a community hospital adult oncology unit as a subculture. This included the effect of physical, physiologic, and psychologic conditions and crises of cancer patients on the intensity and extensity of social relations among nurses, doctors, administrators, patients, families, and others on the ward and in related hospital areas...

Specific attention was given to the various roles that nurses play in this subculture, the problems and stresses they face in this setting, their ways of coping with these problems, and some observed consequences of their socially patterned adaptive behavior. (Germain, 1979, pp. 1–2)

LITERATURE REVIEW

The purpose of a literature review in ethnographic research is to provide background for the study. The researcher is seeking a broad general understanding of the variables to be considered in a specific culture or subculture. Germain, in her review, examined five topics: conflicting hierarchies in the hospital system, intraprofessional issues of nursing, cancer as an illness requiring hospital care, dying and death and ethnographic studies of hospitals.

METHODOLOGY

Gaining Entrance

One of the critical steps in any study is gaining entry into the area being studied. The mechanics of this process may vary greatly, depending on whether one is attempting to gain entrance to another country or into a specific institution. The researcher is responsible at this point for explaining the purposes and methods of the study to those with the power to grant entrance. Germain describes this process clearly in her study.

> The researcher initially contacted the director of nursing... (who) was somewhat hesitant about a field study of the hospital sociocultural system; she stated that the researcher would have to discuss the idea with the hospital administrator, who could not schedule an appointment until six weeks later.
>
> In his well-appointed executive office, the administrator posed some pertinent questions, ... but gave support to the idea of a field study... which involved a minimum of three, three-hour visits per week for one year... Further stipulations included approval of the proposal by the medical director of the Oncology Unit; a written, legal contract between the university and Charles Hospital,... proof of professional licensure; and proof of personal, professional liability insurance. The researcher was to wear a white lab coat and a temporary employee's identification badge, the latter for security reasons.
>
> After these conditions were met, the researcher met with the director of nursing, the supervisor, and the head nurse of the unit to clarify for the head nurse what the researcher's role on the unit would be, primarily with respect to nursing care... The primacy of the research role had to be clarified so that nursing staff and physicians, in particular, did not have unreasonable role expectations of the researcher. Her participation in traditional nursing functions was selective, determined by the goals of the research. She needed to be free from the constraints of an assignment so that she could wander, observe, write notes, or participate in meetings that would not usually be accessible to a member of the staff. (Germain, 1977, pp. 13–14)

Cultural Immersion

The ethnographic researcher becomes very familiar with the culture being studied, by living in it (active participation) and by extensive questioning. The process of becoming *immersed* in the culture involves gaining increasing familiarity with such things as language, sociocultural norms, traditions and other social dimensions such as family, communication patterns (verbal and nonverbal), religion, work patterns and expression of emotion. Immersion also involves gradually increasing acceptance of the researcher into the culture. Germain (1979) describes this process in her study.

Feedback from the staff on the researcher's entry into and role in the subculture was obtained unsolicited as well as solicited on several occasions. For example, the supervisor said, "We told Mrs. Bowman (the director of nursing) that Carol's here, but nobody acts as if she's around." Several months into the study the head nurse remarked, "I can't get over how the staff has accepted you. It's like you're not even an outsider. They pay no attention to you." (pp. 15–16)

Since the research goal was to discover, describe, and explain the nature of the subculture as it was given, the researcher's general policy was non-intervention, so as to disrupt ongoing social processes as little as possible and to minimize the change induced by her presence...

At times, the researcher felt compelled to intervene, as when she had information that might change the staff's view of a patient's situation.

The assumed nursing role seemed natural, for it allowed the researcher to ease in and out of patient care situations. When the researcher was with a patient or responded to a patient's call light when staff were unable to respond as quickly, her usual course was to meet immediate needs for personal, supportive, safety, comfort, or technical care, when these needs were obvious or requested.

Inevitably, as a researcher talks openly with patients, families, or members of the staff in the data-gathering process and listens to their views, complaints, regrets, hopes, or fears, some change occurs, however minimal, that would not have been induced if she were an unseen observer. At times the anthropologist–researcher was also nurse, teacher, counselor, friend, confidante, or helper. It is the researcher's view that these roles enhanced data collection in this subculture. (pp. 21–22)

Acquiring Informants

In order to understand the culture, the researcher seeks out individuals who are willing to interpret the culture to them. These people (who are usually members of the culture) will not be research subjects in the usual sense of the word, but rather colleagues. The researcher must have the support and confidence of these individuals in order to complete the research. Therefore, maintaining these relationships is of utmost importance. Not only will the informants answer questions, they may also have to help formulate the questions, since they understand the culture better than the researcher. Germain (1979) describes this process in her study.

The success of a researcher's entry into a culture can be assessed by the degree to which members share matters that are not usually open to outsiders. During this study, the researcher was invited to join some nursing and medical conferences and social occasions that were closed to outgroup members. A number of individuals voluntarily sought the

> researcher and shared information and/or feelings not shared openly with
> other members of the subculture (p. 19).

Frequently, a member of the culture becomes an assistant to the researcher. Germain employed such an assistant who kept a log of events during a period when the researcher was not available.

Gathering Data (Elicitation Procedures)

The activity of collecting data is referred to as *field research* and requires the taking of extensive notes. The quality of these notes will depend on the expertise of the researcher. A skilled researcher, experienced in qualitative research techniques, will be able to discern more easily what observations need to be noted than will a less experienced researcher or assistant. During observations, the researcher will be bombarded with information. Intuition plays an important role in determining which data to collect. Although researchers must be actively involved in the culture they are studying, they must avoid "going native," which will interfere with both data collection and analysis. In *going native*, the researcher becomes a part of the culture and loses all objectivity and, with it, the ability to observe clearly. Germain (1979) describes her process of data collection as follows:

> In the course of a three-hour period in the field, the researcher would stop several times to write down notes; detailed descriptions of incidents and conversations were written down as soon as possible after they occurred to limit distortion. When it was feasible, she asked individuals or groups about their perceptions of events and their feelings about them shortly after the event. Field notes were typed as soon as possible, and data were roughly categorized concurrently...
>
> A three-hour field visit usually had at least one specific focus, such as observing an individual or group in their daily activities, making rounds with the head nurse or doctors, attending a conference or change-of-shift report, conducting a formal interview, or talking with a patient or family. There was ample time to follow up on ongoing situations or to get involved with new developments. Since the researcher was free to wander, she did not keep a strict schedule, except for appointments, but moved to whatever locations she judged valuable for data collection. The staff were often voluntarily helpful in pointing out events they thought would be valuable for the research. (pp. 16–17)

Analysis of Data

Analysis of data is essentially analysis of the field notes and interviews. The notes themselves may be, in many cases, superficial. However, during the process of analysis, the notes are clarified, extended and interpreted. The abstract thought processes (intuition, introspection and reasoning) are involved in this process. Interpretations are checked out with the informants. The data are then formed into categories and relationships developed between categories. Patterns of behavior are identified.

Germain divided her data into five categories: the Charles Hospital and its administration, the oncology unit, the doctors, the nursing staff and patients and families. Her analysis of data is presented in five chapters of her book. Reading the chapters provides a clear image of the oncology unit and its functioning.

OUTCOMES

The analysis process in ethnography is used to provide detailed descriptions of cultures, develop theories about the culture and/or generate hypotheses from the theories. The results are tested by whether another ethnographer, using the findings of the first ethnographic study, can accurately anticipate human behavior in the studied culture. Although the findings are not usually generalized from one culture or subculture to another, a case may be made for some degree of generalization to other similar cultures (Germain, 1986).

The conclusions of Germain's (1979) study and recommendations for changes, are presented in the final chapter of her book. Her conclusions were organized using six major concepts: work pattern, organization, nurses, professionalism, ideology–reality conflict and patients. Some of the highlights of these conclusions follow, focusing on work pattern, organization, nurses and patients.

WORK PATTERN

The staff usually functioned at a fast pace, fully occupied with their immediate tasks. Urgent physical care requirements often took precedence over other important aspects of care, such as listening to patients. There was neither time nor space for reflective thinking or long-range planning.

Nursing staff at Charles most often acted on the premise that talking, listening, teaching, and providing diversion to patients were activities to be done only if there was time after baths, medications, and treatments. The realities of the staffing pattern sometimes made it necessary for them to set these priorities in their work. (p. 210)

ORGANIZATION

Patient care in the hospital was organized on a part-task, bureaucratic system. Speed, efficiency, cooperation, loyalty to the institution, and adherence to externally imposed rules and regulations were highly valued,... Organizational, professional-bureaucratic, and interpersonal conflicts generated a great deal of tension and job dissatisfaction. (p. 211)

NURSES

Commitment to oncology nursing was associated with job satisfaction and good work performance. Staff who had negative views of cancer tended to have poor job satisfaction. Conflicts among nursing staff occurred over unequal workloads, differing opinions about nursing practice and education, differing education levels and commitment to nursing. Despite the inherent stresses and tensions, there was group solidarity and a general attitude of openness, cooperation, and commitment to patients among the nursing staff. This attitude contributed to the good spirit and stability of the unit, which in turn contributed to stability in the hospital system. Humor, laughter, sarcasm, cooperation, and group support were identified as the group's major coping mechanisms. (Germain, 1979, p. 213)

The major concerns of nurses included feelings of powerlessness, the injustice of being blamed by physicians for situations beyond their control, deference to doctors, and the medical focus of care. Physician anger or the threat of it created tension that disrupted staff morale. When this occurred, nurses avoided spontaneous interaction with physicians, which decreased sharing of patient problems.

PATIENTS

Despite the hospital's statements that individualized patient care was the goal of the institution, patients were usually passive recipients rather than active participants in their program of care. The capriciousness of the disease of cancer and the vagaries of individual response to treatment made powerlessness a fact of life. Patients' place in the system reinforced this. With their own lives in jeopardy, they felt most safe in going along with the system.

Goals of patient care were not discussed; it was all too possible for a patient to have a remission goal, the doctor a research goal, and the nurse a terminal-care goal. (Germain, 1979, p. 222)

Published Ethnographic Studies

Aamodt, A. M. (1986). Discovering the child's view of alopecia: doing ethnography. In P. L. Munhall & C. J. Oiler (Eds.), *Nursing research: a qualitative perspective*. Norwalk, Connecticut: Appleton-Century-Crofts.

Cohen, F. S. (1982). Childbirth belief and practice in a Garifuna (Black Carib) village on the north coast of Honduras. *Western Journal of Nursing Research*, 4(2), 193–208.

Field, P. (1983) An ethnography: four public health nurses' perspectives of nursing. *Journal of Advanced Nursing*, 8(1), 3–12.

Kus, R. (1985). Stages of coming out: an ethnographic approach. *Western Journal of Nursing Research*, 7(2), 177–198.

Macdonald, A. C. (1981). Folk health practices among north coastal Peruvians: implications for nursing. *Image*, 13(2), 51–55.

Parse, R. R., Coyne, A. B. & Smith, M. J. (1985). The experience of aging: an ethnographic study. In R. R. Parse, A. B. Coyne & M. J. Smith (Eds.), *Nursing research: qualitative methods* (Chapter VII). Bowie, Maryland: Brady Communications Company.

Stern, P. N. (1981). Solving problems of cross-cultural health teaching: the Filipino childbearing family. *Image*, 13(2), 47–50.

Tripp-Reimer, T. (1983). Retention of a folk-healing practice (matiasma) among four generations of urban Greek immigrants. *Nursing Research*, 32(2), 97–101.

Historical Research

PURPOSE

Historical research, or historiography, examines events of the past. Although many of us consider history to be boring or unimportant, an often quoted statement of George Santayana warns that those who cannot remember the past are condemned to repeat it. Christy (1978, p. 9) asks "How can we in nursing today possibly plan where we are going when we don't know where we have been nor how we got here?"

One criterion of a profession is that there is a knowledge of the history of the profession that is transmitted to those entering the profession. Until recently, historical nursing research has not been a valued activity and few nurse researchers had the skills or desire to conduct it. Therefore, our knowledge of our past is sketchy. However, there is now a growing interest in the field of historical nursing research.

Some historical research may be simply descriptive. However, in order to be classified as a qualitative research strategy, the following criteria must be met: (1) The research must be conducted within a holistic framework, (2) it's aim must be to examine meaning and (3) the emerging results must be theoretical. In other words, the study must identify concepts, examine relationships, draw inferences and emerge with an increased understanding of the impact of the studied event on the meanings we place on events of the present and our strivings toward the future. In addition to increasing our understanding of our profession, many historians believe that the greatest value of historical knowledge is an increased self-understanding.

METHODOLOGY

The methodology of historical research includes the following components: formulating an idea, developing research questions, developing an inventory of sources, clarifying validity and reliability of data, developing a research outline and conducting data collection and analysis.

Formulating An Idea

The first step in historical research is selecting a topic. Topics appropriate for historical research include the following:

> origins, epochs, events treated as units; movements, trends, patterns over stated periods; history of specific agencies or institutions; broad studies of the development of needs for specialized types of nursing; biographies and portrayals of the nurse in literature, art, or drama. (Newton, 1965, p. 20)

As with many types of research, the initial ideas for historical research tend to be too broad. These ideas must be clearly defined and narrowed to a topic that is precisely defined so that the time required to search for related materials is realistic. In addition to narrowing the topic, it is often important to limit the historical period to be studied. Limiting this time period requires a knowledge of the broader social, political and economic factors that would have an impact on the topic under study.

The researcher may spend much time extensively reading related literature before a final decision is made about the precise topic. Waring (1978) conducted her doctoral dissertation using historical research to examine the idea of the nurse experiencing a "calling" to practice nursing. She described the extensive process of developing a precise topic:

> Originally my idea was to pursue concepts in the area of Puritan social thought and to relate concepts such as altruism and self-sacrifice to nursing. Two years after the formulation of this first idea, I finally realized that the topic was too broad. Reaching that point was slow and arduous but quite essential to the development of my thinking and the prospectus that developed as an outcome.
>
> When I first began the process, it seemed that I might have to abandon the topic "calling." Now, since the clarification and tightening up of my title and the clarification of my study thesis, I open volumes fearing that I will find yet another reference, once overlooked. It is only recently that I have become convinced that there was a needle in the haystack and that I had indeed found it. (pp. 18–19)

In historical research, there frequently is no problem statement. Rather than defining the research topic in a problem statement, it is usually expressed in the title of the study. For example, Waring's title was: "American Nursing and the Concept of the Calling."

Developing Research Questions

After the topic has been clearly defined, the researcher will identify the questions to be examined during the research process. These questions tend to be more general and analytical than those found in quantitative studies. Evans (1978), then a doctoral student, described the research questions she developed for her historical study:

> I propose to study the nursing student. Who was this living person inside the uniform? Where did she come from? What were her experiences as a nursing student? I use the word "experience" in terms of the dictionary definition of "living through." What did she live through? What happened to her and how did she respond, or react, as the case may be? What was her educational program like? We have a pretty good notion of what nurse educators and others thought about the educational program, but what about it from the students' point of view?
>
> What were the functions of rituals and rites of passage such as bed check, morning inspection, and capping?
>
> What kind of person did the nursing student tend to become in

order to successfully negotiate studenthood? What are the implications of this in terms of her own personal and professional development and the development of the profession at large? (p. 16)

Developing an Inventory of Sources

The next step is to determine whether sources of data for the study exist and are available. Many of the materials for historical research are contained within private archives in libraries or are privately owned. One must obtain written permission to gain access to library archives. Private materials are often difficult to ferret out, and, when they are discovered, access may again be a problem. In oral history studies, the individual being studied is interviewed and the proceedings are recorded. Thus, the individuals must be contacted and permission obtained for interviewing. In any type of historical research, the researcher must travel to the source of data. Therefore, access to data must include examination of available funding for travel and sometimes for duplication of materials for further study. Historical materials in nursing are difficult to find. Many materials such as letters, memos, handwritten materials and mementos of significant leaders in nursing are being discarded because no one recognizes their value. The same is true of materials related to the history of institutions and agencies within which nursing has been involved. Christy (1978, p. 9) states: "It seems obvious that interest in the preservation of historical materials will only be stimulated if there is a concomitant interest in the value of historical research." Sometimes when such material is found, it is in such poor condition that many of the data are unclear or completely lost. Christy (1978) describes one of her experiences in searching for historical data:

M. Adelaide Nutting and Isabel M. Stewart are two of the greatest leaders we have ever had, and their friends, acquaintances, and former students were persons of tremendous importance to developments in nursing and nursing education throughout the world. Since both of these women were historians, they saved letters, clippings, manuscripts—primary source materials of inestimable value. Their friends were from many walks of life: physicians, lawyers, social workers, philanthropists—supporters and nonsupporters of nursing and nursing interests. Miss Nutting and Miss Stewart crammed these documents into boxes, files, and whatever other receptacles were available and—unfortunately—some of these materials are this very day in those same old boxes.

When I began my research into the Archives in 1966, the files were broken, rusty, and dilapidated. Many of the folders were so old and ill-tended that they fell apart in my hands, the ancient paper crumbled into dust before my eyes. My research was exhilaratingly stimulating, and appallingly depressing at the same time; stimulating due to the gold mine of data available, and depressing as I realized the lack of care provided for such priceless materials. In addition, there was little or no organization, and one had to go through each document, in each drawer, in each file, piece by piece... The boxes and cartons were worse, for

> materials bearing absolutely no relationship to each other were simply piled, willy-nilly, one atop the other. Is it any wonder that it took me eighteen months of solid work to get through them? (p. 8–9)

Clarifying Validity and Reliability of Data

The validity and reliability concerns in historical research are related to the sources from which data are collected. The most valued source of data is the primary source. A primary source is material most likely to shed true light on the information being sought by the researcher. For example, material written by a person who experienced an event or letters and other mementos saved by the person being studied are primary source material. A secondary source is written by those who have previously read and summarized the primary source material. History books and textbooks are secondary source materials. Primary sources are considered more valid and reliable than secondary sources. "The presumption is that an eyewitness can give a more accurate account of an occurrence than a person not present. If the author was an eyewitness, he is considered a primary source. If the author has been told about the occurrence by someone else, the author is a secondary source. The further the author moves from an eyewitness account, the less reliable are his statements" (Christy, 1975, p. 191). Historiographers use primary sources whenever possible.

The historical researcher must consider the validity and reliability of primary sources used in the study. In order to determine this, the researcher uses principles of historical criticism.

> ...one does not merely pick up a copy of Grandmother's diary and gleefully assume that all the things Grandma wrote were the unvarnished facts. Grandmother's glasses may at times have been clouded, at other times rose-colored. The well-prepared researcher will scrutinize, criticize, and analyze before even accepting its having been written by Grandma! And even after the validity of the document is established, every attempt is made to uncover bias, prejudice, or just plain exaggeration on Grandmother's part. Healthy skepticism becomes a way of life for the serious historiographer. (Christy, 1978, p. 6)

Two strategies have been developed to determine the authenticity and accuracy of the source; these strategies are external and internal criticism. *External criticism* determines the validity of source material. The researcher needs to know where, when, why and by whom a document was written. This may involve verifying the handwriting or determining the age of the paper on which it was written. Christy (1975) describes some difficulties she experienced in establishing the validity of documents:

> An interesting problem presented by early nursing leaders was their frugality. Nutting occasionally saved stationery from hotels, resorts, or steamship lines during vacation trips and used it at a later date. This required double checking as to her exact location at the time the letter was written. When she first went to Teachers College in 1907, she still

wrote a few letters on Johns Hopkins stationery. I found this practice rather confusing in early stages of research. (p. 190)

Internal criticism involves examination of the reliability of the document. The researcher must determine possible biases of the author. To verify the accuracy of a statement, the researcher should have two independent sources that provide the same information. In addition, the researcher should ensure that he or she understands the statements made by the writer, since words and their meanings change across time and across cultures. It is also very possible to read into a document meaning not originally intended by the author. This is most likely to happen when one is seeking to find a particular meaning. Sometimes, words can be taken out of context (Christy, 1975).

Developing a Research Outline

The research outline is a guide for the broad topics to be examined and also serves as a basis for a filing system for classifying collected data. For example, data may be filed by time period. The materials may be cross-referenced for easy access. For example, one piece of data may be filed under several classifications, and the researcher would place a note in one file referring to data stored in another file. The research outline provides a check point for the investigator during the process of data collection and can be used to easily identify gaps in the data collection process.

Data Collection

Data collection may require months or years of dedicated searching for pertinent material. Sometimes, one small source may open a door to an entire new field of facts. In addition, there is no clear, obvious end to data collection. By examining the research guide, the researcher must make the decision to discontinue collection of data. These facets of data collection are described by Newton (1965).

The search for data takes the researcher into most unexpected nooks and corners and adds facet after facet to the original problem. It may last for months or years or a decade. Days and weeks may be fruitless and endless references may be devoid of pertinent material. Again, one minor reference will open the door to the gold mine of facts. The search becomes more exciting when others know of it and bring possible clues to the investigator. The researcher cultivates persistence, optimism, and patience in his long and sometimes discouraging quest. But one real "find" spurs him on and he continues his search. Added to this skill is the training in the most meticulous recording of data with every detail complete, and the logical classification of the data. (p. 23)

Analysis of Data

Analysis of data involves the synthesis of all the data collected. Data must be sifted and choices made about which to accept and which to reject. Sometimes interesting data that do not contribute to the questions of the study are difficult to discard. Conflicting evidence must be reconciled. For example, if two primary sources give opposite information about an incident, the researcher will seek to interpret the differences and determine, as nearly as possible, what actually occurred.

OUTCOMES

Developing a Writing Outline

Before proceeding to write the research report, the researcher must decide the most appropriate means of presenting the data. Some options include a biography, a chronology and a paper organized to focus on issues. If the outline has been well organized and detailed, the writing that follows should flow easily and smoothly.

Writing the Research Report

Historical research reports do not follow the traditional formalized style of much research. The studies are designed to attract the interest of the reader and may appear deceptively simple. The untrained eye may not recognize the extensive work required to write the paper. As explained by Christy (1975),

> The reader is never aware of the painstaking work, the careful attention to detail, nor the arduous pursuit of clues endured by the writer of history. Perhaps that is why so many nurses have failed to recognize historiography as a legitimate research endeavor. It looks so easy. (Christy, 1975, p. 192)

Currently, most historical nursing research has focused on nursing leaders. There seems to have been no examination of historical patterns of nursing practice. Since so much of our nursing knowledge has been transmitted verbally or by role-modeling, we may lose much of the understanding of our roots unless studies are initiated to record them. We have no clear picture of how nursing practice has changed over the years (*e.g.*, when, how and for what reasons have care patterns changed for individuals experiencing diabetes, cardiovascular disease, surgery or stroke?). Changes in nursing procedures such as bed baths, enemas and the feeding of patients could be examined. Procedure manuals, policy books and nurses notes in patient charts are useful sources for examining changes in our nursing practice. Some possible research questions might include: (1) Which of these changes were due to medical actions and which were nursing innovations? (2) What factors in nursing influence changes in nursing practice? (3) What are the time patterns for changes in practice? and (4) Have the time patterns for changes in practice remained fairly consistent, or have they changed over the history of nursing? This type of information might provide increased insight into future directions for nursing practice, research and theory development. However, if quality historical research is to be conducted, those of us in the process of making history must accept responsibility for preserving the sources.

Published Historical Studies

Anderson, N. D. (1981). Ethel Fenwick's legacy to nursing and women. *Image*, 13(2), 32–33.

Ashley, J. (1976). *Hospitals, paternalism, and the role of the nurse.* New York: Teachers College Press.

Baer, E. D. (1985). Nursing's divided house—an historical view. *Nursing Research*, 34(1), 32–38.

Birnbach, N. (1985). The nurse registration movement in Great Britain. *Advances in Nursing Science*, 7(2), 13–19.

Church, O. M. (1985). Emergence of training programs for asylum nursing at the turn of the century. *Advances in Nursing Science*, 7(2), 35–46.

Dennis, K. E. & Prescott, P. A. (1985). Florence Nightingale: yesterday, today, and tomorrow. *Advances in Nursing Science*, 7(2), 66–81.

Donahue, M. P. (1983). Isabel Maitland Stewart's philosophy of education. *Nursing Research*, 32(3), 140–146.

Doona, M. E. (1984). At least as well cared for ... Linda Richards and the mentally ill. *Image*, 16(2), 51–56.

Fitzpatrick, M. L. (1986). An historical study of nursing organization: doing historical research. In P. L. Munhall & C. J. Oiler (Eds.), *Nursing research: a qualitative perspective* (pp. 195–226). Norwalk, Connecticut: Appleton-Century-Crofts.

Kalisch, B. J. & Kalisch, P. A. (1977). An analysis of the sources of physician–nurse conflict, *Journal of Nursing Administration*, 7(1), 50–57.

Kalisch, B. J., Kalisch, P. A. & Belcher, B. (1985). Forecasting for nursing policy: a news-based image approach. *Nursing Research*, 34(1), 44–49.

Kalisch, B. J., Kalisch, P. A. & Young, R. L. (1983). Television news coverage of nurse strikes: a resource management perspective. *Nursing Research*, 32(3), 175–180.

Kalisch, P. A., Kalisch, B. J. & Clinton, J. (1982). The world of nursing on prime time television, 1950 to 1980. *Nursing Research*, 31(6), 358–363.

Krampitz, S. D. (1983). Historical development of baccalaureate nursing education in the American university: 1899–1935. *Western Journal of Nursing Research*, 5(4), 371–380.

Large, J. T. (1976). Harriet Newton Phillips, the first trained nurse in America. *Image*, 8(3), 49–51.

Miller, P. G. (1985). The nurse training act: a historical perspective. *Advances in Nursing Science*, 7(2), 47–65.

Palmer, I. S. (1981). Florence Nightingale and international origins of modern nursing. *Image*, 13(2), 28–31.

Safier, G. (1977). *Contemporary American leaders in nursing: an oral history.* New York: McGraw-Hill Book Company.

Silverstein, N. G. (1985). Lillian Wald at Henry Street, 1893–1895. *Advances in Nursing Science*, 7(2), 1–12.

Wheeler, C. E. (1985). The American journal of nursing and the socialization of a profession, 1900–1920. *Advances in Nursing Science*, 7(2), 20–34.

Summary

Qualitative research is a relatively new approach to nursing research. The concepts and methods of reasoning are very different from those of quantitative research. Some major concepts important to qualitative research include gestalt, sedimented view and open context. A gestalt is a way of viewing the world that is closely related to holism. This view proposes that knowledge about a particular phenomenon is organized into a cluster of linked ideas. It is this clustering and interrelatedness that provide meaning. A gestalt is in some ways like a theory. A sedimented view is seeing things within a specific gestalt, frame of reference or world view. This gives a sense of reality, certainty and, seemingly, control. A sedimented view is a naive and inflexible way of perceiving a phenomenon. The opposite of a sedimented view is an open context. An open context requires deconstruction of the sedimented view, which allows you to see the depth and complexity within the phenomenon being examined. Ihde's work is used as a way of experiencing the jump from a sedimented view to an open context.

The conduct of qualitative research requires the rigorous implementation of techniques such as use of the researcher's personality, bracketing and intuiting. The researcher must use his or her personality to become closely involved in the subject's experience in order to interpret it. The researcher must remain open to the perceptions of the subject. Thus, empathy and intuition are skills that are cultivated by these researchers. In order to accomplish this use of personality in research, the researchers have developed specific strategies, such as bracketing and intuiting. Bracketing is laying aside what is known about an experience being studied and must occur before intuiting. Intuiting is the process of actually "looking at" the phenomenon. During intuiting, the researcher focuses all awareness and energy on the subject of interest. Intuiting and bracketing are methodological strategies used during data collection and analysis.

Four approaches to qualitative research have been described in this chapter: phenomenological, grounded theory, ethnographic and historical. The goal of phenomenological research is to describe experiences as they are lived. Grounded theory is an approach for discovering what problems exist in a social scene and how the persons involved handle them. The research process involves formulation, testing and redevelopment of propositions until a theory is developed. Ethnographic research is the investigation of cultures through an in-depth study of the members of the culture. The ethnographic research process is the systematic collection, description and analysis of data to develop a theory of cultural behavior. Historical research is a narrative description or analysis of events that occurred in the remote or recent past. The data of past events are obtained from records, artifacts or verbal reports. Detailed examples are provided from the literature to demonstrate the process of conducting these types of research.

References

Aamodt, A. M. (1982). Examining ethnography for nurse researchers. *Western Journal of Nursing Research,* 4(2), 209–221.

Andreoli, K. G. & Thompson, C. E. (1977). The nature of science in nursing. *Image,* 9(2), 32–37.

Ashley, J. (1978). Foundations for scholarship: historical research in nursing. *Advances in Nursing Science,* 1(1), 25–36.

Baer, E. D. (1979). Philosophy provides the rationale for nursing's multiple research directions. *Image,* 11(3), 72–74.

Benoliel, J. Q. (1983). The historical development of cancer nursing research in the United States, *Cancer Nursing,* 6(4), 261–268.

Christy, T. E. (1975). The methodology of historical research: a brief introduction. *Nursing Research,* 24(3), 189–192.

Christy, T. E. (1978). The hope of history. In M. L. Fitzpatrick (Ed.), *Historical studies in nursing* (pp. 3–11). New York: Teachers College Press.

Colaizzi, P. (1978). Psychological research as the phenomenologist views it. In R. S. Valle & M. King (Eds.), *Existential phenomenological alternatives for psychology* (pp. 48–71). New York: Oxford University Press.

Conant, L. H. (1967). A search for resolution of existing problems in nursing. *Nursing Research*, 16(2), 114–117.

Crawford, G., Dufault, Sr. K. & Rudy, E. (1979). Evolving issues in theory development. *Nursing Outlook*, 27(5), 346–351.

deChesnay, M. (1983). Cross-cultural research: advantages and disadvantages. *International Nursing Review*, 30(1), 21–23.

Downs, F. S. (1971). This I believe about the dimensions of nursing research. *Nursing Outlook*, 19(11), 719–721.

Eisner, E. (1981). On the differences between scientific and artistic approaches to qualitative research. *Educational Researcher*, 10(4), 5–9.

Evaneshko, V. & Kay, M. A. (1982). The ethnoscience research technique. *Western Journal of Nursing Research*, 4(1), 49–63.

Evans, J. C. (1978). Formulating an idea. In M. L. Fitzpatrick (Ed.), *Historical studies in nursing* (pp. 15–17). New York: Teachers College Press.

Fagerhaugh, S. & Strauss, A. (1977). *Politics of pain management: staff-patient interaction*. Menlo Park, California: Addison-Wesley Publishing Company.

Ferguson, E. S. (1977). The mind's eye: nonverbal thought in technology. *Science*, 197(4306), 827–836.

Field, P. A. (1983). An ethnography: four public health nurses' perspectives of nursing. *Journal of Advanced Nursing*, 8(1), 3–12.

Fitzpatrick, M. L. (1978). *Historical studies in nursing*. New York: Teachers College Press.

Fondiller, S. (1978). Writing the report. In M. L. Fitzpatrick (Ed.), *Historical studies in nursing* (pp. 25–27). New York: Teachers College Press.

Germain, C. P. H. (1979). *The cancer unit: an ethnography*. Wakefield, Massachusetts: Nursing Resources, Inc.

Germain, C. P. H. (1986). Ethnography: the method. In P. L. Munhall & C. J. Oiler (Eds.), *Nursing research: a qualitative perspective* (pp. 147–162). Norwalk, Connecticut: Appleton-Century-Crofts.

Giorgi, A. (1970). *Psychology as a human science: a phenomenologically based approach*. New York: Harper & Row Publishers, Inc.

Glaser, B. G. (1973). *Ward four hundred two*. New York: George Braziller.

Glaser, B. G. (1978). *Theoretical sensitivity*. Mill Valley, California: The Sociology Press.

Glaser, B. G. & Strauss, A. (1965). *Awareness of dying*. Chicago: Aldine.

Glaser, B. G. & Strauss, A. (1967). *The discovery of grounded theory: strategies for qualitative research*. Chicago: Aldine.

Glaser, B. G. & Strauss, A. (1968). *Time for dying*. Chicago: Aldine.

Glaser, B. G. & Strauss, A. (1971). *Status passage*. London: Routledge and Kegan Paul.

Gortner, S. R. (1980). Nursing science in transition. *Nursing Research*, 29(3), 180–183.

Hall, C. & Lindzey, G. (1970). *Theories of Personality*. New York: John Wiley & Sons.

Hodgman, E. C. (1979). Closing the gap between research and practice: changing the answers to the 'who,' the 'where' and the 'how' of nursing research. *International Journal of Nursing Studies*, 16(1), 105–110.

Ihde, D. (1977). *Experimental phenomenology: an introduction*. New York: G. P. Putnam's Sons.

Leininger, M. M. (1985). *Qualitative research methods in nursing*. Orlando: Grune & Stratton, Inc.

Ludemann, R. (1979). The paradoxical nature of nursing research. *Image*, 11(1), 2–8.

Lynch-Sauer, J. (1985). Using a phenomenological research method to study nursing phenomena. In M. M. Leininger (Ed.), *Qualitative research methods in nursing* (pp. 93–107). Orlando: Grune & Stratton, Inc.

Munhall, P. L. (1982a). Ethical juxtapositions in nursing research. *Topics in Clinical Nursing*, 4(1), 66–73.

Munhall, P. L. (1982b). Nursing philosophy and nursing research: in apposition or opposition? *Nursing Research*, 31(3), 176–181.

Munhall, P. L. & Oiler, C. J. (1986). *Nursing research: a qualitative perspective*. Norwalk, Connecticut: Appleton-Century-Crofts.

Newton, M. E. (1965). The case for historical research. *Nursing Research*, 14(1), 20–26.

O'Brien, M. E. (1981). Transcultural nursing research—alien in an alien land. *Image*, 13(2), 37–39.

Oiler, C. (1982). The phenomenological approach in nursing research. *Nursing Research*, 31(3), 178–181.

Omery, A. (1983). Phenomenology: a method for nursing research. *Advances in Nursing Science*, 5(2), 49–63.

Parse, R. R. (1981). *Man-living-health: a theory of nursing*. New York: A Wiley Medical Publication, John Wiley & Sons.

Parse, R. R., Coyne, A. B. & Smith, M. J. (1985). *Nursing research: qualitative methods*. Bowie, Maryland: Brady Communications Company.

Paterson, J. G. & Zderad, L. T. (1976). *Humanistic nursing*. New York: John Wiley & Sons.

Patton, M. (1980). *Qualitative evaluation methods*. Beverly Hills, California: Sage Publications.

Safier, G. (1976). Research Q and A: what is oral history? What are the advantages and disadvantages of oral history? How can it be used in nursing history? *Nursing Research*, 25(5), 383–385.

Schlotfeldt, R. M. (1971). The significance of empirical research for nursing. *Nursing Research*, 20(2), 140–142.

Silva, M. C. (1977). Philosophy, science, theory: interrelationships and implications for nursing research. *Image*, 9(3), 59–63.

Simms, L. M. (1981). The grounded theory approach in nursing research. *Nursing Research*, 30(6), 356–359.

Smith, J. K. (1983). Quantitative versus qualitative research: an attempt to clarify the issue. *Educational Researcher*, 12(3), 6–13.

Stern, P. N. (1980). Grounded theory methodology: its uses and processes. *Image*, 12(1), 20–23.

Strauss, A. L. (1975). *Chronic illness and quality of life*. St. Louis: The C. V. Mosby Company.

Strauss, A. L., Corbin, J., Fagerhaugh, S., Glaser, B. G., Maines, D., Suczek, B. & Wiener, C. L. (1984). *Chronic illness and the quality of life* (2nd ed.). St. Louis: The C. V. Mosby Company.

Strauss, A. & Glaser, B. G. (1970). *Anguish*. Mill Valley, California: Sociology Press.

Swanson, J. M. & Chenitz, W. C. (1982). Why qualitative research in nursing? *Nursing Outlook*, 30(4), 241–245.

Tilden, V. P. & Tilden, S. (1985). The participant philosophy in nursing science. *Image*, 17(3), 88–90.

Van Kaam, A. L. (1966). *Existential foundations of psychology* (vol. 3). Pittsburgh: Duquesne University Press.

Waring, L. M. (1978). Developing the research prospectus. In M. L. Fitzpatrick (Ed.), *Historical studies in nursing* (pp. 18–20). New York: Teachers College Press.

Watson, J. (1979). *Nursing: the philosophy and science of caring*. Boston: Little, Brown and Company.

Watson, J. (1981). Nursing's scientific quest. *Nursing Outlook*, 29(7), 413–416.

II

PLANNING THE RESEARCH PROCESS

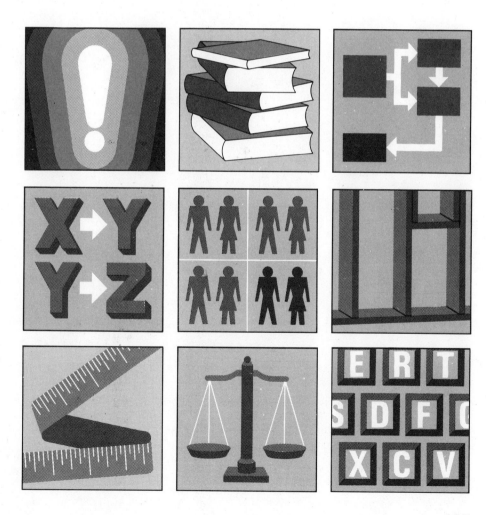

5

Formulating a Research Problem and Purpose

Within our world, we are constantly raising questions to gain a better understanding of ourselves and the world around us. This human ability to wonder and creatively raise questions about behaviors and situations in the real world provides a basis for formulating research problems. Formulating a research problem is the initial and one of the most significant steps in conducting both quantitative and qualitative research. There are a variety of research topics relevant to nursing, and each topic contains numerous potential research problems. However, the abundance of research topics and potential research problems is frequently not apparent to individuals struggling to formulate their first research problem.

This chapter provides information to facilitate the formulation of the research problem and purpose. Definitions of research problem and purpose are provided, and the differences between these terms are discussed. The sources of research ideas and the processes for formulating problem and purpose statements are described. The chapter concludes with examples of quantitative and qualitative research problems and purposes.

What is a Research Problem?

The research problem identifies an area of concern and indicates the concept(s) and population to be studied and the study setting. A problem can be expressed as a statement or a question. Williams, Campbell, Raynor, Musholt, Mlynarczyk and Crane (1985) expressed their problem as a statement: "The extent to which acute confusion can be prevented in patients with hip fractures or in other elderly patients on general hospital units has not been tested" (p. 330). The concepts investigated were acute confusion and prevention measures; the population was patients with hip fractures or other elderly patients. The setting for the study was general hospital units.

Sources of Research Problems

Research problems are developed from many sources. However, one must be astute, imaginative and curious to effectively utilize these sources. The major sources for nursing research problems include nursing practice, researcher and peer interaction, literature review, theory and personal conceptual framework.

NURSING PRACTICE

The practice of nursing must be based on knowledge generated through research. Therefore, clinical practice is an extremely important source for research problems (Diers, 1971; Fuller, 1982). Problems can evolve from clinical observations, such as those concerning the behaviors of a patient and family in crisis and how the nurse might intervene to improve their coping. Chart reviews might reveal concerns or raise questions about practice that might lead to research problems. For example, what is the impact of discharge planning on the cost and quality of patient care? Some students and nurses keep logs or journals of their practice that contain research ideas.

The unanswered questions in clinical practice and the desire to improve nursing interventions have been sources for many nursing studies published in the last 10 years. For example, Nath and Rinehart (1979) studied the effect of relaxation therapy on patients with essential hypertension; and Gerber and Van Ort (1979) studied the effect of topical insulin therapy as a treatment for decubitus ulcers.

In addition to clinical practice, nursing education, nursing administration and societal trends have been sources for many research problems. Merritt (1983) studied learning style preferences of baccalaureate nursing students, and Hanson and Chater (1983) studied role selection made by nurses, which included managerial interests and personal attributes. Nursing practice is constantly evolving in response to consumer needs and the movements in society. The trends and changes in nursing practice are influenced by research and influence the generation of research problems. Some examples of trends that have been researched in nursing are (1) the different types of nursing education (Goldstein, 1980; Munro, 1983; Rosenkoetter & McSweeney, 1983); (2) the development and implementation of the nurse practitioner role (Christensen, Lee & Bugg, 1979; Holzemer, Schleutermann, Farrand & Miller, 1981) and the clinical nurse specialist role (Woodrow & Bell, 1971; Wyers, Grove & Pasterino, 1985); (3) the use of the computer in providing nursing care (White, Wear & Stephenson,

1983); and (4) the increasing focus on prevention of illness and promotion of health (Brown, Muhlenkamp, Fox & Osborn, 1983; Lovejoy, 1980).

RESEARCHER AND PEER INTERACTION

Interaction with researchers and peers is a valuable source for generating research problems. Experienced researchers serve as mentors and share their knowledge with novice researchers in the identification of research topics and the formulation of research problems. For example, nursing educators assist students as they select their research problems. Some health care settings now employ nurse researchers to consult with nurses and other health professionals in identifying research priorities and generating research problems. Peers, including clients as well as nurses and other health professionals, stimulate discussions and thoughts that might lead nurses to identify research topics and/ or raise questions for potential study.

Beveridge (1950) identified four reasons for discussing research ideas with others. One reason is that ideas are clarified, and new ideas are generated when two or more people pool their thoughts. Interactions with others enable the researcher to uncover errors in reasoning and/or information, and these interactions are a source of support in discouraging or difficult times. Lastly, another person provides a refreshing or unique viewpoint, which prevents conditioned thinking or following an established habit of thought. A work place that encourages interaction can stimulate nurses to generate research ideas. Nursing conferences and professional organization meetings also provide excellent opportunities for nurses to discuss their ideas and brainstorm to identify potential research problems. Interactions with others are essential to broaden the perspective and knowledge base of the researcher and to provide support in formulating research problems.

LITERATURE REVIEW

Research topics and potential research problems can be identified by reviewing a variety of nursing publications. Nursing journals such as *Nursing Outlook*, *American Journal of Nursing* and *Topics in Clinical Nursing* contain research ideas, but frequently these ideas are implied. A reader must be oriented toward research and constantly searching for unanswered questions or areas of concern in nursing that are identified in the literature.

Reviewing the research journals *Nursing Research*, *Western Journal of Nursing Research* and *Research in Nursing and Health* will acquaint you with studies conducted in your area of interest. The nursing specialty journals such as *Oncology Nursing*, *Heart and Lung*, *Neurosurgical Nursing* and *MCN* also place a high priority on publishing research findings. From published studies, theses and dissertations, one can identify unresolved questions that can be used to generate research problems. By identifying problems for further study, researchers provide the opportunity for others to build upon their work to generate the knowledge needed in a given area.

Reviewing the literature facilitates the identification of problems that have been studied and gaps that exist in a discipline's knowledge base. The research problems formulated should focus on investigating new phenomena or on refining, expanding or replicating previous studies. Investigating a new phenomenon is referred to as an exploratory or preliminary study. For example, Geden (1982) conducted a preliminary study on the effects of five lifting techniques on 14 normal subjects' energy expenditure. Although lifting techniques have been taught in nursing for years, nursing research has not been conducted to examine the differential effect of various techniques on the nurse's energy expenditure. This study initiated a new dimension of interest for research.

Refining and Expanding Previous Studies

The level of knowledge previously generated on a research topic influences the problems that can be formulated for further research. Therefore, some research problems address the refining and/or expanding of selected studies. For example, Geden's (1982) study could be expanded by investigating problems that focused on the effects of additional lifting techniques in different settings using different populations. Additional research problems can be generated by combining the ideas from two or more studies. For example, one might combine Geden's research problem with Rottkamp's (1976) problem, which focused on body positioning of spinal cord–injured patients. A potential problem is "What are the effects of different lifting techniques on the nurse's energy expenditure in positioning spinal cord–injured patients?"

Replication of Studies

Some researchers replicate, or repeat, the work of other investigators. In replicating a study, researchers are never able to exactly repeat the original study because investigators, settings and subjects change with time. Frequently, a researcher will make modifications to improve the quality of the study. Some researchers replicate studies because they agree with the findings and wonder whether the findings will hold up in different settings and with the passage of time. Others replicate studies because they want to challenge the findings or interpretations of prior studies (Selltiz, Wrightsman & Cook, 1976). Replication is needed to determine whether the information generated from additional studies is consistent with the original study findings. If the findings generated through replications are consistent with original study findings, these findings have a greater probability of being an accurate reflection of the real world and, thus, useful in nursing practice.

Replication should be given a high priority in nursing. Replicating studies would be an excellent learning experience for masters students doing theses. Lindeman and Van Aernam's (1971) study of the effects of structured and unstructured preoperative teaching was replicated by King and Tarsitano (1982). In the original study by Lindeman and Van Aernam (1971), the research questions were

1. What are the effects of a structured and an unstructured preoperative

teaching program upon the adult surgical patient's ability to deep breathe and cough 24 hours postoperatively?

2. What are the effects of a structured and an unstructured preoperative teaching program upon the adult surgical patient's length of hospital stay?

3. What are the effects of a structured and an unstructured preoperative teaching program upon the adult surgical patient's postoperative need for analgesia? (Lindeman & Van Aernam, 1971, p. 321)

King and Tarsitano's (1982) research questions were

1. What are the results of a structured and unstructured preoperative teaching program on the adult surgical patients' postoperative recovery as measured by pulmonary function tests?

2. What are the results of a structured and unstructured preoperative teaching program on the adult surgical patients' length of hospital stay? (King & Tarsitano, 1982, p. 324)

King and Tarsitano (1982) elected to narrow the scope of the problem to exclude the phenomenon of pain, as recommended by the original investigators (Lindeman & Van Aernam, 1971). The researchers also modified the measurement of respiratory function by including pulmonary function tests. They controlled other factors not controlled in the original study:

> ...restricting the sample to patients of three surgeons with similar techniques and to patients having lower or upper abdominal surgery. The structured preoperative teaching was conducted primarily by the principle investigator and associate and a checklist was used to indicate that the patients could perform the deep breathing, coughing and exercises. (King & Tarsitano, 1982, p. 324)

Landmark Studies

Landmark studies are major studies that generate knowledge that influences a discipline and sometimes society in general. These studies are frequently replicated or are the basis for the generation of many additional research problems. For example, Williams (1972) studied the factors that contribute to skin breakdown, and the findings from this study have influenced nursing care for the prevention of skin breakdown. This study has also stimulated the development of additional studies on the prevention and treatment of decubitus ulcers.

THEORY

Theories are an important source for generating research problems because they set forth ideas about events and situations in the real world that require testing. In examining a theory, one notes that it includes a number of propositions and that each proposition is a statement of the relationship of two or more concepts. A research problem could be formulated to explore or describe a concept in a theory, such as a study to explore the concept of self-care in Orem's theory.

In addition, a proposition in a theory can be the basis for generating many research problems. For example, Ketefian (1981) formulated a research problem from a proposition in Kohlberg's theory of moral development. The proposition was that "the degree of intellectual development and the nature of educational preparation will affect the degree to which a person's moral judgment has developed" (Ketefian, 1981, p. 100). The research problem formulated from that proposition was "Is there a relationship between critical thinking, educational preparation, and levels of moral reasoning among selected groups of nurses?" (Ketefian, 1981, p. 98). The proposition was translated into a problem that contained variables (critical thinking, educational preparation and levels of moral reasoning) that could be studied in the real world. Only a limited number of nursing research problems have been generated from theoretical propositions, but the use of theory as a source for research problems is increasing.

PERSONAL CONCEPTUAL FRAMEWORK

All research ideas generated from nursing practice, researcher and peer interaction, literature review and theory are interpreted and evaluated in terms of a researcher's personal framework. A personal conceptual framework is an inner perspective, a person's unique way of organizing knowledge and beliefs that influences the way the person perceives the world (Eells, 1981). Each individual's unique way of perceiving and interacting within the world influences all research problems that individual formulates. Researchers viewing the same situation would identify a variety of research problems because of their personal framework or perspective. Focusing on an individual's framework emphasizes the importance of the human mind in the development of research problems. The creative, dynamic and intuitive qualities of the mind make it the most valuable source in formulating research problems.

Formulating a Researchable Problem

A researchable problem is one that can be studied using quantitative or qualitative research approaches. The exact reasoning process for formulating researchable problems has not been clearly identified because of the abstractness and complexity of the reasoning involved. Formulating research problems involves logical reasoning and also chance happenings or spontaneous realizations (intuition) (Beveridge, 1950). The elements for formulating a research problem include identifying a research topic, generating questions, generating potential nursing research problems and refining the problem statement.

RESEARCH TOPICS

Research topics are broad problem areas that provide the basis for generating questions. Nursing research topics focus on areas that are controlled by nursing and will influence nursing practice. Some of the topics that have been investigated by nurses include coping patterns, developmental changes, teaching or health education, health promotion, rehabilitation, emotional or psychological support, relaxation, biofeedback, physical treatments, oral hygiene, pain control, respiratory patterns, pulmonary hygiene, bowel management, perineal care, intravenous infections, nutritional alterations and skin integrity (O'Connell, 1976; Lindsey, 1982 & 1983). In addition, Gordon (1980) identified nursing diagnoses as study topics, which include such concepts as self-care deficit, impaired home maintenance management, grieving and altered parenting.

TYPES OF QUESTIONS GENERATED FROM RESEARCH TOPICS

Encountering situations in the real world and reading the literature on selected topics stimulate the constant generation of questions. The questions fit into three categories. Some of the questions raised already have a satisfactory answer within nursing's existing body of knowledge, and these answers are available in the literature or from experts in nursing or other disciplines. For example, the answers to questions nurses have about performing certain nursing skills, such as the steps for taking blood pressures or drawing-up medications for injections, are available in procedure manuals. Studying these questions would minimally advance nursing's knowledge base. However, problems that focused on investigating new techniques to improve existing skills, patient responses to techniques or ways to educate patients and families about techniques could add to nursing's knowledge base.

Some of the questions raised can be answered using problem-solving or evaluation projects. Chapter 2 includes a comparison of the problem-solving process and the research process, which indicates when and why to use each process. Many evaluation projects are conducted with minimal application of the rigor and control that are required in conducting the research process. These projects do not fit the criteria of research, and the findings are relevant for a particular situation. For example, quality assurance is an evaluation of client care implemented by a specific health care agency; and the results of this evaluation project are useful and relevant only to the agency conducting the review.

The most important type of question for research is one that requires further knowledge to answer. Research experts have found that asking the right question is frequently much more valuable than finding the solution to a problem. The solution identified in a single study might not withstand the test of time or might be useful only in limited situations. However, one well-formulated question can lead to the generation of numerous research problems, a lifetime of research activities and possibly significant contributions to a discipline's body of knowledge.

Problem Significance

Some of the problems selected for study in nursing might be considered insignificant. For example, a problem might be studied because it appears easy, quick or convenient to study. Some "easy" problems have been studied to the point of diminishing return. For example, problems that focus on the attitudes of nurses regarding job satisfaction have been investigated numerous times with minimal impact on practice.

Every problem investigated should have professional significance and potential or actual significance for society. A research problem is significant when it has the potential to generate or refine knowledge and/or influence nursing practice. The problems that are considered to be significant vary with time and the needs of society. Some currently significant topics for nursing research are (1) the quality of care for a large number of clients, (2) the suffering or severe difficulties of particular clients, (3) access to care, (4) clients' health situations, (5) modification of current health services and (6) the development of effective strategies for maintaining and promoting health. Campbell, Daft and Hulin (1982) indicated that the formation of a significant research problem results from extensive exposure to nursing practice and the literature; the convergence of several streams of thought and ideas; a creative, intuitive ability; and a concern with theoretical understanding and with real-world problems.

Personal Interest

Sometimes individuals fail to follow their research interests because they do not feel competent to identify a significant problem. These individuals might investigate problems that were suggested by instructors or expert researchers. Some researchers are unable to get research subjects or funding for research projects of interest, so they select other problems to investigate. These researchers sometimes lack the commitment of time and energy to complete their studies.

The researcher's personal interest in a problem influences the quality of the problem formulated and the study conducted. A problem of personal interest is one that an individual has pondered for a long time or one that is especially important in the individual's nursing practice or personal life. For example, a researcher who has had a mastectomy may be particularly interested in studying the emotional impact of a mastectomy or strategies for caring for patients experiencing a mastectomy. This personal interest in the topic can become the driving force needed to conduct quality studies (Beveridge, 1950).

GENERATING POTENTIAL NURSING RESEARCH PROBLEMS

Potential nursing research problems emerge from situations in nursing practice. A situation is a significant combination of circumstances that occur at a given time. Inexperienced researchers tend to want to study the entire situation. However, the entire situation is far too complex for the development of a single study. There are multiple problems within a single situation, and each can be developed into a study. The problems that are extracted from the situation will vary with the researcher. Each researcher's perception of what problems exist in the situation depends on that researcher's clinical expertise, theoretical bases, intuition, interests and goals. Some researchers spend years developing different problem statements and new studies from the same clinical situation.

Initial development of the problem begins with identification of research topics and concepts of interest within the situation. Next, consider the questions that come to mind about those concepts. Does the need seem to be to describe them, to know how they are related or to be able to predict or control some event within the situation? What is known and what is not known about the concepts within the situation? What are the most urgent factors to know? Next, the researcher must determine what means are available to measure the concepts (variables) within the situation. Some variables may be easily measured with existing tools, and others may require tool development.

Fantasy and creativity are part of formulating a research problem. Imagine studies that could be done related to the situation, the variables and the measurement tools. Imagine the difficulties likely to occur with each study, but avoid being too critical of potential research problems at this time. Which studies seem the most workable? Which ones appeal intuitively? Which ones seem the most feasible considering the time and money available?

Without narrowing potential problems to only one idea, try some of the ideas out on colleagues. Let them play the devil's advocate, and explore the strengths and weaknesses of each idea. Then begin some preliminary reading in the area of interest. Examine literature related to the situation, the variables within the situation, measurement of the variables and previous studies related to the situation. The literature review will enable you to determine the type of research that needs to be conducted.

REFINING PROBLEM STATEMENTS

The research problem is refined and narrowed as it evolves from a topic to a clear statement. First attempts at writing the problem statement are often frustrating, because it is difficult to put an idea into words. The initial problem statement is modified several times, and each time the statement improves in clarity. As the problem statement is refined, the rest of the study (in particular, the research purpose) begins to emerge in the mind.

Formulating the Research Purpose

The *research purpose* is a statement of "why" the study is being conducted, or the goal of the study. The goal of a study might be to identify or describe a concept or to explain or predict a situation or solution to a situation that indicates the type of study to be conducted (Beckingham, 1974). The purpose statement identifies the variables, population and setting for a study. Every study has an explicit or implicit purpose statement. The purpose in the study by Williams *et al*. (1985) was "to test whether the incidence of confusion in elderly patients with hip fractures, and with no prior history of mental impairment, could be reduced by specific nursing interventions" (p. 330). The goal of this study was to explain the influence of certain interventions on the incidence of confusion in hospitalized patients experiencing fractured hips. The type of study is quasi-experimental.

The research purpose should be stated objectively or in a way that does not reflect particular biases or values of the researcher. Researchers who do not recognize their values might include their biases in their research. This can lead the researcher to generate the answers they want or believe to be true and might add inaccurate information to a discipline's body of knowledge (Kaplan, 1964).

The purpose is generated from the problem statement and clearly focuses the development of the study. For example, Mallick's (1982) study included the following research problem: "Unsupervised dieting occurs partly because promulgation of diets and dispensation of diet aides (appetite suppressants, diet foods) are not regulated by law, and widespread use of various reducing diets and the attendant side effects have not been examined extensively" (p. 167). The purpose of this study was to "examine the characteristics of female adolescent dieters, the types of diets followed and the occurrence of health problems in relation to these diets" (p. 167). The research problem indicates the area of concern, which is dieting and the side effects of dieting. The purpose of this descriptive study was to generate specific knowledge about adolescent dieters, their dieting activities and the occurrence of health problems related to their diets. In the research process, the purpose is usually stated after the problem, supports the problem and clarifies the knowledge to be generated for nursing. As the research problem and purpose increase in clarity and conciseness, the researcher has greater direction in determining the feasibility of a study.

FEASIBILITY

Determining the feasibility of a study involves examining the time and money commitment, the researcher's expertise, availability of subjects, cooperation of others and the study's ethical considerations.

Time

Conducting research frequently takes more time than is anticipated, which makes it difficult for any researcher, especially the novice researcher, to estimate the time that will be involved. In estimating the time commitment, the researcher examines the purpose of the study; the more complex the purpose, the greater the time commitment. An approximation of the time needed to complete a study can be determined by assessing the following factors: (1) the type and number of subjects needed, (2) the number and complexity of the variables to be studied, (3) the methods for measuring the variables (Are instruments available to measure the variables or must they be developed?), (4) the methods for collecting data and (5) the data analysis process. An often overlooked time commitment is the writing of the research report for presentation and publication. The researcher estimates the time needed to complete each of these steps and determines whether the time commitment is reasonable.

Each study that is conducted is done within a designated time period or has a specific deadline. For example, an agency might set a 2-year deadline for studying the turnover rate of staff. The researcher needs to determine whether the identified purpose can be accomplished by the designated deadline; if not, the purpose must be narrowed or the deadline extended. A researcher should be cautious about extending deadlines, because a research project could continue for many months and even years. The individual interested in conducting qualitative research frequently must make an extensive time commitment of months and sometimes years. The time commitment is discussed further in Chapter 16 as part of developing a research plan. Time can be as important as money, and the cost of a study can be greatly affected by the time required to conduct the study.

Money

The problem and purpose selected are influenced by the amount of money available to the researcher. Potential sources for funding should be considered at the time that the problem and purpose are identified (Chapter 14). The cost of a research project can range from a few dollars for a student's small study to hundreds of thousands of dollars for very complex projects. In estimating the cost of a research project, the following questions need to be considered:

1. What will the review of the literature, including computer searches and copying articles, cost?
2. Will the subjects have to be paid for their participation in the study?
3. What will the equipment cost for the study? Can the equipment be borrowed, rented, or bought? Is the equipment available, or will it have to be built?
4. Will assistants and/or consultants be hired to collect and analyze the data and assist with the data interpretation?
5. Will computer time be required to analyze the data? If so, what will be the cost?
6. Will there be any transportation costs?
7. What will be the cost of having the report typed and distributed?

Researcher Expertise

An individual should select a research problem and purpose that is within his or her background to investigate. Initially one might work with another researcher (mentor) to learn the process and then investigate a familiar problem that fits one's knowledge base or experience. Selecting a very difficult, complex problem and purpose can only frustrate and confuse the novice researcher. However, all researchers should formulate problems and purposes that are challenging, and they should seek the assistance of other researchers as needed in order to build their research background. Nurse researchers also need expertise in nursing practice so the problems selected have a potential to influence practice.

Availability of Subjects

In selecting a research purpose, one must consider the type and number of subjects needed. Finding a sample might be difficult if the research problem involves investigating a unique or rare population, such as quadriplegic individuals who live alone. The more specific the population, the more difficult it will be to obtain the sample. The money and time available to the researcher will affect the subjects selected, because with limited time and money, the researcher might want to investigate subjects who are more available and do not require payment for participation. Even if a researcher identifies a population with a large number of potential subjects, these individuals may be unwilling to participate in the study because of the topic selected for study. For example, nurses, as potential subjects, might fear that the investigation of certain nursing interventions could have a negative effect on their jobs.

Cooperation of Others

A research purpose might appear quite feasible, but without the cooperation of others, it is not. Some studies are conducted in laboratory settings and require minimal cooperation of others. However, most nursing studies involve human subjects and are conducted in the settings of those subjects, such as hospitals, clinics, schools, offices or homes. Having the cooperation of people in the research setting, the subjects and the others involved in data collection is essential. People are frequently willing to cooperate with a study if they view the problem and purpose as significant and/or if they are personally interested. For example, nurses and other personnel employed in an institution would probably be very interested in cooperating with a study that would examine the cost-effectiveness of quality nursing care in that institution. Gaining the cooperation of others in a research project is discussed in Chapters 13 and 16.

Ethical Considerations

The purpose selected for investigation must be ethical, which means that the subjects' rights and the rights of the setting are protected. If the purpose appears to infringe upon the rights of the subjects or setting, it should be reexamined and may have to be revised or abandoned. There are usually some risks with every study, but, in general, the value of the knowledge generated should outweigh the risks. The ethical considerations of a study are the focus of Chapter 12.

Quantitative and Qualitative Research Problems

Quantitative and qualitative research approaches enable researchers to investigate a variety of research problems and purposes. The research topics and research problems and/or purposes for the different types of quantitative studies are presented in Table 5–1. Not all published studies clearly express a problem and purpose. The research purpose reflects the type of study that is to be

TABLE 5–1
Research Topics and Quantitative Problems/Purposes

Type of Research	Research Topic	Research Problem/Purpose
Exploratory	Educators, Clinical practice	The purpose of this study was to explore problems of faculty practice with those faculty who are involved in practice and to ascertain the facilitating and/or inhibiting factors that faculty perceive when trying to maintain their clinical skills. (Anderson & Pierson, 1983, p. 129)
Descriptive studies Case study	Cognitive process, Nutrition, Developmental level	Among the many problems presented by a child with mental retardation, certain maladaptive behavior patterns cause significant difficulties for families and caregivers. (Durand, 1975, p. 272)
		This study investigated the extent to which, for a child with Down's Syndrome and severe failure to thrive, a planned program of developmental nursing care effected positive changes in growth and development and in specific maladaptive behaviors. (p. 272)
Survey	Sleep patterns, Aging process	Because of the lack of norms (for changes in sleep patterns with age), nurses and patients tend to evaluate an older person's sleep on the basis of sleep norms for younger adults. (Hayter, 1983, p. 242)
		The purpose of this study was to determine the nature of sleep behaviors among older persons of different ages. (p. 243)
Correlational	PS (Perimenstrual symptoms), Socialization, Menstrual attitude	. . . PS (perimenstrual symptoms) are the primary reason women miss work or school, and these symptoms frequently cause women to seek medical care. (Woods, 1985, p. 145)
		The purpose of this study was to assess the extent to which a woman's environment and socialization influenced her experience of PS, related disability, and menstrual attitudes. (p. 146)
Quasi-experimental	Skin integrity, Intervention	Because decubitus ulcers occur despite preventive measures, methods which are effective and reliable in promoting healing must be found and implemented. (Van Ort & Gerber, 1976, p. 9)
		The purpose of this study was to evaluate the effects of topical application of insulin to promote healing of decubitus ulcers. (p. 10)
Experimental	Cardiac response, Auditory stimulation	Some of the emotional difficulties clinically associated with prematurity, such as restlessness, irritability and lack of attentiveness, emotional lability, and uncontrolled anger, may be the product of understimulation. The rationale is that premature infants may fail to develop a "normal" threshold to stimuli. (Segall, 1972, p. 15)
		The purpose of this study was to determine if there were differences in cardiac responsivity between premature infants who were exposed to the mother's voice while hospitalized and premature infants who did not receive this variation of sensory input. (p. 15)

conducted. The purpose of exploratory and descriptive research is to describe concepts and to identify relationships. The purpose of correlational research is to examine relationships. Quasi-experimental and experimental research is conducted to examine causal relationships. The knowledge level of a particular topic in a discipline determines the purpose stated. If little is known about a topic, the researcher starts with a problem and purpose that requires investigation by an exploratory or descriptive study and progresses to the other types of studies.

The problems of qualitative studies focus on subjective concepts. The research topics, problems and purposes listed in Table 5–2 were the basis for generating the four types of qualitative studies. Phenomenological research seeks an understanding of human experience from an individual researcher's perspective. There are three basic types of research problems that are investigated through phenomenological research. "These are (1) the interpretation of the single, unique event; (2) the interpretation of a single, unique individual; and (3) the interpretation of a general or repetitive psychological process (e.g., anger, learning, etc.)" (Knaack, 1984, p. 111). The problem and/or purpose in grounded theory research identifies the focus of the theory to be developed from the research. In ethnographic research, the problem statement and/or purpose identifies the culture and the specific attribute(s) or aspect(s) of the culture that are to be examined and described. The problem statement and/or purpose in historical research focuses on a specific individual, a characteristic of society, an event or a situation in the past and identifies the time period in the past that will be examined in conducting the research. There are an infinite

TABLE 5–2
Research Topics and Qualitative Problems/Purposes

Type of Research	Research Topic	Research Problem/Purpose
Phenomenological	Restlessness	. . . attempts to identify the behavioral manifestations of restlessness and the nursing significance of this phenomenon. (Norris, 1975, p. 103)
Grounded theory	Critical care nursing	How do critical care nurses determine if a patient is developing cardiogenic shock? What assessment and decision-making processes do they use, and how do they learn them? (Pyles & Stern, 1983, p. 51)
Ethnography	Cultural beliefs, Childbirth	Data on birthing beliefs and practices among the Black Caribs (Garifuna) of Central America is sparse. (Cohen, 1982, p. 193)
		The study reported here describes the beliefs and practices related to pregnancy, delivery, postpartum, and immediate infant care among a population of Garifuna in Rio Tinto, one of 43 Carib settlements located on the north coast of Honduras. (p. 193)
Historical	Nursing education, Baccalaureate	It was the purpose of this research to explore . . . increased specialization and the development of a professional subculture as it relates to the establishment of nursing education in the American University. (Krampitz, 1983, p. 372)

number of qualitative and quantitative problems that require investigation by nurse researchers.

Summary

A research problem is the clear, concise presentation of "what" is to be studied. The problem identifies an area of concern and indicates the concepts(s) to be studied. The major sources for nursing research problems include nursing practice, researcher and peer interaction, literature review, theory and personal conceptual framework. The exact reasoning process for formulating researchable problems has not been clearly identified because of the abstractness and complexity of the reasoning involved. A researchable problem is one that can be studied using quantitative or qualitative research approaches. The elements for formulating a researchable problem include identifying a research topic, generating questions, generating potential nursing research problems and refining the problem statement.

The research purpose is a statement of "why" the study is being conducted or the goal of the study. The goal of a study might be to identify or describe a concept or to explain or predict a situation or solution to a situation. The purpose statement indicates the type of study to be conducted. The purpose is generated from the problem statement and identifies the variables, population and setting of the study. As the research purpose increases in clarity, the researcher has greater direction in determining the feasibility of a study. Determining the feasibility of a study involves examining the time and money commitment, researcher's expertise, availability of subjects, cooperation of others and the study's ethical considerations. The chapter concludes with a description and examples of quantitative and qualitative research problems and purposes.

References

Adebo, E. O. (1974). Identifying problems for nursing research. *International Nursing Review*, 21(2), 53–54, 59.

Anderson, E. R. & Pierson, P. (1983). An exploratory study of faculty practice: views of those faculty engaged in practice who teach in an NLN-accredited baccalaureate program. *Western Journal of Nursing Research*, 5(2), 129–140.

Beckingham, A. C. (1974). Identifying problems for nursing research. *International Nursing Review*, 21(2), 49–52.

Beveridge, W. I. B. (1950). *The art of scientific investigation*. New York: Vintage Books, a division of Random House.

Brown, N., Muhlenkamp, A., Fox, L. & Osborn, M. (1983). The relationship among health beliefs, health values, and health promotion activity. *Western Journal of Nursing Research*, 5(2), 155–163.

Campbell, J. P., Daft, R. L. & Hulin, C. L. (1982). *What to study: generating and developing research questions*. Beverly Hills: Sage Publications.

Christensen, M. G., Lee, C. A. & Bugg, P. W. (1979). Professional development of nurse practitioners as a function of need motivation, learning style, and locus of control. *Nursing Research*, 28(1), 51–56.

Cohen, F. S. (1982). Childbirth belief and practice in a Garifuna (Black Carib) village on the north coast of Honduras. *Western Journal of Nursing Research*, 4(2), 193–208.

Diers, D. (1971). Finding clinical problems for study. *Journal of Nursing Administration*, 1(6), 15–18.

Durand, B. (1975). A clinical nursing study: failure to thrive in a child with Down's syndrome. *Nursing Research*, 24(4), 272–286.

Eells, M. A. W. (1981). The research problem. In S. D. Krampitz & N. Pavlovich (Eds.), *Readings for nursing research* (pp. 3–10). St. Louis: The C. V. Mosby Company.

Fuller, E. O. (1982). Selecting a clinical nursing problem for research. *Image*, 14(2), 60–61.

Geden, E. A. (1982). Effects of lifting techniques on energy expenditure: a preliminary investigation. *Nursing Research*, 31(4), 214–218.

Gerber, R. M. & Van Ort, S. R. (1979). Topical application of insulin in decubitus ulcers. *Nursing Research*, 23(1), 16–19.

Goldstein, J. O. (1980). Comparison of graduating A.D. and baccalaureate nursing students characteristics. *Nursing Research*, 29(1), 46–49.

Gordon, M. (1980). Determining study topics. *Nursing Research*, 29(2), 83–87.

Hanson, H. A. & Chater, S. (1983). Role selection by nurses: managerial interests and personal attributes. *Nursing Research*, 32(1), 48–52.

Hayter, J. (1983). Sleep behaviors of older persons. *Nursing Research*, 32(4), 242–246.

Holmstrom, L. L. & Burgess, A. W. (1982). Low-cost research: a project on a shoestring. *Nursing Research*, 31(2), 123–125.

Holzemer, W. L., Schleutermann, J. A., Farrand, L. L. & Miller, A. G. (1981). A validation study: simulations as a measure of nurse practitioners' problem-solving skills. *Nursing Research*, 30(3), 139–144.

Kaplan, B. A. (1964). *The conduct of inquiry: methodology for behavioral science*. New York: Harper & Row, Publishers.

Ketefian, S. (1981). Critical thinking, educational preparation, and development of moral judgment among selected groups of practicing nurses. *Nursing Research*, 30(2), 98–103.

King, I. & Tarsitano, B. (1982). The effect of structured and unstructured preoperative teaching: a replication. *Nursing Research*, 31(6), 324–329.

Knaack, P. (1984). Phenomenological research. *Western Journal of Nursing Research*, 6(1), 107–114.

Krampitz, S. D. (1983). Historical development of baccalaureate nursing education in the American university: 1899–1935. *Western Journal of Nursing Research*, 5(4), 371–380.

Lindeman, C. A. & Van Aernam, B. (1971). Nursing intervention with the presurgical patient— the effects of structured and unstructured preoperative teaching. *Nursing Research*, 20(4), 319–332.

Lindsey, A. M. (1982). Phenomena and physiological variables of relevance to nursing, review of a decade of work: part I. *Western Journal of Nursing Research*, 4(4), 343–364.

Lindsey, A. M. (1983). Phenomena and physiological variables of relevance to nursing, review of a decade of work: part II. *Western Journal of Nursing Research*, 5(1), 41–63.

Lovejoy, N. C. (1980). Biofeedback: a growing role in holistic health. *Advances in Nursing Science*, 2(4), 83–93.

Mallick, M. J. (1982). Health problems associated with dieting activities of a group of adolescent females. *Western Journal of Nursing Research*, 4(2), 167–177.

Merritt, S. L. (1983). Learning style preferences of baccalaureate nursing students. *Nursing Research*, 32(6), 367–372.

Munro, B. H. (1983). Job satisfaction among recent graduates of schools of nursing. *Nursing Research*, 32(6), 350–355.

Nath, C. & Rinehart, J. (1979). Effect of individual and group relaxation therapy on blood pressure in essential hypertensives. *Nursing Research*, 28(2), 119–126.

Norris, C. M. (1975). Restlessness: a nursing phenomenon in search of meaning. *Nursing Outlook*, 23(2), 103–107.

O'Connell, K. A. (1976). Research in nursing practice: its nature and direction. *Image*, 8(1), 6–12.

Pyles, S. H. & Stern, P. N. (1983). Discovery of nursing gestalt in critical care nursing: the importance of the gray gorilla syndrome. *Image*, 15(2), 51–57.

Rosenkoetter, M. M. & McSweeney, M. (1983). Perceptions of nurse educators regarding ADN and BSN general education. *Western Journal of Nursing Research*, 5(2), 165–177.

Rottkamp, B. C. (1976). A behavior modification approach to nursing therapeutics in body positioning of spinal cord–injured patients. *Nursing Research*, 25(3), 181–185.

Segall, M. A. (1972). Cardiac responsivity to auditory stimulation in premature infants. *Nursing Research*, 21(1), 15–19.

Selltiz, C., Wrightsman, L. S. & Cook, S. W. (1976). *Research methods in social relations*. New York: Holt, Rinehart and Winston.

Van Ort, S. R. & Gerber, R. M. (1976). Topical application of insulin in the treatment of decubitus ulcers: a pilot study. *Nursing Research*, 25(1), 9–12.

White, M. A., Wear, E. & Stephenson, G. (1983). A computer-compatible method for observing falling asleep behavior of hospitalized children. *Research in Nursing and Health*, 6(4), 191–198.

Williams, A. (1972). A study of factors contributing to skin breakdown. *Nursing Research*, 21(3), 238–243.

Williams, M. A., Campbell, E. B., Raynor, W. J. Jr., Musholt, M. A., Mlynarczyk, S. M. & Crane, L. F. (1985). Predictors of acute confusional states in hospitalized elderly patients. *Research in Nursing and Health*, 8(1), 31–40.

Woodrow, M. & Bell, J. A. (1971). Clinical specialization: conflict between reality and theory. *Journal of Nursing Administration*, 1(6), 23–28.

Woods, N. F. (1985). Relationship of socialization and stress to perimenstrual symptoms, disability, and menstrual attitudes. *Nursing Research*, 34(3), 145–149.

Wyers, M. E., Grove, S. K. & Pasterino, C. (1985). Clinical nurse specialist: in search of the right role. *Nursing and Health Care*, 6(4), 202–207.

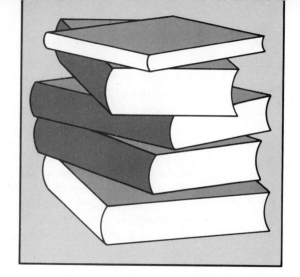

6

Review of Relevant Literature

Conducting a review of relevant literature is a challenging, enlightening experience. Through the literature review, the researcher generates a picture of what is known about a particular situation and the knowledge gaps that exist in the situation. The review of literature bridges the gap between the problem statement and the research subproblems and lays a foundation for the research plan.

Relevant literature refers to those sources that are pertinent or highly important in providing the in-depth knowledge needed to study a selected problem (Batey, 1977). The review of relevant literature is a three-step process: (1) locating a variety of relevant sources, (2) critiquing those sources for significant information and (3) generating a written report of the knowledge gained. This chapter focuses on the purpose, scope, process and end product of the review of relevant literature in the research process.

Purpose for reviewing relevant literature

The primary purpose for reviewing relevant literature is to gain a broad background or understanding of the information that is available related to the research problem of interest. This background enables the researcher to build

127

upon the works of others, which is essential since major breakthroughs or discoveries of new information in a field are always related to previous works (Kaplan, 1964). The researcher's background of the literature should include familiarity with what work (theoretical and empirical) has been done concerning a specific research problem, what is considered to be the current knowledge of the problem and what further research is needed. The literature review will promote the identification of feasible research purposes and subproblems and will direct the development of methodologically sound studies. There are specific purposes for reviewing the literature, depending on whether the study is quantitative or qualitative. The purposes for conducting the review of relevant literature in these different types of studies also determine when the review is done.

PURPOSE OF THE LITERATURE REVIEW IN QUANTITATIVE RESEARCH

The review of relevant literature in quantitative research influences the development of several steps in the research process. In all types of quantitative studies, the literature review is conducted for the same purposes, which are listed in Table 6–1. The literature review is instigated at the beginning of the research process and continues throughout the development of the research plan and proposal.

The initial identification of a research topic frequently evolves from a clinical nursing experience; however, a topic may be identified and clarified through the literature review. The research problem, which emerges from the research topic, is initially very broad and general. The problem is refined and clarified many times throughout the literature review. With a background in the relevant literature, the researcher ultimately is able to formulate the research purpose, one that is clearly focused, significant for nursing and feasible to study (Chapter 5). The significance, or importance, of the problem and purpose in generating and/or refining nursing knowledge are clarified by examining relevant sources.

The researcher gains essential information from existing studies and

TABLE 6–1
Purposes of the Literature Review in Quantitative Research

Clarify the research topic
Clarify the research problem
Verify the significance of the research problem
Specify the purpose of the study
Identify relevant studies
Identify relevant theories
Clarify research subproblems
Develop definitions of major variables
Identify limitations and assumptions
Select a research design
Identify instruments or tool(s) of measurement
Direct data collection and analysis
Interpret findings

theories through a literature review. This information is logically organized and presented in the review of literature section of the research proposal and the final research report. Theories are reviewed to clarify the definitions of concepts and to develop the framework for the study (Chapter 7). Specific research subproblems are identified, and variables to be studied are operationally defined using information from the literature (Chapter 8). The limitations and assumptions for a study are identified or become clearer after determining those identified by other researchers in the literature.

The design selected for a study should reflect a thorough understanding of the designs used by other researchers who have studied the same or similar problems (Chapter 10). The researcher examines the designs of previous studies to identify the designs used, to clarify the flaws in these designs, and, ultimately, to develop an improved design. Reviewing relevant studies can also reveal promising measurement tool(s) and provide useful information to increase the effectiveness of data collection and analysis (Chapters 11, 16 and 17). Lastly, the findings from previous studies are a basis for comparison when interpreting the findings from the proposed study.

PURPOSE OF THE LITERATURE REVIEW IN QUALITATIVE STUDIES

The review of literature in qualitative studies is different in both purpose and timing (Table 6–2). Phenomenologists believe that the literature should be reviewed after data collection so that the information in the literature will not influence the researcher's objectivity. Thus, the researcher's description of a real-world phenomenon should include only what is seen in the real situation and not what is read in the literature. For example, if a researcher decided to describe the phenomenon of a "dying person," the review of literature would reflect Kubler-Ross' (1969) five stages of grieving. Knowing these five stages could influence the way the researcher viewed the phenomenon. The researcher might not really be able to observe the real world phenomenon of a "dying person" using an open context. After data are collected and analyzed, the information from the literature is compared with findings from the present study to determine similarities and differences (Oiler, 1982). The literature and

---

TABLE 6–2
Purpose of the Literature Review in Qualitative Research

Type of Qualitative Research	Purpose of Literature Review
Phenomenological research	Compare the findings from the study with the information in the literature.
Grounded theory research	Combine the information in the literature with the theory generated in the study.
Ethnographic research	Review the literature to provide a background for conducting the study.
Historical research	Review of literature is used to develop research questions and is a source of data.

study findings are combined to determine the current knowledge of a phenomenon.

Grounded theory research is a five-step process: (1) collection of empirical data, (2) concept formation, (3) concept development, (4) concept modification and integration and (5) production of the research report. In this type of research, a minimal review of relevant studies is conducted at the beginning of the research process. This review is only a means of making the researcher aware of what studies have been conducted, but the information from these studies is not used to direct the collection of empirical data or the development of theory from that data. The main review of literature is conducted in step three, concept development. The literature is used to define certain concepts and to further verify the relationships in the theory developed from the empirical data (Stern, 1980).

The purpose and time for conducting the review of literature in ethnographic research is similar to that of quantitative research. The literature is reviewed early in the research process after the culture and the variables to be studied have been identified (Aamodt, 1982). The information obtained from the literature provides a background for conducting the study, and the findings from the study are compared with the findings from previous studies. The intent of the research is to generate new insights regarding the culture studied, which would add to the current knowledge about that culture.

Historical research requires an extensive review of relevant literature. The relevance of the sources obtained determine the quality of the research conducted. An initial literature review occurs early in the research process after the development of research questions and provides a background for investigating the research questions (Christy, 1975). The information gained from the sources reviewed is analyzed to explain how an identified phenomenon has evolved over a particular time period.

Scope of the Literature review

The scope of the literature review should be broad enough for the researcher to be knowledgeable of the research problem and narrow enough to include predominantly relevant sources. In determining the scope of a literature review, the researcher should evaluate three areas: (1) the different types of information available, (2) the depth and breadth of the literature review and (3) the time frame for conducting the review.

TYPES OF INFORMATION

Two types of information are covered in the review of literature: theoretical and empirical. Other types of information such as opinions, beliefs, clinical impressions and narrations of a situation or event are usually not included in the review of literature because of their subjectivity (Selltiz, Wrightsman & Cook, 1976). To gain theoretical information, the researcher reviews theories, conceptual frameworks and models that lend support to a selected research problem. Theoretical and conceptual sources are included to demonstrate the current knowledge of the research problem and to provide direction in defining the research variables and selecting the study design. No matter what problem is selected for study, there are theoretical works that will provide a background for the problem; these might be the works of nurse theorists or theorists in related fields. The empirical information is generated from previous studies conducted on the selected research problem and from related studies. The studies reviewed include published studies in journals and books and unpublished studies, such as master's theses and doctoral dissertations.

The information included in the review of literature depends on the problem, purpose and type of study selected. A research problem and/or purpose that is timely (currently being investigated by a number of researchers) or one that has been investigated frequently in the past will have a more extensive base of empirical information than will a new or unique problem. For example, many studies have been conducted on nurses' stress levels, whereas little research (empirical information) is available on the impact of the computer on nursing activities such as making nursing diagnoses. Some problems have been the focus of more theorists than researchers, such as the problem of "What is health to a human being?"; therefore, the literature review for this problem is predominantly theoretical.

The type of study undertaken will influence the information available for review. In quantitative research, an exploratory study is considered the initial investigation of a research problem, so there are few studies available on the problem. The review of literature would include primarily theoretical information and relevant related studies. The information reviewed in a descriptive study is similar to that of the exploratory study, although there may be more studies available on the problem selected. In correlational, quasi-experimental and experimental studies, the information reviewed is both theoretical and empirical, with a more extensive number of studies available on the selected problem.

The information reviewed in qualitative research is predominantly theoretical, with some empirical information that is usually generated from related studies. Qualitative research is relatively new in nursing; therefore, the empirical information is frequently obtained from literature in related fields. However, even in other fields, prior studies on many qualitative research problems relevant to nursing are limited.

DEPTH AND BREADTH OF THE LITERATURE REVIEW

The depth of a literature review refers to the number and quality of the sources that are examined on a topic. The breadth is determined by the number of topics examined. If the literature review is too broad, the researcher will be examining many irrelevant sources. When the review lacks sufficient depth and/ or breadth, there is a great chance of omitting some important information. The depth and breadth of the literature review depends on the background of the researcher, the complexity of the research project and the amount of literature available on a selected research problem.

Researcher's Background

When a research topic is new to an investigator, an extensive review of the literature is needed to gain the in-depth knowledge necessary to conduct the study. Some researchers spend their lives studying a specific research topic or even one specific problem, and they are aware of the information available on a selected topic and/or problem. However, these researchers continue to review the literature to update their knowledge. An experienced researcher with a broad background regarding a research problem can be very helpful to beginning researchers by directing their review of relevant sources.

Complexity of the Research Project

The major research projects that involve numerous variables and complex methodologies require a more extensive review of literature than does a study that focuses on one or two variables and includes simple methodology. A doctoral dissertation is frequently a complex research project, and the academic professor usually requires an extensive review of the literature. This extensive literature review is carried out to provide the student with the necessary background to conduct the study and to provide the instructor with some understanding of the literature available on a selected problem.

Availability of Sources

A research topic or problem that has been studied frequently in the past or that has been the focus of many theorists' works will require reviewing numerous sources. Some individuals believe that "nothing" has been published on their research problem. No problem is so unique that no literature is available. In examining the sources that are available, the concern should be with quality rather than with quantity. The intent is to provide a background for the research problem and purpose. Many sources will be reviewed but only relevant sources will be included in the review of literature section of a written proposal or study report.

TIME FRAME FOR THE LITERATURE REVIEW

The time required to review the literature is influenced by the problem studied, sources available and goals of the researcher. The amount of information available is astronomical, and no researcher can read every piece of information that makes some reference or is somewhat related to a selected problem. If researchers attempt to read all the information related to their research topic, they will be well read but will probably never begin conducting their studies. Some people believe that they do not know enough about the area they are studying, so they continue to read; but this really becomes an excuse for not progressing with their research. If the review of literature continues for an extremely long time, researchers might forget what they read and will have to reread and update themselves on what has been recently written regarding their research problem. The opposite of this is the researcher who wants to move rapidly through the review of literature to get on with the "important" part of conducting the study. In both situations, the researcher has not been able to set a realistic time frame for conducting a review of relevant literature.

There is no set length of time for reviewing the literature, but there are guidelines for directing the review process. A problem with a very narrow focus will require less time for reviewing the literature. The difficulty in identifying, locating and obtaining sources and the number of sources to be located will influence the time involvement. Another factor that influences the time spent reviewing the literature is the researcher's goals. If a researcher plans to conduct a study within a set time frame, the review of literature will have to be limited in order to meet the deadline. For example, when a researcher receives funds from an outside agency, there is frequently a time limit set for completing the study. In a study to be conducted within 1 year, the review of literature will probably take a minimum of a month but should not exceed 3 months. The intensity of the effort will determine the time required to complete the review. Only through experience do researchers become knowledgeable about the time frame for the literature review. Beginning researchers frequently underestimate the time needed to review the literature and should plan twice the amount of time originally projected.

Process of Reviewing the Literature

The quality (accuracy and completeness) of the review of literature depends on the researcher's knowledge of the reviewing process and organization in conducting this process. The process of reviewing the literature involves (1) using the library, (2) identifying and locating sources, (3) reading sources and (4) recording notes. The literature review process is the same for conducting quantitative and qualitative research.

USING THE LIBRARY FACILITIES

Using the library is essential for conducting research and requires current knowledge of the available library resources. There are essentially three categories of libraries: (1) public, (2) academic and (3) special (Strauch & Brundage, 1980). The public libraries serve the needs of the communities where they are constructed, and these libraries frequently do not contain the sources needed for research.

Academic libraries are located within institutions of higher learning and contain numerous resources for researchers. However, if you are unable to find a source, most academic libraries have an interlibrary loan department. This department locates books and articles in other libraries and provides the book or copy of the article requested. There is a network of seven Regional Medical Libraries that contain relevant sources for health care providers and researchers. With this type of library network available, nursing researchers can obtain almost any source they need. These libraries can be contacted directly or through a local librarian. For easy reference, the name, location and phone numbers of these regional libraries are included in Table 6–3.

The special library contains a collection of materials on a specific topic or for a specialty area, such as nursing or medicine. Large hospitals, health care centers and health research centers frequently have special libraries that contain sources that are relevant to health care providers and researchers.

When using a library for the first time, a formal orientation to the facility is helpful. This orientation provides information on identifying and locating the resources and sources that are available in the library. A researcher should be

---

TABLE 6–3
Regional Libraries

Greater Northeastern Regional Medical Library Program
The New York Academy of Medicine
2 East 103rd Street
New York, New York 10029
Phone: 212/876–8763

Southeastern/Atlantic Regional Medical Library Services
University of Maryland
Health Sciences Library
111 South Greene Street
Baltimore, Maryland 21201
Phone: 301/528–7637

Region 3—Regional Medical Library
University of Illinois at Chicago
Library of the Health Sciences
Health Sciences Center
P.O. Box 7509
Chicago, Illinois 60680
Phone: 312/996–2464

Midcontinental Regional Medical Library Program
University of Nebraska
Medical Center Library
42nd Dewey Avenue
Omaha, Nebraska 68105
Phone: 402/559–4326

South Central Regional Medical Library Program
University of Texas
Health Science Center at Dallas
5323 Harry Hines Blvd.
Dallas, Texas 75235
Phone: 214/688–2085

Pacific Northwest Regional Health Sciences Library Service
Health Sciences Library
University of Washington
Seattle,Washington 98195
Phone: 206/543–8262

Pacific Southwest Regional Medical Library Service
UCLA Biomedical Library
Center for the Health Sciences
Los Angeles, California 90024
Phone: 213/825–1200

familiar with the following library resources: the library personnel, interlibrary loan department, circulation department, reference department, audiovisual department, computer search department and photocopy services. The circulation department provides information on the library's borrowing policies, and some libraries provide interlibrary loan cards that make it possible to check out books and materials from other libraries. The library personnel in the reference department are familiar with the library's collections and operations and can provide assistance in using the catalog, indexes, abstracts and other reference materials in the facility. The common sources of interest to nurse researchers in the library include dictionaries, encyclopedias, books, journals, monographs, conference proceedings, bibliographies, directories, government documents, audiovisuals, master's theses, doctoral dissertations, research in progress and publications of the American Nurses' Association and National League for Nursing (Binger & Jensen, 1980; Interagency Council on Library Resources for Nursing, 1978).

IDENTIFYING AND LOCATING SOURCES

Searching the literature involves identifying and locating sources. Conducting an organized search of the literature involves four steps: (1) clarifying a research topic; (2) searching the catalog, indexes, abstracts and bibliographies for relevant sources; (3) conducting a computer search; and (4) locating relevant sources.

Clarifying a Research Topic

A researcher selects a topic for study and then proceeds to clarify and narrow that topic by identifying synonymous terms and appropriate subheadings for the topic. Synonymous terms can be found in thesauruses, such as the International Nursing Index's Nursing Thesaurus. Subheadings can be located in the Cumulative Index to Nursing & Allied Health Literature's Nursing Subject Headings and the National Library of Medicine's Medical Subject Headings. Frequently, dictionaries and encyclopedias are helpful in identifying relevant synonymous terms and subheadings. The synonymous terms and subheadings for the research topic postoperative experience are outlined in Table 6–4.

TABLE 6–4
Clarifying a Research Topic

Research Topic	Synonymous Terms	Subheadings
Postoperative experience	Postsurgical experience Surgical recovery Postoperative recovery Postoperative care Surgical care	Postoperative pain Postoperative teaching Postoperative ambulation Postoperative attitude Postoperative complications Postoperative hospitalization

Searching the Catalog, Indexes, Abstracts and Bibliographies

The research topic, synonymous terms and subheadings identified are used to guide the search of the catalog listings, indexes, abstracts and bibliographies for relevant sources. The search for relevant sources starts with the most recent sources and works backward until the sources related to a specific topic have been exhausted. Frequently, research on a topic is cyclic, which means that one might find a number of sources related to a specific research topic in the 1980s, almost no sources in the 1960s and 1970s, and a number of sources in the 1950s. When starting a search of the literature, do not prematurely limit the number of years of publications to be examined.

Catalog □ The catalog identifies what is available in the library; these listings may be on cards (card catalog), in a book or on an on-line computer. The catalog listings are usually organized in one of two ways: split catalog or a dictionary catalog. The split catalog usually contains the authors and titles in one section and the subjects in another or separates all three categories. The dictionary catalog interfiles the authors, titles and subjects together in alphabetic order (Strauch & Brundage, 1980). The catalog listings include books, monographs, conference proceedings, audiovisuals, theses and dissertations. Those new to research sometimes overlook the value of books, because they believe the content is too old. However, books are excellent sources of theoretical information and frequently contain in-depth information on a specific topic. Most books also include extensive bibliographies that might direct the researcher to other relevant sources.

Monographs and conference proceedings usually contain current empirical and theoretical information, but the content included is frequently limited to an abstract or a brief paper. For more information, the researcher or theorist can be contacted. Audiovisuals might contain useful information for the review of literature for a study, or the methodology step might include the use of audiovisuals. Theses and dissertations frequently provide a complete review of relevant literature for a specific research problem and an extensive bibliography.

Indexes □ In an index, a number of sources are referenced under different divisions and subdivisions. An index provides assistance in identifying journal articles and other publications that contain a topic that is part of the index's headings. Many indexes are available that will aid researchers in identifying sources for a selected research topic. Some of the key indexes used by nursing researchers are *Cumulative Index to Nursing & Allied Health Literature, International Nursing Index, Nursing Studies Index, Index Medicus, Hospital Literature Index* and *Current Index to Journals in Education*. The content, availability and use of these indexes are described briefly.

Cumulative Index to Nursing & Allied Health Literature (CINAHL) (formerly, Cumulative Index to Nursing Literature). This index is usually consulted first by nurse researchers, because it is published frequently, references a large number of relevant nursing sources and is the original index for nursing literature. *CINAHL* was first published in 1956 and is currently published in five bimonthly issues and a cumulative annual bound volume. The index references approximately 300 nursing, allied health and health-related journals and includes more than 2600 pertinent articles from the biomedical journals indexed in *Index Medicus*, as well as relevant publications from popular journals. This index includes the following: an explanation of how to use the index, criteria for selection of materials, *CINAHL* services, regional medical libraries, new journals indexed, U.S. Government publications, subject section, author section and appendix (audiovisual materials, book reviews and pamphlets).

Indexes are organized in a similar manner and include two major sections: subject and author. Knowing how to use one index will assist you in using all indexes; the *Cumulative Index to Nursing & Allied Health Literature* is used as an example. The first step is to read the section on "How to use the index," which can save you time and aggravation. Once the topic, synonymous terms and subheadings have been identified, these terms are used to guide the search through the subject section of the index. The subject section includes headings and subheadings, and under these headings, several publications are listed, which are predominantly articles. These publications are listed under more than one subject heading and/or subheading for easy access by the researcher. For example, a qualitative nursing study of adolescents with chronic pain might be listed under the subject headings of pain, adolescent and nursing research and under the subheadings of chronic pain and qualitative nursing research. The indexing of each publication includes the following information: title, first author (if more than one), journal title abbreviated, date of issue, volume number, issue number, pages and bibliographic references. An example of an index listing is provided in Figure 6–1.

If you are familiar with the names of key researchers for a specific research topic or problem, you can search the author section of the index to identify recent publications by these researchers. The author section is organized alphabetically by the first author's name; no more than three authors are listed. The second and third authors' names appear as cross-references to the full citation under the first author's name. The author(s)' name(s) are followed by the same bibliographic content that is described above for the subject section.

Using an index is a fairly easy task, but many researchers are not organized or thorough in their review of indexes. The complete citation for a

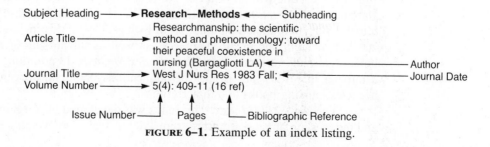

FIGURE 6–1. Example of an index listing.

Index Reviewed: Cumulative Index to Nursing and
                   Allied Health Literature

Subject Headings	Years				
	1987	1986	1985	1984	1983
Postoperative Experiences					
Postoperative Pain					
Postoperative Teaching					
Postoperative Attitude					
Postoperative Ambulation					
Postoperative Complications					

FIGURE 6–2. Record of indexes reviewed.

source must be recorded in order to locate that source; this complete citation includes spelling out the entire name of the journal, which is included in the index. The complete citation should be recorded on note cards or in a notebook, not on scraps of paper. A file of the citations should then be developed for easy access. As the sources are obtained, the researcher should systematically record them in the file to decrease duplication of citations and prevent omission of important sources. The researcher should also keep an organized list of the indexes that have been reviewed, including the names and years of the indexes and the subject headings and subheadings. Note cards such as the one outlined in Figure 6–2 might be kept on each index. There are several other indexes available to nurse researchers; five of these additional indexes are presented in order of importance and are described briefly.

International Nursing Index (INI). This index was first published in 1966 by the American Journal of Nursing Company in cooperation with the National Library of Medicine (NLM). *INI* is published quarterly, and the fourth issue is an annual cumulation of listings. This index includes more than 200 nursing journals in all languages, as well as all nursing articles in non-nursing journals currently indexed for *Index Medicus.* In addition, *INI* includes a nursing thesaurus and listings of publications of nursing organizations and agencies, nursing books and dissertations.

Nursing Studies Index. This index was developed by Virginia Henderson and indexes the nursing literature from 1900 to 1959. The *Nursing Studies Index* includes publications from several fields, including nursing, medicine, public health, education, sociology, psychology and anthropology. This index is a guide to reported studies, research in progress at the time that the index was published, research methods, historical materials in periodicals, books and pamphlets published in English.

Index Medicus (IM). *IM* is the oldest health-related index and was first published in 1879. This index cites articles from approximately 2600 domestic and foreign journals. *IM* is published monthly and has a bound annual volume of cumulated listings. This index also includes listings of books related to biomedicine and publications from selected proceedings.

Hospital Literature Index (HLI). This index is published quarterly, and the fourth issue is the annual cumulation of listings. *HLI* was first published in 1945 by the American Hospital Association in cooperation with the National Library of Medicine. This index includes citations from more than 600 English language journals and relevant listings from *Index Medicus*. The listings in *HLI* focus on the administration and delivery of health care in hospitals.

Current Index to Journals in Education (CIJE). This index includes articles from more than 700 journals, as well as other publications. *CIJE* was first published in 1969 and is currently published monthly, with semiannual cumulations. This index is published in cooperation with the Educational Resources Information Center (ERIC). The listings in this index represent several specialized fields: adult education, administration, teacher education, special education for handicapped as well as nursing education.

Abstracts □ Another essential resource used in identifying relevant publications is abstracts. Abstracts include the same bibliographic data as indexes, and, in addition, they include a brief, objective summary (abstract) of the content covered in the publication. Abstracts are helpful in determining whether sources are relevant to the research problem identified. Some of the important abstracts used in nursing research include *Nursing Abstracts, Psychological Abstracts, Sociological Abstracts, Dissertation Abstracts* and *Masters Abstracts*. The searching of abstracts is very similar to the searching of indexes and involves starting with the most recent publications and working backward.

Nursing Abstracts. This resource was first published in 1979 and is currently published bimonthly, with an annual cumulation. The abstracts included in this publication are generated from the articles in 53 nursing journals. *Nursing Abstracts* is indexed by subject, author and journal. An example of a listing from this resource is presented below.

Title: A Comparison of Rectal and Axillary
              Temperatures By Electronic Thermometer
              Measurement in Preschool Children
Author: Barrus, Dorothy H.
Publ: Pediatr Nurs, 9:6, Nov./Dec. 83, pp 424–425
Preschool children often perceive rectal temperature–taking as intrusive and frightening. The author recommends axillary temperature-taking as more acceptable. The accuracy of axillary temperatures was documented by this study comparing axillary and rectal temperatures as measured by an IVAC 821 electronic thermometer.

Psychological Abstracts (PA). This resource was first published in 1927 and is currently published monthly, with semiannual cumulative bound volumes. *PA* covers 950 journals and publications in psychology, education, sociology, psychiatry, physiology, anthropology and pharmacology. *PA* is organized into two sections: author and subject; and the abstracts included in *PA* are available through the computer search PSYCHOLOGICAL ABSTRACTS.

Sociological Abstracts (SA). This index covers more than 1000 publications in sociology and related topics in the behavioral and social sciences. *SA* was first published in 1952 and is currently published in April, June, August, October and December, with an annual cumulative index. *SA* is indexed by subject, author and source; and some of the subject headings include health, illness and health care systems that might be relevant to nurse researchers. These abstracts are also available through the computer search SOCIOLOGICAL ABSTRACTS.

Dissertation Abstracts International (DAI). This resource includes abstracts of the doctoral dissertations from more than 400 institutions in the United States and Canada. *DAI* was first published in 1938 and is currently published monthly, with an annual cumulative author index. The authors determine under which heading(s) and subheading(s) their dissertations will be listed. Some of the nurses indexed their dissertations under "Nursing" in the HEALTH SCIENCES section; however, many other nurse-authored dissertations are indexed under other headings. This requires searching a variety of headings to locate relevant dissertations.

Masters Abstracts (MA). This resource includes abstracts of master's theses from a variety of fields, including science, social sciences and humanities. This index was first published in 1962/1963 and is currently a quarterly publication with a cumulative subject and author index annually. Very few abstracts of the nursing master's theses have been included in *MA*. Therefore, many of the master's level studies are relatively unavailable to researchers and have essentially been lost to nursing's body of knowledge.

Bibliographies □ A bibliography is a list of publications for a specific topic, such as nursing research on nutrition, or a specialty area, such as cancer nursing. This list contains a variety of sources, including articles, books, conference proceedings, monographs, letters to the editor, editorials, government documents and dissertations. The length of a bibliography is limited by the specific time period it covers. Some excellent bibliographies have been compiled that are useful for nurse researchers. Taylor (1975) published a "Bibliography on nursing research, 1950–1974," including references compiled from the *Cumulative Index to Nursing & Allied Health Literature, International Nursing Index* and *Nursing Studies Index*. This bibliography includes 1004 sources and is organized into 22 broad classifications.

Sparks (1984), an educational specialist at the National Library of Medicine in Bethesda, Maryland, described the availability of a Specialized Bibliography Series at this facility. These bibliographies cover a broad scope of topics and were generated through manual and computerized searches. Some of the topics covered include nursing diagnosis, failure to thrive, acquired immune deficiency syndrome (AIDS), hospices, deinstitutionalization, non–insulin-dependent (type 2) diabetes, and food and drug interaction. These bibliographies are available on request from Literature Search Program, Reference Section, National Library of Medicine, 8600 Rockville Pike, Bethesda, Maryland 20209.

Two valuable bibliographies for historical research were developed by Thompson: *A Bibliography of Nursing Literature 1859–1960* and *A Bibliography of Nursing Literature 1961–1970* (Binger & Jensen, 1980, p. 226). The initial bibliography of the nursing literature contains nearly 4600 books and journal articles, and the second bibliography contains nearly 7000 publications. Some useful bibliographies are available through the American Nurses' Association and the National League for Nursing, as well as through specialty groups such as the Critical Care Nurses, Nurse Practitioners and Clinical Nurse Specialists.

Research articles, books, theses and dissertations also include valuable bibliographies. For example, Fernsler, Holcombe and Pulliam (1984) published an article entitled "A survey of cancer nursing research, January 1975–June 1982," which contained an extensive bibliography. The bibliography of this article was generated through a descriptive study and included 70 cancer nursing studies that were identified by examining 9 journals. Knowledge of the bibliographies that exist on selected research topics or problems can greatly reduce the time spent searching the literature.

Conducting a Computer Search

The previous section focused on how to search the literature manually. Another method of searching the literature is the computer search. The advancement of technology has made this type of search readily available and reasonably affordable. Computer searches have become invaluable with the rapid expansion of published materials in nursing. A computer search is used to generate a list of references with complete bibliographic information; for many of the references, abstracts are also available if requested. The sources in a computer are indexed by specific terms that are similar to the indexes described. The indexing system for each type of computer search is recorded in a manual that is kept by the computer search librarian.

The usefulness or quality of a computer search will depend on the expertise of the person requesting the search and the efficiency of the computer system that searches the literature. A computer search does not spontaneously generate a list of relevant sources; it takes a knowledgeable, persistent person to conduct a useful computer search.

Conducting a computer search requires a request that is specific, has a clear focus and limits the topic and the years searched. Frequently, a search is limited to the last 5 years if the research topic is current; however, a much more extensive search is needed for a topic studied frequently over many years. Examining indexes and abstracts briefly will help to further specify the focus of a search by clarifying the years and topics to be covered. A computer search can be further limited by restricting the language(s) of the sources and the countries where the sources are published. With this background, you are now ready for a discussion with library personnel about conducting a search. This presearch preparation will frequently save money (by narrowing the search conducted) and time (by decreasing the number of irrelevant references that would have to be examined).

The usefulness of a computer search is also limited by the efficiency of the automated literature search mechanisms that are available. Fox and Ventura (1984) studied the efficiency of automated literature techniques by investigating three questions: (1) Is the search reproducible? (2) Does it locate the most important articles pertaining to a particular topic? and (3) Can a system be developed that can efficiently determine which articles in a search should actually be obtained? They found that the National Library of Medicine literature search was reproducible but that the list of sources obtained was only a small proportion of the studies available. In addition, the studies cited did not include a high proportion of the critical or key studies for the selected research topic (nurse practitioners). The authors did determine that, based on a classification system of the sources' titles, a system could be developed to identify those articles in a computer search that are relevant and should be retrieved. This study reinforces the importance of conducting both manual and computerized searches to identify relevant sources for a selected research topic. In addition, computer searches require further sophistication if they are to identify the critical sources that should be reviewed by a researcher.

A computer search can be used to generate a list of references immediately on-line or can print these references off-line, which is less expensive. Generating a list of references on-line means that the computer system is up, or on, and the person conducting the search can interact with the system and request lists of certain references. These reference lists appear on the computer screen and can be visually reviewed for relevance. An off-line list of references can be obtained by identifying the references related to a research topic on-line and instructing the computer to print these references off-line to provide the researcher with a hard copy, or a printed copy, of the references (Grobe, 1984). Obtaining a list of references off-line usually takes longer but is also less expensive. The majority of the cost for a computer search is determined by the time that is spent on-line, with a minimal cost for printing the references off-line. Consult the librarian about the potential cost of the search, and identify the amount of money to be spent. The cost of a computer search should not be left to chance.

There are several databases (computerized lists of references) pertinent to nursing. Conducting a computer search involves identifying which databases to search to generate the references for a selected research problem. Some of the most useful databases for nurse researchers and what they have to offer are described here. There are also databases available for personal computers. For example, the Apple has some databases available for selected topics.

1. CINAHL (Nursing & Allied Health)—This database is the on-line version of the *Cumulative Index to Nursing and Allied Health Literature*. Over 300 English-language nursing publications and approxi-

mately 3200 biomedical journals are indexed. The materials are indexed using *CINAHL's* annually updated thesaurus, which is adapted from the U.S. National Library of Medicine's Medical Subject Headings (MeSH). No abstracts are included. The database was started in 1983 and is updated every 2 months with a current file of more than 24,600 sources.

2. MEDLINE (MEDical Literature Analysis and Retrieval System onLINE)—This database is supplied by the National Library of Medicine and covers the biomedical, dental and nursing literature. The information obtained includes author, title, abstract (since 1975 for some citations), language and indexing terms. The MEDLINE includes about 3000 journals, 200 of which are nursing journals, from all over the world. This database covers the time period from 1966 to the present and is updated every month.

3. CATLINE (CATalog onLINE)—This database contains about 500,000 references for books and serials catalogued at the National Library of Medicine. The information obtained includes author, title, source, language, indexing terms and other data such as edition, series, title and notes. CATLINE was originated in 1965 and is currently updated weekly.

4. AVLINE (AudioVisual catalog onLINE)—This database includes more than 11,000 audiovisual packages covering a broad range of health related subjects, such as nurse–patient relationships, nursing care, nursing audit and legal aspects of nursing. The supplier of AVLINE is the National Library of Medicine; it covers the last 5 years and is updated every month. The information obtained includes title, media type, authorship, physical description, indexing terms, run time, audience level, review rating and date, reviewer, learning method, abstract, continuing education credit note, price and source for purchase or loan (Binger & Jensen, 1980).

5. HEALTH (Health Planning and Administration)—This database contains more than 200,000 references and is supplied by the National Library of Medicine and the American Hospital Association. The subjects covered include management, health planning, organization, financing, manpower, patient education, accreditation and other related subjects (Sparks, 1984). The database covers the time period from 1975 to the present and is updated every month. The information obtained includes author, title, abstract, language and indexing terms.

6. BIOETHICSLINE—This database covers citations that deal with ethical questions arising in health care or biomedical research, such as human experimentation, patients' rights, death and dying and resources allocation. The supplier of BIOETHICSLINE is the National Library of Medicine and the Kennedy Institute of Ethics. This database covers the time period from 1973 to the present and is updated three times a year. The information obtained is the author, title, source, indexing terms, language and type of publication.

7. CANCERLIT—This database contains more than 300,000 references from over 3000 journals, books, conference proceedings, theses and reports. The supplier of CANCERLIT is the National Library of Medicine and the Cancer Institute. This database covers all aspects of cancer from 1963 to the present and is updated monthly. The information obtained is author, author's affiliation, title, abstract, language, type of publication and indexing terms.

LOCATING SOURCES

After identifying sources through a manual and/or computerized search of the literature, the journals, books and other publications containing these sources must be located. The process of locating sources involves the following steps: (1) organizing the list of identified sources, (2) searching the library for those sources, (3) systematically recording the sources located and not located and (4) determining additional ways to locate the sources not found.

The list of identified sources can be organized in several ways to facilitate locating them within the library. Journal sources might be efficiently organized by journal name and year, author and/or title (subject). The organization by journal and year can greatly reduce the time spent wandering from journal to journal in the library. The researcher can methodically locate all relevant sources for a research problem that are published within a specific journal and then proceed to another journal. Sources included in the library catalog (such as books, monographs, organizational publications and conference proceedings) can be organized by author and/or subject. This organization will not only make it easier to find these sources in the library but will also assist the researcher in eliminating any duplicated references.

Searching the library for the identified sources is facilitated by a discussion with library personnel to determine the classification system; the availability of resources and publications; and the location of journals, books, dictionaries, indexes and abstracts in the library. In locating books, the library call number should be recorded in case you need to find the source a second time. Persistence is required to find sources in the library. The researcher should not mark a source off the list simply because it was not easily located on the first search.

When a journal article is located, the article should be copied. Although some journals record the complete bibliographic reference at the bottom or top of the first two pages of an article, some do not. If the information is not recorded on the article, a complete bibliographic reference should be recorded on the article at the time that it is copied. If the article is obtained from interlibrary loan, the complete bibliographic citation is stapled to the article and should be kept. Computerized lists of sources usually contain complete citations for sources and should be filed for future use.

The bibliographic information on a source should be recorded in a systematic manner, according to the writing style format that will be used in writing the review of literature section and in developing the bibliography. Many journals and academic institutions use the American Psychological

Association (APA) (1983) writing style format. An example of the APA format for citing a source in the bibliography is presented below.

Rudy, E. B., & Estok, P. J. (1983). Intensity of jogging: Its relationship to selected physical and psychological variables in women. *Western Journal of Nursing Research*, 5(4), 325–336.

The systematic recording of references is demanding but can save time that might be lost in searching for misplaced references. Almost every researcher has lost or misplaced important references and spent hours relocating these sources. Or they might have inaccurately documented a source in a paper or inaccurately referenced a source in the bibliography. Anyone reviewing the literature has at some time been frustrated by inaccurate references in publications.

The process of locating sources also requires a systematic method of recording the researcher's activities in attempting to locate sources. The recording method should identify the sources that were located in the available library(ies), the sources that are available in the library but were not found, and those sources that are unavailable. If certain sources cannot be located in the local library facilities, the researcher should attempt to locate them through the interlibrary loan department. Locating a source might also require contacting the author when a journal article is incomplete or when requesting reprints of a study, instrument or other relevant information.

The bibliographies of the journal articles are an important source for locating additional references. The citations in the bibliographies should be compared with the sources already identified to detect additional references. The review of the literature is an additive process, in which identifying and locating sources leads to further identification and location of sources until the relevant sources related to a selected problem or topic are exhausted.

READING SOURCES

Reading sources in a systematic way will promote comprehension of the source's content. This comprehension is essential for effective use of the content in developing the research proposal. Four levels of reading are necessary for reviewing relevant literature in research: skimming, comprehending, analyzing and synthesizing.

Skimming Sources

Skimming is a quick review of a source to gain a broad overview of the content. The reader frequently reads the title, author's name and an abstract or introduction for the source. Then the major headings are read and sometimes one or two sentences under each heading. Lastly, the conclusion or summary is reviewed. Skimming enables the reader to make a preliminary judgment about the value of a source and to determine whether it is a primary or secondary source. At this point, the reader does a preliminary sort of the sources into specific content areas. The reader also initially identifies the value of sources and discards the sources considered not valuable.

Primary and Secondary Sources □ A *primary source* is written by the person who originated or is responsible for generating the ideas published. In research publications, a primary source is written by the person or persons who conducted the research. In theoretical publications, a primary source is written by the theorist who developed the theory or conceptual content. A *secondary source* summarizes and/or quotes content from primary sources. Thus, authors of secondary sources present the works of other researchers or theorists, which are paraphrased in their own words. The problem with secondary sources is that the author has interpreted the works of someone else, and this interpretation is influenced by that author's perception and bias. The sources included in a review of literature for research should be predominantly primary. Secondary sources should be used only if primary sources cannot be located or if the secondary source provides creative ideas and/or a unique organization of information not found in a primary source.

Comprehending Sources

Comprehending a source requires that the entire source be read carefully. The reader focuses on understanding major concepts and the logical flow of ideas within a source. The content that is considered significant is highlighted and sometimes ideas are recorded in the margins. The notes on the source might indicate where the information will be useful in the research process or possible categories for organizing the content of a source. These notes might also include creative ideas about content that develop while one is reading. At this point, the reader begins identifying relevant categories for sorting and organizing sources. These categories will ultimately serve as a guide for writing the review of literature section, and some may even be major headings in this section.

Analyzing Sources

During analysis of a source, the reader determines its value for a particular study. The content of the source is broken into parts, and the parts are examined in depth. An in-depth examination of a source involves determining the accuracy, completeness, uniqueness of information, organization and relevance of each part of the source for the study to be conducted. At this point, the reader is able to clearly identify relevant content in sources and to sort these sources into a sophisticated system of categories. Conducting an analysis of sources to be used in a research proposal requires that the reader have some knowledge of the subject to be critiqued, some knowledge of the research process and the ability to exercise judgment in evaluation (Fleming & Hayter, 1974). Additional information on the analysis of research literature is presented in Chapter 20.

Synthesis of Source Content

Through synthesis, the reader is able to cluster and interrelate ideas from several sources to form a new gestalt. Synthesis involves clarifying the meaning obtained from the source as a whole. This meaning should then be paraphrased. Paraphrasing involves expressing clearly and concisely the ideas of an author in your own words. The meaning of these sources must then be connected to the proposed study. Lastly, the meanings obtained from all sources are combined, or "chunked," to determine the current knowledge of a proposed research problem. Synthesis is the basis for writing the review of literature section of a proposal.

MECHANICS OF RECORDING NOTES

There are a variety of ways researchers can record and later reorganize notes on sources. It is better to record notes on 3" × 5" or 5" × 8" cards than on sheets of notebook paper, which are hard to organize and easily misplaced. Computers are also very handy for easy storage, retrieval and rearrangement of notes. Some researchers record notes on the copies of articles.

There are specific notes that should be recorded concerning theoretical and empirical literature. These notes are based on comprehension, analysis and synthesis of source content. The notes recorded about theoretical sources should include relevant concepts, definitions of those concepts and relationships among the concepts. The researcher should also generate notes connecting the information from sources to the proposed study.

The notes recorded on the empirical literature should include relevant information about the researcher (Is this a key researcher of a selected problem and what other studies has this researcher conducted?), research problem, study purpose, framework, major research variables, study design, implementation of the study, study findings and application of this information to the proposed study. You may wish to record quotations (including page numbers) that might be used in the review of literature section. The decision to paraphrase these quotes can then be made later. While collecting notes on a variety of sources, systematically organize these notes according to an identified category system. The note cards developed should be labeled in some way so that the researcher can refer back to the original source. One quick way to do this is to cite the author and the year on each note card. The complete, organized file of notes provides the basis for writing the review of literature.

Writing the Review of Literature

If the literature review is conducted in a thorough and organized way, it will greatly facilitate the writing of the review of literature section. Writing the review of literature section involves the selection of sources, organization of information and the mechanics of writing the review.

SELECTION OF RELEVANT SOURCES

The sources are selected for inclusion in the review of literature section based on their relationship to the problem statement and purpose of the proposed study. If a source focuses on the selected research topic but has no implications for developing the steps in a particular study, it should not be included. The literature included should build a case for the proposed study.

ORGANIZATION OF SOURCES

The relevant sources (theoretical and empirical) identified for inclusion in the research proposal are organized according to where they will be presented in the research process. The sources to be included in the review of literature section of the proposal are further organized to reflect the current knowledge of the research problem. The researcher will designate which sources support the significance of the research problem and what source will provide the framework for the study. Other relevant sources become the basis for defining the research variables and for identifying assumptions and limitations. Sources will direct the development of the research design, guide implementation of the study and influence interpretation of the findings. At this point, many researchers are beginning to get a complete picture of their study and are excited about the study's potential. In addition, they are probably more confident about their knowledge of the research problem and their ability to make the study a reality.

The review of literature in published studies has been organized in different ways. The literature review may be organized into two sections: empirical and theoretical. In other studies, the literature review is organized by concepts and subconcepts that are relevant to the problem investigated. The theoretical and empirical literature is then organized under the appropriate concepts.

Organization of Empirical and Theoretical Literature

When a quantitative approach is being used and previous research has been conducted on the research problem, the researcher should closely examine the techniques and quality of past studies. To reflect this examination, the following guidelines are suggested for the literature review section.

1. Critique of Studies. Each study should be critiqued using the guidelines suggested in Chapter 20. Discussion should not be limited to the findings but should examine the validity of the findings. In many cases, the studies can be presented in an historical fashion, demonstrating the progressive development of knowledge related to a specific problem. Sources can also be organized to present the least relevant source first and move to the most relevant sources to build a case for the problem studied.

2. Summary of Critiques. The researcher should summarize previous approaches to studying the research problem, evaluate their effectiveness and identify needed improvements. Such elements as measurement, design and analysis should be addressed. A summary of findings from previous work in the area can be clustered to provide a picture of the present state of knowledge. Gaps in this knowledge should be identified.

3. Theoretical Literature. Theoretical ideas related to the problem are explored. The conceptual definitions of variables are presented, and relationships between the concepts are proposed. Operational definitions of the variables should emerge from the conceptual definitions. The theoretical section of the review of literature provides a basis for the development of the theoretical framework. The theoretical framework should be presented separately from the literature review. Development of the framework is discussed in Chapter 7.

4. Related Clinical Literature. For some research problems, clinical literature is significant for the development of the study and should be examined. This section often validates the problem and purpose of the study.

The review of literature for qualitative studies and exploratory and descriptive quantitative studies might be organized in the manner previously described. However, some researchers choose to organize the sources under major concepts. The empirical and theoretical literature is then presented under each major concept. The empirical literature presented should include a critique of the previous studies and summarize study methodology as well as findings. The theoretical literature should include the works (concepts and relationships among concepts) of relevant theorists. The theoretical literature provides the basis for the development of the study framework.

MECHANICS OF WRITING THE REVIEW OF LITERATURE

Writing the review of literature requires the development of a detailed outline that will be used as a guide in the writing. The review of literature section will begin with an introduction, will include a presentation of empirical and theoretical sources and will provide a summary of relevant ideas. The introduction describes the organization and purpose of the review of literature. Conciseness is essential in providing a clear direction to the reader.

In writing the main section of the literature review, the researcher must present empirical and theoretical content from sources in a concise and accurate manner. The content from these sources should be paraphrased or summarized in the researcher's own words whenever possible. If a direct quote is used, it should be kept short to promote the flow of the content. Long quotes are often unnecessary and may interfere with the reader's train of thought. Long quotes can also disturb the flow of the content, because the author quoted will always have a different writing style than the researcher writing the review.

The researcher should discuss in depth those studies that are most relevant in guiding the investigation. Studies with similar methodology and/or findings should be discussed in relation to each other to show similarities and differences and to prevent repetition. Some beginning researchers tend to randomly list sources, with a paragraph about each source. This strategy indicates no analysis and synthesis of the meaning obtained from various sources. The findings from the studies should logically build on each other so that the reader can see how the body of knowledge in a particular research area developed.

There are ethical issues to consider in the presentation of sources in the review of literature (Gunter, 1981). The content from sources should be honestly presented, not distorted to support the selected problem. A researcher will frequently read studies and wish that the authors had studied a slightly different problem or that the study had been designed or conducted differently. The researcher must recognize that these are his or her opinions and be objective in the presentation of information from each source. The defects of a study should be included, but it is not necessary to be highly critical of another researcher's work. The criticisms should only focus on the content that is in some way relevant to the proposed study. Criticisms should be stated as possible or plausible explanations, so that they are more neutral and scholarly than negative and blaming. Researchers must accurately document another author's work to differentiate it from their own. The bibliography should include only those sources that have been read and used to develop the study.

The final step in writing the review of literature is the summary. The summary should be concise and not repetitive. The summary should include discussion of the quality of the literature reviewed, should identify knowledge gaps that currently exist and should indicate the directions for further research.

Example of the Review of Literature

A review of literature section from a published study follows in order to reinforce the points that were addressed in this chapter. The research article is on the compliance of cancer patients to therapy (Itano, Tanabe, Lum, Lamkin, Rizzo, Wieland & Sato, 1983); only selected content from this review of literature is presented to demonstrate the introduction, organization of empirical and theoretical information under concepts and the summary.

INTRODUCTION

Health professionals have recognized for some time that to assist patients in health promotion they must be skilled in helping patients adhere to the regimes for prevention or treatment of disease. Numerous variables related to compliance have been studied... The following literature review is divided into sections on specific variables related to compliance: locus of control, self-esteem, anxiety, patient's understanding of illness, severity of symptoms, and patient's perception of nurses' care and concern. (pp. 5–6)

LOCUS OF CONTROL

The concept of health locus of control has its origin in social learning theory (Rotter, 1966). Rotter's theory is that individuals, through a learning process, come to expect that certain outcomes are a result of either their actions or forces external to them. The Health Locus of Control Scale (HLC) was constructed...

Several studies have used these scales to show that people who believe that their health outcome is contingent upon their behavior (internals) are more likely to engage in behaviors that facilitate physical well-being than are people who believe their health is primarily contingent upon luck or chance (externals). (p. 6)

SELF-ESTEEM

Lum *et al.* (1978) defined self-esteem as the affirmation or acceptance of the self despite weakness or deficiencies and the affirmation of self because of worth or strength. In their study, the more complete the content or information given the patient about his or her treatment and care regimen, and the better the quality of the explanation, the higher the patient's self-esteem... (p. 7)

ANXIETY

Anxiety is an unpleasant and uncanny experience perceived as a result of an environmental change and experienced as a threat to one's security (Lucente & Fleck, 1972). Lum *et al.* (1978) show that the lower the patient's anxiety, the greater was the importance of maintaining contact with others and the less the patient viewed himself as a burden to others... (p. 7)

PATIENT'S UNDERSTANDING OF ILLNESS

Studies conducted about the effect of the patients' knowledge and understanding of their disease and therapeutic regime on their compliance to treatment were conflicting (Sackett & Haynes, 1976). Studies indicated either no association or a positive relationship... (p. 7)

SEVERITY OF SYMPTOMS

Studies on symptoms and their effects on compliance also showed variable results (Sackett & Haynes, 1976). Physical symptoms probably exert an elevating or realistic effect on perceived severity,... (p. 8)

PATIENT'S PERCEPTION OF NURSES' CARE AND CONCERN

Sackett and Haynes (1976) found a positive association between degree of supervision and compliance. Hospitalized patients were more compliant than outpatients. Compliance improved when the frequency of outpatient visits was increased... (p. 8)

SUMMARY

Despite the voluminous literature on compliance, the investigators found no studies specific to compliance among cancer patients except for studies on reasons for delay in seeking care (Robbins, 1950; Gold, 1964). A search of the literature revealed no information on compliance rates for cancer patients or any possible determinants of compliance among cancer patients. (p. 8)*

SUMMARY

The review of literature enables the researcher to generate an image of what is known about a particular situation and the knowledge gaps that exist in the situation. The literature review focuses on relevant literature, which includes those sources that are pertinent or highly important in providing the in-depth knowledge needed to study a selected problem. The review of relevant literature is a three-step process: (1) finding a variety of relevant sources, (2) critiquing those sources for significant information and (3) generating a written report of the knowledge gained. The primary purpose for reviewing the literature is to gain a broad background or understanding of the information that is available related to the research topic of interest. This background enables the researcher to build upon the works of others.

The scope of the literature review should be broad enough for the researcher to be knowledgeable of the research topic and narrow enough to include predominantly relevant sources. The researcher should evaluate (1) the different types of information available, (2) the depth and breadth of the review desired and (3) the time frame for conducting the review.

The process of reviewing the literature involves (1) using the library, (2) identifying and locating sources, (3) reading sources and (4) recording notes. Sources can be identified by computer searches and manual searches of the catalog, indexes, abstracts and bibliographies. The process of locating sources involves organizing a list of identified sources, searching the library for those sources and systematically recording the sources located. There are four levels of reading necessary for reviewing the literature in research: skimming, comprehending, analyzing and synthesizing. In reading the empirical and theoretical literature, the researcher should systematically record notes on the sources.

Writing the review of literature involves the selection of sources, the organization of information and the incorporation of the mechanics of writing a review. An example of a review of literature selection from a published study has been provided to demonstrate the development of a literature review.

REFERENCES

Aamodt, A. M. (1982). Examining ethnography for nurse researchers. *Western Journal of Nursing Research*, 4(2), 209–221.
Abdellah, F. G. & Levine, E. (1979). *Better patient care through nursing research* (2nd ed.). New York: Macmillan Publishing Co., Inc.

---

*Itano et al.: Compliance of Cancer Patients to Therapy. Western Journal of Nursing Research, 5(1):5,6,7,8, Winter 1983. Copyright 1983 by Western Journal of Nursing Research. Reprinted by permission of Sage Publications, Inc.

American Psychological Association. (1983). *Publication manual of the American Psychological Association* (3rd ed.). Washington, D. C.: American Psychological Association.

Batey, M. V. (1977). Conceptualization: knowledge and logic guiding empirical research. *Nursing Research*, 26(5), 324–329.

Binger, J. L. & Jensen, L. M. (1980). *Lippincott's guide to nursing literature: a handbook for students, writers, and researchers*. Philadelphia: J. B. Lippincott Company.

Christy, T. E. (1975). The methodology of historical research: a brief introduction. *Nursing Research*, 24(3), 189–192.

Fernsler, J., Holcombe, J. & Pulliam, L. (1984). A survey of cancer nursing research: January 1975–June 1982. *Oncology Nursing Forum*, 11(4), 46–52.

Fleming, J. W. & Hayter, J. (1974). Reading research reports critically. *Nursing Outlook*, 22(3), 172–175.

Fox, R. N. & Ventura, M. R. (1984). Efficiency of automated literature search mechanisms. *Nursing Research*, 33(3), 174–177.

Glasser, B. G. & Strauss, A. L. (1966). The purpose and credibility of qualitative research. *Nursing Research*, 15(1), 56–61.

Grobe, S. J. (1984). *Computer primer & resource guide for nurses*. Philadelphia: J. B. Lippincott Company.

Gunter, L. (1981). Literature review. In S. D. Krampitz & N. Pavlovich (Eds.), *Readings for nursing research* (pp. 11-16). St. Louis: The C. V. Mosby Company.

Interagency Council on Library Resources for Nursing. (1978). Reference sources for nursing. *Nursing Outlook*, 26(5), 325–329.

Itano, J., Tanabe, P., Lum. J. L. J., Lamkin, L., Rizzo, E., Wieland, M. & Sato, P. (1983). Compliance of cancer patients to therapy. *Western Journal of Nursing Research*, 5(1), 5–16.

Kaplan, A. (1964). *The conduct of inquiry: methodology for behavioral science*. New York: Chandler Publishing Company.

Kubler-Ross, E. (1969). *On death and dying*. New York: Macmillan Publishing Company.

Newton, M. E. (1965). The case for historical research. *Nursing Research*, 14(1), 20–26.

Oiler, C. (1982). The phenomenological approach in nursing research. *Nursing Research*, 31(3), 178–181.

Selltiz, C., Wrightsman, L. S. & Cook, S. W. (1976). *Research methods in social relations* (3rd ed.). New York: Holt, Rinehart and Winston.

Sparks, S. M. (1984). Research notes—the national library of medicine's bibliographic databases: tools for nursing research. *Image*, 16(1), 24–27.

Stern, P. N. (1980). Grounded theory methodology: its uses and processes. *Image*, 12(1), 20–23.

Strauch, K. P. & Brundage, D. J. (1980). *Guide to library resources for nursing*. Norwalk, Connecticut: Appleton-Century-Crofts.

Taylor, S. D. (1975). Bibliography on nursing research, 1950–1974. *Nursing Research*, 24(3), 207–225.

7

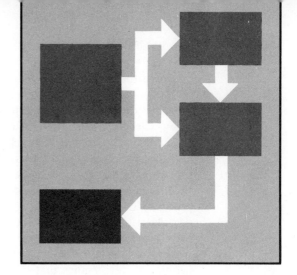

Developing a Frame of Reference

A *frame of reference*, or *framework*, for a particular study is the abstract, logical structure (frame) that enables the researcher to link the findings (reference) to nursing's body of knowledge. A frame of reference can be derived from an existing theory (theoretical framework) or developed by the researcher through identifying and defining the concepts of interest and proposing relationships among them (conceptual framework). The purpose of a framework is to organize the development of a study and provide a context for interpretation of the findings. In interpreting the findings, a framework provides a mechanism for abstractly generalizing the findings beyond the situation of a specific study. The findings are abstractly generalized as they are used to clarify the meaning of concepts and explain relationships among concepts within the study frame of reference. As this process adds theoretical information to the body of knowledge, the increased abstract meaning influences nursing practice in a variety of settings. Without a framework, the findings are limited to a concrete situation (the sample of the study) and remain concrete facts. Although these facts may be of some use, science and a body of knowledge cannot be made from scattered pieces of facts from various studies. The facts must be organized, explained and given meaning through a framework. Therefore, a frame of reference is important beyond the study itself, because it allows the development of new theory or improvement of existing theory.

155

In the past, nurse researchers either decided a frame of reference was unnecessary or were awed by its importance. At present, there is an increasing emphasis on the value of an integrated frame of reference within each nursing study. Clearly, a framework is essential to both the conduct and utilization of research. Consumers of research need to comprehend and critique the frames of reference used in studies to determine appropriate applications of study findings. Beginning researchers must learn how to develop frames of reference for specific studies from existing theories or from concepts of interest to nursing practice. To provide this background, this chapter explains relevant terminology, describes the development of a frame of reference and identifies strategies for integrating a frame of reference within a study. Examples of theorists' works that are useful in the development of frames of reference are provided in this chapter; studies that have incorporated these theorists' works are also included.

Understanding Frames of Reference

Both quantitative and qualitative research require the use of a frame of reference. The primary purpose of quantitative research is to test theory, and the theory to be tested should be explicitly stated in the study framework. Even if a published study has not expressed a framework, it is implicitly present and influences the development of the study. In qualitative research, the researcher initially avoids a specific theoretical orientation in order to maintain an open context and develops the study with a broad overriding framework of ideas. For example, the concept of culture and the factors that constitute a culture are the framework of ethnographic research. Qualitative studies develop a more specific framework during the data collection and analysis process. In the following section, the two types of frames of reference, the elements of a frame of reference, the problems related to frames of reference and the process of constructing a frame of reference are described.

TYPES OF FRAMES OF REFERENCE

There are two types of frames of reference: conceptual and theoretical. The two types have not been clearly delineated in the literature, and the two terms are sometimes used interchangeably. A *conceptual framework* for research is an organization or matrix of concepts that provides a focus for inquiry (Newman, 1979). In research, a conceptual framework is often loosely constructed, has not been presented in the literature previously and/or has not been tested. Its concepts may have been taken from various sources, and the relationships might have been proposed by the researcher for a study. A *theoretical framework* is a general, abstract explanation of the interrelationships of the concepts in a theory to be investigated (Silva, 1981). A theoretical framework emerges from one theory that has previously been published and has conceptually defined concepts and propositions that can be tested. Usually, only a portion of a theory is used as the theoretical framework for a study.

ELEMENTS OF A FRAME OF REFERENCE

A frame of reference is an abstract conceptualization that places the study within a context of meaning. This context of meaning forms a gestalt, which is a way of viewing a phenomenon. The framework or way of viewing a phenomenon must be clearly developed within a study. The development of a frame of reference involves identification of its basic elements: concepts and relationships among the concepts.

Concepts

A *concept* is a word or idea to which abstract meaning is attached. Concepts can be considered at several different levels of abstractness. The most abstract form of a concept is a broad, general idea that is likely to include most meanings for the concept. Frames of reference for studies usually contain abstract forms of concepts. The concepts that constitute a frame of reference may be selected from one theorist's work, several theorists' works, previous research or personal experience.

The concepts within a frame of reference must be refined or conceptually defined for use in a study. A *conceptual definition* differs from the denotative or dictionary definition of a word. A conceptual definition clarifies the personal knowledge (connotative) meaning of the word. These meanings are often difficult to express; the meaning is "known" but not easily put into words. Conceptual definitions can be generated through concept analysis or obtained from theorists' works.

A *concept analysis* is a strategy that involves examining the attributes or characteristics of a concept (Walker & Avant, 1983). This process involves a specialized search of the literature, introspection and reasoning to identify the various meanings attached to a concept. These meanings are organized into a conceptual definition. The steps of this process are explained by Walker and Avant (1983) in their book entitled *Strategies for theory construction in nursing*.

A number of concept analyses have been published in the nursing literature. For example, Gaut (1983) analyzed the concept of "caring" and stated:

> Caring, whether used in common word usage or scholarly literature, seems to involve at least three senses: (1) disposition or feeling within the carer, (2) the doing of certain activities regarded as caring activities, or (3) a combination of both attitude and action in which the caring about the other (as a value, or responsibility, or commitment) disposes the person to care for another through the doing of certain activities. (p. 316)

This description of caring could be used in the development of a conceptual definition for a theory or for research. The idea of conceptual definitions is further discussed in Chapter 8.

Relationships Among Concepts

All the concepts used within a study must be linked together (related). In a frame of reference, possible relationships, the strength of these relationships and/or the directions (positive or negative) of these relationships are proposed. When the type of relationship is made specific, it is referred to as a *proposition*. Examples of propositions are given below, using A and B to indicate the concepts. Further explanation of relationships and propositions is available in Newman (1979).

1. A and B occur simultaneously and vary in intensity together. For example, A and B both increase, but the increase of one does not lead to or cause the increase in the other.

2. If A occurs, B probably will occur.

$$A \xrightarrow{\ ?\ } B$$

3. An increase in A leads to an increase in B. A decrease in A leads to a decrease in B. On a diagram, these relationships are often indicated by a + symbol.

$$\uparrow A \xrightarrow{\ +\ } \uparrow B \qquad \downarrow A \xrightarrow{\ +\ } \downarrow B$$

4. An increase in A leads to a decrease in B. A decrease in A leads to an increase in B. On a diagram, these relationships are often indicated by a − symbol.

$$\uparrow A \xrightarrow{\ -\ } \downarrow B \qquad \downarrow A \xrightarrow{\ -\ } \uparrow B$$

5. A causes B.

$$A \longrightarrow B$$

Relationships in a framework are often clarified by using a model. A *model* is a pictorial demonstration, using illustrations or mathematical formulas, that helps clarify the relationships being tested. Things that can be seen visually often help one to pull together ideas that are more difficult to understand from written explanations. Burckhardt (1985) developed a model of the framework used in studying the impact of arthritis on quality of life (Fig. 7–1). This hypothetical causal model clearly demonstrates what relationships exist and the direction of these relationships.

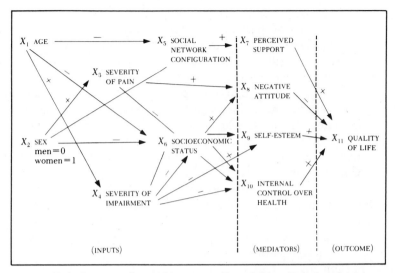

FIGURE 7–1. Impact of arthritis on quality of life. (Reprinted with permission from Burckhardt, C. S.: The impact of arthritis on quality of life. Nursing Research, *34*(1):12, Jan/Feb 1985; Copyright 1985 American Journal of Nursing Company.)

CONSTRUCTING A FRAME OF REFERENCE

Nursing studies often emerge from identified nursing problems, and the idea for a study comes from a search for ways to solve that problem. The nurse's knowledge of the problem originates from both clinical practice and previous nursing education. During nursing education, theoretical ideas from many disciplines are taught, including theories from medicine, biology, chemistry, sociology, psychology and physics, as well as from nursing. The initial development of the frame of reference for a study can emerge from these sources of knowledge.

There are two limitations in using the knowledge from basic nursing education for developing frameworks. First, frequently the information is not presented as theories; therefore, the student may make no connection between the knowledge obtained and theory. The student may consider the theoretical statements from classroom lectures to be "facts." Second, only fragments of the theory may be presented, leaving the student unaware of the logic underlying the theory or the relationships proposed by the theory. Portions of theories taught in classrooms are intermingled with clinical practice strategies. Therefore, most basic nursing students cannot differentiate whether the source of their personal knowledge came from theory, clinical experience or research. This difficulty in identifying theoretical knowledge seriously limits efforts to generate frames of reference.

Constructing a frame of reference involves gaining increased insight into the meanings that have been incorporated into personal knowledge. Often, the researcher begins formulating the framework by identifying fragmented pieces of personal knowledge incorporated from nursing education and practice and seeking ways to identify the theory within them. It is then necessary to obtain a more complete understanding of the identified theories. This is usually accomplished as part of the literature review. When theories from related disciplines have been selected, it may then be necessary to translate them into a form that will enable their incorporation into a nursing framework. To construct a theoretical framework, the concepts of interest in the theory are identified and defined according to the theorist's work. One or more propositions from the theory that explain the relationships among the selected concepts are stated. Hypotheses are generated from the propositions.

Often, phenomena of concern in nursing have not been expressed theoretically. Sometimes the phenomenon has not even been previously isolated or named. In this case, to formulate a conceptual framework, the researcher must describe the phenomenon, name it, analyze the concepts within the idea, and, from experience, identify expected relationships. In these situations, the literature search will focus on clinical practice and empirical findings of research. Conceptual examination of nursing phenomena, now beginning to appear in the literature, will be helpful in constructing frames of reference for these phenomena.

PROBLEMS RELATED TO THE FRAME OF REFERENCE

If the researcher fails to rigorously construct a frame of reference, problems with the framework emerge. The problems related to the frame of reference are actually problems related to the researcher and are usually indicative of insufficient research experience and/or education. The most commonly occurring problems are inappropriate framework, disconnected framework, multiple frameworks and unidentified framework.

Inappropriate Framework

An inappropriate framework is one that does not "fit" the study. There may be a logic gap between the framework and the study, or the framework may be only tangentially connected to the study. An inappropriate framework can occur for various reasons. Sometimes researchers identify a research problem and then try to make a theory fit the problem. Their intent is to fulfill the requirement of having a framework without going through the rigor of adequately developing one. Additionally, they may not have developed the skills of assessing the logical flow between the framework and the rest of the study. Lastly, some researchers have limited knowledge of available theories and tend to select from those they are familiar with, whether they fit or not. These problems are apparent in a critique of the published study. An inappropriate framework is useless in interpreting the findings of the study.

Disconnected Framework

A disconnected framework exists when the researcher has selected and/or developed an appropriate framework but has failed to connect it to the rest of the study. This usually happens when researchers do not know what to do with the framework once it is developed, possibly because it was suggested to them by another researcher or an instructor. This type of framework is essentially useless because it has no meaning within the study.

Multiple Frameworks

In some studies, multiple frameworks or multiple theories are presented. This has the same effect as a disconnected framework, because the researcher cannot logically link multiple theories throughout the components of a study. Researchers might include multiple frameworks in their studies to demonstrate their extensive knowledge of relevant theories (or more likely because they do not know the true purpose of a framework). The framework is again useless and adds no meaning to the study. If concepts from various theories are used or if a broad overriding nursing framework is joined with a more specific non-nursing theory, these theoretical ideas must all be logically connected and the relationships clearly indicated in a model.

Unidentified Framework

Some researchers believe that the framework is not important or that no framework fits the area of their study; thus, their frameworks are unidentified. In these studies, the frameworks exist implicitly—the researchers have failed to identify them. These researchers tend to be concrete thinkers who have little use for abstract or theoretical thinking. They derive satisfaction from the precise, detailed methods of actually conducting the research. Although the conduct of the research might be precise, the findings lack meaning and cannot easily be added to nursing's body of knowledge without a framework. All research has a framework, and, if the framework is not identified, the reader must pull the material out of the literature review or attempt to read between the lines of the research report to identify it.

Conceptual Framework

Purpose

The major goals of a conceptual framework are to clarify the concepts used in the study and to propose relationships between the concepts. The conceptual framework also provides meaning within which to interpret the research findings. A conceptual framework is used for studies in which existing theory is not available or sufficient. This is a common situation in new fields of knowledge such as nursing. Until our body of knowledge is better developed, many of the studies conducted must be exploratory or descriptive and use a conceptual framework rather than a theoretical framework. These conceptual frameworks and the findings of the studies using the frameworks can eventually be developed into theory that is useful to nursing practice.

Constructing a Conceptual Framework

The development of a conceptual framework is a two-step process. The first step involves identifying the concepts to be examined within the study and examining the meaning of each concept in the context of the study (conceptual definition). Concept analysis can be used to develop some of the conceptual definitions in the framework, while other concepts may be extracted from a theory and defined in the same manner as the theorist defined them. In this manner, the meanings of multiple concepts may be examined. In exploratory and descriptive studies, the concepts identified in the framework are operationalized and described.

In the second step in constructing a conceptual framework, which involves examining the proposed relationships between these concepts, the relationships may be clarified by illustrating them in a model. This is a very important step, because it is the relationship, not the concept, that is tested in a study. A descriptive study may examine multiple possible relationships among concepts. A correlational study tests the strength of identified relationships.

Chiriboga, Jenkins and Bailey (1983) used a conceptual framework in their study of stress and coping among hospice nurses. Their contention was that knowledge about effective coping strategies was incomplete and unsystematic. They developed their own framework from previous research findings and a theory of a transactional stress process proposed by Lazarus. Stress was defined as external or internal demands that exceed adaptive resources. The concepts identified by the researchers were conditioning factors, environmental and internal demands, stress appraisal, coping strategies, social resources and adaptive status. In this study, the relationships between the concepts were clearly described and a model of the framework (Fig. 7–2) was presented.

Using a Conceptual Framework to Guide a Study

To be useful, the conceptual framework must organize all other components of the study. Each concept must be operationally defined. This means that the researcher must find a means to measure that idea that is in keeping with the

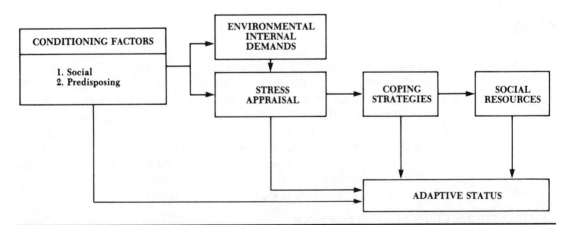

FIGURE 7–2. Revised psychological model of stress. (Reprinted with permission from Chiriboga et al.: Stress and coping among hospice nurses: Test of an analytic model. Nursing Research, 32(5):295, Sept/Oct 1983. Copyright 1983 American Journal of Nursing Company.)

conceptual definition. The measurement (which is concrete) can never completely capture the essence of the concept (which is abstract) but the closer the fit, the greater the meaning of the research findings.

Chiriboga, Jenkins and Bailey (1983) developed conceptual and operational definitions for their concepts; the definitions for one concept are given below.

COPING STRATEGIES

Conceptual Definition:...behaviors directed at modifying the stressors, redefining the situation, or reducing distress. (p. 295)
Operational Definition: Modified Lazarus Ways of Coping Scale. (p. 296)

The relationships between the concepts identified in Figure 7–2 were examined through statistical analysis. Statistical procedures in this study included correlation, factor analysis and regression.

Interpreting Results in The Context of the Conceptual Framework

Findings of the statistical analysis are examined in light of the conceptual framework. In this study, the researchers reported the following findings:

> Hospice nurses who reported fewer experiences with death prior to entry, higher initial work stresses, or who saw themselves as having a more comfortable financial status seemed to do better. Among the coping and resource variables, there was also evidence that adaptive status could be predicted. Nurses who had the most favorable outcome employed a professional orientation as a coping style, expressed their emotional responses to job-related stresses, and resorted to more cognitive or rational coping strategies. Finally, nurses who found their spouses and the staff to be supportive seemed to have the most favorable outcomes. Somewhat surprisingly, however, the presence of supportive friendships was not related to outcome. (Chiriboga, Jenkins & Bailey, 1983, pp. 296–297)

The researchers then examined the meaning of their findings in terms of their framework. Although many of the relationships could not be clarified by this single test of the model, the researchers did find that stress appraisals and coping strategies were the best predictors of adaptive status. Although social resources exerted an influence, it was more of an indirect influence than a direct influence. Further research is required to examine the conceptual framework more completely.

Theoretical Framework

Purpose

A theoretical framework is used when the intent of a study is to test a theory. The framework may be designed to describe the major components of the theory or may include only those segments of the theory being tested. One study seldom tests an entire theory, because theories are a compilation of complex relationships (propositions). In fact, the focus of many studies is on one proposition within a theory.

It is important to note that some metatheorists (people who study theories) are very rigid in their definition of a theory. They will not classify an abstract formulation as a theory unless it meets very specific criteria, including having been previously tested. Any logically organized abstract formulations that do not meet these criteria may be classified by these metatheorists as conceptual frameworks or models and not as theoretical frameworks.

Components of a Theory

In order to test a theory, one must first be able to analyze the theory to identify the various concepts and the logical links between these concepts.

Concepts □ The basic elements of a theory are its concepts. Each major concept within a theory has usually been conceptually defined by the theorist to have a specific meaning that is often unique to that theory. Even though the same word may be used in other theories or in our common language, these meanings of the concept often differ from that of the selected theory.

Relationships □ The linkage between two concepts is called a *relationship*. Ideally, all the concepts within a theory should be linked together in some way.

Propositions □ A proposition is an abstract statement that further clarifies the relationship between two concepts. Some refined theories include clearly stated propositions. In many cases, however, the person analyzing the theory must infer the propositions intended by the theorist. Propositions, like concepts, range from broad and general (abstract) to specific (concrete). Well-developed theories, especially those that have been empirically tested, tend to have several layers of propositions. One broad, general proposition can lead to a number of more specific propositions. This specificity lends itself to facilitating studies to test the theory. Generally, nursing theories have not reached the stage of having specific propositions for research. However, Roy & Roberts (1981) have developed levels of propositions for Roy's theory. For example:

GENERAL PROPOSITION

The magnitude of the internal and external stimuli will positively influence the magnitude of the physiological response of an intact system. (p. 90)

SPECIFIC PROPOSITIONS

1. An environment conducive for eating will positively influence the level of anorexia or nausea. (p. 110)
2. The level of hydration achieved will positively influence the level of fluid and electrolyte balance. (p. 156)

3. The level of alveolar-capillary exchange and perfusion will positively influence the level of oxygen and circulatory balance. (p. 181)

The proposition of a theory is tested in research; the theory itself is not tested. Many propositional statements within theories are not clearly identified. Thus, the researcher must be skilled in extracting propositions crucial to the essence of the theory. Newman (1979) provides a useful guideline for extracting propositions from theories. The following example, from Newman's work, illustrates the extraction of one proposition from the review of literature.

EXCERPT FROM THE LITERATURE

...simple withdrawal is a fundamental type of reaction of stress...in addition to withdrawing physically, the individual may withdraw in various psychological ways...

DERIVED PROPOSITION

Stress leads to physical and psychological withdrawal. (p. 26)

Relationships Between Propositions □ All the propositions within a theory should be logically linked together. Through analysis, these linkages between propositions must be identified. A study will sometimes test more than one proposition and the relationship between the propositions.

Empirical Generalizations □ If a researcher is testing a theory, it is important to identify previous research that has tested that theory. More refined theories have had many propositions tested. If multiple studies have been conducted to test a specific proposition and have failed to disprove it, this proposition becomes an *empirical generalization*. Empirical generalizations become part of science and the nursing body of knowledge. Research also provides the theorist with additional information to modify the theory for a better fit with reality. A theory cannot be proved through testing; rather, the intent is to cast doubt on the theory's propositions. This process requires multiple studies.

Developing Hypotheses From Propositions

In order to test a proposition, it must be translated from abstract to concrete terms. This is achieved by expressing the abstract proposition as a concrete, more specific hypothesis. The process of formulating hypotheses is discussed in Chapter 8; however, an example at this point will illustrate the conversion from proposition to hypothesis.

Yonkman (1982) used Cole's theory of heat and water exchange in the respiratory tract in her study entitled "Cool and heated aerosol and the measurement of oral temperature." Cole's theory emerges from the application of physics principles to physiology. A possible model of the theory is presented in Figure 7–3.

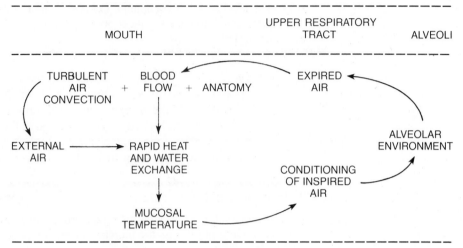

FIGURE 7–3. Model of relationships in Cole's theory. Theoretical framework in Yonkman's study derived from written description by Yonkman.

The propositions generated by Yonkman (1982) are:
1. The mouth assists in warming and cooling the air. (p. 354)
2. Air in the oral cavity is turbulent and allows for rapid heat and water exchange. (p. 354)
3. The same factors that affect heat and water exchange in the inspiratory cycle (anatomy, air flow and blood blow) also affect the expiratory cycle in a slightly reversed manner. (p. 354)
4. Expired air "encounters the cooler mucosa of the upper respiratory tract and with turbulent convection causes heat and water to return to the cooler mucosa." (p. 354)

Two empirical generalizations are noted related to the theory:
1. When the expiratory cycle begins, air exits the alveolar environment at 37°C and at a relative humidity of 100 per cent. (p. 354)
2. The conditioning of inspired air is complete before it enters the trachea. (p. 355)

From these propositions, Yonkman developed the hypothesis that "the accuracy of body temperature as measured by oral thermometer is not significantly affected by the presence of heated or cool aerosol delivered by face mask" (p. 355).

Operationalizing Theoretical Concepts

To test hypotheses, the concepts within them must be operationalized. Yonkman (1982) operationalized external air as cool or heated aerosol, and mucosal temperature was measured by an electronic thermometer.

Interpreting Results in the Context of a Theory

The real impact of using a theoretical framework becomes apparent during data analysis. In addition to the exciting experience of knowing the results of the study, one is able to link the concrete findings back to the abstract ideas of the theory. In reporting the study, the link between the findings and the theory must be made clear; otherwise, a key purpose of the study is lost.

Yonkman's (1982) study did not support her hypothesis. She found a statistically significant difference in temperatures taken when the aerosol mask was in place. However, the differences in temperature were so slight that she questioned whether they were clinically significant, since the greatest difference was 0.3°C. Yonkman's (1982, p. 357) findings of "little temperature variation when mean values are compared for both treatments (cool and heated aerosol mist)" are consistent with previous studies testing this theory.

Testing Nursing Theories

Although single studies designed to test portions of a theory are useful, the process of theory testing is most efficiently conducted by a group of researchers who identify the critical propositions in the theory and develop a plan to test them. Multiple studies must be conducted in order to determine how well a theory describes reality and thus how useful it is for guiding clinical practice.

Nursing theories are relatively new in the scientific realm. Many of them are in early stages of development. Concepts and relationships are not always well defined, propositions either have not been stated or are general, and little or no research has been conducted to test them. These theorists' works must be tested and refined through research to render them useful in clinical practice.

In the following section, a brief summary of four nursing theories is presented, which includes a model of each theory, propositions, ideas for research and studies using the theories for frameworks. Currently, most published nursing research designed to test theory is using theory borrowed from other fields. Nursing is now ready to build its own body of knowledge by testing nursing theory and translating tested theory from related sciences into a nursing body of knowledge.

ROGERS—SCIENCE OF UNITARY MAN

Rogers (1970, 1980) sees unitary man as the primary concern of nursing. She views unitary man in a holistic way, seeing man as more than and different from the sum of his parts. Thus, it is impossible to study a part of unitary man and then relate it to man as a whole. Unitary man and environment are considered open systems that are constantly in interaction. Both unitary man and environment are forms of energy expressed in wave forms. She sees life as evolving irreversibly along a space-time continuum. Thus, she views unitary man within a four-dimensional structure. Rogers sees health as change and growth, not adaptation, and she calls this process homeodynamics. Life increases in complexity throughout man's development. As unitary man evolves, pattern and organization reflect his wholeness. She sees man as having "the capacity for abstraction and imagery, language and thought, sensation and emotion" (Rogers, 1970, p. 73). The relationships of Rogers' (1980, p. 332) concepts of environmental field are illustrated in Figure 7–4.

Rogers has identified three concepts that further explain the life process of unitary man. These are helicy, resonancy and complementarity. She has developed principles that explain the relationship of these concepts to her description of unitary man.

PRINCIPLES FROM ROGERS' THEORY (1980)

1. *Principle of Helicy*: The nature and direction of human and environmental change is continuously innovative, probabilistic, and characterized by increasing diversity of human field and environmental field pattern and organization emerging out of the continuous, mutual, simultaneous interaction between the human and environmental fields and manifesting nonrepeating rhythmicities.

2. *Principle of Resonancy*: The human field and the environmental field are identified by wave pattern and organization manifesting continuous change from lower-frequency, longer wave patterns to higher-frequency, shorter wave patterns.

3. *Principle of Complementarity*: The interaction between human and environmental fields is continuous, mutual, simultaneous. (p. 333)

Rogers' theoretical ideas are very abstract. Some researchers consider her ideas difficult to operationalize in such a way that the theory can be tested. For example, Rogers sees man as unitary and as an energy field in constant interaction with the environment, which is also an energy field. It is difficult to measure man as a unity or measure energy fields and wave patterns that are necessary in order to test her theory. Reeder (1984) and Wilson and Fitzpatrick

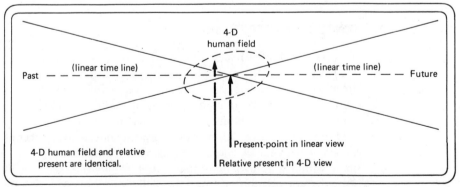

FIGURE 7–4. 4-D environmental field. (From Rogers, M. E.: Nursing: A science of unitary man. *In* Riehl, J. P., and Roy, C. (Eds.) Conceptual Models for Nursing Practice, 2nd ed. Norwalk, Connecticut, Appleton-Century-Crofts, 1980; with permission.)

(1984) suggest that qualitative research approaches may be more effective means than quantitative approaches to test Rogers' theory. Rogers (1970) has developed several questions to direct the testing of her theory.

SUGGESTED QUESTIONS FOR STUDIES

1. Where does the individual perceive his boundary to be? (Rogers, 1970, p. 113)
2. What are some implications of differences that may occur between an individual's perceived boundary and his visible mass which is identified as physical man? (p. 113)
3. In what ways and under what conditions do perceptual boundaries vary in size and shape? (p. 113)
4. Do human field boundaries take on increased definitiveness in the process of growth? (p. 113)
5. Is motion a significant factor in man's patterning and organization? (p. 114)
6. Could there be a relationship between the nature and speed of motion and the coherence and integrity of the individual? (p. 114)
7. How might motion be related to such factors as longevity and rhythmic phenomena? (114)
8. How are sound waves related to pattern formation and transformation of the human field? (p. 114)
9. Is there an association between the nature and speed of sound and the nature and speed of the aging process? (p. 114)
10. What are the natures of the human field pattern and the simultaneous environmental field pattern that are coincident with thought transmission by extrasensory means? (p. 115)
11. Are there identifiable field correlates of thought transmission? (p. 115)
12. What is the relationship between environmental sound rhythms and the rhythms of the individual? (p. 115)
13. Is the speed with which time is perceived to be passing an index of the speed with which the aging process is occurring? (p. 115)
14. What is the nature of the relationship between time perception and the integrity of the human field? (p. 115)
15. Is perception of the passing of time a rhythmical phenomenon? (p. 115)
16. How does man perceive space? (p. 116)
17. What are the environmental space needs of people? (p. 116)
18. Does the sleep-wake rhythm reflect a facet of the space-time dimension? (p. 118)
19. Are there patterns of variability in sleep-wake rhythms that correlate with health and illness, with the process of aging, with developmental patterns? (p. 118)
20. What are the implications for interpreting disease incidence, distribution, susceptibility, prognosis, and seemingly causal factors coupled with anatomical, biological, sociocultural,

psychological and physical, etc., deviations occurring within the context of holistic patterning? (p. 119–120)

Studies Using Rogers' Theory as a Framework

Fawcett, J. (1975). The family as a living open system: an emerging conceptual framework for nursing. *International Nursing Review*, 22(4), 113–116.

Fawcett, J. (1977). The relationship between identification and patterns of change in spouses' body images during and after pregnancy. *International Journal of Nursing Studies*, 14(4), 199–213.

Fitzpatrick, J. J. (1980). Patients' perceptions of time: current research. *International Nursing Review*, 27(5), 148–153, 160.

Fitzpatrick, J. J. & Donovan, M. J. (1978). Temporal experiences and motor behavior among the aging. *Research in Nursing and Health*, 1, 60–68.

Gill, B. P. & Atwood, J. R. (1981). Reciprocy and helicy used to relate mEGF and wound healing. *Nursing Research*, 30(2), 68–72.

Quinn, J. F. (1984). Therapeutic touch as energy exchange: testing the theory. *Advances in Nursing Science*, 6(2), 42–49.

Smith, M. J. (1984). Temporal experience and bed rest: replication and refinement. *Nursing Research*, 33(5), 298–302.

OREM—SELF-CARE

Orem (1985) focuses on the domain of nursing practice and on what nurses actually do when they practice nursing. She proposes that individuals generally know how to take care of themselves (self-care). If they are dependent in some way, such as a child, or aged or handicapped, other responsible family members take on this responsibility (dependent care). If individuals are ill or have some defect (such as diabetes or a colostomy), these individuals or their family members acquire special skills to provide that care (therapeutic self-care). Nursing care is provided only when there is a deficit in the self-care or dependent care that the individual and his or her family cannot provide (self-care deficit). In this case, the nurse or nurses develop a nursing system to provide the needed care. This system involves prescribing, designing and providing the needed care. The goal of nursing care is to facilitate resumption of self-care by the person and/or family.

Orem breaks her formulations down into three segments: (1) a theory of self-care deficits, (2) a theory of self-care and (3) a theory of nursing systems. Orem (1985, p. 32) has developed the following model of her ideas (Fig. 7–5). Orem's ideas are much more concrete than Rogers' and thus may be easier to test. Propositions from her theory, questions for research and published studies testing her theory follow:

PROPOSITIONS—SELF-CARE DEFICIT THEORY

1. Persons who take action to provide their own self-care or care for dependents have specialized capabilities for action.
2. The individual's abilities to engage in self-care or dependent

FIGURE 7–5. A conceptual framework for nursing (R = relationship; < = deficit relationship, current or projected). (From Orem, D. E.: Nursing: Concepts of Practice, 3/e. Copyright 1985. Reproduced with permission from McGraw-Hill Co., New York.)

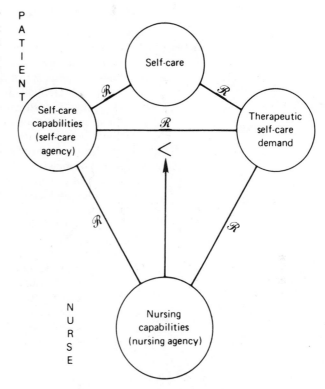

care are conditioned by age, developmental state, life experience, sociocultural orientation, health, and available resources.

3. The relationship of individuals' abilities for self-care or dependent care to the qualitative and quantitative self-care or dependent-care demand can be determined when the value of each is known.

4. The relationship between care abilities and care demand can be defined in terms of equal to, less than, more than.

5. Nursing is a legitimate service when (a) care abilities are less than those required for meeting a known self-care demand (a deficit relationship), or (b) self-care or dependent-care abilities exceed or are equal to those required for meeting the current self-care demand but a future deficit relationship can be foreseen because of predictable decreases in care abilities, qualitative or quantitative increases in the care demand, or both.

6. Persons with existing or projected care deficits are in, or can expect to be in, states of social dependency that legitimate a nursing relationship. (Orem, 1985, p. 35)

PROPOSITIONS—THEORY OF SELF-CARE

1. Self-care and care of dependent family members are learned within the context of social groups by human interaction and communication.
2. Self-care and care of dependent family members are deliberate actions sequentially performed to meet known needs for care.
3. Requisites for self-care have their origins in human beings and their environments.
4. Some requisites for self-care are common to all human beings; others are specific to the developmental and health states of individuals.
5. Universal self-care requisites and ways of meeting them may be modified by the age, sex, or developmental or health state of individuals.
6. A specific process or technology (a way to achieve a purpose) or a specific set of processes or technologies is necessary to meet each self-care requisite.
7. Self-care (or dependent care) as a process or system results from the individual's deliberate use of conceptualized processes or technologies to meet known self-care requisites.
8. A system of self-care or care for dependent family members may be composed of courses of action to meet universal care requisites and requisites associated with developmental and health states.
9. Existing self-care or dependent-care systems are made up of the discrete actions individuals select and perform in sequence in order to meet their particular self-care needs.
10. Knowledge of actual self-care or dependent-care systems results from the deliberate recall and ordering of the discrete actions that were performed or from observing the care actions of others. (Orem, 1985, pp. 36–37)

PROPOSITIONS—THEORY OF NURSING SYSTEMS

1. Nurses relate to and interact with persons who occupy the status of nurse's patient.
2. Legitimate patients have existent and projected continuous self-care requisites.
3. Legitimate patients have existent or projected deficits for meeting their own self-care requisites.
4. Nurses determine the current and changing values of patients' continuous self-care requisites, select valid and reliable processes or technologies for meeting these requisites, and formulate the courses of action necessary for using selected processes or technologies that will meet identified self-care requisites.
5. Nurses determine the current and changing values of patients' abilities to meet their self-care requisites using specific processes or technologies.
6. Nurses estimate the potential of patients to (a) refrain from

engaging in self-care for therapeutic purposes, or (b) develop or refine abilities to engage in self-care now or in the future.

7. Nurses and patients act together to allocate the roles of each in the production of patients' self-care and in the regulation of patients' self-care capabilities.

8. The actions of nurses and the actions of patients (or nurses' actions that compensate for the patients' action limitations) that regulate patients' self-care capabilities and meet patients' self-care needs constitute nursing systems. (Orem, 1985, p. 38)

SUGGESTED QUESTIONS FOR RESEARCH

1. What self-care functions are necessary to perform in order to meet the need for rest and activity?
2. What is the correlation between age and the amount of rest and activity required?
3. If a person does not get enough rest, will illness occur?
4. Exactly what nursing measures will meet the need for rest and activity in the elderly client? (Thibodeau, 1983, p. 137)

Studies Using Orem's Theory as a Framework

Backscheider, J. E. (1971). The use of self as the essence of clinical supervision in ambulatory patient care. *Nursing Clinics of North America*, 6(4), 785–794.

Backscheider, J. E. (1974). Self-care requirements, self-care capabilities, and nursing systems in the diabetic management clinic. *American Journal of Public Health*, 64(12), 1138–1146.

Clinton, J. F., Denyes, M. J., Goodwin, J. O. & Koto, E. M. (1977). Developing criterion measures of nursing care: case study of a process. *Journal of Nursing Administration*, 7(7), 41–45.

Dickson, G. L. & Lee-Villasenor, H. (1982). Nursing theory and practice: a self-care approach. *Advances in Nursing Science*, 5(1), 29–40.

Osguthorpe, N., Roper, J. & Saunders, J. (1983). The effect of teaching on medication knowledge. *Western Journal of Nursing Research*, 5(3), 205–216.

Pridham, K. F. (1971). Instruction of a school-age child with chronic illness for increased responsibility in self-care, using diabetes mellitus as an example. *International Journal of Nursing Studies*, 8, 237–246.

Woods, N. F. (1985). Self-care practices among young adult married women. *Research in Nursing & Health*, 8(3), 227–233.

ROY—ADAPTATION

Roy views the individual as an adaptive system. The person has two internal processor subsystems, which are mechanisms for adapting: the regulator and the cognator. There are four adaptive modes of the individual: physiological, self-concept, role function and interdependence.

Physiologic needs involve the body's basic needs and ways of dealing with adaptation...Self-concept is the composite of beliefs and feelings that one holds about oneself at a given time... Role function is the performance of duties based on given positions in society... The interdependence mode involves one's relations with significant others and support systems. (Roy & Roberts, 1981, pp. 43–44)

The regulator and the cognator act in relation to the adaptive modes to effect adaptation. The regulator subsystem is composed of the neural, endocrine and perception-psychomotor components of the adaptive system. The cognator subsystem is composed of "the psychosocial pathways and apparatus for: (1) perceptual/information processing, (2) learning, (3) judgment, and (4) emotion" (Roy & Roberts, 1981, p. 63). The goal of nursing is to promote adaptation. Nursing activities are carried out within the framework of the nursing process.

Roy's theory, partly based on the medical model, has relatively concrete concepts that are easily operationalized for research. The recent update of her theory has included carefully developed models and propositions that should generate increased testing of her theory. The models Roy has developed include the adaptive system, the regulator subsystem, the cognator subsystem, self-concept system, role function system and interdependence intersystem. Propositions are presented in Roy and Roberts (1981) for each of these systems. Two of the models (Figs. 7–6 and 7–7) and related propositions are presented in this text (Roy & Roberts, 1981, p. 61 & 255).

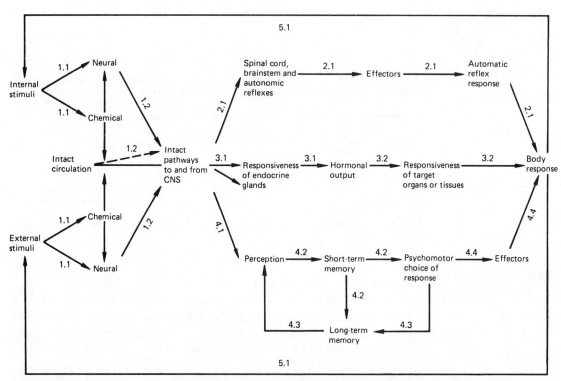

FIGURE 7–6. Regulator subsystem (numbers refer to propositions listed on p. 175). (From Roy, Sr. C., and Roberts, S. L.: Theory Construction in Nursing: An Adaptation Model. Englewood Cliffs, N.J., Prentice-Hall, Inc., 1981; with permission.)

FIGURE 7–7. Self Concept System (numbers refer to propositions listed below). (From Roy, Sr. C., and Roberts, S. L.: Theory Construction in Nursing: An Adaptation Model. Englewood Cliffs, N.J., Prentice-Hall, Inc., 1981; with permission.)

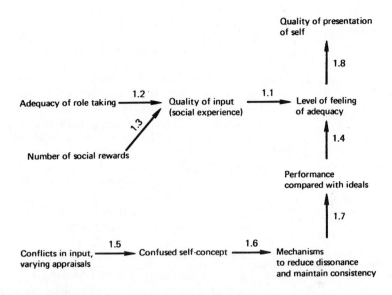

PROPOSITIONS—REGULATOR SUBSYSTEM

1.1. Internal and external stimuli are basically chemical or neural; chemical stimuli may be transduced into neural inputs to the central nervous system.

1.2. Neural pathways to and from the central nervous system must be intact and functional if neural stimuli are to influence body response.

2.1. Spinal cord, brain stem, and autonomic reflexes act through effectors to produce automatic, unconscious effects on the body responses.

3.1. The circulation must be intact for chemical stimuli to influence endocrine glands to produce the appropriate hormone.

3.2. Target organs or tissues must be able to respond to hormone levels to effect body responses.

4.1. Neural inputs are transformed into conscious perceptions in the brain (process unknown).

4.2. Increase in short-term or long-term memory will positively influence the effective choice of psychomotor response to neural input.

4.3. Effective choice of response, retained in long-term memory, will facilitate future effective choice of response.

4.4. The psychomotor response chosen will determine the effectors activated and the ultimate body response. (Roy & Roberts, 1981, p. 62)

PROPOSITIONS—SELF-CONCEPT SYSTEM

1.1. The positive quality of social experience in the form of others' appraisals positively influences the level of feelings of adequacy.

1.2. Adequacy of role-taking positively influences the quality of input in the form of social experience.

1.3. The number of social rewards positively influences the quality of social experience.

1.4. Negative feedback in the form of performance compared with ideals leads to corrections in levels of feelings of adequacy.

1.5. Conflicts in input in the form of varying appraisals positively influences the amount of self-concept confusion experienced.

1.6. Confused self-concept leads to activation of mechanisms to reduce dissonance and maintain consistency.

1.7. Activity of mechanisms for reducing dissonance and maintaining consistency (*e.g.*, choice) tends to lead to feelings of adequacy.

1.8. The level of feelings of adequacy positively influences the quality of presentation of self. (p. 255)

SUGGESTED HYPOTHESES FOR STUDIES

Roy and Roberts (1981) have identified not only general propositions, but specific propositions and hypotheses for research. An example is presented below.

General Proposition

The magnitude of the internal and external stimuli will positively influence the magnitude of the physiological response of an intact system.

Specific Proposition

The amount of mobility in the form of exercising positively influences the level of muscle integrity.

Hypothesis

If the nurse helps the patient maintain muscle tone through proper exercising, the patient will experience fewer problems associated with immobility. (Roy & Roberts, 1981, p. 90)

Studies Using Roy's Theory as a Framework

Norris, S., Campbell, L. A. & Brenkert, S. (1982). Nursing procedures and alterations in transcutaneous oxygen tension in premature infants. *Nursing Research*, 31(6), 330–335.

Wagner, P. (1976). Roy adaptation model: testing the adaptation model in practice. *Nursing Outlook*, 24(11), 682–685.

KING—GOAL ATTAINMENT

King's (1981) goal attainment theory was developed within an open systems framework that includes personal systems, interpersonal systems and social systems. Within this framework, human beings are perceived as total persons who make transactions with individuals and things in the environment. Perception is an essential part of living, and it takes place in each person's concrete world. Interaction is the perception and communication among persons and their environment. Transactions involve interactions in which each person is an active participant and is changed by the experience. King suggests that there is purposeful interaction of nurses with clients to mutually establish goals and to explore and agree upon means of goal achievement. Transactions involve bargaining, negotiating and social exchange. When transactions are made, goals are achieved. A model of the relationships in King's (1981, p. 157) theory is presented in Figure 7–8.

King's propositions are broad and general. More specific propositions must be developed from the theory to stimulate theory testing. Concepts are not well operationalized in her writing and will require operationalization by the researcher.

KING'S IDENTIFIED PROPOSITIONS

1. If perceptual accuracy is present in nurse–client interactions, transactions will occur.
2. If nurse and client make transactions, goals will be attained.
3. If goals are attained, satisfactions will occur.
4. If goals are attained, effective nursing care will occur.
5. If transactions are made in nurse–client interactions, growth and development will be enhanced.
6. If role expectations and role performance as perceived by nurse and client are congruent, transactions will occur.
7. If role conflict is experienced by nurse or client or both, stress in nurse–client interactions will occur.
8. If nurses with special knowledge and skills communicate appropriate information to clients, mutual goal setting and goal attainment will occur. (King, 1981, p. 149)

KING'S IDENTIFIED HYPOTHESES

1. Perceptual accuracy in nurse–patient interactions increases mutual goal setting.

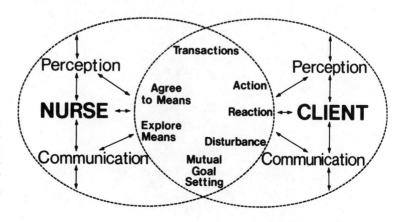

FIGURE 7–8. Schematic diagram of a theory of goal attainment. (From King, I. M.: A Theory for Nursing: Systems, Concepts, Process. New York, John Wiley & Sons, 1981; with permission.)

2. Communication increases mutual goal setting between nurses and patients and leads to satisfactions.
3. Satisfactions in nurses and patients increase goal attainment.
4. Goal attainment decreases stress and anxiety in nursing situations.
5. Goal attainment increases patient learning and copying ability in nursing situations.
6. Role conflict experienced by patients, nurses, or both decreases transactions in nurse–patient interactions.
7. Congruence in role expectations and role performance increases transactions in nurse–patient interactions. (King, 1981, p. 156)

Studies Using King's Theory as a Framework

King, I. M. (1981). *A theory for nursing: systems, concepts, process*. New York: John Wiley & Sons, pp. 150–156.

Summary

A frame of reference is the abstract, logical structure that enables the researcher to link the findings to nursing's body of knowledge. The purpose of a framework is to organize the development of a study and provide a context for interpretation of the findings. The development of a framework involves identification of its basic elements: concepts and relationships between the concepts. A concept is a work or idea to which abstract meaning is attached. All concepts used within a study should be linked together or related. A study's framework can state possible relationships, the strength of a relationship and/or the direction of a relationship. When the type of relationship is made specific, it is referred to as a proposition. The interrelationships among the concepts within a framework are sometimes illustrated with models. A model is a pictorial demonstration, using illustrations or mathematical formulas, that helps clarify the relationships being explained.

The frame of reference for the study begins to evolve at an early stage of research development. The process of constructing a frame of reference involves gaining increased insight into the meanings that have been incorporated into personal knowledge. In addition, literature searches need to be conducted that focus on existing theories, clinical practice ideas and empirical findings from research. The construction of a framework requires the rigorous clarification of concepts and their relationships in the framework and demonstration of the logical flow between the framework and the rest of the study. If a framework is not developed properly, problems arise related to the framework, including inappropriate frameworks, disconnected frameworks, multiple frameworks and unidentified frameworks.

There are two types of frames of reference: conceptual and theoretical. A conceptual framework is an organization or matrix of concepts that provides a focus for inquiry. A conceptual framework is usually seen as loosely constructed, not previously presented in the literature and/or not tested. A theoretical framework is a general, abstract explanation of the interrelationships of the concepts in a theory to be investigated. A theoretical framework emerges from one theory that has been previously published, has conceptually defined concepts and has propositions that can be tested. The purpose, construction and use of conceptual and theoretical frameworks have been presented in this chapter, and examples have been provided.

Nursing is beginning to test nursing theory and to incorporate these tested theories into nursing's body of knowledge. The works of four nursing theorists, Rogers, Orem, Roy and King, have been presented. Models of the theories, propositions, ideas for research and studies using these theories for frameworks have been identified.

References

Abdellah, F. G. & Levine, E. (1979). *Better patient care through nursing research* (2nd ed.). New York: Macmillan Publishing Co., Inc.

Allison, S. E. (1973). A framework for nursing action in a nurse-conducted diabetic management clinic. *Journal of Nursing Administration*, 3(4), 53–60.

Anna, D. J., Christensen, D. G., Hohon, S. A., Ord, L. & Wells, S. R. (1978). Implementing Orem's conceptual framework. *Journal of Nursing Administration*, 8(11), 8–11.

Atwood, J. R. & Gill-Rogers, B. P. (1984) Metatheory, methodology, and practicality: issues in research uses of Rogers' science of unitary man. *Nursing Research*, 33(2), 88–91.

Batey, M. V. (1977). Conceptualization: knowledge and logic guiding empirical research. *Nursing Research*, 26(5), 324–329.

Becker, C. H. (1983). A conceptualization of concept. *Nursing Papers*, 15(2): 51–58.

Blalock, H. J., Jr. (1982). *Conceptualization and measurement in the social sciences*. Beverly Hills: Sage Publications.

Brown, M. I. (1964). Research in the development of nursing theory: the importance of a theoretical framework in nursing research. *Nursing Research*, 13(2), 109–112.

Burckhardt, C. S. (1985). The impact of arthritis on quality of life. *Nursing Research*, 34(1), 11–16.

Chinn, P. L. & Jacobs, M. K. (1983). *Theory and nursing: a systematic approach*. St. Louis: The C. V. Mosby Company.

Chiriboga, D. A., Jenkins, G. & Bailey, J. (1983). Stress and coping among hospice nurses: test of an analytic model. *Nursing Research*, 32(5), 294–299.

Dubin, R. (1978). *Theory building*. New York: The Free Press.

Fawcett, J. (1975). The family as a living open system: an emerging conceptual framework for nursing. *International Nursing Review*, 22(4), 113–116.

Fawcett, J. (1983). Contemporary nursing research: its relevance for nursing practice. In N. L. Chaska (Ed.), *The nursing profession: a time to speak* (pp. 169–182). New York: McGraw-Hill Book Company.

Fitzpatrick, J. J. (1980). Patients' perceptions of time: current research. *International Nursing Review*, 27(5), 148–153.

Gaut, D. A. (1983). Development of a theoretically adequate description of caring. *Western Journal of Nursing Research*, 5(4), 313–324.

Howland, D. (1977). Models in nursing research. In P. J. Verhonick (Ed.), *Nursing Research II* (pp. 135-148). Boston: Little, Brown and Company.

King, I. M. (1975). A process for developing concepts for nursing through research. In P. J. Verhonick (Ed.), *Nursing Research I* (pp. 25–43). Boston: Little, Brown and Company.

King, I. M. (1981). *A theory for nursing: systems, concepts, process*. New York: John Wiley & Sons.

Krueger, J. C., Nelson, A. H. & Wolanin, M. O. (1978). *Nursing research: development, collaboration, and utilization*. Germantown, Maryland: Aspen Systems Corporation.

Newman, M. A. (1979). *Theory development in nursing*. Philadelphia: F. A. Davis Company.

Orem, D. E. (1985). *Nursing: concepts of practice* (3rd ed.). New York: McGraw-Hill Book Company.

Quinn, J. F. (1984). Therapeutic touch as energy exchange: testing the theory. *Advances in Nursing Science*, 6(2), 42–49.

Reeder, F. (1984). Philosophical issues in the Rogerian science of unitary human beings. *Advances in Nursing Science*, 6(2), 14–23.

Reynolds, P. D. (1971). *A primer in theory construction*. Indianapolis: The Bobbs-Merrill Company, Inc.

Rogers, M. E. (1970). *An introduction to the theoretical basis of nursing*. Philadelphia: F. A. Davis Company.

Rogers, M. E. (1980). Nursing: a science of unitary man. In J. P. Riehl, & Sr. C. Roy (Eds.), *Conceptual models for nursing practice* (2nd ed.)(pp. 329-337). Norwalk, Connecticut: Appleton-Century-Crofts.

Roy, Sr. C. & Roberts, S. L. (1981). *Theory construction in nursing: an adaptation model*. Englewood Cliffs, New Jersey: Prentice-Hall, Inc.

Schlotfeldt, R. M. (1975). The need for a conceptual framework. In P. J. Verhonick (Ed.), *Nursing Research I* (pp. 3–24). Boston: Little, Brown and Company.

Silva, M. C. (1977). Philosophy, science, theory: interrelationships and implications for nursing research. *Image*, 9(3), 59–63.

Silva, M. C. (1981). Selection of a theoretical framework. In S. D. Krampitz & N. Pavlovich (Eds.), *Readings for nursing research* (pp. 17–28). St. Louis: The C. V. Mosby Company.

Silva, M. C. & Rothbart, D. (1984). An analysis of changing trends in philosophies of science on nursing theory development and testing. *Advances in Nursing Science*, 6(2), 1–13.

Stevens, B. J. (1984). *Nursing theory: analysis, application, evaluation* (2nd ed.). Boston: Little, Brown and Company.

Thibodeau, J. A. (1983). *Nursing models: analysis and evaluation*. Monterey, California: Wadsworth Health Sciences Division.

Walker, L. O. & Avant, K. C. (1983). *Strategies for theory construction in nursing*. Norwalk, Connecticut: Appleton-Century-Crofts.

Williams, C. A. (1979). The nature and development of conceptual frameworks. In F. S. Downs & J. W. Fleming (Eds.), *Issues in nursing research* (pp. 89–106). Norwalk, Connecticut: Appleton-Century-Crofts.

Wilson, L. M. & Fitzpatrick, J. J. (1984). Dialectic thinking as a means of understanding systems-in-development: relevance to Rogers's principles. *Advances in Nursing Science*, 6(2), 24–41.

Wooldridge, P. J., Leonard, R. C. & Skipper, J. K., Jr. (1978). *Methods of clinical experimentation to improve patient care*. St. Louis: The C. V. Mosby Company.

Yonkman, C. A. (1982). Cool and heated aerosol and the measurement of oral temperature. *Nursing Research*, 31(6), 354–357.

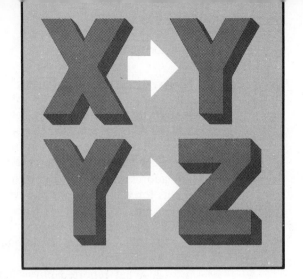

8

Formulating Research Subproblems and Defining Major Variables

The statement of a research problem is broad and provides limited guidance for the investigation of that problem in the real world. The statement of the purpose is more narrow and specific in focus than is the problem. However, even more specificity is often needed to guide the actual development of a study. Therefore, researchers identify subproblems that close the gap between the more abstractly stated research problem and what is actually to be studied in a real-life situation.

The subproblems identify the major variables to be studied, and these variables require clear definition before they can be investigated in the real world. The researcher needs to develop both conceptual and operational definitions for the variables identified within the subproblems. In this chapter, the term subproblem is defined, the types of subproblems formulated in quantitative and qualitative research are identified and the formulation of different types of subproblems is described. The different types of variables are discussed, and the development of conceptual and operational definitions are described.

What Are Research Subproblems?

Research subproblems are the specific or more concrete subparts of a research problem. Subproblems can be stated as objectives, questions or hypotheses. The specific variables, relationships among the variables and population to be studied are clarified in the research subproblems. Rudy and Estok's (1983) study addressed the problem of limited knowledge concerning health risks and benefits for women who jog. The "purpose of this study was to investigate the relationship of jogging to selected physical and psychosocial variables in women" (p. 328), and five subproblems (research questions) were identified.

1. What physical symptoms are reported most frequently by female joggers?
2. What reported physical symptoms of female joggers are related to the intensity of jogging?
3. Is the level of self-esteem of female joggers related to the intensity of jogging?
4. Is the level of anxiety of female joggers related to the intensity of jogging?
5. Is a change in the quality of interpersonal relationship with others (husband/family) related to the intensity of jogging in female joggers? (p. 328)

The subproblems identified in this example are more concise and provide greater direction for conducting this study than the research purpose. Subproblems identify the target population or the specific population to be studied, which, in this example, is female joggers. The subproblems clarify the major variables (underlined in the previous example) that are to be observed, surveyed and/or manipulated in conducting a study. The variables identified in the subproblems are defined in a way that renders them measurable in the real world (operational definition).

Selecting Research Subproblems

The researcher must select subproblems appropriate to the type of study to be conducted. Subproblems are stated as objectives when the intent of the study is to identify or describe characteristics of variables. Objectives are often used in exploratory (quantitative and qualitative) and descriptive research (Table 8–1). Subproblems are stated as questions when the intent of the study is to identify and describe variables and/or to determine the existence of relationships among variables. Questions can be used in exploratory and descriptive research and are frequently used in correlational research. The researcher identifies hypotheses when the relationships or results of a study can be anticipated or predicted. Hypotheses may be identified in correlational research and are used in quasi-experimental and experimental research.

Some types of quantitative research may not include subproblems (Table 8–1). Some experienced researchers can clearly focus and develop their selected

TABLE 8–1
Research Subproblems for Different Types of Research

Types of Research	Research Subproblems
Exploratory research (quantitative and qualitative)	Objectives, questions or no subproblems
Descriptive research	Objectives, questions or no subproblems
Correlational research	Questions or hypotheses
Quasi-experimental research	Hypotheses
Experimental research	Hypotheses

study without the statement of subproblems. In these studies, a specific research purpose might be stated to direct the implementation of the research process.

In qualitative research, some researchers recommend not identifying subproblems. The specification of subproblems might limit the scope of the study and the methods of data collection and analysis. Discovery is important in qualitative research, and sometimes the "research questions may be unclear, the objectives ambiguous and the final outcome uncertain." The use of "hypotheses and detailed accounts of precise research strategies are not necessary nor desirable in a well constructed qualitative design" (Aamodt, 1983, p. 399).

The researcher selects subproblems based on (1) the number and quality of relevant studies conducted on a selected problem (existing knowledge base), (2) the frame of reference developed for the study and (3) the personal experience the researcher has with the problem in the real world. If minimal or no research has been conducted on a problem, frequently investigators will state objectives or questions because inadequate knowledge is available to formulate an hypothesis. In developing the frame of reference for a study, the researcher indicates whether the intent of the study is to develop theory or to test theory. Objectives and questions are usually stated to guide theory development, and the focus of an hypothesis is to test theory. From personal experience, the researcher may wish to describe a variable, identify relationships among variables or examine causality between two variables.

The subproblems designated for study frequently indicate a pattern that the researcher uses in conducting investigations. Problems can be investigated in a variety of ways; some researchers start at the core of a problem and work their way outward. Other investigators study a problem from the outside edge and work to the core (Kaplan, 1964). Researchers can select a variety of subproblems and state these subproblems in different ways to direct their investigation of a problem. In identifying subproblems, it is important to remember that they must flow logically from and provide direction for answering the research problem. The subproblems developed should also indicate that there is order in the researcher's investigations, which means that the researcher has an established pattern for studying a problem area. This pattern of investigation will affect the quality and quantity of the knowledge generated and/or refined in a problem area.

Formulating Research Objectives

Objectives are clear, concise, declarative statements that are expressed in the present tense. For clarity, an objective should focus on only one or two variables. Objectives state which characteristics of a variable are to be identified (identification) and which are to be described (description). Infrequently, research objectives focus on the determination of relationships or associations among variables (relational). The objectives stated in studies might be worded as follows:

1. The objective of this study is to identify the elements or characteristics of variable X in a specific population.
2. The objective of this study is to describe the existence of variable X in a specified population.
3. The objective of this study is to determine or identify the existence of a relationship between variable X and variable Y in a specific population.

Objectives are developed from the research problem and purpose, and they clarify the variables to be studied and the population to be observed or surveyed. An exploratory study by Carrieri, Stotts, Murdaugh, Levinson and Holzemer (1982) demonstrates the logical flow from research problem, to the research purpose and then to the research objectives.

RESEARCH PROBLEM

Recent teaching experiences in both academic and continuing education programs prompted the investigators to question whether nurses who have been taught physical assessment were using their skills in the work setting. (p. 6)

RESEARCH PURPOSE

The primary purpose of this survey was to evaluate whether registered nurses who had been taught cardiopulmonary assessment skills were using these skills in their clinical setting. (p. 6)

RESEARCH SUBPROBLEMS—OBJECTIVES

...to determine:

1. the parts of the cardiopulmonary examination used on a regular basis;
2. the major obstacles practicing nurses perceive as deterrents to the use of their skills; and
3. the relationship between the frequency of skill performance and educational level, type of position and setting, requirements for recording, and type of course. (p. 6)

The first objective focused on identification of the parts of the cardio-pulmonary examination used regularly. The second objective focused on identification and description of major obstacles practicing nurses perceived. The third objective focused on the determination of relationships between frequency of skill performance and the variables of educational level, position, setting, requirements for recording and type of course. The outcomes from this study can include relational statements that can be used to formulate hypotheses to direct further research.

Formulating Research Questions

A *research question* is a concise, interrogative statement that is worded in the present tense and usually includes one or two variables. Research questions frequently focus on what variable(s) are to be described and what relationships might exist among variables. Research questions might be worded as follows:

1. How is variable X perceived in a population?
2. What is the response of a specific population to variable X?
3. Is there a relationship between variable X and variable Y in a specific population?
4. What is the relationship between variable X and variable Y in a specific population?

A descriptive study conducted by McKeever and Galloway (1984) included research questions to direct their investigation.

RESEARCH PROBLEM

The incidence of menstrual cycle length alterations following surgery has not been described in the professional literature. (p. 42)

RESEARCH PURPOSE

This study was undertaken to determine the nature and frequency of menstrual cycle alterations following nongynecological surgery in adolescent and adult females. (p. 42)

RESEARCH SUBPROBLEMS—QUESTIONS

1. How is menstrual cycle length affected by surgery performed under general anesthesia in adolescent and adult females?
2. What is the relationship between menstrual cycle phase at the time of surgery and the onset of the first postoperative menses?
3. What is the relationship between the extent to which hospitalization is stressful and postoperative menstrual cycle length alterations?
4. How do women perceive menstrual cycle length alterations following nongynecological surgery? (p. 42)

The first and fourth questions focus on description of variables, and the second and third questions focus on determination of relationships among variables. The research questions stated in qualitative studies are frequently broader in focus but are otherwise similar to the questions generated in quantitative studies. An historical study by Krampitz (1983) focused on the development of baccalaureate education in the American university from 1899 to 1935.

RESEARCH PURPOSE

It was the purpose of this research to explore... increased specialization and the development of a professional subculture as it related to the establishment of nursing education in the American University. (p. 372)

RESEARCH SUBPROBLEMS—QUESTIONS

1. What forces within society and the nursing profession were instrumental in the development of functional specialization?
2. What was the relationship between the development of a professional subculture and the movement of the profession to formal affiliation with colleges and universities?
3. What factors were significant in the establishment of baccalaureate nursing programs as integral parts of American colleges and universities? (Krampitz, 1983, p. 372)

The first and third questions focused on description of variables; the second question focused on determining a relationship between variables.

Formulating Hypotheses

An *hypothesis* is the formal statement of the expected relationship(s) between two or more variables. The hypothesis translates the research problem and purpose into a clear explanation or prediction of the expected results or outcomes of the study. The statement of an hypothesis implies theory testing and is derived from a proposition. The number of nursing studies containing hypotheses is increasing, and there appears to be a "trend away from descriptive and fact-finding studies toward efforts to establish relationships between variables and to test hypotheses" (Brown, Tanner & Padrick, 1984, p. 31).

The increasing use of hypotheses in research could indicate that an increased level of knowledge has been generated in selected problem areas and could also indicate the increasing sophistication of nurse researchers. However, Brown, Tanner & Padrick (1983) noted in the studies they reviewed that only 51 per cent of these studies included explicitly stated hypotheses and the other studies had implicit or implied hypotheses. The formulation of explicit hypotheses is a valuable mechanism for directing the implementation of the research process. The novice researcher must be familiar with the purpose, sources, elements, characteristics and types of hypotheses. This knowledge provides a basis for formulating and testing hypotheses.

PURPOSE OF HYPOTHESES

The purpose of an hypothesis is similar to that of the other research subproblems. The hypothesis includes the variables to be studied, identifies the population to be examined and indicates the type of research to be conducted. In addition, hypotheses direct the measurement of variables; the selection of the study design, including the sampling technique and the methods of data collection and analysis; and the interpretation of the findings.

Hypotheses differ from other subproblems because they predict the outcomes of a study, and the findings from the study indicate the "acceptance" or "nonacceptance" of the hypotheses. Testing hypotheses is a means of generating knowledge through the testing of theoretical propositions. The ultimate purpose of an hypothesis is to suggest new experiments or new observations, for hypotheses are tools for uncovering ideas rather than ends in themselves (Beveridge, 1950). All hypotheses are productive in generating new ideas, whether they are accepted or not in a particular investigation.

SOURCES OF HYPOTHESES

Hypotheses are generated by observing a particular phenomenon or problem in the real world, analyzing theory and reviewing the literature. Hypotheses are frequently initially formulated from real-life experiences. A researcher observes events in the real world and identifies relationships among these events (theorizing), which is the basis for formulating hypotheses. For example, in the clinical setting, you may have noted that the patient who complains the most receives the most pain medicine. The relationship identified is a prediction or speculation about events in the real world that has the potential for empirical testing. Through a literature review, the researcher can identify theory from which these ideas evolved. Fagerhaugh and Strauss (1977) developed a theory of pain management that identified a relationship between pain management and expression of pain. This theoretical relationship may be useful in developing an hypothesis for the relationship observed in clinical practice. The proposition in a theory and clinical experience provide the basis for the generation of hypotheses. A possible hypothesis is "The hospitalized adult female with a higher number of verbal complaints is administered more frequent doses of analgesic medications than is the hospitalized adult female with a low number of verbal complaints." A prediction that was made based on experience and theory now has potential for testing through research.

In caring for clients, nurses are constantly formulating nursing diagnoses, and these diagnoses can be used in the development of hypotheses. The development of hypotheses from nursing diagnosis requires that the theoretical formulations from which the diagnosis was derived be identified. For example, the theoretical relationships identified in Orem's (1985) theory of self-care and the self-care nursing diagnoses could serve as the basis for the generation of hypotheses. Testing relationships identified in clinical practice is a valuable means of generating and refining nursing knowledge.

Some hypotheses are initially generated from theory. The primary intent of the researcher is to test elements of the theory that will ultimately have an impact on nursing practice. The propositions stated in theory include numerous relationships that can be formulated into hypotheses. For example, the proposition "If there is a high level of sociability, there is decreased personal space" is the basis for generating the hypothesis "Persons low in sociability prefer more personal space than persons high in sociability" (Newman, 1979, pp. 36–37).

Hypotheses can be generated by reviewing the literature. A researcher might restate an hypothesis that was tested previously by another researcher and focus on a different variable. For example, the hypothesis stated by Lim-Levy (1982, p. 150) "Oxygen inhalation by nasal cannula of up to 6 LPM (liters per minute) does not effect oral temperature measurement taken with an electronic thermometer" might be restated as "oxygen inhalation by face mask of up to 6 LPM does not effect oral temperature measurement taken with an electronic thermometer." A researcher could also choose to replicate the study and test the original hypothesis of Lim-Levy. In reviewing the literature, researchers analyze the findings from different studies and synthesize the findings or relate the findings in one study with those of another study. The relationships identified from synthesis of study findings are valuable sources for generating hypotheses.

ELEMENTS OF HYPOTHESES

The elements of an hypothesis are the population(s), variables and relationships of variables. The relationships identified in hypotheses are associative or causal. An *associative relationship* includes research variables and states the covariation of these variables in the real world. A format for expressing an associative hypothesis follows: Variable X is related to variable Y in a specified population. *Causal relationships* include independent and dependent variables. The *independent variable* (treatment or experimental variable) is manipulated by the researcher in order to examine the effects on the dependent variable. The *dependent variable* (outcome variable) is measured by the researcher to examine its relationship with the independent variable. A format for stating a causal hypothesis follows: The population that experiences the independent variable demonstrates a greater change as measured by the dependent variable than the subjects not exposed to the independent variable.

CHARACTERISTICS OF HYPOTHESES

An hypothesis that is clearly and concisely stated provides the greatest direction in conducting a study. For clarity, hypotheses are expressed as declarative statements written in the present tense. Thus, hypotheses should not include the wording "There will be a positive relationship...," because the future tense refers to the sample being studied. Hypotheses are statements of relationships about populations, not about study samples. According to mathematical theory related to generalization, one cannot generalize to the future.

Phrases such as "significant difference," "testing a relationship" or "measuring a variable" should not be included in an hypothesis statement. For example, hypotheses should not contain statements such as "There is no significant difference...," because the level of significance is only a statistical technique applied to sample data (Armstrong, 1981). A statement of an hypothesis should not identify methodological points such as techniques of sampling, measurement and data analysis (Kerlinger, 1973). Therefore, statements such as "measured by", "in a random sample of" or "using ANOVA" are not acceptable. The statement of an hypothesis should not be limited to the variables, methodology and sample identified for one study. The researcher must state an hypothesis that is reflective of the variables and population outlined in the research purpose.

A well-formulated hypothesis clearly identifies the relationship between the variables to be studied. A study by Beck (1983) contained the following hypothesis: "During the active phase of labor, women who receive analgesics have higher Speed of Time Passing scores than women who do not receive analgesics" (p. 286). The hypothesis identifies a relationship between receiving analgesics (independent variable) and the Speed of Time Passing scores (dependent variable). For clarity, novice researchers and many expert researchers state a simple, concise hypothesis that identifies one relationship between variables. A study might contain as few as one or as many as 15 hypotheses. There is no set number of hypotheses that are needed to direct the study of a problem. The number of hypotheses stated is usually reflective of the researcher's expertise and the complexity of the problem studied. However, most studies include one to four hypotheses, and the relationships identified in these hypotheses set the limits for the study.

The value of an hypothesis is ultimately derived from whether or not it is testable in the real world. A *testable hypothesis* is one that contains variables that are observable or measurable in the real world. A testable hypothesis was formulated by Heidt (1981).

HYPOTHESIS

In subjects receiving intervention by therapeutic touch, there is a reduction in post-test A-state anxiety scores. (p. 33)

INDEPENDENT VARIABLE—THERAPEUTIC TOUCH

Conceptual Definition: A derivative of laying-on of hands that uses the hands to direct excess body energies from a person in the role of healer to another for the purpose of helping or healing that individual. Although derived from the laying-on of hands, it differs from it in that TT (therapeutic touch) is not performed within a religious context. The person in the role of healer does the act of TT while in a meditative state and is motivated by an interest in the needs of the patient. (p. 33)

Operational Definition: In intervention by TT the nurse performs the following operational steps:

1. Makes the intention mentally to assist the subject therapeutically.
2. Centers himself or herself in an act of self-relatedness and becomes aware of himself or herself as an open system of energies in constant flux.
3. Moves the hands over the body of the subject from head to feet attuning to the condition of the subject by becoming aware of changes in sensory cues in the hands.
4. Redirects areas of accumulated tension in the subject's body by movement of the hands.
5. Concentrates attention on the specific direction of these energies, using the hands as focal points.
6. Directs this energy to the subject by placing hands on the solar plexus area of the body (just above the waist) and leaving them in this area for approximately 90 seconds.
   The total time for this intervention is 5 minutes. (p. 35)

DEPENDENT VARIABLE—A-STATE ANXIETY SCORES

Conceptual Definition: A-state anxiety is a transitional emotional state of the human organism that varies in intensity and fluctuates over time. A-state anxiety is differentiated from A-trait anxiety in that the latter is defined as a relatively stable personality trait, characterized by feelings of diffuse apprehension and proneness to experience stressful events. (p. 33)

Operational Definition: The A-state anxiety score was measured by the Self-Evaluation Questionnaire... It was administered pre- and postintervention. (p. 33)

A testable hypothesis must also predict a relationship that can be accepted or rejected based on the data collected. In the study by Heidt (1981), the hypothesis stated a relationship between therapeutic touch and A-state anxiety. An analysis of the pre- and post-test A-state anxiety scores revealed a highly significant difference. "Subjects in this group (therapeutic touch) experienced a decrease in anxiety, supporting the first hypothesis" (Heidt, 1981, p. 35).

TYPES OF HYPOTHESES

Many types of hypotheses appear in published studies. For clarity, the types of hypotheses are described using four categories: (1) simple versus complex, (2) nondirectional versus directional, (3) associative versus causal and (4) statistical versus research.

Simple Versus Complex Hypotheses

Depending on the theoretical proposition and the variables to be manipulated or measured in a study, the researcher will state simple or complex hypotheses.

A *simple hypothesis* states the relationship between two variables. The mathematical representation for a simple, associative hypothesis is:

$$X \updownarrow Y$$

This indicates that variable X is related to, or associated with, variable Y but is not the cause of variable Y. The mathematical representation of a simple, causal hypothesis is $X \longrightarrow Y$, which means that X is the cause of Y.

A complex hypothesis predicts the relationship between two (or more) independent variables and/or two (or more) dependent variables. Therefore, any hypothesis that contains more than two variables is a complex hypothesis. The mathematical expression of a complex, causal hypothesis with two independent variables (X_1 and X_2) and one dependent variable (Y) is:

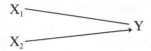

Although complex hypotheses include more than one relationship, only one prediction is made in each hypothesis.

A quasi-experimental study about the compliance of cancer patients to therapy included simple and complex hypotheses (Itano, Tanabe, Lum, Lamkin, Rizzo, Wieland & Sato, 1983). Table 8–2 includes four of the study's hypotheses, which are labeled as simple or complex; the independent and

TABLE 8–2
Simple and Complex Hypotheses

Simple Hypotheses	Independent Variable	Dependent Variable
There will be a greater compliance rate among cancer patients with an increased understanding of their illness than among those who have less understanding of their illness.	Understanding of illness	Compliance rate
There will be a greater compliance rate among cancer patients who perceive greater severity of symptoms than among those who perceive less severe symptoms. (Itano *et al.*, 1983, p. 10)	Perceived severity of symptoms	Compliance rate
Complex Hypotheses	**Independent Variable**	**Dependent Variable**
There will be a greater compliance rate among cancer patients with high self-esteem and low anxiety level compared with those with low self-esteem and high anxiety level.	Self-esteem and anxiety	Compliance rate
There will be a greater compliance rate among cancer patients who perceive that nurses are caring and concerned as compared with those who do not perceive nurses as caring and concerned. (Itano *et al.*, 1983, p. 10)	Nurses' caring and concern	Compliance rate

dependent variables of these hypotheses are identified. These hypotheses might have been more reflective of the population studied rather than the sample if they had been expressed in the present tense (there is) rather than the future tense (there will be).

Nondirectional Versus Directional Hypotheses

A *nondirectional hypothesis* states that a relationship exists but does not predict the exact nature of the relationship. If the relationship being studied is not clear in clinical practice, the theoretical literature or the empirical literature, the researcher has no clear indication of the nature of the relationship. In this situation, the statement of a nondirectional hypothesis is necessary. An example of a simple, nondirectional hypothesis follows: "The increasing age of the postoperative patient is related to the amount of analgesic medication that is administered during the first 48 hours following surgery." This hypothesis states that a relationship exists but does not indicate the nature of the relationship. The intent of the study is to determine whether a positive or negative relationship exists between the variables of increasing age and the amount of medication administered.

A *directional hypothesis* states the specific nature of the relationship between two or more variables. As the knowledge on which the study is based increases, the researcher is capable of making a prediction about the nature of a relationship between the variables being studied. If an hypothesis is based on a theoretical proposition that specifies the nature of a relationship, a directional hypothesis must be stated and should reflect the relationship expressed in the proposition. An example of a simple, directional hypothesis is: "With increasing age, less analgesic medication is administered during the first 48 hours following abdominal surgery" (Faherty & Grier, 1984, p. 369). This hypothesis predicts a negative or inverse relationship between the variables.

Associative Versus Causal Hypotheses

The relationship stated in an hypothesis can be *associative* or *causal*. An hypothesis that states an associative relationship identifies variables that occur or exist together in the real world (Reynolds, 1971). In an associative relationship, when one variable varies or changes in the relationship, the other variable changes. A directional, associative relationship between variables can be either positive or negative. An example of an hypothesis that states a positive association is: "The strength of the marital relationship as perceived by the expectant father during gestation is positively associated with the level of a father's attachment to the fetus" (Weaver & Cranley, 1983, p. 69). This simple, directional, associative hypothesis predicts that with stronger marital relationships, there is a greater attachment of the father to the fetus. The two variables are predicted to vary together in the same direction (positive relationship).

The hypothesis in Weaver and Cranley's (1983) study could also be stated with a negative association among the variables: "The strength of the marital conflict as perceived by the expectant father during gestation is negatively associated with the level of a father's attachment to the fetus." This hypothesis predicts that strong marital conflict decreases the father's attachment to the fetus. The variables in this hypothesis are predicted to vary together but in opposite directions (negative or inverse relationship).

The hypothesis in Weaver and Cranley's (1983) study could be stated as a nondirectional hypothesis. For example, the hypothesis might be "the strength of the marital relationship as perceived by the expectant father during gestation is associated with the level of a father's attachment to the fetus." This nondirectional, associative hypothesis identifies a relationship between two variables but does not indicate the direction (positive or negative) of this relationship. For example, one is left with uncertainty as to whether a strong marital relationship is associated with high- or low-level attachment to the fetus.

Roberts (1983) developed a model illustrating the relationships among the variables infant behavior, effects on transition to parenthood and parental perceptions of the infant. This model was the basis for the generation of eight directional hypotheses (Fig. 8–1). These hypotheses identified both positive and negative associations among the variables in the model. Examine the model and see whether you can identify the hypotheses that were used in conducting this study; compare your findings with the actual study hypotheses listed below. Hypotheses proposed for the relationships in the model were:

1. The amount of obligatory infant behavior is negatively related to ease of role transition and to the parents' perception of the infant. (Complex, Associative Hypothesis)
2. The amount of obligatory infant behavior is positively related to the amount of normative change. (Simple, Associative Hypothesis)
3. The amount of normative change is negatively related to the ease of

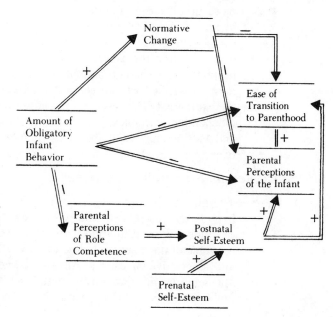

FIGURE 8–1. A model for infant behavior effects on transition to parenthood and parental perceptions of the infant. (Reprinted with permission from Roberts, F. B.: Infant behavior and the transition to parenthood. Nursing Research, 32(4):214, July/August 1983. Copyright 1983 American Journal of Nursing Company.)

role transition and to the parents' perception of the infant. (Complex, Associative Hypothesis)

4. The ease of role transition is positively related to the parents' perception of the infant. (Simple, Associative Hypothesis)
5. The amount of obligatory infant behavior is negatively related to parental perceptions of role competence. (Simple, Associative Hypothesis)
6. Parental perceptions of role competence are positively related to postnatal self-esteem. (Simple, Associative Hypothesis)
7. Prenatal self-esteem is positively related to postnatal self-esteem. (Simple, Associative Hypothesis)
8. Postnatal self-esteem is positively related to the ease of transition and to parents' perception of the infant. (Complex, Associative Hypothesis) (Roberts, 1983, p. 214)

Some hypotheses identify causal or cause-and-effect relationships among variables. This means that one variable (independent variable) is thought to cause or create an effect on a second variable (dependent variable), which indicates direction. Therefore, all causal hypotheses are directional. An example of a simple, causal hypothesis is: "Patients who receive preadmission booklets containing specific exercise instructions achieve higher exercise performance scores during hospitalization than patients who receive the preadmission booklets containing nonspecific instructions" (Rice & Johnson, 1984, p. 148). Rice and Johnson predicted that preadmission booklets with specific exercise instructions (independent variable) cause higher exercise performance scores (dependent variable) for hospitalized patients.

In real-life situations, there are often many variables that cause an event to occur. Therefore, complex rather than simple causal hypotheses are really more predictive of real-life events. For example, a possible complex, causal hypothesis is: "Patients who receive preadmission booklets containing specific exercise instructions and receive positive reinforcement from family members in carrying out the exercises achieve higher exercise performance scores during hospitalization than do patients who receive the preadmission booklets containing nonspecific instructions and whose family members are nonsupportive of the exercises." The researcher is now studying the interaction between the two independent variables, preadmission booklets with specific exercise instructions and family support of exercises, and the effect these variables have on the dependent variable of exercise performance score.

Statistical Versus Research Hypotheses

The null hypothesis (H_o) is also referred to as a *statistical hypothesis*. A null hypothesis is used for the purpose of statistical testing and interpreting statistical outcomes. Even if the null hypothesis is not stated, it is implied, since it is the converse of the research hypothesis. A null hypothesis can be simple or complex and associative or causal. An associative, null hypothesis states that there is "no relationship between the variables." An example of a simple, associative, null hypothesis is: "There is no relationship between the number of experiences performing a developmental assessment skill and learning of the skill, as measured by clinical performance test scores" (Koniak, 1985, p. 85).

A causal, null hypothesis states that "there is no effect of one variable on another" or "there is no difference in the effect of the independent variable on two or more samples of the dependent variable." A simple, causal, null hypothesis directed the study of Lim-Levy (1982, p. 151): "Oxygen inhalation by nasal cannula of up to 6 LPM (liters per minute) does not affect oral temperature measurement taken with an electronic thermometer."

A *research hypothesis* is the alternative hypothesis (H_1) for the null hypothesis. The research hypothesis states that there is a relationship between two or more variables. A research hypothesis can be simple or complex, nondirectional or directional and associative or causal. An example of a complex, nondirectional, associative, research hypothesis is: "Adherence to the medical regimen 6 to 9 months posthospitalization is related to one's attitudes and intentions during hospitalization" (Miller, Wikoff, McMahon, Garrett & Ringel, 1985, p. 269). All example hypotheses presented in this chapter except for the two null hypotheses are research hypotheses.

There is debate among researchers about when to state a research hypothesis and when the null hypothesis should be used. Some researchers state the null because it is more easily interpreted from the findings of statistical analysis than is the research hypothesis. There are valid reasons for stating the hypothesis as a research hypothesis. A research hypothesis is used if the researcher desires to make a prediction about the existence or direction of a relationship between variables to be studied. The prediction in a research hypothesis can be based on a theoretical proposition, previous research findings or experience in clinical practice.

FORMULATING HYPOTHESES

Formulating hypotheses requires inductive and deductive thinking. Most people have a predominant way of thinking and will follow that thinking pattern in the development of hypotheses. An inductive thinker has the tendency to focus on the specific relationships that are observed in clinical practice and will synthesize these observations to formulate a general statement about the relationships observed. For example, the inductive thinker might have noted in several clinical situations that the elderly patients who were not instructed in the reasons for early ambulation following surgery made no effort to get out of bed.

A deductive thinker examines more abstract relational statements from theories or previous research and then formulates a specific hypothesis for study. A deductive thinker might translate a proposition such as "people who receive instruction in self-care are more responsible in caring for themselves" into a relational statement.

Neither the inductive nor the deductive thinker has completed the process of formulating an hypothesis. The inductive thinker must link the relational statement that was formulated with a theoretical framework to increase the usefulness of the study results. This requires deductive thinking. The deductive thinker must use inductive thinking to determine whether the relationship of events in the real world of clinical practice is accurately predicted in the theoretical proposition. Without this real-world experience, the selection of subjects and the identification of ways to measure the variables would be unclear. An example hypothesis, including both inductive and deductive thinking, might be: "Elderly who receive no self-care instruction on early ambulation remain in bed longer following surgery than do elderly patients who receive self-care instruction on early ambulation."

In formulating an hypothesis, a researcher has several decisions to make. These decisions will be directed by the problem studied and the expertise of the researcher. The researcher must decide whether the problem to be studied is best investigated using simple or complex hypotheses. Complex hypotheses frequently require complex methodology and the outcomes may be difficult to interpret. The researcher must also decide whether an associative or causal relationship is to be studied. Testing an hypothesis that states a causal relationship requires expertise in controlling variables. Another decision involves the formulation of a research hypothesis or a null hypothesis. This decision must be made based on what the researcher believes is the most accurate prediction of the relationship between the variables being studied.

TESTING HYPOTHESES

An hypothesis is evaluated with statistical analyses. If the hypothesis states an associative relationship, correlational analyses are conducted to determine the existence, type and degree of the relationship between the variables studied. The hypothesis that states a causal relationship is analyzed using inferential statistics. It is the null hypothesis (stated or implied) that is tested. The intent is to determine whether the independent variable caused a significant effect on the dependent variable. The level of significance ($p = 0.05, 0.01, 0.001$) is set following the generation of the causal hypotheses. Further discussion of testing an hypothesis is included in Chapter 17.

In describing the results obtained from a tested hypothesis, certain terminology is used to accurately reflect the outcome of a study. Hypotheses are not proved "true" or "false" by the findings from one study. Hypotheses are statements of relationships or differences in populations; the findings from one study do not prove an hypothesis. Even after a series of studies, the word "proved" is not used in scientific language because of the tentative nature of science.

If the researcher is testing a null hypothesis, the hypothesis is either rejected or accepted. Accepting the null indicates that there was no relationship or effect found among the variables. Rejecting the null hypothesis indicates the possibility that a relationship or difference exists. Research hypotheses are described as being supported or not supported in a study. One study may only lend support to the existence of a relationship and does not determine whether or not that relationship exists in the real world.

Defining Major Variables

The research problem and subproblems identify the variables to be examined in a study. This section defines the concept variable, identifies the types of variables and describes the process of operationalizing variables.

WHAT IS A RESEARCH VARIABLE

Variables are qualities, properties and/or characteristics of persons, things or situations that are studied in research. Variables are concepts that have been concretely defined to facilitate observation or measurement within a study. Concepts are labels for abstract ideas; highly abstract concepts are sometimes called *constructs* (Chinn & Jacobs, 1983). Constructs contain elements or less abstract concepts. Through concept analysis, the researcher is able to select variables for research and develop conceptual and operational definitions of these variables (Fig. 8–2).

The variables in quantitative research are narrow and specific in focus and are capable of being quantified (converted to numbers). These variables are objectively defined to decrease researcher bias. Variables in qualitative research are more abstract than quantitative variables and are often defined in broader, more general terms. In many cases in qualitative research, the phenomena being examined are not named until the data analysis step. Thus, some variables may not be identified and/or defined until late in the study.

TYPES OF RESEARCH VARIABLES

Variables have been classified into a variety of types to explain their use in research. In research, some variables are manipulated, others are controlled. Some variables are identified but not measured, others are measured with very refined measurement devices. The variables to be described are independent, dependent, research, extraneous and attribute variables.

Independent and Dependent Variables

The most frequently discussed variables in research are the independent and dependent variables. The relationship between the independent and dependent variables is the basis for formulating hypotheses for correlational, quasi-experimental and experimental studies. An *independent variable* is a stimulus or activity that is manipulated or varied by the researcher to create an effect

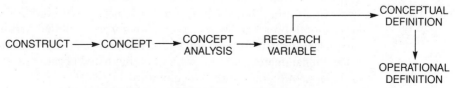

FIGURE 8–2. Process of identifying and defining research variables.

on the dependent variable. An independent variable is also known as a treatment or experimental variable.

A *dependent variable* is the response, behavior or outcome that the researcher wants to predict or explain. Changes in the dependent variable are presumed to be caused by the independent variable. A dependent variable is also called an effect variable or a criterion measure.

The hypothesis tested by Lim-Levy (1982) is used to demonstrate independent and dependent variables. The hypothesis was: "Oxygen inhalation by nasal cannula of up to 6 LPM (liters per minute) does not affect oral temperature measurement taken with an electronic thermometer" (p. 150). The independent variable is oxygen inhalation by nasal cannula, and the oxygen was administered at three levels: 2 LPM, 4 LPM and 6 LPM. The dependent variable was oral temperature that was measured by an electronic thermometer. The independent variable of administration of oxygen was manipulated by the researcher to produce an effect on the dependent variable, oral temperature.

Research Variables

Qualitative studies and some quantitative (exploratory, descriptive and some correlational) studies involve the investigation of research variables. *Research variables* are the qualities, properties and/or characteristics identified in research problems and subproblems (objectives and questions) that are to be identified, described or measured in a study. Krampitz (1983) conducted an historical study of baccalaureate nursing education in the American university. The study included the following subproblem: "What forces within society and the nursing profession were instrumental in the development of functional specialization?" (p. 372). The research variables studied were "forces within society," "forces in nursing" and "functional specialization." In studies that have associative hypotheses, research variables are investigated, not independent and dependent variables.

Extraneous Variables

Extraneous variables exist in all studies and can affect the measurement of the study variables and examination of the relationships within a study. Extraneous variables interfere with obtaining a clear understanding of the relational or causal dynamics within a study situation. These variables are primarily of concern in quantitative research. Extraneous variables are classified as controlled or uncontrolled and recognized or unrecognized. The researcher should attempt to identify and control as many extraneous variables as possible within a study. Quasi-experimental and experimental designs have been developed to control the influence of extraneous variables (Chapter 10). Lim-Levy (1982) controlled some of the extraneous variables in her study. The subjects who were mouth breathing or hyperventilating were excluded because these human characteristics might have influenced the oral temperature. Any subjects with a local inflammatory process were also eliminated because of the possible effect of inflammation on the oral temperature.

The extraneous variables that have not been recognized are sometimes referred to as *confounding* or uncontrolled variables. Some confounding variables are recognized but cannot be controlled. Sometimes these variables can be measured during the study and controlled statistically during analysis. However, in other cases, measurement of the confounding variable is not possible and thus limits the interpretation of findings. As control decreases in a quantitative study, the potential influence of recognized and unrecognized confounding variables increases. In a study of the impact of social support on adherence to a treatment protocol, variables such as stage of illness, knowledge of treatment, attitudes of health care professionals, home environment and the value placed on health by the patient could be confounding.

Environmental variables are types of extraneous variables. Environmental variables constitute factors that make up the setting where the study is conducted; examples of these variables include climate, family, health care system and governmental organizations. If a researcher is studying humans in an uncontrolled or natural setting, it is impossible to control all the extraneous variables.

Attribute Variables

Attribute variables are characteristics or elements of the human subject that are collected to describe the sample. Some common attribute variables are age, gender, educational level, income, race, socioeconomic status and job classification. These variables are sometimes referred to as *demographic variables*. Foxall, Ekberg and Griffith (1985) studied the adjustment patterns of chronically ill middle-aged persons and their spouses. The characteristics of the sample are described below.

> The 30 ill subjects consisted of 18 males and 12 females, aged 36 to 67 years (median 56.5 years). Twelve had completed high school, and 14 reported some type of formal education beyond high school. The majority (N = 19) identified the work done most of their lives as skilled or semi-skilled. Of the 18 employed subjects, 10 were receiving disability benefits and 5 were retired. (p. 431–432)
>
> The 30 spouses consisted of 12 males and 18 females, aged 32 to 65 years (median 56.5 years). Fourteen had completed high school, and 10 indicated some type of formal education beyond high school. Seventeen identified the work done most of their lives as skilled or semi-skilled. Twenty were employed full-time and 2 part-time. (p. 432)
>
> The majority of couples were caucasian (N = 26) and reported their annual household income as $20,000 or more per year (N = 19). The median length of marriage was 29.5 years. (p. 432)

OPERATIONALIZING VARIABLES

Operationalizing a variable involves developing conceptual and operational definitions. The *conceptual definition* is the broad, abstract meaning of a concept. This definition is derived from a theorist's definition of a concept or is developed by the researcher through concept analysis. The framework of a study reflects the conceptual definitions of the variables. Conceptual definitions of variables provide the basis for formulating operational definitions.

An *operational definition* is derived from a set of procedures or progressive acts that a researcher performs to receive sensory impressions (such as sounds, visual or tactile impressions) that indicate the existence or degree of existence of a variable (theoretical concept) (Reynolds, 1971). Operational definitions should be independent of time and setting, so that variables can be investigated at different times and in different settings using the same operational definitions. An operational definition is developed so that a variable can be measured in a concrete situation and the knowledge gained from studying the variable will increase the understanding of the theoretical concept that variable represents.

Murdaugh and Hinshaw (1986) developed a preventive behavior model to direct their study (Fig. 8–3). "The purpose of this research was to determine the influence of perceived barriers and benefits and value orientations on undertaking preventive behaviors of regular aerobic exercise and smoking behaviors" (p. 19). These authors identified constructs (psychological situation, reinforcement value and behavior) and concepts (benefits, barriers, health value orientation and health care activities) and instruments used to measure these concepts in their model. The conceptual and operational definitions for the study variables of benefits, barriers, health value orientation and health care activities follow:

BENEFITS

> *Conceptual Definition:*... benefits are beliefs about the positive aspects that arouse motives to carry out health care activities. (Murdaugh & Hinshaw, 1986, p. 19)
> *Operational Definition*: Benefit Scales

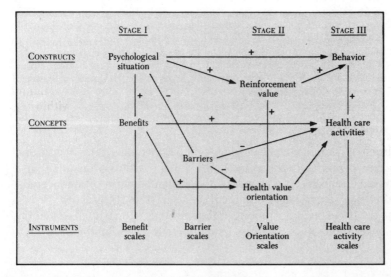

FIGURE 8–3. Preventive behavior model. (From Murdaugh, C., and Hinshaw, A. S.: Theoretical model testing to identify personality variables affecting preventative behaviors. Nurs Res, *35*:19, 1986; with permission.)

BARRIERS

Conceptual Definition:... barriers are beliefs about the negative aspects or costs of health actions that arouse conflicting motives of avoidance. (p. 19)
Operational Definition: Barrier Scales

HEALTH VALUE ORIENTATION

Conceptual Definition: Health value orientations are those aspects of individuals' principles that commit them to personally prefer well-being as opposed to a situation in which they are not able to make a choice. (p. 20)
Operational Definition: Value Orientation Scales

HEALTH CARE ACTIVITIES

Conceptual Definition: Health care activities included participation in a regular exercise program or being a nonsmoker. (p. 20)
Operational Definition: Health Care Activity Scales

Operationalizing Variables in Qualitative Studies

Some researchers believe that qualitative studies do not require operational definitions, because sensitizing or experiencing the real situation rather than operationalizing the concepts is most important (Benoliel, 1984). Operational definitions are thought to limit the focus of the investigation so that a phenomenon such as pain or a characteristic of a culture such as the health practices of a culture are not completely experienced or understood from the investigation. However, broadly stated operational definitions that identify the procedures the researcher will use to determine the existence of a variable are sometimes used.

An ethnographic study of the folk-healing practice among four generations of urban Greek immigrants by Tripp-Reimer (1983) provides an example of the operational definitions for the variables in a qualitative study. The purpose of this study was to "provide baseline qualitative data concerning the description of matiasma as practiced by a specific Greek immigrant community ... and to quantify the distribution of these beliefs and practices within the population" (p. 97). The following terms were defined:

Matiasma: The configuration of beliefs and practices surrounding the prevention, diagnosis, and treatment of the evil eye.

Greek immigrant: A person living in the United States having at least one parent of full Greek ancestry, who self-affiliates with the Greek community.

Generation of immigration: The number of successive filial stages since the first lineal Greek ancestor arrived in the United States (immigrant group = first generation). (pp. 97–98)

Summary

Research subproblems are the specific or more concrete subparts of the research problem and purpose. The specific variables, relationships among the variables and population to be studied are clarified in the research subproblems. Subproblems can be stated as objectives, questions or hypotheses. Objectives are clear, concise, declarative statements that are expressed in the present tense. Objectives state which characteristics of a variable are to be identified and which are to be described. Infrequently, objectives focus on the determination of relationships or associations among variables. A research question is a concise, interrogative statement that is worded in the present tense and usually includes one or two variables. Research questions frequently focus on what variables are to be described and what relationships might exist among variables.

An hypothesis is the formal statement of the expected relationship(s) between two or more variables. The hypothesis translates the research problem and purpose into a clear explanation or prediction of the expected results or outcomes of the study. Hypotheses are generated by observing a particular phenomenon or problem in the real world, analyzing theory and reviewing the literature. The elements of an hypothesis are the population(s), variables and relationships of variables. The types of hypotheses are described using four categories: (1) simple versus complex, (2) nondirectional versus directional, (3) associative versus causal and (4) statistical versus research. An hypothesis is formulated using inductive and deductive thinking and is evaluated with statistical analysis.

The research subproblems (objectives, questions and hypotheses) identify the variables to be examined in a study. Variables are qualities, properties and/or characteristics of persons, things or situations that are studied in research. Variables are concepts that have been concretely defined to facilitate observation or measurement within a study. The common types of variables include independent, dependent, research, extraneous and attribute variables. Independent variables are stimuli or activities that are manipulated or varied by the researcher to create an effect on the dependent variable. A dependent variable (outcome variable) is measured by the researcher to examine its relationship with the independent variable. Research variables are the qualities, properties and/or characteristics included in research subproblems that are to be identified, described or measured in a study. Extraneous variables exist in all studies and can affect the measurement of the study variables and examination of the relationships within a study. Attribute variables are characteristics or elements of the human subject that are collected to describe the sample. The major variables in a study are operationalized by developing conceptual and operational definitions. Conceptual definition is the broad, abstract meaning of a concept. Operational definition is derived from a set of procedures or progressive acts that a researcher performs to receive sensory impressions that indicate the existence or degree of existence of a variable.

References

Aamodt, A. M. (1983). Problems in doing nursing research: developing a criteria for evaluating qualitative research. *Western Journal of Nursing Research*, 5(4), 398–402.

Armstrong, R. L. (1981). Hypothesis formulation. In S. D. Krampitz & N. Pavlovich (Eds.), *Readings for nursing research* (pp. 29-39). St. Louis: The C. V. Mosby Company.

Beck, C. T. (1983). Parturients' temporal experiences during the phases of labor. *Western Journal of Nursing Research*, 5(4), 283–300.

Benoliel, Q. (1984). Advancing nursing science: qualitative approaches. *Western Journal of Nursing Research*, 6(3), 1–8.

Beveridge, W. B. (1950). *The art of scientific investigation*. New York: Vintage Books, A Division of Random House.

Brown, J. S., Tanner, C. A. & Padrick, K. P. (1984). Nursing's search for scientific knowledge. *Nursing Research*, 33(1), 26–32.

Carrieri, V., Stotts, N., Murdaugh, C., Levinson, J. & Holzemer, W. L. (1982). The use of cardiopulmonary assessment skills in the clinical setting. *Western Journal of Nursing Research*, 4(1), 5–17.

Chinn, P. L. & Jacobs, M. K. (1983). *Theory and nursing: a systematic approach*. St. Louis: The C. V. Mosby Company.

Fagerhaugh, S. Y. & Strauss, A. (1977). *Politics of pain management*. Menlo Park, California: Addison-Wesley Publishing Company.

Faherty, B. S. & Grier, M. R. (1984). Analgesic medication for elderly people post-surgery. *Nursing Research*, 33(6), 369–372.

Foxall, M. J., Ekberg, J. Y. & Griffith, N. (1985). Adjustment patterns of chronically ill middle-aged persons and spouses. *Western Journal of Nursing Research*, 7(4), 425–444.

Heidt, P. (1981). Effect of therapeutic touch on anxiety level of hospitalized patients. *Nursing Research*, 30(1), 32–37.

Itano, J., Tanabe, P., Lum, J. L. J., Lamkin, L., Rizzo, E., Wieland, M. & Sato, P. (1983). Compliance of cancer patients to therapy. *Western Journal of Nursing Research*, 5(1), 5–16.

Kaplan, A. (1964). *The conduct of inquiry: methodology for behavioral science*. New York: Harper & Row, Publishers.

Kerlinger, F. N. (1973). *Foundations of behavioral research* (2nd. Ed.). New York: Holt, Rinehart and Winston.

Koniak, D. (1985). Autotutorial and lecture-demonstration instruction: a comparative analysis of the effects upon students' learning of a developmental assessment skill. *Western Journal of Nursing Research*, 7(1), 80–100.

Krampitz, S. D. (1983). Historical development of baccalaureate nursing education in the American university: 1899-1935. *Western Journal of Nursing Research*, 5(4), 371–380.

Lim-Levy, F. (1982). The effect of oxygen inhalation on oral temperature. *Nursing Research*, 31(3), 150–152.

McKeever, P. & Galloway, S. C. (1984). Effects of nongynecological surgery on the menstrual cycle. *Nursing Research*, 33(1), 42–46.

Miller, P. Sr., Wikoff, R. L., McMahon, M., Garrett, M. J. & Ringel, K. (1985). Indicators of medical regimen adherence for myocardial infarction patients. *Nursing Research*, 34(5), 268–272.

Murdaugh, C. & Hinshaw, A. S. (1986). Theoretical model testing to identify personality variables affecting preventive behaviors. *Nursing Research*, 35(1), 19–23.

Newman, M. (1979). *Theory development in nursing*. Philadelphia: F. A. Davis Company.

Orem, D. E. (1985). *Nursing: concepts of practice* (3rd Ed.). New York: McGraw-Hill Book Company.

Reynolds, P. D. (1971). *A primer in theory construction*. Indianapolis: The Bobbs-Merrill Company, Inc.

Rice, V. H. & Johnson, J. E. (1984). Preadmission self-instruction booklets, postadmission exercise performance, and teaching time. *Nursing Research*, 33(3), 147–151.

Roberts, F. B. (1983). Infant behavior and the transition to parenthood. *Nursing Research*, 32(4), 213–217.

Rudy, E. B. & Estok, P. J. (1983). Intensity of jogging: its relationship to selected physical and psychosocial variables in women. *Western Journal of Nursing Research*, 5(4), 325–336.

Tripp-Reimer, T. (1983). Retention of a folk-healing practice (matiasma) among four generations of urban Greek immigrants. *Nursing Research*, 32(2), 97–101.

Weaver, R. H. & Cranley, M. S. (1983). An exploration of paternal-fetal attachment behavior. *Nursing Research*, 32(2), 68–72.

9

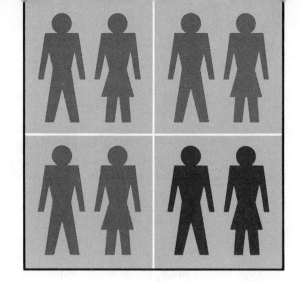

SAMPLING

One tends to enter the field of research with preconceived notions about samples and sampling, many of which are acquired through television advertisements, polls of public opinion, market researchers in shopping centers and newspaper reports of research findings. The commercial boasts that four of five doctors recommend their product; the newscaster announces that John Jones is predicted to win the senate election by a margin of 3 to 1; the newspaper reports that scientists have now shown that treatment of early breast cancer with lumpectomy and radiation is as effective as mastectomy.

All of the aforementioned examples use sampling techniques. However, some of the outcomes are more valid than others. The differences in validity are due, in part, to the sampling techniques used. In most instances, television, newspapers and advertisements do not explain their sampling techniques. We may hold certain opinions about the adequacy of their techniques, but there is inadequate information from which to make a judgment.

In research, it is critical that the sampling component of the research process be carefully thought out and clearly described. This requires knowledge of the techniques of sampling and the reasoning behind it. This chapter examines sampling theory, sampling plans, sample size, the process of acquiring a sample and the implications it has for nursing research.

Sampling Theory

Sampling involves selecting a group of people, events, behaviors or other elements with which to conduct a study. *Sampling* defines the process of making

205

the selections; *sample* defines the selected group of elements. Decisions made related to sampling have a major impact on the meaning that can be applied to the findings.

Sampling theory was developed to mathematically determine the most effective way of acquiring a sample that would accurately reflect the population under study. Many sampling techniques have been developed and refined by researchers conducting surveys. The theoretical mathematical rationale for decisions related to sampling was derived from the experiences of these researchers. One of the most important surveys that stimulated improvements in survey techniques was the national census.

The assumptions of sampling theory have been adopted by researchers and incorporated within the logic of the research process. Researchers need to know these assumptions and understand the rationale behind them. In this section, key concepts of sampling theory are focused upon, and the assumptions within the theory are discussed. With this knowledge, one can make more intelligent decisions about sampling.

SAMPLING CONCEPTS

Many of the terms used in relation to sampling were developed by survey researchers. Familiarity with these terms provides a basis for understanding the logic of sampling theory. Many of the terms are common ones, but they have special meanings within sampling theory. The concepts examined include target population, elements of the population, sampling frame, accessible population, representativeness, randomization, statistics, parameters, precision, sampling errors and systematic bias.

Target Population and Elements of the Population

The first step of the sampling process is the identification of the population from which the sample will be drawn. This population is identified to some extent in the problem and purpose statements and the research subproblems. However, at this point in the research process, the description of the population requires clarification and refinement. The *population* is the entire set of individuals or elements defined by the sampling criteria established for the study. The sample is then chosen from the study population, which is commonly referred to as the *target population*. The findings are generalized to the target population. Generalizing means that the findings are expected to describe not only the sample but also the target population from which the sample was taken.

The individual units of a population are called *elements*. An element can be a person, event, behavior or any other single measurement unit of a study. When elements are persons, they are referred to as subjects.

Randomization

From a sampling theory point of view, the sample should be randomly selected from the target population, with each individual in the population having equal opportunity to be selected for the sample. This equal opportunity is referred to as *randomization*. The purpose of randomization is to ensure that the sample is representative of the target population. Methods of achieving randomization are described later in the chapter.

Sampling Frame and Accessible Population

In order for each person in the target population to have an opportunity for selection in the sample, each person in the population must be identified. To accomplish this, a listing of every member of the target population must be acquired, using the sample criteria to define membership. This listing is referred to as the *sampling frame*. A sampling frame could be extremely large if the target population was national or international.

Randomly selecting subjects from a target population is an ideal. Realistically, time and cost factors limit the possibilities of achieving this ideal. Because of this difficulty, an accessible population has also been defined. An *accessible population* is the portion of the target population to which the researcher has reasonable access. The accessible population might be elements within a state, city, hospital or nursing unit. In this case, the sample is obtained from the accessible population, and findings are generalized first to the accessible population and then, more abstractly, to the target population.

Representativeness and Randomization

Whether the sample is derived from the target population or the accessible population, representativeness is extremely important. *Representativeness* means that the sample must be like the population in as many ways as possible. The sample must be representative in relation to the variables being examined in the study and other factors that may influence the study variables. For example, if the study examined attitudes toward X, the sample should be representative of the distribution of attitudes toward X that exists in the population. In addition, a sample needs to be representative of such character-istics as age, gender, ethnicity, income and education, which often influence study variables. The most effective way to achieve representativeness is ran-domization.

Statistics, Parameters and Precision

Representativeness is usually evaluated by comparing sample means with target population means. A measure or numerical value of a sample is called a *statistic*. A measure or numerical value of a population is called a *parameter*. The accuracy with which the population parameters have been estimated within a study is referred to as precision. Precision is extremely important in increasing control in certain quantitative studies. For example, studies of the effect of drugs on human beings require a high degree of precision.

Sampling Error

The difference between a sample statistic and a population parameter is called the *sampling error* (Fig. 9–1). A large sampling error means that the sample is

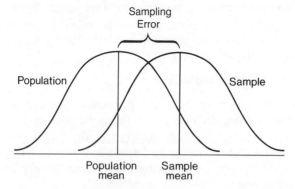

FIGURE 9–1. Sampling error.

not providing an accurate picture of the population; it is not representative. The sampling error is usually larger with small samples and decreases as the sample size increases. Thus, a large sample is usually more representative than a small sample.

The greatest risk of sampling error occurs in situations in which the parameters of a population are not known, because the extent of the sampling error is not known. Suppose that a study examined hope in the cancer patient and the researcher did not know how much hope most cancer patients felt. In this case, it would not be possible to determine whether the sample's mean score was lower or higher than the mean hope score of the population of cancer patients.

Systematic Bias

Sampling error may be due to random variation in scores of subjects from a population or may be due to systematic variation. *Random variation* is the expected difference that occurs when one examines different subjects from the same population. The difference is random because the score of each subject is likely to vary in a different direction. Thus, the scores will be randomly scattered around the mean. Some scores will be higher and others will be lower than the population mean.

Systematic variance, or systematic bias, is a consequence of selecting subjects whose scores are different, or vary, in some specific way from the population at large. Because the subjects have something in common, their scores tend to be similar. The scores do not vary randomly around the population mean. The variation from the mean is all in the same direction; it is systematic. All the scores may tend to be higher or lower than the mean. Because of systematic variance, the sample mean is different from the population mean. The extent of the difference is the sampling error. If a sample has systematic bias, increasing the sample size will not decrease the sampling error.

When the intent of a study is to examine the influence of a treatment on the experimental group's scores, the researcher will compare the experimental group's scores to the population mean. When the sample mean is different from the population mean, the researcher might think that the treatment has made a difference when, in actuality, the scores would be different even without the treatment. The differences are due to systematic bias as a consequence of sampling techniques. Systematic variation is most likely to occur when the sampling process is not completely random.

Sampling Plan

A sampling plan is developed to increase representativeness, decrease systematic bias and decrease the sampling error. To accomplish this task, sampling theory has devised strategies that optimize sample selection. These strategies increase precision and confidence in the statistical measures of the sample. There are two main types of sampling plans: probability sampling and non-probability sampling.

PROBABILITY SAMPLING

Probability sampling plans have been developed to ensure some degree of precision in accurately estimating the population parameters. Thus, probability samples reduce sampling error. Probability sampling is also referred to as random sampling. The term *probability sample* refers to the fact that *every* member (element) of the population has a probability higher than zero of being selected for the sample. Inferential statistical analyses are based on the assumption that the sample from which data were derived have been obtained randomly. Such a sample is more likely to be representative. All the subsets of the population, which may differ from each other but contribute to the parameters of the population, have a chance to be represented in the sample. There is no opportunity for systematic bias in the selection of subjects. For example, the researcher cannot decide that person X will be a better subject for the study than person Y. In addition, researchers cannot exclude a subset of people from being selected as subjects because they do not agree with them, do not like them or find them hard to deal with. Random sampling leaves the selection to chance.

To obtain a probability sample, the researcher must know every element in the population. A sampling frame must be developed, and the sample must be randomly selected from the sampling frame. Thus, it is not possible to randomly select a sample from a population that cannot be clearly defined. Five sampling designs have been developed to achieve probability sampling: simple random sampling, stratified random sampling, cluster sampling, systematic sampling and random assignment.

Simple Random Sampling

Simple random sampling is the most basic of the probability sampling plans. To achieve simple random sampling, elements are selected at random from the sampling frame. This can be accomplished in a variety of ways, limited only by the imagination of the researcher. If the sampling frame is small, names can be written on slips of paper, placed in a container, mixed well and then drawn out one at a time until the desired sample size has been reached. Each name in the sampling frame can be assigned a number. In large population sets, elements may already have assigned numbers. For example, numbers are assigned to medical records, organizational memberships and licenses. Numbers then are selected randomly to obtain a sample.

There are some differences in the probability for the selection of each element, depending on whether the selected element's name or number is replaced before the next name or number is selected. Selection with replacement, the most conservative random sampling approach, provides exactly equal opportunities for each element to be selected. For example, if the researcher draws names out of a hat to obtain a sample, each name must be replaced prior to drawing the next name to ensure equal opportunities for each subject. Selection without replacement gives each element differing levels of probability of selection. For example, if the researcher is selecting 10 subjects from a population of 50, the first name has a 1 in 5 chance, or a 0.2 probability, of being selected. If the first name is not replaced, the second name has a 9 in 49 chance, or a 0.18 probability, of being selected. As further names are drawn, the probability of being selected decreases.

There are many ways of achieving random selection. For example, a computer, bingo wheel or roulette wheel could be used. The most common method of random selection is a table of random numbers. A section from a random numbers table is presented in Table 9–1. To use a table of random numbers, a pencil or the finger is placed on the random table with the eyes closed. That is the starting place. Then moving up, down, right or left, numbers are used in order until the desired sample size is obtained.

Using the table of random numbers in Table 9–1, if the pencil were initially placed on 58, which is the 4th column across from the left and 4th row down, if five subjects were to be selected from a population of 100, and a decision was made to go across the column to the right, the subject numbers would be 58, 25, 15, 55, 38. This table is only useful if the population number is less than 100. However, tables are available for larger populations. A larger random numbers table is available in Appendix A. With very large populations in which the sampling frame has been computerized, the simplest approach is to write a computer program to randomly select subjects.

Riffee (1981) used a simple randomized sample in her study of "Self-esteem changes in hospitalized school-age children." Riffee describes her sample selection as follows:

> Two groups of hospitalized subjects and one group of nonhospitalized subjects were randomly selected. Potential hospitalized subjects were identified from the

TABLE 9–1
Section From a Random Numbers Table

06	84	10	22	56	72	25	70	69	43
07	63	10	34	66	39	54	02	33	85
03	19	63	93	72	52	13	30	44	40
77	32	69	58	25	15	55	38	19	62
20	01	94	54	66	88	43	91	34	28

daily lists of scheduled admissions to a 220-bed university-affiliated pediatric hospital in a large midwestern city. Subjects in the nonhospitalized group were identified from class lists of an elementary school in a neighboring community.

To be eligible for subject selection, the child had to: be 9 through 12 years 11 months of age; have not been hospitalized during the year prior to participation in this investigation; have no disability or terminal illness; and have experienced no family crisis during the one-month interval between two data collection sessions...

Meeting the stated criteria were 26 surgical, 25 nonsurgical, and 28 nonhospitalized subjects. Originally, a total of 95 subjects responded. Seven were excluded because their pets died during the one-month interval between data-collection sessions, and five were excluded because a family member was hospitalized during the one-month interval. Two in the nonhospitalized group were excluded because they were absent on the second data-collection day, and two were excluded because their lie scores were greater than five. (pp. 94–95)

Stratified Random Sampling

Stratified random sampling is used in situations in which the researcher knows some of the variables in the population that are critical to achieving representativeness. The variables used to stratify should be correlated with the variables being examined in the study. In order for stratification to be effective, the stratified layers of the sample must be more "homogeneous" in relation to the variable used for stratification than the population as a whole. This means that their scores on the variables being examined will be more alike than the scores of subjects in the population as a whole. Variables commonly used for stratification include age, gender, race, socioeconomic status, diagnosis, geographic region, type of institution, type of care and site of care. In stratified random sampling, the sample is divided into strata using the identified variables. The population is then classified into these strata, and samples of each strata are randomly selected. One problem with stratification is that in order to stratify the sample, the researcher must have sufficient knowledge of the population to select appropriate parameters by which to stratify.

Stratification ensures that all levels of the identified variables will be adequately represented in the sample. Stratification allows the researcher to use a smaller sample size and achieve the same degree of representativeness as a large sample acquired through simple random sampling. Smaller samples usually decrease the cost of the study. If the same sample size is used as would be used for a simple random sample, precision is increased and sampling error is decreased.

One question that arises in relation to stratification is whether each stratum should have equivalent numbers of subjects in the sample (disproportionate sampling) or whether the numbers of subjects should be selected in proportion to their occurrence in the population (proportionate sampling). For example, if stratification were being achieved by ethnicity and the population was 60 per cent Caucasian, 20 per cent Black, 15 per cent Mexican–American and 5 per cent Oriental, the researcher would have to decide whether to select equal numbers of each ethnic group or calculate a proportion of the sample. There are good arguments for both approaches. The stratification is not as useful if one stratum contains only a small number of subjects. In the above situation, if proportions are used and the sample size is 50, the study would only include 2 Orientals, hardly enough to be representative. If equal numbers of each group are used, each group will contain at least 12 subjects; however, the Caucasian group will be underrepresented. In this case, mathematically "weighting" the findings from each stratum can equalize the representation to ensure proportional contributions of each stratum to the total score of the sample.

Norbeck (1981) used stratified random sampling in her study "Young children's ability to conserve facial identity when facial emotion varies." The subjects were stratified by age and gender. The following is her description of her sample.

> The subjects were 60 middle-class, Caucasian children ages 3 years, zero months, to 5 years, 11 months. Ten boys and ten girls were tested at each age level (3 years, 4 years, 5 years). The mean age for each group was 5.5 months beyond the year, and the range, 10 to 11 months. Children with previously identified perceptual, learning, or emotional handicaps were not included.
>
> Consent forms were sent home with each child from urban and suburban nursery school and kindergarten classes. Names were drawn randomly from the returned forms until each age group was filled for each sex. Children were asked whether they wanted to participate: four refused, one began but did not complete testing. (p. 330)

Cluster Sampling

Cluster sampling is used in two situations. The first situation is when a simple random sample would be prohibitive in terms of travel time and cost. Imagine trying to make personal contacts with 100 people, each in a different part of the United States. The second situation is in cases in which the individual elements making up the population are not known, thus preventing the development of a sampling frame. For example, there is no list of all the open–heart surgery patients in the United States. In these cases, it is often possible to obtain lists of institutions or organizations with which the elements of interest are associated.

In *cluster sampling*, a sampling frame is developed that includes a list of all the states, cities, institutions or organizations with which elements of the identified population would be linked. A randomized sample of these states, cities, institutions or organizations would then be used in the study. In some cases, this randomized selection continues through several stages and is then referred to as multistage sampling. For example, the researcher might first randomly select states, then randomly select cities within the sampled states. Then hospitals within the randomly selected cities might be randomly selected. Within the hospitals, nursing units might be randomly selected. At this level, all the patients on the nursing unit who fit the criteria for the study might be included, or patients could be randomly selected.

Cluster sampling provides a means for obtaining a larger sample at a lower cost. However, there are some disadvantages. Data from subjects associated with the same institution are likely to be correlated and, thus, not completely independent. This can lead to a decrease in precision and an increase in sampling error. However, these disadvantages can be offset by a larger sample. Appropriate statistical analysis of the data is also more complicated in cluster sampling. Nonetheless, the design is frequently used by survey researchers.

Kirchhoff and Kviz (1981) used cluster sampling in their study: "A strategy for surveying nursing practice in institutional settings." They described their sampling technique as follows.

A national survey of critical-care nurses practicing in acute medical-surgical hospitals was conducted during the winter and spring of 1979 with the purpose of assessing the frequency and perceived importance of performing certain coronary-care nursing practices generally known as coronary precautions.

Sample

First Stage □ Criteria for inclusion in the population of institutions were: (a) accreditation by the Joint Commission on the Accreditation of Hospitals, (b) designation as an acute medical-surgical hospital, and (c) presence of an intensive or coronary-care unit (ICU/CCU). Although the focus of the study was on coronary care, ICUs were included as well as CCUs because many large hospitals combine coronary-care patients with other critically ill medical patients in an ICU.

An up-to-date, computer-generated list of hospitals that satisfied the criteria for inclusion in the study was obtained from the American Hospital Association (AHA). This list contained 3,864 hospitals arranged according to bed capacity. The hospitals were then grouped into six strata according to size (number of beds): less than 100, 100 to 199, 200 to 299, 300 to 399, 400 to 499, and 500 or more. Hospitals with less than 100 beds comprised approximately 25% of the population; hospitals with 100 to 199 beds, approximately 30%; and the four strata containing the largest hospitals comprised approximately 45% when combined. This meant that either a simple random sample or a proportional, stratified sample selected from the AHA list would have yielded a relatively large number of small hospitals but insufficient numbers of larger hospitals for the analysis. The selection of few large hospitals was of particular concern because the variance observed between larger institutions tends to be large. Variance within a stratum can be reduced by increasing the sample size within the stratum. Therefore, we decided to select an equal number of hospitals from each of the six strata.

Sudman recommended 200 as the minimum sample size for a national sample of institutions. To obtain a final sample of 200 institutions, assuming a cooperation rate of 87.5% (obtained in a pilot study), we estimated that approximately 230 institutions would have to be selected in the sample. Therefore, 40 hospitals were selected from each stratum for a total sample of 240 hospitals.

Five of the selected hospitals, however, were considered ineligible for inclusion in the study because it was learned during data collection that they had recently closed their ICU/CCUs. These ineligible hospitals were from the two strata containing the smallest hospitals (three from the less-than-100-beds stratum and two from the 100-to-199-beds stratum). Thus, the final sample consisted of 235 eligible hospitals, distributed across 42 states and two U.S. territories (one in Guam and two in Puerto Rico).

Second Stage □ A list of critical-care nurses practicing at each hospital selected in the first stage of sampling was requested from the head nurse of each ICU/CCU. The criteria for inclusion in the list of staff nurses were: (a) registered nurse with at least one year of experience in the unit, (b) at least 75% of the nurse's time must be spent in providing patient care, (c) full-time employment at the hospital, and (d) assignment to the day or evening shift. The first three criteria were included to ensure familiarity with unit practices; the fourth criterion was included because the practices to be assessed in the survey occur primarily on the day and evening shifts. However, these criteria were relaxed to include night shift and part-time nurses at 25 hospitals because less than two eligible staff nurses were listed.

A list of staff nurses was obtained from 202 (86%) of the 235 eligible hospitals. The second-stage sampling design called for the random selection of two staff nurses from each hospital. This would have yielded a sample of 404 staff nurses. But four hospitals listed only one staff nurse. Additionally, five staff-nurse questionnaires were returned because the nurses were no longer employed in the ICU/CCU or at that hospital by the time the questionnaires were mailed. A replacement was selected for the latter group from the list of remaining eligible staff nurses for all but one hospital where no replacement was available. Therefore, the final sample consisted of 399 staff nurses.

The head nurse of each unit was also included in the sample so that comparisons could be made between responses obtained from staff and head nurses. Because there was no head nurse in the ICU/CCU at one hospital, the head-nurse sample consisted of 201 head nurses. The total number of nurses contacted was 600. (pp. 310–311)

Systematic Sampling

Systematic sampling can be conducted when an ordered list of all members of the population is available. The process involves selecting every kth individual on the list, using a starting point selected randomly. If the initial starting point is not random, it is not a probability sample.

In order to use this design, the researcher must know the number of elements in the population and the size of the sample desired. The population size is divided by the desired sample size, giving "k," the size of the gap between elements selected from the list. For example, if the population size was $N = 1242$ and the desired sample size was $n = 50$, then $k = 24$. Every 24th person on the list would be included in the sample. There is argument that this procedure does not truly give each element an opportunity to be included in the sample, certainly not an equal chance.

Care must be taken to determine that the original list has not been set up with any ordering that could be meaningful in relation to the study. The assumption is being made that the order of the list is random in relation to the variables being studied. If the order of the list is related to the study, it would introduce a systematic bias. In addition to this risk, computation of the sampling error using this design is difficult.

Random Assignment

Random assignment is used in studies in which several groups, such as experimental and control or comparison groups, will be involved. Subjects selected for the study are randomly assigned to the treatment or control groups. In some cases, but not all, the group itself has been randomly selected. If the original group was selected randomly, the findings can be generalized to the population from which the original sample was derived. In other situations, the original sample was not selected by random means, and some investigators question referring to this as a randomized method. However, Kerlinger (1973), usually conservative, classifies this as a probability sample in spite of the initial lack of randomization.

According to sampling theory, if the original sample was not randomized, the population to which the findings can be generalized must be considered the sample itself. In many of these cases, as Kerlinger points out, the researcher is not attempting to estimate parameters of the population, but rather to examine interactions of variables, cause and effect, with an eye toward prediction and control. The researcher is using a specific population as one instance of the occurrence of the phenomenon under study. Random assignment without random selection lacks the strength of full randomization. If the sample from which the random assignment to groups is made is biased, the groups will be biased.

Ziemer (1983) used random assignment in her study on the "Effects of information on postsurgical coping." She describes her sample as follows.

> Patients' names were obtained from operating room schedules the evening before surgery and each patient was contacted by a registered nurse research assistant, who asked patients to participate in a study designed to explore patients' responses to surgery. If they agreed, they signed an informed consent and were provided with a tape-recorded message corresponding to a randomly assigned information condition. (p. 283)

NONPROBABILITY SAMPLING

In *nonprobability sampling*, not every element of the population has an opportunity for selection in the sample. There is no sampling frame. The parameters of the population may not be known. In fact, in many cases, there is no clearly identified population. In some cases, a hypothetical population is defined. A hypothetical population assumes the presence of a population that cannot be defined by traditional means. For example, individuals who successfully lose weight would be a hypothetical population. The number of individuals in the population, who they are, how much weight they have lost, how long they have kept it off or how they achieved the weight loss is unknown. In some studies, the population is not identified until the study is completed.

This may seem like poor science. However, there are many areas in which there has not been sufficient theory and research to clearly define populations. In other areas, the population is elusive and constantly changing. For example, listing all women in active labor in the United States would not be possible. Defining a population of people experiencing a grief reaction to the loss of a loved one would also be impossible. These individuals are not members of a common organization and are not being cared for by an institution. How does one define the population of people coming into an emergency room? These are hypothetical populations.

In other situations, institutions or circumstances will not allow random selection of subjects because of the possible disruption. In some cases, the number of subjects may be too small for randomization, or randomization may be too costly. And yet it is critical that there be acceptable ways to collect samples in these circumstances. Actually, most nursing studies use nonprobability sampling. In the past, they have simply been viewed as inferior in design. But are they? Does this sampling method simply serve a different purpose? Some studies are not designed to generalize to a population. The variables, not the subject, are the primary area of concern. The pattern in studies using nonprobability sampling is often to examine the same variables in several studies with differing populations. The specific population used may be incidental.

There are several types of nonprobability sampling designs. Each addresses a different research need. The four nonprobability designs included are accidental sampling, quota sampling, purposive sampling and network sampling.

Accidental Sampling

Accidental sampling is sometimes called *convenience sampling* or *incidental sampling*. In accidental sampling, subjects are included in the study because they happened to be in the right place at the right time. Available subjects are simply entered into the study until the desired sample size is reached. Multiple biases may be in action in the sample, some of which may be subtle and unrecognized. However, serious biases are not always present in accidental samples. The researcher should identify and describe known biases in the sample. Biases that tend to be present in this type of sample include subjects who are different because they have chosen to enter a treatment program. For example, obese individuals who chose to enter a program to lose weight may differ from those who did not enter a program. Those who have volunteered to participate in a study may differ from those not interested. Studies conducted in private hospitals usually exclude the poor. Other settings could exclude the elderly or the undereducated. Subjects in research centers and the care they receive are different from patients in community hospitals, public hospitals or veteran hospitals. Uncooperative or noncompliant patients who are not as likely to be included in an accidental sample are different from cooperative, compliant patients.

The circumstance of sample selection should be carefully described to allow others to identify possible biases. In addition, as much data as possible should be collected about the sample. These data can be used to compare the sample with other populations and are useful in developing parameters of populations not previously studied.

There are many strategies for selecting an accidental sample. A classroom of students might be used. Patients who attend a clinic on a specific day, subjects who attend a support group, patients currently admitted to a hospital with a specific diagnosis or nursing problem and every fifth person who enters the emergency room are examples of types of frequently selected accidental samples.

Accidental samples are inexpensive, accessible and usually require less time to acquire. They provide means to conduct studies on topics that could not be examined at all using probability sampling. They provide means to acquire information in unexplored areas. As Kerlinger stated (1973): "used with reasonable knowledge and care, it (accidental sampling) is probably not as bad as it has been said to be" (p. 129). Kerlinger does recommend using this type of sampling only if the possibility of obtaining any other type is not available. Riesch and Munns (1984) used accidental sampling in their study "Promoting awareness: the mother and her baby." The following is a description of their sample selection.

> All women who delivered their neonates without complication at two university-affiliated urban medical centers in a midwestern city during the study period were eligible for the term study. Sample criteria excluded high-risk or ill mothers and infants. Thus mothers with chronic diseases, teen mothers (aged 17 years and under), or mothers who required a cesarean birth were excluded. Although 169 mother-infant dyads met the criteria during the study period and agreed to participate, only 108 formed the study sample. Most potential subjects were lost due to early discharge, unforeseen complications such as phototherapy or feeding problems, and scheduling mishaps between the investigators and subjects. (p. 272)

Quota Sampling

Quota sampling uses an accidental sampling technique with an added feature, a strategy to ensure the inclusion of subject types that are likely to be underrepresented in the accidental sample. Subgroups likely to be underrepresented include females, minority groups, the aged, the poor, the rich and the undereducated. In each study, the researcher needs to examine their sample for possible underrepresented subgroups.

The goal of quota sampling is to replicate the proportions of subgroups present in the population to which the researcher desires to generalize the findings. The technique is similar to that used in stratified random sampling. If necessary, mathematical weighting can be used to adjust sample values so that they are in keeping with the proportion of subgroups found in the population of interest. Mathematical weighting is described in Chapter 17. Quota sampling offers an improvement over accidental sampling and tends to decrease the biases that can occur. In most cases in which accidental samples are used, quota sampling could be used and should be considered.

Murphy (1984) used quota sampling in her study "Stress levels and health status of victims of a natural disaster." Her study also demonstrates network sampling, described in this chapter. She described her sample selection as follows.

> Subjects were needed to represent each of the five magnitudes of loss: (a) presumed death bereavement, (b) confirmed death bereavement, (c) loss of a permanent residence, (d) loss of a leisure residence, and (e) no disaster-related loss. It was expected that adequate samples for both types of property loss and control subjects could be obtained, but obtaining representative bereaved samples of adequate size was a potential problem for several reasons. First, there was a finite population from which to select. Of the 60 persons reported dead or missing, 31 adults were presumed dead while 20 adults were confirmed dead. The remaining 9 persons were either children or adults whose next of kin did not apply for provisional death certificates. Next, death certificates were unavailable for the 31 presumed dead, making it difficult to contact next of kin. As a result, a unique sampling plan was developed.
>
> For both the presumed and confirmed bereaved groups, a close relative and a close friend who enjoyed a central relationship with the deceased victim was selected... Of the 62 potential subjects for the presumed group of bereaved 45 (73%) were contacted, and 39 (87%) of those contacted participated. Of the 40 potential subjects from the confirmed dead bereaved group, 36 (90%) were contacted and 30 (83%) of those contacted participated. The permanent property loss group consisted of 21 persons or 54% of 39 persons contacted whose residences were destroyed. Potential subject names were randomly selected from local telephone listings because tax assessment records were not available. The recreational property loss group consisted of 15 persons or 58% of persons randomly selected from a recreational home-owners list. Finally, a control group of 50 persons was selected. These persons had suffered no disaster-related loss but were similar to the 105 loss subjects in occupation, age, sex and geographic location. The total number of subjects, then, was 155. (pp. 206–207)

Purposive Sampling

Purposive sampling is sometimes referred to as judgmental sampling. Purposive sampling involves the conscious selection by the researcher of certain subjects or elements to include in the study. Efforts might be made to include "typical" subjects or typical situations. Examples of good care and poor care, good patients and bad patients might be used. This approach is often used in qualitative studies. The strategy has been criticized because there is no way to evaluate the precision of the researcher's judgment. How does one determine that the patient or element was typical, good, bad, effective or ineffective? However, this sampling method may be a way to get some beginning ideas about an area not easily examined using other sampling techniques.

Forsyth, Delaney and Gresham (1984) used purposive sampling in a study entitled "Vying for a winning position: management style of the chronically ill." Their description of sample selection is as follows.

Initially, chronically ill patients presenting a wide range of diseases were interviewed at a large midwestern teaching medical center hospital. Early analysis revealed substantial differences related to the nature of the illness. Differentiation between patients commonly called chronically ill thus was necessary. Final criteria for subjects limited inclusion to those with a progressive chronic disease which could not be controlled with medication or diet, who faced an ambiguous disease process involving considerable intrusion, and which held the threat of progression to greater levels of distress. Persons with multiple sclerosis, arthritis, Parkinsonism, chronic obstructive pulmonary disease (COPD) and varied neurological diseases (amyotrophic lateral sclerosis and fibrocitis) became the subjects. By design, respondents had various characteristics of age (29 to 85), sex, ethnicity, economic status, and education. In 8 months 50 patients were interviewed: 30 in the medical center and 20 in two community hospitals. Those interviewed had similar histories representing both early and long-standing illness as well as first-time and multiple hospitalizations for diagnosed chronic illness. (p. 182)

Network Sampling

Network sampling, sometimes referred to as snowballing, holds promise for locating samples difficult or impossible to obtain in other ways. Network sampling takes advantage of social networks and the fact that friends tend to hold characteristics in common. When the researcher has found a few subjects with the needed criteria, they are asked for their assistance in getting in touch with others with similar characteristics. This strategy is particularly useful for finding subjects in socially devalued populations such as alcoholics, child abusers, sex offenders, drug addicts and criminals. These individuals are seldom willing to make themselves known to others. Other groups such as widows, grieving siblings, successful dieters or those successful at life style changes can be located using this strategy. These individuals are outside the existing health care system and are difficult to find. Obviously there are biases built into the sampling process, since the subjects are not independent of each other.

Sample Size

One of the most frequent questions asked by researchers is "What size sample should I use?" Unfortunately, there are no absolute answers to this question. There are so many qualifiers that, to some extent, the answer must be specific to the study. The most general rule is to make the sample as large as possible. Overall, large samples are better approximations of the target population than small samples. Sampling error decreases as sample size increases. The possibility of achieving statistical significance is greater with a large sample. However, practical restraints such as time, money and availability of potential subjects must enter into the decision. Factors that must be considered in making decisions about sample size include the type of study, the number of variables, the sensitivity of the measurement tools, the data analysis techniques and the expected effect size.

Type of Study

Exploratory studies, both qualitative and quantitative, and case studies tend to use very small samples. Known target populations with a sampling frame and known parameters do not usually exist for subjects selected for these studies. Problems related to sampling error and generalization have little relevance for these studies. A small sample size may better serve the researcher who is usually interested in examining the situation in depth from various perspectives.

Descriptive surveys and correlational studies often use large samples. In these studies, large numbers of variables may be examined, and extraneous variables are likely to affect subject response to the variables under study. In addition, subjects are likely to be heterogeneous in terms of demographic variables, and measurement tools are sometimes not adequately refined. Although target populations may have been identified, sampling frames may not be available, and parameters have not usually been well defined. Data from these studies may be used in the process of developing population parameters.

Quasi-experimental and experimental studies often use smaller samples than descriptive and correlational studies. As control in the study increases, the sample size can decrease and still approximate the population. Instruments in these studies tend to be more refined. In these studies, the researcher needs to conduct a power analysis to determine the sample size. Power analysis is discussed in the section entitled Expected Effect Size in this chapter.

Number of Variables

As the number of variables under study increases, the needed sample size increases. To determine sample size, it is helpful to develop a matrix of all variables included in the study. Each compartment in the matrix is called a *cell*. The minimum number of subjects for each cell category should be 5. No cell should be empty. Although the minimum number is 5, 10 or 20 per cell is more desirable and will provide much better information.

Gierszewski (1983) conducted a study of the relationship of weight loss, locus of control and social support. Weight loss was measured using a "reduction index (RI)," which was calculated mathematically. This is shown on the example matrix as high RI, medium RI and low RI. The locus of control tool was divided into three categories: internal, external/powerful others and external/chance. Social support was grouped into four categories: no support, minimal support, moderate support and a lot of support. The matrix shown in Table 9–2 indicates the needed sample size for this study.

In Table 9–2, there are four dimensions of one variable (Social Support) and three dimensions of two variables (RI and Locus of Control), which create a 36-cell matrix. When a sample of at least 5 subjects is placed in each cell, the total sample must be at least 180. Gierszewski's initial sample totaled 229. However, her sample mortality was high, and only 64 subjects completed the 6-month follow-up. Most of her findings did not reach statistical significance. Trends in some of the data were in opposite directions from the hypotheses. Reliability and validity were not well established for the measuring instruments, suggesting the possibility of a great deal of variance in measures. Possibly a larger sample or a sample with lower mortality would have provided a clearer picture of the dynamics in action in this situation.

TABLE 9–2
Matrix of Needed Sample Size

Social Support	RI High			RI Medium			RI Low		
	Locus of Control			*Locus of Control*			*Locus of Control*		
	I	*E/P*	*E/C*	*I*	*E/P*	*E/C*	*I*	*E/P*	*E/C*
No Support	5	5	5	5	5	5	5	5	5
Minimal Support	5	5	5	5	5	5	5	5	5
Moderate Support	5	5	5	5	5	5	5	5	5
A Lot of Support	5	5	5	5	5	5	5	5	5

I = Internal; E/P = External/Powerful Others; E/C = External/Chance;
RI = Reduction Index
Minimum total sample size = 180

Measurement Sensitivity

Well-developed instruments measure the phenomenon being examined with precision. A thermometer, for example, measures body temperature precisely. Tools measuring psychosocial variables tend to be less precise. However, a tool with strong reliability and validity tends to measure more precisely than a tool that is less well developed. Scores from less well-developed tools are likely to vary somewhere around the actual occurrence. In other words, the variance would be higher in a less well-developed tool than in one that is well developed. For example, if anxiety were being measured and the actual anxiety score of several subjects was 80, the subjects' scores on a less well-developed tool might range from 70 to 90, whereas a well-developed tool would tend to show a score closer to 80 for each subject. If scores vary from the actual situation, a larger sample size is needed to gain an accurate understanding of the phenomenon under study.

Data Analysis Techniques

Data analysis techniques vary in ability to detect differences in the data. Statisticians refer to this as the "power" of the statistical analysis. Overall, parametric statistical analyses are more powerful in detecting differences than are nonparametric techniques if the data meet criteria for parametric analysis. However, in many cases, nonparametric techniques are more powerful when a small sample has been used. There is a wide range of difference among the parametric techniques in their capacity to distinguish fine differences in the data. There is also an interaction between the measurement sensitivity and the power of the data analysis technique. Larger samples should be used when the power of the planned statistical analysis is weak. Parametric and nonparametric analyses are discussed in Chapter 17.

Expected Effect Size

In some studies, the treatment given to the experimental group is expected to make a large difference in scores. In other studies, the expected difference may be small but still meaningful. This is referred to as the *expected effect size*. The hypothesis is an expression of the effect expected within an experiment. The size of the effect influences the ability of statistical analyses to detect any real difference between groups. A large effect is easier to detect statistically than a small effect. The power of a statistical analysis is associated with the expected effect size as well as the sample size. Effect size is usually smaller with a small sample and is thus more difficult to detect. Increasing the sample size also increases the effect size, making it more likely that the effect will be detected and will be statistically significant.

Determining Sample Size By Power Analysis

Cohen (1977) has developed a mathematical technique called *power analysis* to determine needed sample size. The technique uses three parameters of the study: the significance level, the expected effect size and the desired level of power. Power is the capacity of a statistical test to reject a null hypothesis that is false. Cohen's (1977) book, *Statistical Power Analysis for the Behavioral Sciences*, contains formulas for calculating the effect size and tables for many types of statistical tests that show the needed sample size.

Using power analysis is not difficult and can provide a more rational way to determine sample size. In some cases, the researcher may decide not to conduct a study when the power analysis indicates that, because of the small available sample, the study is unlikely to detect significance that may be present. In many published studies, the researcher concludes that no significance exists. But, in truth, the sample was too small to have detected any significance that did occur. This is a Type II error. In the current stage of nursing theory development, a Type II error may have more serious consequences to understanding nursing phenomena than a Type I error (indicates a difference that does not exist). If a study does not have the power to detect a difference that exists, it should not be conducted. Type I errors, Type II errors and power analysis are discussed more completely in Chapter 17.

Acquiring and Retaining Subjects

Once a decision has been made about the size of the sample, the next step is to develop a plan for actually acquiring the sample. The sampling process is initiated at the beginning of data collection. This process is almost always more difficult than was expected. The problems encountered are usually associated with human interaction rather than with the sampling plan. In some cases, the problems involve the data collector rather than the subject. The effectiveness of acquiring subjects depends on the initial approach by the researcher. Retaining acquired subjects is critical to the study and requires consideration of the effects of data collection on subject mortality (loss of subjects).

Approaching Subjects

There are two aspects to the process of approaching subjects: (1) determining which subjects to approach, and (2) using effective interactive skills during the initial contact with a potential subject. The sampling plan should direct selection of subjects. If data collectors are being used in the study, the researcher should verify that they are following the sampling plan, especially in random samples. When the data collectors encounter difficult subjects or are unable to easily make contact, they may simply shift to the next person without informing the principal investigator. This behavior could violate the rules of random sampling and bias the sample. If the data collector does not understand or believe in the importance of randomization, there are multiple ways that their decisions and actions can undermine the intent of the sampling plan. Thus, data collectors should be carefully selected and thoroughly trained. A plan should be developed for the supervision and follow-up of the actions of data collectors, increasing their sense of accountability.

The initial approach to a potential subject usually strongly affects his or her decision about participating in the study. Therefore, the approach should be pleasant and positive. The importance of the study should be explained, and the researcher should make clear exactly what the subject will be asked to do, how much time will be involved for the subject and what the time range of the study will be. Subjects are extremely valuable resources. The recognition of this value should be communicated to the potential subject. High pressure techniques, such as insisting that the subject make an instant decision to participate in a study, usually lead to resistance and increased refusals. The researcher should accept refusals to participate gracefully—in terms of body language as well as words. The actions of the researcher can influence the decision of other potential subjects who are observing or who may hear about the encounter at a later time. Studies in which a high proportion of individuals refuse to participate have a serious validity problem. The sample is likely to be very biased because usually only a certain type of individual has agreed to participate. Therefore, records should be kept of the numbers of persons who refuse and, if possible, their reasons for refusal. The actual process of obtaining informed consent is discussed in Chapter 12.

RETAINING SUBJECTS

One of the serious problems in many studies is subject retention. Often, subject loss cannot be avoided. Subjects move, die or withdraw from treatment. However, if subjects have a personal investment in the study, they are more likely to continue. This investment occurs through interactional processes with the researcher. A combination of the subject's personal belief in the significance of the study and the nurturing of the subject during data collection by the researcher may diminish subject mortality.

The process of collecting data takes time. The researcher must always keep in mind that the subject's time is valuable and must be used frugally. During data collection, it is easy to begin taking the subject for granted. Taking time for social amenities with subjects may pay off. However, one must take care that these interactions do not influence the data being collected. Beyond that, nurturing subjects participating in the study is critical. In some situations, providing refreshments and pleasant surroundings is helpful. During the data collection phase, often there are others interacting with the subjects who also need to be nurtured. These may be volunteers, family, staff, students or other professionals. It is important to maintain a pleasant climate for the data collection process, which will pay off in the quality of data collected and the retention of subjects. Planning and implementing data collection are presented in Chapter 16.

Implications of Sampling Theory for Nursing Research

As mentioned earlier, sampling theory was developed for use in survey research. The purpose of the sampling techniques is to facilitate representativeness so that findings can justifiably be generalized to the target population. These techniques have been effective strategies for accomplishing the desired goals for survey research.

Sampling theory offers a strategy that can be successfully used in specific types of nursing studies to strengthen the significance of the findings. Current statistical analysis techniques have been developed based on the assumptions of sampling theory. Nurse researchers must wisely use this theory in ways that will facilitate the generation of knowledge for nursing practice.

However, one must question the appropriateness of sampling theory for all nursing research. Most nursing studies are not survey research as defined in sampling theory. To what extent is generalization a major goal of a single nursing study? Are conditions of randomization necessary in order to justify generalization? Is it necessary to have a clearly identified target population with a sampling frame to which one can generalize? Is true randomization possible in clinical nursing studies? These are important questions to consider, because a commitment to the randomization and target population tenets of sampling theory limit the phenomena of interest that can be studied in nursing.

It seems that sampling theory confronts nursing with a paradox. Sampling theory is both very important and not as important as some would propose. Researchers cannot rigidly adhere to sampling theory under all circumstances and cannot ignore the concerns expressed by the theory. Generalization of nursing research findings is important. In nursing, this will require the development of nursing science beyond its present stage.

Generalization occurs by inductive reasoning. First, findings are generalized from known samples to known populations. Then through inference, generalization moves from the known population to populations defined in theories. These generalizations occur in a present time frame and a future time frame. The present time frame makes broad inferences to theoretical populations. The future time frame moves from generalization to forecasting for populations that do not yet exist.

When generalization moves from the known to broad inferences and forecasting, it goes beyond the realms of sampling theory and generalizes from the findings to an abstract idea. This abstraction involves the use of intuition and abstract reasoning and is best done within the context of theory and theory development. Abstractions from the concrete findings of research can be easily examined for implications in a wide range of phenomena. Generalization in nursing must go beyond the concrete generalization that is proposed in sampling theory and move to abstract, theoretical generalization that can be understood and applied in multiple dimensions of nursing situations with many varied populations.

Summary

Sampling involves selecting a group of people, events, behaviors or other elements with which to conduct a study. Sampling defines the process of making the selections; sample defines the selected group of elements. Sampling theory was developed to mathematically determine the most effective way of acquiring a sample that would accurately reflect the population under study. Important concepts in sampling theory include target population, elements of the population, randomization, sampling frame, accessible population, representativeness, statistics, parameters, precision, sampling errors and systematic bias.

A sampling plan is developed to increase representativeness, decrease systematic bias and decrease the sampling error. There are two main types of sampling plans: probability sampling and nonprobability sampling. Probability sampling plans have been developed to ensure some degree of precision in accurately estimating the population parameters. Thus, probability samples reduce sampling error. To obtain a probability sample, the researcher must know every element in the population. A sampling frame must be developed and the sample randomly selected from the sampling frame. Five sampling designs have been developed to achieve probability sampling: simple random sampling, stratified random sampling, cluster sampling, systematic sampling and random assignment.

In nonprobability sampling, not every element of the population has an opportunity for selection in the sample. There is no sampling frame. There are several types of nonprobability sampling designs. Each addresses a different research need. Four nonprobability designs are included in this text: accidental sampling, quota sampling, purposive sampling and network sampling.

A major concern in conducting a study is determining the size of a sample. The most general rule is to make the sample as large as possible. Sampling error decreases as sample size increases. Factors that must be considered in making decisions about sample size include the type of study, the number of variables, the sensitivity of the measurement tools, the data analysis techniques and the expected effect size.

Another concern in conducting a study is acquiring and retaining subjects in a study. This process is almost always more difficult than was expected. The problems encountered are usually associated with human interaction rather than with the sampling plan. Acquiring subjects effectively depends on the initial approach by the researcher. Retaining acquired subjects is critical to the study and requires consideration of the effects of data collection on subject mortality.

References

Abdellah, F. G. & Levine, E. (1979). *Better patient care through nursing research*. New York: Macmillan Publishing Co., Inc.

Beck, C. T. (1984). Subject mortality: is it inevitable? *Western Journal of Nursing Research*, 6(3), 331–339.

Cochran, W. G. (1977). *Sampling techniques* (3rd ed.). New York: John Wiley & Sons.

Cohen, J. (1977). *Statistical power analysis for the behavioral sciences*. New York: Academic Press.

Deming, W. E. (1950). *Some theories of sampling*. New York: John Wiley & Sons.

Forsyth, G. L., Delaney, K. D. & Gresham, M. L. (1984). Vying for a winning position: management style of the chronically ill. *Research in Nursing and Health*, 7(3), 181–188.

Friday, F. A. (1967). *The elements of probability and sampling*. New York: Barnes & Noble.

Gierszewski, S. A. (1983). The relationship of weight loss, locus of control, and social support. *Nursing Research*, 32(1), 43–47.

Goodwin, L. D. (1984). The use of power estimation in nursing research. *Nursing Research*, 33(2), 118–120.

Hajek, J. & Dupac, V. (1981). *Sampling from a finite population*. New York: Marcel Dekker, Inc.

Hansen, M. H., Hurwitz, W. N. & Madow, W. G. (1953). *Sample survey methods and theory*. New York: John Wiley & Sons.

Kenneth, H. & Gortner, S. R. (1984). Researchmanship: some issues in gaining access to subject participants for clinical nursing research. *Western Journal of Nursing Research*, 6(2), 256–258.

Kerlinger, F. N. (1973). *Foundations of behavioral research* (2nd ed.). New York: Holt, Rinehart and Winston.

Kilpatrick, S. J. Jr. (1973). *Statistical principles in health care information*. Baltimore: University Park Press.

Kirchhoff, K. T. & Kviz, F. J. (1981). A strategy for surveying nursing practice in institutional settings. *Research in Nursing and Health*, 4(3), 309–315.

Levy, P. S. & Lemsbow, S. (1980). *Sampling for health professionals*. Belmont, California: Lifetime Learning Publications.

Murphy, S. A. (1984). Stress levels and health status of victims of a natural disaster. *Research in Nursing and Health*, 7(3), 205–215.

Neale, J. M. & Liebert, R. M. (1980) *Science and behavior: an introduction to methods of research* (2nd ed.). Englewood Cliffs, New Jersey: Prentice-Hall, Inc.

Norbeck, J. S. (1981). Young children's ability to conserve facial identity when facial emotion varies. *Nursing Research*, 30(6), 329–333.

Riesch, S. K. & Munns, S. K. (1984). Promoting awareness: the mother and her baby. *Nursing Research*, 33(5), 271–276.

Riffee, D. M. (1981). Self-esteem changes in hospitalized school-age children. *Nursing Research*, 30(2), 94–97.

Selltiz, C., Wrightsman, L. S. & Cook, S. W. (1976). *Research methods in social relations* (3rd ed.). New York: Holt, Rinehart and Winston.

Slonim, M. J. (1960). *Sampling: a quick, reliable guide to practical statistics*. New York: Simon and Schuster.

Tuckman, B. W. (1978). *Conducting educational research*. New York: Harcourt Brace Jovanovich, Inc.

Volicer, B. J. (1984). *Multivariate statistics for nursing research*. New York: Grune & Stratton, Inc.

Waltz, C. & Bausell, R. B. (1981). *Nursing research: design, statistics and computer analysis*. Philadelphia: F. A. Davis Company.

Williams, B. (1978). *A sampler on sampling*. New York: John Wiley & Sons.

Yates, F. (1981). *Sampling methods for censuses and surveys*. New York: Macmillan Publishing Company, Inc.

Ziemer, M. M. (1983). Effects of information on postsurgical coping. *Nursing Research*, 32(5), 282–287.

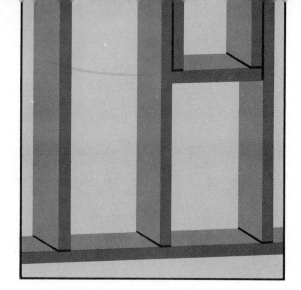

10

Selecting A Research Design

Selecting a research design involves following paths of logical reasoning. A calculating mind is needed to explore all the possible consequences of taking a particular action in design selection. In some ways, selecting a design is like thinking through the moves in a chess game. One must carefully think through the consequences of each option. The research design organizes all the components of the study in a way that is most likely to lead to valid answers to the subproblems that have been posed.

The following discussion of research design focuses on the purpose of design and links the design with the study's frame of reference and research plan. Selecting a design requires an understanding of certain concepts: causality, bias, manipulation, control and validity. The chapter concludes with a discussion of designs for nursing research, including designs for exploratory (quantitative and qualitative), descriptive, correlational, quasi-experimental and experimental studies.

What is a Research Design?

The term *research design* is used in two ways. Some consider research design to be the entire strategy for the study, from identifying the problem to final plans for data collection. Others limit design to clearly defined structural frameworks within which the study is implemented. In this text, the former is referred to as methodology and the latter as design. The design is the structural framework for a study. Design has been addressed in the literature primarily from the point of view of quantitative research.

PURPOSE

The research design directs the researcher in planning and implementing the study in a way is most likely to achieve the intended goal. Research design is a blueprint for the conduct of a study that maximizes control over factors that could interfere with the desired outcomes from studies. The control provided by the design increases the probability that the study results are telling us what we think they are telling us. Skill in selecting and implementing research design is important to improving the quality of the study and thus the usefulness of the findings.

RELATIONSHIP BETWEEN RESEARCH DESIGN FRAMEWORK AND FRAME OF REFERENCE

The theoretical or conceptual framework and the design framework are both critical to the study and are interlinked in their functions. The two must be compatible, and each must complement the other. Both frameworks provide logical connections that intertwine throughout the study. Through the interactions of the two frameworks, all the components of the study merge into a meaningful whole. Both frameworks direct the process of the study, and findings are interpreted within the context of both. For example, if one were examining a theoretical proposition that stated a positive relationship between variable A and variable B, a design that allowed the examination of relationships or correlations between variables would need to be selected rather than one that examined differences or causality. Correlational statistics would be used, and findings would be interpreted in terms of relationships between the two variables.

LINK BETWEEN DESIGN AND PLAN

As a blueprint, the design is not specific to a particular study. The design is a broad pattern or guide that can be applied to many studies. Just as the blueprint for a house must be linked to the specific house being built, so must the design be made specific to a study. Using the statement of problem, frame of reference, subproblems and clearly defined and operationalized variables, a research plan can then be devised for data collection and analysis that is in keeping with the design. This research plan specifically directs the implementation of the study design. Developing a research plan is discussed in Chapter 16.

Concepts Important to Design

There are many terms used in discussing research design that have special meanings within this context. An understanding of the meaning of these concepts is critical to understanding the purpose of a specific design. Some of the major concepts used in relation to design are causality, bias, manipulation, control and validity.

CAUSALITY

The first assumption one must make in examining causality is that things have causes and that causes lead to effects. Some of the ideas related to causation emerged from the logical positivist philosophical tradition. Hume, a positivist, proposed that there were three conditions that must be met in order to establish causality: (1) There must be a strong correlation between the proposed cause and the effect, (2) the proposed cause must precede the effect in time and (3) the cause has to be present whenever the effect occurs. Cause, according to Hume, is not directly observable but must be inferred. Another philosophical group, essentialists, proposed that two concepts must be considered in determining causality: necessary and sufficient. The proposed cause must be necessary for the effect to occur. (The effect cannot occur unless the cause first occurs.) The proposed cause must also be sufficient (requiring no other factors) for the effect to occur. This leaves no room for a variable that may sometimes, but not always, serve as the cause of an effect. John Stuart Mill, another philosopher, added another idea related to causation. He suggested that in addition to the above criteria for causation, there could be no alternative explanations for why a change in one variable seemed to lead to a change in a second variable (Cook & Campbell, 1979).

Causes are frequently expressed within the propositions of a theory. Testing the accuracy of these theoretical statements indicates the usefulness of the theory. A theoretical understanding of causation is considered important because it improves the ability to predict and, in some cases, to control events in the real world. The purpose of an experimental design is to determine cause and effect. The independent variable in a study is expected to be the cause, and the dependent variable is expected to reflect the effect of the independent variable.

Multicausality

A more recent idea related to causality is the recognition that a number of interrelating variables can be involved in causing a particular effect. Because of the complexity of causal relationships, a theory is unlikely to identify every variable involved in causing a particular phenomenon. A study is unlikely to identify every component influencing a particular change or effect. Cook and Campbell (1979) have suggested three levels of causal assertions that must be considered in establishing causality. Molar causal laws relate to large and complex objects. Intermediate mediation considers causal factors operating in between molar and micro levels. Micromediation examines causal connections at the level of small particles such as atoms. Cook and Campbell (1979) use the example of turning on a light switch "causing" the light to come on (molar). An electrician would tend to explain the cause of the light coming on in terms of wires and electrical current (intermediate mediation). However, the physicist would explain the cause of the light coming on in terms of ions, atoms and subparticles (micromediation).

The essentialists' ideas of necessary and sufficient do not hold up well when one views a phenomenon from the perspective of multiple causation. The light switch may not be necessary to turn on the light if the insulation has worn off the electrical wires. Additionally, the light will not come on even though the switch is turned on if the light bulb is burned out. Although this is a rather concrete example, it is easy to relate to common situations in nursing.

Very few phenomena in nursing can be clearly pinned down to a single cause and a single effect. However, the greater the proportion of causal factors that can be identified and explored, the clearer the understanding of the phenomenon. This greater understanding will increase the ability to predict and control. For example, currently, nurses have only a limited understanding of patients' preoperative attitudes, knowledge and behaviors and their effects on postoperative attitudes and behaviors. Nurses assume that high preoperative anxiety leads to less healthy postoperative responses and that providing information before surgery will improve healthy responses in the postoperative period. Many nursing studies have examined this particular phenomenon. However, the causal factors involved are complex and have not been clearly delineated. This lack of knowledge limits the effectiveness of nursing actions in facilitating the most healthy response to the surgical experience.

Probability

The original criteria for causation required that a variable "cause" an identified "effect" each time the "cause" occurred. Although this may occur in the basic sciences, such as chemistry or physics, it is unlikely to occur in health sciences or social sciences. Because of the complexity of nursing's field, we deal in probabilities. Causality, then, becomes relative rather than absolute. The cause will not produce a specific effect each time that particular cause occurs. What is being examined in nursing research is the probability that a specific effect will occur. Reasoning changes when one thinks in terms of probabilities. Rather than seeking to prove that A causes B, a researcher would state that if A occurred, there was a 50 per cent probability that B would occur. The reasoning behind probability is more in keeping with the complexity of multicausality. Using the surgical example, nurses could seek to predict the probability of unhealthy patient outcomes postoperatively when anxiety levels are high preoperatively.

Causality and Nursing Philosophy

Traditional theories of prediction and control are built on theories of causality. Nursing science must be built within a philosophical framework of multicausality and probability. The strict sense of single causality and of "necessary and sufficient" are not in keeping with the progressively complex, holistic philosophy of nursing. Acquiring an understanding of multicausality and increasing the probability of being able to predict and control the occurrence of an effect will require an understanding of both wholes and parts. Nursing knowledge for practice will require understanding of molar, intermediate mediational and micromediational aspects of a particular phenomenon. A variety of differing approaches, such as qualitative and quantitative, exploratory and experimental research are necessary to develop a knowledge base for nursing. Explanation and causality have been seen by some as different and perhaps opposing forms of knowledge, yet these forms of knowledge must be joined, sometimes within the design of a single study, to acquire the knowledge needed for nursing practice.

BIAS

The term *bias* means to slant away from the true or expected. A biased opinion has failed to include both sides of the question. Cutting fabric on the bias means to cut across the grain of the woven fabric. A biased witness is one who is strongly for or against one side of the situation. A biased scale is one that does not measure accurately.

Bias is of great concern in research because of the potential effect on the meaning of the study findings. Any component of the study that deviates or causes a deviation from true measure leads to distorted findings. Many factors related to research can be biased: the researcher, the measurement tools, the individual subjects, the sample, the data and/or the statistics. Thus, an important concern in designing a study is to identify possible sources of bias and eliminate or avoid them. Designs, in fact, are developed to reduce the possibilities of bias.

MANIPULATION

In nursing, manipulation tends to have a negative connotation and is associated with one person underhandedly causing another person to behave in a desired way. To manipulate means to move around or to control the movement of, such as manipulating a syringe. In research, manipulation is used in experimental or quasi-experimental research and is sometimes called the "treatment." Thus, in a study on preoperative care, preoperative teaching might be "manipulated" so that one group received the treatment and another did not. In a study on oral care, the frequency of care might be "manipulated." In nursing research, when experimental designs are used to explore "causal" relationships, the nurse must be free to manipulate the variables under study. If the freedom to manipulate a variable (*e.g.*, pain control measures) is under the control of someone else, a bias is introduced into the study. In exploratory (quantitative and qualitative), descriptive and correlational studies, no attempt is made to manipulate. Instead, the purpose is to describe a situation as it exists.

CONTROL

Control means having the power to direct or manipulate factors to achieve a desired outcome. We think of a "control" tower at an airport, "controlling" our temper and "controlling" the temperature of a baby's bath water. The idea of control is very important in research, particularly in experimental and quasi-experimental studies. The greater the amount of control of the researcher over the study situation, the more credible the study findings. The purpose of research designs is to maximize control factors in the study situation. Statistical analyses are sometimes planned to achieve greater control; this is called *statistical control*. Statistical control is discussed in Chapter 17.

One means of achieving control is in the selection of subjects for the study. In many studies, "control" groups are selected whose members will receive no treatment or a lesser treatment, to allow comparison between groups. Subjects in the control group and the experimental group should be as similar as possible in characteristics not under study.

The most desirable way to maximize the likelihood that the groups are similar is through randomization. In randomization, the subjects are selected for the treatment and control groups in a random way, to avoid bias. Another strategy to achieve control is matching. Subjects who are to receive the "treatment" are matched with another subject, using variables such as age, gender, diagnosis or other factors considered important in a particular study. Methods of achieving randomization and matching are discussed in Chapter 9.

VALIDITY

Validity is a measure of the truth or accuracy of a claim and is an important concern throughout the research process. Questions of validity refer back to the propositions from which the study was developed. Thus, validity is an examination of the approximate truth or falsity of the propositions (Cook & Campbell, 1979). Is the theoretical proposition an accurate reflection of reality? Was the study designed well enough to provide a valid test of the proposition? Validity is a very complex idea and has been examined from various perspectives by several authors. These ideas are important to the researcher and to those who read and consider using the findings in their practice. Critical analysis of research involves being able to think through threats to validity that have occurred and make judgments about how seriously these threats affect the integrity of the findings. Validity provides a major basis for making decisions about which findings are useful for patient care. The classification developed by Cook and Campbell (1979) is used to explain validity.

Cook and Campbell (1979) have described four types of validity: statistical conclusion validity, internal validity, construct validity and external validity. When conducting a study, the researcher is confronted with major decisions regarding the four types of validity. In order to make decisions about validity, a variety of questions must be addressed.

1. Is there a relationship between the two variables?

2. Given that there is a relationship, is it plausibly causal from one operational variable to the other or would the same relationship have been obtained in the absence of any treatment of any kind?

3. Given that the relationship is plausibly causal and is reasonably known to be from one variable to another, what are the particular cause and effect constructs involved in the relationship?

4. Given that there is probably a causal relationship from construct A to construct B, how generalizable is this relationship across persons, settings, and times? (p. 39).

Statistical Conclusion Validity

The first step in inferring cause is to determine whether the independent and dependent variables are related. The determination of a relationship (co-variation) is made through statistical analysis. *Statistical conclusion validity* is concerned with whether the conclusions about relationships and/or differences drawn from statistical analysis are an accurate reflection of the real world. The second step is to identify differences between groups. However, there are reasons why false conclusions can be drawn about the presence or absence of a relationship or difference. The reasons for the false conclusions are called threats to statistical conclusion validity. These threats include the following:

1. *Low Statistical Power.* Low statistical power increases the probability of concluding that there is no significant difference between samples when actually there is a difference (Type II error). A Type II error is most likely to occur when the sample size is small or when the power of the statistical test to determine differences is low. The concept of statistical power and strategies to improve it are discussed in Chapter 17.

2. *Violated Assumptions of Statistical Tests.* Most statistical tests have assumptions about the data being used such as assuming that the data are interval data, or that there is a normal distribution of scores to be analysed. If these assumptions are violated, the statistical analysis may provide inaccurate results.

3. *Fishing and the Error Rate Problem.* A serious concern in research is incorrectly concluding that a relationship or difference exists when it does not (Type I error). The risk of Type I error increases when the researcher conducts multiple statistical analyses of relationships or differences. This is referred to as fishing. When fishing is used, a given portion of the analyses will show significant relationships or differences simply by chance. For example, commonly, the t test is used to make multiple statistical comparisons of mean differences in a single sample. This procedure increases the risk of a Type I error because some of the differences found in the sample occurred by chance and are not actually present in the population. Multivariate statistical techniques have been developed to deal with this error rate problem (Goodwin, 1984). Fishing and error rate problems are discussed in Chapter 17.

4. ***The Reliability of Measures.*** The technique of measuring variables must be reliable if true differences are to be found. A measure is reliable if it gives the same result each time the same situation or factor is measured. For example, a thermometer would be reliable if it showed the same reading when tested repeatedly on the same patient. If a scale is used to measure anxiety, it should give the same score if repeatedly given to the same person in a short period of time (unless, of course, repeatedly taking the same test caused anxiety to increase or decrease).

5. ***The Reliability of Treatment Implementation.*** If the method of administering a research treatment varies from one person to another, the chance of detecting a true difference decreases. The lack of standardization in administering the treatment must be controlled during the planning phase by ensuring that the treatment will be provided in exactly the same way each time it is administered.

6. ***Random Irrelevancies in the Experimental Setting.*** Environmental (extraneous) variables in complex field settings can influence scores on the dependent variable. These variables will increase the difficulty of detecting differences. Consider the activities occurring on a nursing unit. The numbers and variety of staff, patients, crises and work patterns merge into a complex arena for the implementation of a study. Any of the dynamics of the unit can influence manipulation of the independent variable or measurement of the dependent variable.

7. ***Random Heterogeneity of Respondents.*** Subjects in a treatment group can differ in ways that are correlated with the dependent variable. This difference can have an influence on the outcome of the treatment and prevent detection of a true correlation between the treatment and the dependent variable. For example, subjects may vary in response to preoperative attempts to lower anxiety because of unique characteristics associated with differing levels of anxiety.

Internal Validity

Internal validity is the extent to which the effects detected in the study are a true reflection of reality, rather than being the result of the effects of extraneous variables. Although internal validity should be a concern in all studies, it is addressed more frequently in relation to studies examining causality than in other studies. In studies examining causality, the researcher must attempt to determine whether the independent and dependent variables may have been caused by a third, often unmeasured, variable. Any study can contain threats to internal validity, and these validity threats can lead to a false-positive or false-negative conclusion. The following question must be considered: "Is there another reasonable (valid) explanation for the finding other than that proposed by the researcher?" Threats to internal validity include the following:

1. ***History.*** This is an event that is not related to the planned study but occurs during the time of the study. History could influence the responses of subjects to the treatment.

2. **Maturation.** In research, maturation is defined as growing older, wiser, stronger, hungrier, more tired or more experienced during the study. These unplanned and unrecognized changes can influence the findings of the study.

3. **Testing.** Sometimes, the effect being measured can be due to the number of times the subject's responses have been tested. The subject may remember earlier inaccurate responses that can be modified, thus altering the outcome of the study. The test itself may influence the subject to change attitudes or increase the subject's knowledge.

4. **Instrumentation.** Effects can be due to changes in measurement instruments between the pretest and the post-test rather than an effect of the treatment. For example, a scale, accurate when the study began, could weigh subjects 2 lb less than they actually weigh on the post-test. Instrumentation is also involved when people serving as observers or data collectors become more experienced between the pretest and the post-test, thus altering in some way the data they collect.

5. **Statistical Regression.** Statistical regression is the movement or regression of extreme scores toward the mean in studies using a pretest–post-test design. The process involved in statistical regression is more difficult to understand. When a test or scale is used to measure a variable, some subjects will achieve very high or very low scores. In some studies, subjects are selected to be included in a particular group because their scores on a pretest are high or low. A treatment is then performed, and a post-test is administered. However, with no treatment, subjects who initially achieve very high or very low scores will tend to have more moderate scores when retested. Their scores will "regress" toward the mean. The treatment did not necessarily cause the change. If the pretest scores were low, the post-test may show statistically significant differences (higher scores) from the pretest, leading to the conclusion that the treatment "caused" the change (Type I error). If the pretest scores were high, the post-test scores would tend to be lower (because of a tendency to regress toward the mean) even with no treatment. In this situation, the researcher may mistakenly conclude that there is no difference "caused" by the treatment (Type II error).

6. **Selection.** Selection addresses the phenomenon of which subjects take part in a study and how subjects are grouped within a study. A selection threat is more likely to occur in studies in which randomization is not possible. In some studies, people selected for the study may differ in some important way from people not selected for the study. In other studies, the threat is due to differences in subjects selected for study groups. For example, people included in the control group could be different in some important way from people included in the experimental group. This difference in selec-

tion could lead to the two groups reacting differently to the treatment, rather than the treatment causing the differences in group responses.

7. *Mortality.* This threat is due to subjects who drop out of a study before completion. Mortality becomes a threat when those who drop out of a study are a different type of person than those who remain in the study, or when there is a difference in the kinds of people who drop out of the experimental group and the control group.

8. *Interactions with Selection.* The aforementioned threats can interact with selection to further complicate the validity of the study. The threats most likely to interact with selection include history, maturation and instrumentation. For example, if a control group selected for the study has a different history than the experimental group, responses to the treatment may be due to this interaction rather than to the treatment.

9. *Ambiguity About the Direction of Causal Influence.* This threat occurs most frequently in correlational studies that address causality. In a study in which variables are measured simultaneously and only once, it may be impossible to determine whether A "caused" B, B "caused" A or the two variables interact in a noncausal way.

10. *Diffusion or Imitation of Treatments.* This threat occurs when the control group gains access to the treatment intended for the experimental group or a similar treatment available from another source. For example, suppose a study examined the effect of teaching specific information to hypertensive patients as a treatment and then measured the effect of the teaching on blood pressure readings and adherence to treatment protocols. Suppose the control group patients communicated with the experimental patients and the teaching information was shared. The control group patients' responses to the outcome measures may show no differences from those of the experimental group when the teaching actually did make a difference (Type II error).

11. *Compensatory Equalization of Treatments.* When the experimental group receives a treatment that is seen as desirable, such as a new treatment for cancer, administrative people and other health professionals may not tolerate the difference and insist that the control group receive the treatment. If this occurs, the researcher no longer has a control group and cannot document the effectiveness of the treatment through the study. In health care, this has ethical implications on both sides.

12. *Compensatory Rivalry by Respondents Receiving Less Desirable Treatments.* In some studies, the design and plan of the study are publicly known. The control group subjects then know the expected difference between their group and the experimental group and may attempt to reduce or reverse the difference. This phenomenon may have occurred in the National Hospice Study, funded by the Health

Care Financing Administration and conducted by Brown University (Greer, Mor, Sherwood, Morris, & Birnbaum, 1983). In this study, 26 hospices were temporarily reimbursed through Medicare while a comparison of the care between hospices and hospitals were examined. The study made national headlines and was widely discussed in Congress. Health policy decisions related to reimbursement of hospice care hinged on the findings of the study. The study found no significant differences in care between the two groups although there were cost differentials. In addition to a selection threat (hospitals providing poor care to dying cancer patients were unlikely to agree to participate in the study), health care professionals in the hospitals selected may have been determined to counter the criticism that the care they provided was poor in quality. The rivalry in this situation could have influenced the outcomes of the study and thus threatened the validity.

13. ***Resentful Demoralization of Respondents Receiving Less Desirable Treatments.*** If control group subjects believe that they are receiving less desirable treatment, they may react by withdrawing, giving up or becoming angry. Changes in behavior resulting from this reaction rather than from the treatment can lead to differences that cannot be attributed to the treatment.

Construct Validity

Construct validity examines the fit between the conceptual definitions and operational definitions of variables. Theoretical constructs or concepts are defined within the theoretical framework (conceptual definitions). These conceptual definitions provide the basis for the development of operational definitions of the variables. Operational definitions (methods of measurement) need to validly reflect the theoretical constructs. Examination of construct validity determines whether the instrument actually measures the theoretical construct it purports to measure. The process of developing construct validity for an instrument often requires years of scientific work. When selecting methods of measurement, the researcher needs to determine previous development of instrument construct validity. The threats to construct validity are related both to previous instrument development and to the development of measurement techniques as part of the methodology of a particular study. Threats to construct validity include the following:

1. ***Inadequate Preoperational Explication of Constructs.*** Measurement of a construct stems logically from a concept analysis of the construct, either by the theorist who developed the construct or by the researcher. The conceptual definition should emerge from the concept analysis, and the method of measurement (operational definition) should clearly reflect both. A deficiency in the conceptual or operational definitions leads to low construct validity.

2. ***Mono-Operation Bias.*** Mono-operation bias occurs when only one method of measurement is used to measure a construct. When only

one method of measurement is used, fewer dimensions of the construct are measured. Construct validity is greatly improved if the researcher uses more than one instrument. For example, if anxiety was a dependent variable, more than one measure of anxiety could be used. More than one measurement of the dependent variable can often be accomplished with little increase in time, effort or cost. However, increasing numbers of measures of independent variables is more complex and may involve altering the design of the study.

3. *Mono-Method Bias.* In mono-method bias, the researcher uses more than one measure of a variable, but all measures use the same method of recording. Attitude measures, for example, may all be paper and pencil scales. Attitudes that are personal and private may not be detected using paper and pencil tools. Paper and pencil tools may be influenced by feelings of nonaccountability for responses, acquiescence or social desirability. For example, construct validity would be improved if anxiety were measured by a paper and pencil test, verbal messages of anxiety and observer recording of incidence and frequency of behaviors that have been validly linked with anxiety.

4. *Hypothesis-Guessing Within Experimental Conditions.* Many subjects within a study can guess the hypotheses of the researcher. The validity concern is related to behavioral changes that may occur in the subjects as a consequence of knowing the hypothesis. The extent to which this modifies study findings is not presently known.

5. *Evaluation Apprehension.* Subjects wish to be seen in a favorable light by researchers. They want to be seen as competent and psychologically healthy. Their responses in the experiment may be due to this desire rather than an effect of the independent variable.

6. *Experimenter Expectancies.* The expectancies of the researcher can bias the data. For example, if the researcher expected a particular intervention to be effective in pain relief, the data may reflect this expectation. If another researcher who did not believe the intervention would be effective had collected the data, results could be different. The extent to which this actually influences studies is not known. Because of this concern, some researchers are not involved in the data collection process. In other studies, data collectors do not know which subjects are assigned to treatment and control groups. Another way to control this threat is to design the study so that data collectors differ in expectations. If the sample size is large enough, comparisons could be made in data collected by the different data collectors. Failing to determine a difference in the data collected by the two groups would verify construct validity.

7. *Confounding Constructs and Levels of Constructs.* When developing the methodology of a study, the researcher makes decisions about the intensity of a variable that will be measured or provided as a treatment. The intensity of the variable measured influences the

level of the construct that will be reflected in the study. These decisions can affect validity, since the method of measuring the variable influences the outcome of the study and the understanding of the constructs in the theoretical framework. For example, the researcher might find that variable A does not affect variable B when, in fact, it does, but not at the level of A that was manipulated, or perhaps not at the level of B that was measured. This is particularly a problem when A is not linearly related to B or when the effect being studied is weak. Control of this threat involves including several levels of A in the design and measuring many levels of B. For example, if A is preoperative teaching and B is anxiety, the instrument being used to measure anxiety may measure only high levels of anxiety. The preoperative teaching may be provided for 15 minutes when 30 minutes or an hour is required to cause significant changes in anxiety.

In some cases, there is confounding of variables, which leads to mistaken conclusions. Few measures of a construct are pure measures. Rather, a selected method of measuring a construct can measure a portion of the construct and also other related constructs. Thus, the measure can lead to confusing results, since the variable measured does not provide an accurate reflection of the construct.

8. *Interaction of Different Treatments.* The interaction of different treatments is a threat if subjects receive more than one treatment in a study. For example, a study might examine the effectiveness of pain relief measures, and subjects might receive medication, massage, distraction and relaxation strategies. In this case, each one of the treatments will interact with the others, and the effect of any single treatment on pain relief would be impossible to extract. The findings cannot be generalized to any situation in which patients did not receive all four pain treatments.

9. *Interaction of Testing and Treatment.* In some studies, pretesting the subject is thought to modify the effect of the treatment. In this case, the findings can be generalized only to subjects who have been pretested. Although there is some evidence that "pretest sensitivity" does not have the extent of impact that was once feared, it must be considered in examining the validity of the study. One design, the Solomon Four-Group Design (discussed later in the chapter) tests this threat to validity. Repeated post-tests can also lead to an interaction of testing and treatment.

10. *Restricted Generalizability Across Constructs.* When designing studies, the researcher must consider the impact of the findings on constructs other than those originally conceived in the problem statement. Often, by including another measure or two, the generalization of the findings to clinical settings and the translation back to theoretical dimensions can be much broader.

External Validity

External validity is concerned with the extent to which study findings can be generalized beyond the sample used in the study. The most serious threat would lead to the findings being meaningful only for the group being studied. To some extent, the significance of the study is dependent on the number of types of people and situations to which the findings can be applied. Sometimes, the factors influencing external validity are subtle and may not be reported in research papers; however, the researcher must be responsible for these factors. Generalization is usually more narrow for a single study than for multiple replications of a study using different samples, perhaps from different populations, in different settings. The threats to the ability to generalize the findings (external validity) in terms of study design include the following:

1. *Interaction of Selection and Treatment.* Seeking subjects who are willing to participate in a study can be difficult, particularly if the study requires extensive amounts of time or other types of investment by subjects. If a large number of the persons approached to participate in a study decline to participate, the sample actually selected tends to be limited in ways that might not be evident at first glance. Only the researcher knows the subjects well. Subjects might tend to be volunteers, do-gooders or those with nothing better to do. In this case, generalizing the findings to all members of a population such as all nurses, all hospitalized patients or all persons experiencing diabetes is not easy to justify.

   The study should be planned to limit the investment demands on subjects in order to increase participation. The number of persons who were approached and refused to participate in the study should be reported so that threats to external validity can be judged. As the percentage of those who decline to participate increases, external validity decreases. Sufficient data should be collected on the subjects so that the researcher can be familiar with the characteristics of subjects and, to the extent possible, the characteristics of those who decline to participate. Handwritten notes of verbal remarks made by those who decline and observations of behavior, dress or other significant factors can be very useful in determining selection differences.

2. *Interaction of Setting and Treatment.* Bias exists in settings and organizations who will agree to participate in studies. This bias has been particularly evident in nursing studies. For example, some hospitals welcome nursing studies and encourage employed nurses to conduct studies. Others are very resistant to the conduct of research. These two types of hospitals may be very different in important ways; thus, there might be an interaction of setting and treatment that limits the generalizability of the findings. This factor should be considered in making statements about the population to which the findings can be generalized.

3. *Interaction of History and Treatment.* The circumstances during which a study was conducted (history) influence the treatment and thus the ability to generalize findings. Logically, one can never generalize to the future; however, replication of the study during various time periods gives further strength to the usefulness of findings across time. In critiquing studies, one must always consider the period of history during which the study was conducted and the impact of nursing practice and societal events during that time period on the reported findings.

Designs for Nursing Research

Designs have been developed by researchers to meet unique research needs as they emerged. The first experimental designs were developed in the 1930s by Sir Ronald A. Fisher (1935) and published in a book entitled *The Designs of Experiments*. However, most work on design has been conducted in the last 30 years (Abdellah & Levine, 1979). During this time, designs have become much more sophisticated and varied.

The purpose of designs is to achieve greater control and thus improve the validity of the study in solving the research problem. Originally, only experimental designs were considered of value. In addition, many believe the only setting in which an experiment can be conducted is a laboratory, which allows much stricter controls to be maintained than does a field setting. This is appropriate for the natural sciences but not for the social sciences. From the social sciences have emerged additional quantitative designs (exploratory, descriptive, correlational and quasi-experimental) and qualitative designs.

At present, nursing research is using designs developed by other disciplines that met the needs of that discipline for adding to nursing's knowledge base. These designs are a useful starting point, but nurse scientists must go beyond these designs to develop designs that will more appropriately meet the needs of nursing's knowledge base. To go beyond the present designs, nurse scientists must have a working knowledge of available designs and the logic on which they are based. Designs created to meet nursing needs must be congruent with nursing philosophy. They must provide means to examine dimensions of nursing within a holistic framework and allow examination of nursing dimensions across time. Designs must be developed that can seek answers to important nursing questions rather than answering only questions that can be examined by existing designs.

Innovative design strategies are beginning to appear within nursing research. For example, designs are being developed that facilitate examination of a phenomenon both qualitatively and quantitatively within the same study. The use of time series analysis strategies (described later in the chapter) holds great promise for examining important dimensions of nursing. Designs in the area of prevention also have great potential for exploring aspects of nursing. However, nurse researchers must see themselves as credible scientists in order to dare to develop new design strategies that facilitate examination of little understood aspects of nursing. Developing a new design requires careful consideration of possible threats to validity and ways to diminish them. Design development requires a willingness to risk the temporary failures that are always inherent in developing something new.

The following section describes designs commonly used in nursing studies. There is no universal standard for categorizing designs. Names of designs change as they are discussed by various authors. The list of designs described is intended to be more instructive than exhaustive. Sometimes, several designs are merged to meet the research needs of a particular study. From these, new designs sometimes emerge. A presentation of "pure" designs is hard to find in the research literature, since the listed designs have been artificially separated to increase clarity. In this text, designs have been categorized by types of studies for which they would be appropriate, using the categorization of studies described in Chapter 2. The designs need to be examined with thought to the threats to validity controlled by the design and threats that will continue to influence the validity of the findings.

EXPLORATORY STUDY DESIGNS

Exploratory studies are conducted in areas about which nursing has little knowledge, theoretical or factual. The researcher is exploring the field to learn what is there, what meanings are attached to the discoveries and how the meanings can be organized. Intuition and insight play important roles in this process. The researcher must feel free to follow through on a new lead and move the study into new areas in the middle of the study process. Therefore, these studies tend to have less design structure than other types of studies. The design is very flexible; the researcher functions somewhat as a detective, searching out clues to factors in the situation that may be significant. Designs for exploratory studies are not frequently discussed, and, when they are, the design is not specifically delineated. In a sense, each researcher must develop an exploratory design uniquely suited to the research problem and purpose. In addition to the importance of design flexibility, the researcher must rigorously design the study to maximize the accuracy (reliability) of the evidence collected and minimize bias and threats to the validity of the findings. These actions increase the probability that if the study were repeated, similar findings would result, thus adding credibility to the study (Selltiz, Wrightsman & Cook, 1976).

Exploratory designs can be either qualitative or quantitative. The classification of the study depends on two factors: (1) Whether the data are numeric or in words, and (2) whether the intent of the study is to develop theory or to develop the knowledge of a field to the point that more controlled quantitative designs can be used. Qualitative approaches have data expressed as words, and the intent of these studies is to develop theory. Phenomenologic, grounded theory, ethnography and historical research have specific exploratory designs that are presented in Chapter 4. The quantitative approach usually assumes that initial studies will be exploratory and then progress through descriptive, correlational, quasi-experimental and experimental as knowledge is gained. An example of a quantitative exploratory design is Chen, Barkauskas and Chen's (1984) study "Health problems encountered by nurse practitioners and physicians in general medicine clinics." The design is illustrated by the following excerpt from the abstract of the study.

> Distribution of health problems encountered by nurse practitioners and physicians in general/adult medicine clinics was studied. Proportional samples by clinics were selected from a total of 13,039 patient visits made to four clinics during an 18-week period in 1978. A Patient Encounter Form was used as the instrument and the ICD-9-CM as the coding system. (p. 79)

DESCRIPTIVE STUDY DESIGNS

Descriptive studies are designed to gain more information about characteristics within a particular field of study. Their purpose is to provide a picture of situations as they naturally happen. A descriptive design may be used for the purpose of developing theory, identifying problems with current practice, justifying current practice, making judgments or determining what others in similar situations are doing (Waltz & Bausell, 1981). No manipulation of variables is involved. Dependent and independent variables should not be used within a descriptive design because there is no attempt to establish causality. Although causally oriented studies are more highly valued in the scientific community, in many aspects of nursing, there is a need for a clearer delineation of the phenomenon before causality can be examined.

Descriptive designs vary in levels of complexity. Some contain only two variables, whereas others may include multiple variables. The relationships between variables are identified to obtain an overall picture of the phenomenon being examined, but examination of types and degree of relationships is not the primary purpose of a descriptive study. To use a descriptive design, the existing body of knowledge must contain more information about the variables to be examined than would be known when an exploratory design is used. Greater protection against bias is required in a descriptive design than in an exploratory design, because the researcher is attempting to achieve a clearer picture of the phenomenon than will be obtained using an exploratory design. Protection against bias is achieved through (1) conceptual and operational definitions of variables, (2) sample selection, (3) valid and reliable instruments and (4) data collection procedures that achieve some environmental control.

Typical Descriptive Study Design

The most commonly used design within the category of descriptive studies is presented in Figure 10–1. The design is used to examine characteristics of a single sample. The design includes identifying a phenomenon of interest, identifying the variables within the phenomenon, developing conceptual and operational definitions of the variables and describing the variables. The description of the variables leads to an interpretation of the theoretical meaning of the findings and the development of hypotheses.

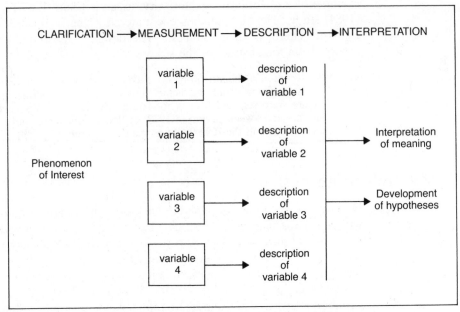

CLARIFICATION → MEASUREMENT → DESCRIPTION → INTERPRETATION

FIGURE 10–1. Descriptive study design.

Very few studies are purely descriptive; however, many contain descriptive components. An example of a descriptive design is Gill, White and Anderson's (1984) study "Transitional newborn infants in a hospital nursery: from first oral cue to first sustained cry." The following is an excerpt from this study.

> This research was done in the newborn nursery of a large teaching hospital. The sample consisted of 15 clinically normal transitional newborn infants who were products of an uncomplicated pregnancy, labor, and delivery... Two instruments were used in this research: The Senders, Signals, and Receivers (SSR) System and the Cry Scale... The investigator sat by the crib and encoded the infant's behavior onto the SSR System keyboard... Observations were encoded without interruption until the infant reached a sustained cry... (pp. 214–215)

Comparative Descriptive Design

The comparative descriptive design examines and describes differences in variables in *two* or more groups that occur naturally in the setting. Descriptive statistics and statistical analyses may be used to examine differences between or among groups. The results obtained from these analyses are frequently not generalized to a population. An example of this design is Flaskerud's (1984) study "A comparison of perceptions of problematic behavior by six minority groups and mental health professionals." The following is an excerpt from the abstract of the study.

> This study compared the perceptions of problematic behavior and the suggested management of those behaviors by six minority groups and mental health

professionals. Minority respondents (N = 159) included Chinese-Americans, Mexican-Americans, Filipino-Americans, Native-Americans, Black-Americans, and Appalachians. Mental health professional respondents (N = 68) were from Pennsylvania, Louisiana, and California. All respondents were interviewed using a structured interview schedule. Groups were compared on responses to 10 vignettes. (p. 190)

Time Dimensional Designs

Time dimensional designs were developed within the discipline of epidemiology, which studies the occurrence and distribution of disease among populations. These designs examine sequences and patterns of change, growth or trends across time. The dimension of time, then, becomes an important factor. Within the field of epidemiology, the samples in time dimensional studies are called *cohorts*. Cohorts were originally age categories; however, the idea has been expanded to include many other variables. Other means of classifying populations that have relevance in relation to time include time of diagnosis, point of entry into a treatment protocol, point of entry into a new life style, or age at which the subject started smoking. An understanding of temporal sequencing is an important prerequisite to examining causality between variables. Thus, the results of these designs lead to the development of hypotheses and are often forerunners to experimental designs.

Epidemiological studies that use time dimensional designs are developed to determine the risk factors or causal factors of illness states. Cause determined in this manner is called *inferred causality*. The best known studies in this area are those on smoking and cancer. Because of the strength of multiply repeated studies, the causal link is strong. The strategy is not as powerful as experimental designs in supporting causality; however, in this situation, as in many others, one can never ethically conduct a true experiment.

Epidemiologists use two strategies to examine a situation across time: retrospective studies and prospective studies. The norm in epidemiologic studies is to use the term cohort in reference to groups of subjects in prospective studies; but the term cohort is generally not used in retrospective studies. In retrospective studies, both the proposed cause and the proposed effect have already occurred. For example, the subjects could have a specific type of cancer and the researcher could be searching for commonalities among subjects that may have led to the development of that type of cancer. In a prospective study, causes may have occurred, but the proposed effect has not. The Framingham Study is the best known example of a prospective study. In this study, members of a community were followed by researchers for 20 years who examined such variables as dietary patterns, exercise, weight and blood lipid levels. As the subjects developed illnesses, such as heart disease, hypertension or lung disease, their illnesses could be related to previously identified variables. Prospective studies are considered more powerful than retrospective studies in inferring causality, because it can be demonstrated that the risk factors occurred prior to the illness and are positively related to the illness. These are important designs for use in nursing studies because a person's responses to health situations are patterns that developed long before the health situation occurred (Newman, 1979). These patterns then influence responses to nursing interventions. Several designs are used to conduct time dimensional studies: longitudinal, cross-sectional, trend and treatment partitioning.

Longitudinal Designs □ These designs examine changes in the same subjects over an extended period of time. This design is sometimes called a *panel design* (Fig. 10–2). Longitudinal designs are expensive and require researcher and subject commitment over a long period of time. The area to be studied, the variables and their measurement must be clearly identified before data collection begins. There is often a bias in selection of subjects because of the requirement for a long-term commitment. In addition, loss of subjects (mortality) can be high and can lead to decreased validity of findings. An example of a longitudinal design is Ellison's (1983) study "Parental support and school-aged children." The following is an excerpt from that study.

> This study explores the concept of parental support as it relates to psychosocial adjustment of school-aged children and their parents... The Family Peer Relationship Questionnaire (FPRQ) was developed to measure both the quality of the child's relationship with parents and with peers... Data collection consisted of administering the FPRQ to 101 primarily middle class mothers and their children, living in a northwest metropolitan area. It was part of a longitudinal, multimeasure, multimethod investigation on the early prediction of problems in the intellectual, physical, and psychological development of children. (pp. 145–148)

Cross-sectional Designs □ These designs are used to examine groups of subjects in various stages of development simultaneously (Fig. 10–3). The assumption is that the stages are part of a process that will progress across time. Selecting subjects at various points in the process will provide important information about the totality of the process, even though the same subjects are not followed through the entire process. The processes of development selected for the study might be related to age, position in an educational system, growth pattern or stages of maturation or personal growth (if these could be clearly enough defined to develop criteria for inclusion within differentiated groups). Subjects are then categorized by group, and data on the selected variables are collected at a single point in time. For example, one might wish to study grief reactions at various periods after the death of a spouse. Using a cross-sectional design, a group of individuals whose spouse had died 1 week ago could be tested, another whose loss was 6 months ago, another 1 year, another 2 years and another 5 years. All these groups could be studied at one time period, but

Time 1	Time 2	Time 3	Time 4	Time..n
measure variables	measure variables	measure variables	measure variables	measure variables
Sample 1	Sample 1	Sample 1	Sample 1	Sample 1

FIGURE 10–2. Longitudinal design.

FIGURE 10–3. Cross-sectional study design.

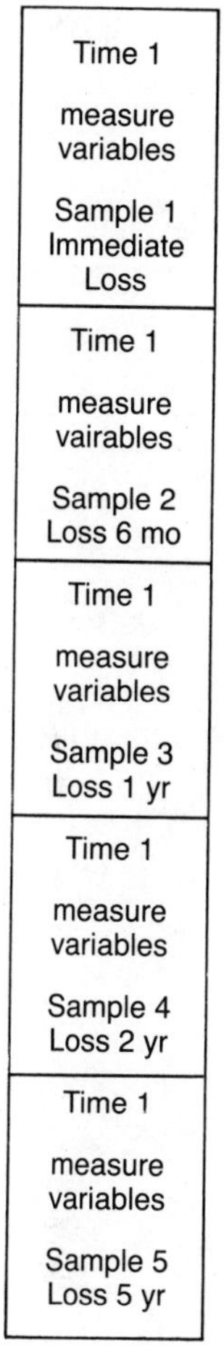

Time 1 measure variables Sample 1 Immediate Loss
Time 1 measure vairables Sample 2 Loss 6 mo
Time 1 measure variables Sample 3 Loss 1 yr
Time 1 measure variables Sample 4 Loss 2 yr
Time 1 measure variables Sample 5 Loss 5 yr

a pattern of grief reactions over a 5-year period could be described. The design is not as strong as the longitudinal design but allows some understanding of the phenomenon over time when time allowed for the study is limited. An example of this design is Penckofer and Holm's (1984) study "Early appraisal of coronary revascularization on quality of life." The following is an excerpt from the abstract of that study.

> In order to assess earlier impact (of bypass surgery) two groups of bypass patients—alike in terms of preoperative physical activity, angina level, and type of revascularization—were compared in terms of quality of life and related areas. Seventeen patients were 3 to 5 months (88–141 days) postoperative and 17 patients were 6 to 8 months (161–222 days) postoperative. They were asked to rate themselves on Cantril's Self-Anchoring Scale in relation to past, present, and future life satisfaction. (p. 60)

Trend Designs □ Trend designs examine changes in the general population in relation to a particular phenomenon (Fig. 10–4). Different samples of subjects

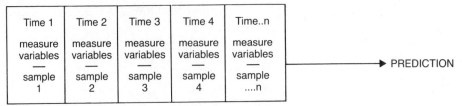

FIGURE **10–4.** Trend study design.

are selected from the same population at preset intervals of time, and, at each selected time, data are collected from that particular sample. The researcher must be able to justify generalizing from the samples to the population under study. Analysis will involve strategies to predict future trends from examination of past trends. An example of this design is Greenleaf's (1983) study "Labor force participation among registered nurses and women in comparable occupations." The following example is excerpted from the abstract of the study. The purpose of that study was

> To compare factors related to nurses' labor force participation with those for women in similar fields... Data were gathered in interviews with national samples using a standardized interview schedule... Included in the data are demographic items, behavioral items, personal evaluations of satisfaction with a number of items, and attitude measures on a broad spectrum of issues. The surveys, conducted during February, March, and April of each year from 1972 through 1978 and 1980, involved an independently drawn sample of approximately 1,500 English-speaking persons over 18 years of age, non-institutionalized, who were living within the continental United States. (p. 308)

Event Partitioning Designs □ A merger of the cross-sectional or longitudinal and trend designs is used in some cases to increase sample size and to avoid the effects of history on the validity of findings. Cook and Campbell (1979) refer to these as cohort designs with treatment partitioning (Figs. 10–5 and 10–6). The term *treatment* is used loosely here to mean a key event that is thought to lead to change. In a descriptive study, the researcher would not "cause" or "manipulate" the key event, but rather clearly define it so that when it occurred naturally it would be recognized. If the "treatment" were controlled or manipulated and subjects selected to receive the treatment, the design would be quasi-experimental.

For example, the event partitioning design could be used to study subjects who have completed programs to stop smoking. Smoking behaviors and incidence of smoking-related diseases might be measured at intervals of 1 year for a 5-year period. However, the number of subjects available at one time period might be insufficient for adequate analysis of findings. Therefore, subjects from several programs offered at different times could be used. Data would be examined in terms of the relative length of time since the subjects' completion of the stop smoking program, not the absolute length of time. Data are assumed to be comparable, and a larger sample size is available for analysis of changes across time. An example of this design is Davis's (1978) study "ODWIN expansion program: a study in success." The purpose of this study

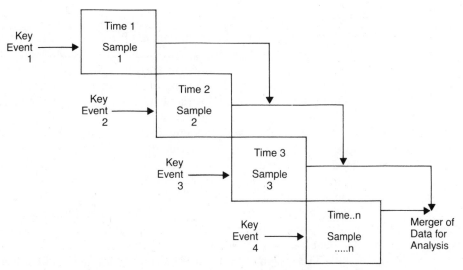

FIGURE 10–5. Cross-sectional study with treatment partitioning.

was to examine the effectiveness of the ODWIN (Open Doors Wider In Nursing) expansion program in improving the successful completion of nursing programs by marginal students. The "treatment" (key Event) was the ODWIN program.

> The population considered was restricted to the 182 students who successfully completed the Expansion program and enrolled in schools of nursing upon recommendation by the ODWIN staff... Each summer from 1966 through 1970 an eight-week ODWIN Expansion prenursing program for marginal students was taught at the College of Basic Studies, Boston University... Class size did not exceed 12 students... (p. 230)

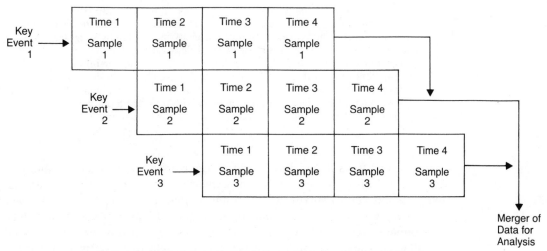

FIGURE 10–6. Longitudinal design with treatment partitioning.

Case Study Design

The case study design involves an intensive exploration of a single unit of study: a person, family, group, community or institution or a very small number of subjects who are examined intensively. Although the number of subjects tends to be small, the number of variables involved is usually large. In fact, it is important to examine all variables that might have an impact on the situation being studied.

Case studies were a commonly used design in nursing 30 years ago but appear in the literature less frequently today. Well-designed case studies are a good source of descriptive information and can be used as evidence for or against theories. They are also useful in demonstrating the effectiveness of specific therapeutic techniques. In fact, the reporting of a case study can be the vehicle by which the technique is introduced to other practitioners. The case study design also has important potential for revealing important findings that can generate new hypotheses for testing.

The design of a case study is dependent on the circumstances of the case but usually includes an element of time. History and previous behavior patterns are usually explored in detail. As the case study proceeds, the researcher may become aware of components important to the phenomenon being examined that were not originally built into the study. Because there is an exploratory element to case studies, these components should be incorporated into the study design. Although analysis of data includes descriptive statistics, intuition and insight are also important. Organizing the findings of a case study into a coherent whole is a difficult but critical component of the study. Major insights of the study emerge through the integrative thought processes. An example of a case study design is presented in Durand's (1975) study "A clinical nursing study: failure to thrive in a child with Down's syndrome." The following is an excerpt from the abstract of that study:

> A five-year-old child with Down's syndrome and severe failure to thrive, given a program of individually tailored developmental nursing care, showed substantial improvement as evidenced by changes in seven of nine criteria chosen for measurement. When investigation of the child and his family suggested that the failure to thrive was the result of masked deprivation, a study was designed to measure the effect of a 17-day program of developmental nursing care on specific parameters of growth and behavior—height, weight, amount of sleep, caloric intake, active mobility, awareness of the environment, prelanguage vocalizations, self-stimulation behavior, and play activity with toys. Data on these criteria were gathered before, during, and after the nursing care program. (p. 272)

Surveys

There are two ways in which the term *survey* is used within scientific thought. It is used in a broad sense to mean any exploratory, descriptive or correlational study. In this sense, survey tends to mean nonexperimental. In a narrower sense, survey is used to describe a technique of data collection in which questionnaires (collected by mail or in person) or personal interviews are used to gather data about an identified population. Data gathered in this manner must address variables that can be acquired through self-report. Because of this limitation in data, some researchers view surveys as rather shallow and as contributing in a limited way to scientific knowledge. This belief has led to a bias in the scientific community against survey research. However, surveys can be an extremely important source of data. In this text, the term *survey* is used to designate a data collection technique, not a design. Surveys can be used within many designs, including exploratory, descriptive, correlational or quasi-experimental.

CORRELATIONAL STUDIES

Correlational studies examine relationships between variables. This examination can occur at several levels. The researcher can seek to describe a relationship, predict relationships among variables or test the relationships proposed by a theoretical proposition. In any correlational study, a representative sample needs to be selected for the study. The sample should reflect the full range of scores possible on the variables being measured. In correlational designs, a large variance in the variable scores is necessary to determine the existence of a relationship. Therefore, correlational designs are unlike experimental designs, in which variance in variable scores is controlled (limited). In correlational designs, if the range of scores is truncated, the obtained correlation will be artificially depressed. Truncated means that the lowest scores and the highest scores are not measured or are condensed and merged with less extreme scores. For example, if an attitude scale were scored from a low score of 1 to a high score of 50, truncated scores might only indicate scores in the range from 10 to 40. More extreme scores would be combined with scores within the designated range. If this occurs, the researcher may not find a correlation when the variables are actually correlated.

Researchers tend to make two serious errors with correlational studies. First, they often attempt to establish causality by correlation, reasoning that if two variables are related, one must cause the other. Second, they confuse studies in which differences are examined with studies in which relationships are examined. Examining differences and examining relationships are two sides of the same coin with important distinctions. The existence of a difference assumes the existence of a relationship. However, when designing a study and when conducting data analysis, the researcher must clearly understand whether differences or relationships are being examined. When one is examining two or more groups in terms of one or more variables, one is examining differences between groups as reflected in scores on the identified variables. When one is examining a single group in terms of two or more variables, one is examining relationships between variables. In a correlational study, the relationship examined is that between two research variables within an identified situation.

Descriptive Correlational Design

The purpose of a descriptive correlational design is to examine the relationships that exist in a situation. Using this design will facilitate the identification of

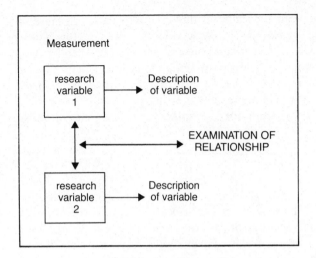

FIGURE 10–7. Descriptive correlational design.

many interrelationships in a situation in a short period of time (Fig. 10–7). The study may examine variables in a situation that has already occurred or a currently occurring situation. No attempt is made to control or manipulate the situation. As with descriptive studies, variables must be clearly identified and defined. An example of a descriptive correlational design is Newman and Gaudiano's (1984) study examining the relationship between depression and subjective time in the elderly.

> Subjects were volunteers from a congregate meal program in central Pennsylvania. The sample (N = 8) was restricted to women over 65 years of age. All subjects were ambulatory and lived at home. Depression was measured by the Beck Depression Inventory. Subjective time was determined by having the subject give a production estimate of an interval of 40 seconds. Analysis of data, which showed a correlation coefficient of 0.35 (p < 0.002) between depression and subjective time, supports the hypothesis that depression is related to decreased subjective time. (p. 137)

Predictive Design

Predictive designs are developed to predict the value of one variable based on values obtained in another variable(s). Prediction is one approach to examining causal relationships between variables. Since causal phenomena are being examined, the terms *dependent* and *independent* are used to describe the variables. One variable is classified as the dependent variable and all other variables as independent variables. The aim of a predictive design (Fig. 10–8) is to predict the level of the dependent variable from the independent variables.

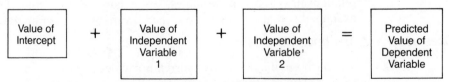

FIGURE 10–8. Predictive design.

Independent variables most effective in prediction are highly correlated with the dependent variable but not highly correlated with other independent variables used in the study. Predictive designs require the development of a theory-based mathematical hypothesis proposing variables expected to effectively predict the dependent variable. The hypothesis is then tested using regression analysis.

Carney and Burns' (1985) study of hospice care used a predictive design to predict the total minutes of care (dependent variable) from days of hospice enrollment (independent variable). The equation expressing the hypothesis is

$$TM = a + b \, DURATION$$

where TM is total minutes and DURATION is the days of hospice enrollment (p. 296). The equation was derived from economic theory. The sample consisted of 266 patients who died in hospice care. Data were analysed using regression analyses (see Chapter 17).

Theory Testing Correlational Designs

The propositions in a theory are statements of relationships. Correlational designs can be used to test the accuracy of propositions. In fact, several correlational designs require a clear theoretical explanation of relational patterns before the study can proceed. These include the partial correlation design, the cross-lagged panel design and path analysis.

Partial Correlation Design □ In some cases, a relationship that has been obtained is partially a consequence of the influence of a third variable, called an *intervening variable*. A partial correlation design is developed to eliminate the influence of the third variable and determine the magnitude of the relationship between the two remaining variables. In order to determine the magnitude of the relationship, the operation of the intervening variable must be specified theoretically. Selection of appropriate statistical analysis techniques is dependent on the variable's theoretical clarity. In a partial correlational design, data are collected on all three variables. The effect of the intervening variable is held constant mathematically, and the correlation of the other two research variables is examined (Fig. 10–9).

An example of partial correlation design is Parsons and Beek's (1982)

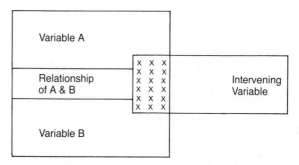

FIGURE 10–9. Partial correlation design.

study "Sleep-awake patterns following cerebral concussion." An excerpt from that study follows.

> This study compared sleep-awake patterns in clients following head injury with their sleep-awake patterns prior to head injury. Data were collected from 75 subjects who had experienced a minor head injury with a disturbance in consciousness three months prior to filling out a questionnaire... Data were collected over a period of one year from all subjects. Three months following their injuries, the clients were asked by a research assistant to participate in a study by answering questions related to the head injury experienced as well as questions about each individual's sleep-awake pattern before and after injury... Partial correlation coefficients were used to determine the degree of significant relationship between length in time of consciousness disruption (research variable) and post-traumatic sleep pattern values (research variable) adjusted for pre-injury sleep pattern values (intervening variable). (pp. 260–261)

Cross-Lagged Panel Design □ This design involves collecting data on two variables at two or more time periods using the same subjects for all measures (Fig. 10–10). When this design was first developed, correlational analysis was conducted on all variables. At present, statistical analyses using multiple regression techniques are used to provide a more powerful examination of data. This design is a strategy for examining inferred causality extracted from theoretical statements. By allowing a time lag, the assertion that a proposed causal variable occurs first in time before a second variable (purported to be the effect) is strengthened (Neale & Liebert, 1980).

Path Analysis Design □ Path analysis design was specifically developed to determine the accuracy of a theoretical model. A hypothesized causal model is developed based on a theoretical model. Using the path analysis design, all major variables within the model are measured, and relationships are determined (Fig. 10–11). The analysis determines whether or not the data are consistent with the model.

Variables are classified into three categories: exogenous variables, endogenous variables and residual variables. Exogenous variables are within the

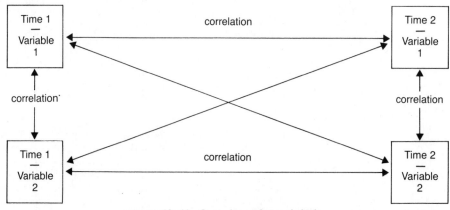

FIGURE 10–10. Cross-lagged panel design.

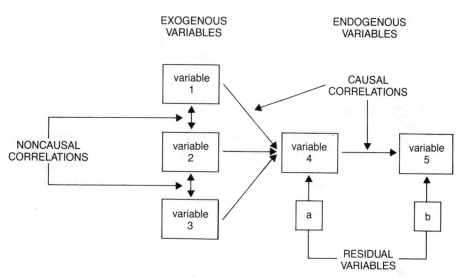

FIGURE 10–11. Path analysis.

theoretical model but are caused by factors outside of this model. Endogenous variables are those whose variation is explained within the theoretical model. Exogenous variables influence the variation of endogenous variables. Residual variables indicate the effect of unmeasured variables not included in the model. These variables explain some of the variance found in the data but not the variance within the model (Waltz & Bausell, 1981).

In Figure 10–11, paths are drawn demonstrating directions of cause and effect. The arrows (paths) from the exogenous variables 1, 2 and 3 lead to the endogenous variable 4, indicating that variable 4 is theoretically proposed to be "caused" by variables 1, 2 and 3. The arrow (path) from endogenous variable 4 to endogenous variable 5 indicates that variable 4 causes variable 5. Exogenous and endogenous variables are measured by collecting data from the experimental subjects, and the accuracy of the proposed paths are analyzed by using a series of regression analyses. Path coefficients are calculated that indicate the effect one variable has on another. The amount of variance explained by the model as well as the fit between the path coefficients and the theoretical model indicate the accuracy of the theory. Variance not accounted for in the statistical analysis is attributed to residual variables (variables a and b) not included in the analyses. An example of this design is Magilvy's (1985) study "Quality of life of hearing-impaired older women." The following is an excerpt from that study.

> A survey of 66 hearing-impaired older women aged 54 to 96 years interviewed at home examined major influences on quality of life experienced by 27 prevocationally deaf and 39 later onset subjects. A causal model was specified;... The exogenous variables, age and hearing loss group were not influenced by other variables in the model. All other variables were endogenous (financial adequacy, social hearing handicap, perceived health, quality of life and functional social support), i.e., hypothesized to have some effect on the other identified

variables. Residuals, representing other impinging variables, were not directly measured and were assumed to be independent.

The direct relationships between variables were then hypothesized [Fig. 10–12] with arrows symbolizing direction of relationships and plus and minus signs indicating the nature of the hypothesized relationships. (pp. 140–141)

QUASI-EXPERIMENTAL STUDY DESIGNS

The purpose of quasi-experimental and experimental designs is to examine causality. The power of the design to accomplish this purpose is dependent on the degree to which the actual effects of the experimental treatment (the independent variable) can be detected by measurement of the dependent variable. Obtaining an understanding of the true effects of an experimental treatment requires action to control threats to the validity of the findings. Threats to validity are controlled through selection of subjects, manipulation of the treatment and reliable measurement of the dependent and independent variables.

Experimental designs with their strict control of variance are the most powerful method of examining causality. However, in social science research, for many reasons—ethical and practical—experimental designs cannot be used. Quasi-experimental designs were developed to provide alternate means for examining causality in situations not conducive to experimental controls. Quasi-experimental designs were first described as a group by Campbell and Stanley in 1963 at a time when only experimental designs were considered of any worth. The quasi-experimental designs facilitated the search for knowledge and examination of causality in situations in which complete control is not possible. These designs have been developed to control as many threats to validity as possible in a situation in which at least one of the three components of true experimental design (randomization, control groups and manipulation of the treatment) is lacking.

Each of the designs described below is ineffective in controlling variance

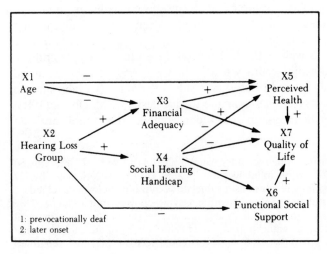

FIGURE 10–12. Hypothesized causal model illustrating influences on the quality of life of older hearing-impaired women. (Reprinted with permission from Magilvy, J.K.: Quality of life of hearing-impaired older women. Nursing Research, *34* (3):141, May/June 1985. Copyright 1985 American Journal of Nursing Company.)

and thus has increased threats to validity. Some achieve greater amounts of control than others. When choosing designs, one should select the design that offers the greatest amount of control possible within the study situation. Even the first designs described in this section, which have very low power in terms of proving causality, can provide useful information on which to design later studies.

Nonequivalent Control Group Designs

Random selection is the only acceptable way of maximizing the probability of equivalence between groups. A nonequivalent control group is one in which the control group is not selected by random means. Some groups are more nonequivalent than others. Some quasi-experimental designs involve using groups (control and treatment) that evolved naturally rather than being developed randomly. These groups cannot be considered equivalent because the individuals in the control group may be different from individuals in the treatment group. Individuals have selected the group in which they are included rather than being selected by the researcher. Thus, selection becomes a threat to validity.

The approach to statistical analysis is problematic in quasi-experimental designs. Although many researchers use the same approaches to analysis used for experimental studies, the selection bias inherent in nonequivalent control groups makes this a questionable practice. Reichardt (1979) recommends using multiple statistical analyses to examine the data from various perspectives and to compare levels of significance obtained from each analysis. The researcher must carefully assess the potential threats to validity in interpreting statistical results since statistical analysis cannot control for threats to validity. The following are examples of nonequivalent control group designs.

The One-Group Post-Test–Only Design □ This design is the weakest of the quasi-experimental designs and is usually inadequate for making causal inferences (Fig. 10–13). In this design, no attempt is usually made to control the selection of those who receive the treatment (the experimental group). Generalization of findings beyond those tested is difficult to justify. The group is not pretested; therefore, there is no direct way to measure change. The researcher cannot claim that the post-test score was a consequence (effect) of the treatment when scores before the treatment are unknown. Because there is no control group, one does not know whether groups not receiving the treatment would have similar scores on the dependent variable. This one-group post-test–only design is commonly used by the inexperienced researcher to evaluate a program of a nursing intervention.

Cook and Campbell (1979) suggest situations in which the one-group post-test–only design is very appropriate and adequate for inferring causality. For example, this design could be used to determine that a single factory's use of vinyl chloride is causing an increase in neighborhood and employee cancers. The incidence of cancer in the community at large is known. The fact that vinyl chloride causes cancer and the types of cancer caused by it are also known.

Manipulation of independent variable	Measurement of dependent variable(s)
TREATMENT ────────────────⟶	POST-TEST

Treatment—often ex post facto

Experimental Group—those who receive the treatment and the post-test

Pretest—inferred—norms of measures of dependent variable(s) of population from which pretreatment experimental group taken

Control Group—implied—norms of measures of dependent variable(s) of population from which experimental group taken

Findings: • comparison of post-test scores with inferred norms
           • confident inferences about change

Example: Lamb (1979). Effect of positioning of postoperative fractured-hip patients as related to comfort.

Uncontrolled   • no link between treatment and change
Threats   • no control group
to Validity: • maturation
               • undetected confounding variables
               • inability to assess threats to validity

FIGURE 10–13. One-group post-test-only design.

These norms would then take the place of the pretest and the control group. Thus, in order to intelligently use this design, one must know a great deal about causal factors interacting within the situation.

The Post-Test–Only Design with Nonequivalent Groups ☐ This design offers an improvement in the previous design, with the addition of a nonequivalent control group (Fig. 10–14). However, this addition can lead to a false confidence in the validity of the findings. Selection threats are a problem with both groups. The lack of a pretest remains a serious impediment to defining change. Differences in post-test scores between groups can be caused by the treatment or by differential selection processes.

The One-Group Pretest–Post-Test Design ☐ This design is one of the more frequently used designs but has such serious weaknesses that findings are often uninterpretable (Fig. 10–15). Pretest scores cannot adequately serve the same function as a control group. Events can occur between the pretest and post-test that alter responses to the post-test. These events then serve as alternate hypotheses to the proposal that the change in post-test scores is due to the treatment. Post-test scores might be altered by (1) maturation processes, (2) administration of the pretest and (3) changes in instrumentation. Additionally, subjects in many studies using this design are selected based on high or low scores on the pretest. Thus, there is an additional threat that changes in the post-test may be due to regression toward the mean. The addition of a nonequivalent control group, as described in the next design, can greatly strengthen the validity of the findings.

	Manipulation of independent variable	Measurement of dependent variable(s)
Experimental Group ————→TREATMENT	——————————————————→	**POST-TEST**
Nonequivalent Control Group	——————————————————→	**POST-TEST**

Treatment—often ex post facto
   may not be well defined

Experimental Group—those who receive the treatment and the post-test

Pretest—inferred—norms of measures of dependent variable(s) of population from which
   pretreatment experimental group taken

Control Group—not randomly selected—tend to be those who naturally in the situation do
   not receive the treatment

Findings: • comparison of post-test scores of experimental and control groups
            • comparison of post-test scores with norms

Example: Marut and Mercer (1979). Comparison of primiparas' perceptions of vaginal and
          cesarean births.

Uncontrolled   • no link between treatment and change
Threats   • no pretest
to Validity: • selection

FIGURE 10–14. Post-test-only design with nonequivalent groups.

	Measurement of dependent variable(s)	Manipulation of independent variable	Measurement of dependent variable(s)
Experimental Group ————→	**PRETEST** ————→	**TREATMENT** ————→	**POST-TEST Group**

Treatment—greater researcher control
   usually not ex post facto

Experimental Group—greater researcher control

Control Group—pretest scores of treatment group
   expected to serve as control

Findings: comparison of pretest and post-test scores

Examples: Dittmar and Dulski (1977). Early evening administration of sleep medication to
           the hospitalized aged: A consideration in rehabilitation.

Uncontrolled   • history
Threats   • statistical regression
to Validity: • maturation
               • testing
               • instrumentation

FIGURE 10–15. One-group pretest–post-test design.

The Untreated Control Group Design with Pretest and Post-Test □ This is the most frequently used design in social science research (Fig. 10–16). This quasi-experimental design is the first design discussed that is generally interpretable. The uncontrolled threats to validity are primarily due to the nonequivalent control group. For the researcher planning to use this design, the effects of these threats on interpreting study findings are discussed in detail by Cook and Campbell (1979). Variations in this design include using proxy pretest measures (a different pretest that correlates with the post-test), separate pretest and post-test samples and pretest measures at more than one time interval. The first two variations weaken the design, but the latter variation greatly strengthens it.

The Nonequivalent Dependent Variables Design □ At first glance, the nonequivalent dependent variables design would seem to be equivalent to the single group pretest–post-test design in which two dependent variables are measured (Fig.10–17). This design is used in situations in which only one study group is available. The key difference is in the selection of two theoretically linked concepts as dependent variables that are expected to react differently to the planned treatment. The contrasting of patterns of change and no-change in a theoretical context is critical to the effectiveness of the design. The design can be expanded into one that examines broader pattern-matching and that has

	Measurement of dependent variable(s)	Manipulation of independent variable	Measurement of dependent variable(s)
Experimental Group ———→	PRETEST ———————→	TREATMENT ——————→	POST-TEST
Nonequivalent Control Group →	PRETEST ————————————————————→		POST-TEST

Treatment—experimental group
        control group not treated

Control Group—not randomly selected

Findings: • comparison of control and experimental pretest
          • comparison of pretest and post-test
          • comparison of control and experimental post-test

Example: King and Tarsitano (1982). The effect of structured and unstructured preoperative teaching: A replication.

Uncontrolled • selection–maturation
Threats to   • instrumentation
Validity: • differential statistical regression
              • interaction of selection and history

FIGURE 10–16. Untreated control group design with pretest and post-test.

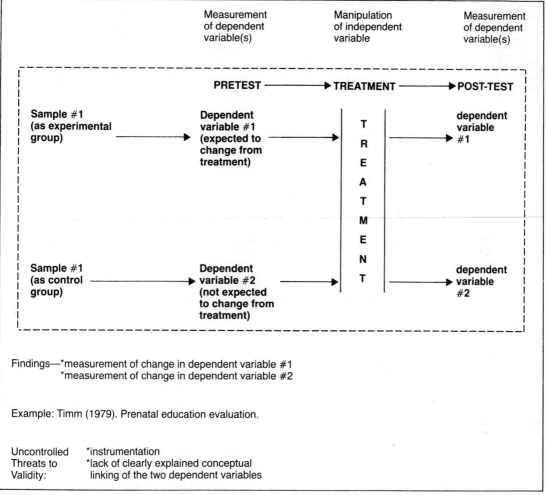

Measurement of dependent variable(s)	Manipulation of independent variable	Measurement of dependent variable(s)

PRETEST ⟶ TREATMENT ⟶ POST-TEST

Sample #1 (as experimental group)

Dependent variable #1 (expected to change from treatment)

T R E A T M E N T

dependent variable #1

Sample #1 (as control group)

Dependent variable #2 (not expected to change from treatment)

dependent variable #2

Findings—*measurement of change in dependent variable #1
        *measurement of change in dependent variable #2

Example: Timm (1979). Prenatal education evaluation.

Uncontrolled Threats to Validity: *instrumentation
*lack of clearly explained conceptual linking of the two dependent variables

FIGURE 10–17. Nonequivalent dependent variables design.

been carefully planned to rule out alternative interpretations. The primary usefulness of this design and expansions of it is in theory testing.

The Removed-Treatment Design with Pretest and Post-Test □ In some cases, gaining access to even a nonequivalent control group is not possible. The removed-treatment design with pretest and post-test creates conditions that approximate the conceptual requirements of a control group receiving no treatment. The design is basically a one-group pretest–post-test design. However, after a delay of time, a third measure of the dependent variable is taken, followed by an interval of time in which the treatment is removed, followed by a fourth measure of the dependent variable (Fig. 10–18). The period of time between each measure must be equivalent. In nursing situations, the ethics of removing an effective treatment must be considered. Even if it is ethically

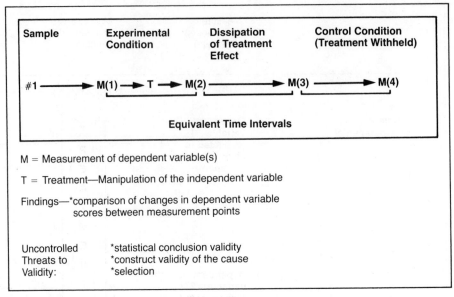

FIGURE 10–18. Removed-treatment design with pretest and post-test.

acceptable, the response of subjects to the removal may make interpreting changes difficult.

The Repeated-Treatment Design □ This design builds on the previous design and allows a treatment to be introduced, withdrawn and then reintroduced (Fig. 10–19). Skinner's research on stimulus-response characteristics used this design. The study from which the Hawthorne effect emerged was also based on this design. In the past, researchers who have used the design have held a disdain for statistical analysis. In addition, outcomes are difficult to interpret. In using this design, large samples, careful statistical analysis, unobtrusive measures of the dependent variable and a long delay between the treatment and its reintroduction are recommended.

The Reversed-Treatment Nonequivalent Control Group Design with Pretest and Post-test □ This design introduces two independent variables: one expected to produce a positive effect, and one expected to produce a negative effect (Fig. 10–20). There are two experimental groups, each exposed to one of the treatments. The design tests differences in response to the two treatments. This design is more useful for theory testing than the no-treatment control group design because of its high construct validity of the cause. The theoretical causal variable must be rigorously defined to allow differential predictions of directions of effect. In order to be maximally interpretable, two additional groups should be added: a placebo control in which the treatment is not expected to affect the dependent variable, and a no-treatment control group to provide a baseline. The use of this design in nursing practice situations may be limited because of the undesirability of intentionally causing a negative effect.

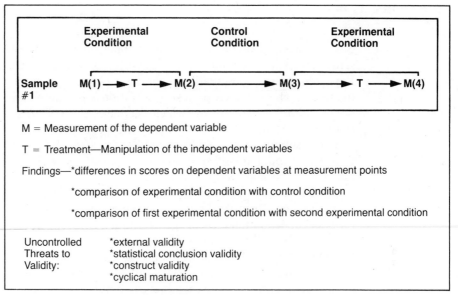

M = Measurement of the dependent variable

T = Treatment—Manipulation of the independent variables

Findings—*differences in scores on dependent variables at measurement points

　　　　　*comparison of experimental condition with control condition

　　　　　*comparison of first experimental condition with second experimental condition

Uncontrolled　*external validity
Threats to　　*statistical conclusion validity
Validity:　　　*construct validity
　　　　　　　*cyclical maturation

FIGURE 10–19. Repeated treatment design.

	Measurement of dependent variable(s)	Manipulation of independent variable	Measurement of dependent variable(s)
Experimental Group #1 ——→	PRETEST ——→	proposed positive effect treatment ——→	POST-TEST
Experimental Group #2 ——→	PRETEST ——→	proposed negative effect treatment ——→	POST-TEST

Findings:　• comparison of group #1 and group #2 pretest
　　　　　• comparison of group #1 and group #2 post-test
　　　　　• comparison of changes between pretest and post-test between groups

Example:　Hartfield, Cason, and Cason (1982). Effects of information about a threatening procedure on patients' examinations and emotional distress.

Uncontrolled　• statistical conclusion validity
Threats to
Validity:

FIGURE 10–20. The reversed-treatment nonequivalent control group design with pretest and post-test.

Interrupted Time-Series Designs

The interrupted time-series designs are similar to descriptive time designs except that a treatment is applied at some point in the observations. Time-series analyses have some advantages over other quasi-experimental designs. Repeated pretest observations can assess trends in maturation before the treatment. The repeated pretest observations also allow measures of trends in scores before the treatment, which decreases the risk of statistical regression leading to misinterpretation of findings. If records are kept of events that could influence subjects in the study, the researcher can determine whether historical factors that could modify responses to the treatment were in operation between the last pretest and the first post-test.

There are, however, threats that are particularly problematic in time-series designs. Record-keeping procedures and definitions of constructs used for data collection tend to change over time. Thus, maintaining consistency can be a problem. The treatment can cause attrition so that the sample before treatment may be different in important ways from the post-treatment group. Seasonal variation or other cyclical influences can be interpreted as treatment effects. Therefore, identifying cyclical patterns that may be occurring and controlling for them is critical to the analysis of study findings. McCain and McCleary (1979) suggest the use of the ARIMA statistical model (described in Chapter 17) to analyze time-series data. ARIMA is a relatively new model but has some distinct advantages over regression analysis techniques. For adequate statistical analysis, at least 50 measurement points are needed; however, Cook and Campbell (1979) believe that even small numbers of measurement points can provide information greater than that obtained in cross-sectional studies. Numbers of measures shown in the illustrated designs are limited by space and are not meant to suggest limiting measures to the numbers shown.

Simple Interrupted Time Series □ This design is similar to the descriptive study, with the addition of a treatment that occurs or is applied at a given point in time (Fig. 10–21). The treatment, which in some cases is not completely under the control of the researcher, should be clearly defined. The use of multiple methods to measure the dependent variable greatly strengthens the design. Threats that are well controlled by this design include maturation and statistical regression.

Interrupted Time Series With A Nonequivalent No-Treatment Control Group Time Series □ The addition of a control group to this design greatly strengthens the validity of the findings. The control group allows examination of differences in trends between groups after the treatment and the persistence of treatment effects over time (Fig. 10–22). Although the treatment may continue (*e.g.*, a change in nursing management practices or patient teaching strategies) the initial response to the change may differ from later responses.

Interrupted Time Series with Nonequivalent Dependent Variables □ The capacity for theory testing is a major strength of this design (Fig. 10–23). Whether or not theory testing is the primary purpose of the study, the two variables

Measurement of dependent variable(s)				Manipulation of independent variable		Measurement of dependent variable(s)			
PRETESTS ————————→TREATMENT ————————→POST-TESTS									
Experimental Group M(1)	M(2)	M(3)	M(4)	T	M(5)	M(6)	M(7)	M(8)	

Subjects: may remain the same across the study or different individuals may be selected at each measurement period (as in the descriptive time dimensional designs)

Pretest Dependent Variable Measures: In addition to researcher initiated tools, measures may be obtained from archival data sources such as patient records, scores available in student records or employee records.

Treatment: may be a key event occurring at one specific point in time that is expected to modify subject responses to the dependent variable, *e.g.*, curriculum change, administrative change, change in nursing care of particular type of patient. The treatment tends to continue after implementation rather than occurring and then being withdrawn.

Findings: changes in trends of scores before and after treatment

Example: Norris, Campbell, and Brenkert (1982). Nursing procedures and alterations in transcutaneous oxygen tension in premature infants.

Uncontrolled Threats to Validity:
- history
- seasonal trends
- instrumentation
- selection
- mono-operation bias
- cyclic influences interpreted as treatment effects

FIGURE 10–21. Simple interrupted time series.

must be conceptually related, with one expected to change with the treatment, and the other not expected to change with the treatment. The design allows for the examination of the effects of history without the use of a control group. As with all quasi-experimental studies, attempts to rule out alternate explanations of the causal construct are important.

Interrupted Time Series With Removed Treatment □ This design is basically two interrupted time series (Fig. 10–24). The treatment is administered from M(5) to M(7). The first time series, from M(1) to M(7), examines the effects of the presence of the treatment. The second time series, from M(5) to M(11), assesses the effects of the absence of the treatment. The most powerful effect would be a change in one direction between M(4) and M(5) and a change in the opposite direction between M(7) and M(8). The design reduces the threats of history, selection and instrumentation. The design is more interpretable when the treatment has low salience (value, importance) to the subjects, thus leading to less confounding responses by subjects to withdrawal of the treatment. In addition to the ethical constraints of removing an effective treatment, caution should be taken in withdrawing a treatment. Withdrawing a treatment

Measurement of dependent variable(s)				Manipulation of independent variable		Measurement of dependent variable(s)			
PRETESTS ———————————→TREATMENT ———————————→POST-TESTS									
Experimental Group	M(1)	M(2)	M(3)	M(4)	T	M(5)	M(6)	M(7)	(M(8))
Control Group	M(1)	M(2)	M(3)	M(4)		M(5)	M(6)	M(7)	M(8)

Subjects: may remain the same across the study or may be part of a group in which some individuals may change (*e.g.,* class, work group, patient teaching, or patient care group)

Pretest Dependent Variable Measures: In addition to researcher initiated tools, measures may be obtained from archival data sources.

Treatment: may be key event occurring at one specific point in time that is expected to modify experimental subjects' responses to dependent variable measures. Treatment tends to continue after implementation rather than occurring and then being withdrawn.

Findings: • changes in trends of scores before and after treatment
• comparison of trends in experimental and control groups
• temporal persistence of treatment effects

Example: Farr, Keene, Samson, and Michael (1984). Alterations in circadian excretion of urinary variables and physiological indicators of stress following surgery.

Uncontrolled Threats to Validity: • selection and history interaction
• as experimental and control groups increase in noncomparability, threats to validity increase
• interaction of populations and treatment
• cyclical influences interpreted as treatment effects

FIGURE 10–22. Interrupted time series with a nonequivalent no-treatment control group time series.

will interfere with statistical analysis of the effects of treatment application as a result of the shortened series. The statistical analyses used to examine time-series studies are more powerful with a long series of measurements. Removing the treatment shortens the series of measurements of a trend in a particular direction. If removing the treatment has an effect, the trend will shift to another direction, preventing adequate examination of the first trend.

Interrupted Time Series With Multiple Replications ◻ This is a very powerful design for inferring causality (Fig. 10–25). It requires greater researcher control than is usually possible in social science research outside closed institutional settings. The studies that led to the adoption of behavior modification techniques used this design. In order for significant differences to be interpretable, the pretest and post-test scores must be in different directions. Within this design, treatments can be modified, substituting one treatment for another or combining two treatments and examining interaction effects.

Measurement of dependent variable(s)	Manipulation of independent variable	Measurement of independent variable(s)
PRETESTS ⟶ TREATMENT ⟶ POST-TESTS **Single Sample** M(1ab) M(2ab) M(3ab) M(4ab) T M(5ab) M(6ab) M(7ab) M(8ab) **a = variable theoretically expected to change with treatment** **b = variable theoretically not expected to change with treatment**		
Subjects: Single subjects may be followed throughout the study or may be separate individuals representing the population under study.		
Dependent Variable Measures: Design requires that dependent variables be extracted from theoretical formulation in which one variable is predicted to change with the treatment and one variable is not expected to change with the treatment.		
Treatment: may be key event not under control of researcher		
Findings: • changes in trends in variable a after treatment • changes in trends in variable b after treatment • comparison in trends in the two variables		
Uncontrolled Threats to Validity: • instrumentation • selection • cyclical influences interpreted as treatment effects		

FIGURE **10–23.** Interrupted time series with nonequivalent dependent variables.

Interrupted Time Series With Switching Replications □ This is a very powerful design that controls most threats to internal validity, extends external and construct validity and facilitates examination of delayed causal effects (Fig. 10–26). The design is feasible to implement in any situation in which a time-series design with a no-treatment control group is possible. It simply provides the treatment to the no-treatment control group nearer the end of the study.

Measurement of dependent variable(s)	Manipulation of independent variable	Measurement of dependent variable(s)
PRETESTS ⟶ TREATMENT ⟶ POST-TESTS **Single Sample** M(1) M(2) M(3) M(4) T M(5) M(6) M(7) T M(8) M(9) M(10) M(11)		
Treatment: applied across a period of time and then withdrawn		
Dependent Variable(s): measured before the treatment, at several points during the treatment and after the treatment		
Findings: • the effects of the presence of a treatment • the effects of the absence of a treatment • change in trends in relation to treatment time		
Uncontrolled Threats to Validity: • resentful demoralization at treatment withdrawal • selection-maturation interaction • instrumentation		

FIGURE **10–24.** Interrupted time series with removed treatment.

```
PRETEST ──→ T ──→ POST-TEST ──→ PRETEST ──→ T ──→ POST-TEST etc
Single Sample
M(1)  M(2)  T  M(3)  M(4)  T  M(5)  M(6)  T  M(7)  M(8)  T  M(9)  M(10)
```

Treatment: provided repeatedly
            effects must dissipate rapidly
            should be scheduled randomly

Findings: • powerful for inferring causal effects
           • differences in pretest and post-test scores must be in opposite directions to be
             interpretable

Example: Parsons and Wilson (1984). Cerebrovascular status of severe closed head–
          injured patients following passive position changes.

FIGURE 10–25. Interrupted time series with multiple replications.

EXPERIMENTAL STUDY DESIGNS

Experimental designs are set up to provide the greatest amount of control possible in order to more closely examine causality. To examine cause, one must eliminate all factors influencing the dependent variable other than the cause (independent variable) being studied. Other factors are eliminated by controlling them. The study is designed to prevent any other element from intruding into observation of the specific cause and effect that the researcher wishes to examine. The three essential elements of experimental research are (1) randomization, (2) researcher controlled manipulation of the independent variable and (3) researcher control of the experimental situation, including a control or comparison group. Experimental designs exert much effort to control variance. Characteristics of subjects included in the study are narrowly defined, the independent variable is provided in a precisely defined way, the dependent variables are carefully operationalized and the situation in which the study is conducted is rigidly controlled to prevent the interference of unstudied factors from modifying the dynamics of the process being studied.

Measurement of dependent variable(s)	Manipulation of independent variable	Measurement of dependent variable(s)

```
PRETESTS ──────→ TREATMENT ──────→ POST-TESTS

Experimental Group 1
M(1)  M(2)  M(3)  M(4)  M(5)  M(6)  M(7)  T  M(8)  M(9)  M(10)

Experimental Group 2
M(1)  M(2)  M(3)  T  M(4)  M(5)  M(6)  M(7)  M(8)  M(9)  M(10)
```

Samples: nonequivalent; each group serves as control to the other group

Findings: • probing delayed causal effects

Uncontrolled   • controls for most threats to internal validity
Threats to Validity: • extends external and construct validity

FIGURE 10–26. Interrupted time series with switching replications.

Pretest–Post-test Control Group Design ☐ This design is the most commonly used experimental design (Fig. 10–27). The experimental and control groups are both randomly selected. Comparison of pretest scores allows evaluation of the effectiveness of randomization in providing equivalent groups. The treatment is under control of the researcher. The dependent variable is measured twice, before and after the manipulation of the independent variable. As with all well-designed studies, the dependent and independent variables will be conceptually linked, conceptually defined and operationalized. Instruments used to measure the dependent variable will clearly reflect the conceptual meaning of the variable. Often, more than one means to measure the dependent variable is advisable to avoid mono-operation and mono-method bias.

Multiple groups (both experimental and control) can be used to great advantage in the pretest–post-test design and the post-test–only design. For example, one control group could receive no treatment while another control group could receive a placebo treatment. Multiple experimental groups could receive varying levels of the treatments, such as differing frequency, intensity or length of nursing care measures. These additions greatly increase the generalizability of the study findings.

Post-Test–Only Control Group Design ☐ In some studies, the dependent variable cannot be measured before the treatment. For example, it is not possible to meaningfully measure responses to interventions designed to control nausea from chemotherapy prior to the beginning of chemotherapy treatment. Additionally, in some cases, subjects' responses to the post-test can be due, in

Measurement of dependent variable(s)	Manipulation of independent variable	Measurement of dependent variable(s)
Randomly Selected Experimental Group	PRETEST ──────→ TREATMENT ──────────→ POST-TEST	
Randomly Selected Control Group	PRETEST ──────────────────────────────→ POST-TEST	

Treatment: under control of researcher

Findings: • comparison of pretest and post-test scores
          • comparison of experimental and control groups
          • comparison of pretest–post-test differences between samples

Example: Ventura, Young, Feldman, Pastore, Pikula, and Yates (1984). Effectiveness of health promotion interventions.

Uncontrolled • testing
Threats to   • instrumentation
Validity: • mortality
            • restricted generalizability as control increases

FIGURE 10–27. Pretest–post-test control group design.

part, to learning from or subjective reaction to the pretest (pretest sensitization). If this is a concern in a specific study, the pretest may be eliminated and a post-test–only control group design can be used (Fig. 10–28). However, this elimination prevents the use of many powerful statistical analysis techniques within the study. Additionally, the effectiveness of randomization in obtaining equivalent experimental and control groups cannot be evaluated.

Solomon Four-Group Design ☐ This design is rather cumbersome but was developed to test the effects of pretesting on post-test scores (Fig. 10–29). The Solomon four-group design is a stronger design than the post-test–only design but requires more complicated statistical analyses. Four groups are used, two experimental groups and two control groups. One experimental group and one control group are pretested and post-tested. The other two groups receive only the post-test. This strategy allows multiple comparisons between groups and an assessment of the effect of the pretest on post-test scores.

Randomized Block Design ☐ This design uses the two-group pretest–post-test pattern or the two-group post-test pattern with one addition, a blocking variable. The blocking variable, if uncontrolled, is expected to confound the findings of the study. To prevent confounding the findings, the subjects are rank ordered in relation to the blocking variable. For example, if effectiveness of a nursing intervention to relieve post-chemotherapy nausea was the independent variable, severity of nausea could confound the findings. Subjects would be ranked according to severity of nausea. The two subjects with the most severely classified nausea would be identified and randomly assigned, one to the experimental group and one to the control group. The two subjects next in rank would then be identified and randomly assigned. This pattern would be

	Manipulation of independent variable	Measurement of dependent variable
Randomly Selected Experimental Group	TREATMENT————————————→	POST-TEST
Randomly Selected Control Group	————————————→	POST-TEST

Treatment: under control of researcher

Findings: • comparison of experimental and control groups

Example: Ziemer (1983). Effects of information on postsurgical coping.

Uncontrolled • instrumentation
Threats to • mortality
Validity: • limited generalizability as control increases

FIGURE 10–28. Post-test only control group design.

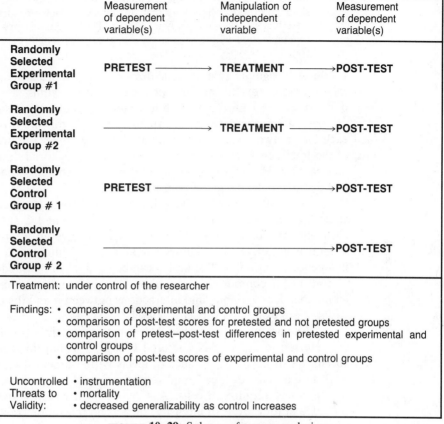

	Measurement of dependent variable(s)	Manipulation of independent variable	Measurement of dependent variable(s)
Randomly Selected Experimental Group #1	**PRETEST** ⟶	**TREATMENT** ⟶	**POST-TEST**
Randomly Selected Experimental Group #2	⟶	**TREATMENT** ⟶	**POST-TEST**
Randomly Selected Control Group # 1	**PRETEST** ⟶		**POST-TEST**
Randomly Selected Control Group # 2	⟶		**POST-TEST**

Treatment: under control of the researcher

Findings: • comparison of experimental and control groups
• comparison of post-test scores for pretested and not pretested groups
• comparison of pretest–post-test differences in pretested experimental and control groups
• comparison of post-test scores of experimental and control groups

Uncontrolled   • instrumentation
Threats to   • mortality
Validity: • decreased generalizability as control increases

FIGURE 10–29. Solomon four-group design.

followed until the entire sample was randomly assigned as matched pairs. This procedure ensures that the experimental group and the control group are equal in relation to the potentially confounding variable. The effect of blocking can also be accomplished statistically (using Analysis of Covariance) without categorizing the confounding variable into discrete components. However, for this analysis to be accurate, one must be careful not to violate the assumptions of the statistical procedure (Spector, 1981). An example of this design is Powers and Wooldridge's (1982) study "Factors influencing knowledge, attitudes, and compliance of hypertensive patients." The following excerpt describes the study design:

> ...four aspects of an educational program for 160 hypertensive patients were manipulated: number of meetings, patient responsibility and participation, directiveness of the intervention, and emphasis on negative consequences of uncontrolled hypertension... The 160 subjects who participated in the educational program were from five clinical settings: inner city health facility (n = 62), community health center (n = 20), private hospital clinic (n = 34), university hospital clinic (n = 27), and private physician's office (n = 17)... The resulting sample was more heterogeneous than found in most studies conducted within a

single setting, thus potentially enhancing the generalizability of the findings. It should be noted, however, that an unusually high proportion of the patients were black (72%) and women (70%)... The assignment procedure incorporated randomization with blocking on sex, race, and length of time since diagnosis. (pp. 171–173)

Factorial Designs □ In a factorial design, two or more different characteristics, treatments, or events are independently varied within a single study. This design is a very logical approach to examining multiple causality. The simplest arrangement is one in which two treatments or factors are involved, and, within each factor, two levels are manipulated (for example, the presence or absence of the treatment). This is referred to as a 2 × 2 factorial design. This design is illustrated in Figure 10–30, using the two independent variables of relaxation and distraction as means of pain relief.

A 2 × 2 factorial design produces a study with four cells. Each cell must contain an equivalent number of subjects. Cells B and C allow examination of each separate intervention. Cell D subjects receive no treatment and serve as a control group. Cell A allows examination of interaction between the two independent variables. The design can be used, as in the random blocks design, to control for confounding variables. The confounding variable is included as an independent variable, and interactions between it and the other independent variable are examined (Spector, 1981).

Extensions of the factorial design to more than two levels of variables are referred to as M × N Factorial Designs. Within this design, independent variables can have any number of levels within practical limits. Note that a 3 × 3 design involves 9 cells and requires a much larger sample size. A 4 × 4 design would require 16 cells. A 4 × 4 design would allow relaxation to be provided at four levels of intensity, such as no relaxation, relaxation 10 minutes twice a day, 15 minutes three times a day and 20 minutes four times a day. Distraction would be provided in similar levels. Factorial designs are not limited to two independent variables; however, interpretation of larger numbers becomes more complex, and increased knowledge of statistical analysis is required. Factorial designs do allow the examination of theoretically proposed interrelationships between multiple independent variables. However, very large samples are required. An example of this design is Rice and Johnson's study (1984) "Preadmission self-instruction booklets, postadmission exercise performance, and teaching time." An excerpt from that study follows:

The relative effects of preadmission self-instructional information on levels of performance and time needed to achieve level of mastery of exercise behaviors were examined using a sample of 130 presurgical cholecystectomy and herniorrhaphy patients... A 3 × 2 factorial design was used with preadmission exercise instructions as the experimental factor and type of surgery (cholecystectomy or herniorrhaphy) as the second factor. Clients were randomly assigned to one of the three levels of preadmission instruction—specific exercise instructions, non-specific exercise instructions, and no exercise instructions—for coughing, deep breathing, ambulatory activity, and leg movements. (pp. 147–148)

Nested Designs □ In some experimental situations, the researcher wishes to consider the effect of variables that are found only at some levels of the

FIGURE 10–30. Example of factorial design.

Level of Relaxation	Level of Distraction	
	Distraction	No Distraction
Relaxation	A	B
No Relaxation	C	D

independent variables being studied. Variables found only at certain levels of the independent variable are called *nested variables*. Possible nested variables include gender, race, socioeconomic status and education or may be such factors as patients who are cared for on specific nursing units or at different hospitals. The statistical analysis is then conducted as though the unit or hospital was the subject, rather than the individual patient. Figure 10–31 illustrates the nesting design. In actual practice, nursing units used in this manner would have to be much larger in number than those illustrated, since each unit would be considered a subject and randomly assigned to a treatment. The following excerpt from Harris and Hyman's (1984) study "Clean vs. sterile

Pain Control Management		Primary Nursing Care							
		Primary Care				No Primary Care			
		Unit A	Unit B	Unit C	Unit D	Unit E	Unit F	Unit G	Unit H
Traditional Care PRN Medication	Unit A								
	Unit B								
	Unit C								
	Unit D								
New Approach "around the clock" medication	Unit E								
	Unit F								
	Unit G								
	Unit H								

FIGURE 10–31. Design using nesting.

tracheotomy care and level of pulmonary infection," is an example of this design:

> The purpose of this research was to determine if clean tracheotomy care was more effective than sterile as measured by levels of postoperative pulmonary infection. Ten hospitals with large Head and Neck/ENT services were selected as data collection sites... To increase external validity, possible unique effects associated with hospitals were controlled by use of a nested design–hospital nested within treatment procedure... At these centers a minimum of 15 tracheostomy patient charts were reviewed pre and postoperatively for clinical and laboratory data related to infection. Patient level of infection was defined using the Weighted Level of Pulmonary Infection Tool, which was constructed for this study. (pp. 80–83)

Multivariate Designs □ Multivariate designs involve multiple variables. Any experimental design can be expanded to a multivariate version. This strategy allows the examination of complex relationships among variables, which is in keeping with the idea of multicausality. Multiple measures and multiple methods of measuring are used to examine the dependent variables. Powerful multivariate statistical techniques are used to analyze the complex data. The techniques are relatively recent, and results are difficult for the novice to interpret. An example of this design is Goldberg and Fitzpatrick's (1980) study "Movement therapy with the aged." The following is an excerpt from the abstract of that study:

> This study examined effect of participation in a movement therapy group on morale and self-esteem in a population of institutionalized aged persons. Control group subjects participated in the usual treatment program at the nursing home, and experimental group subjects participated in a series of movement therapy sessions. Scores on morale and self-esteem scales were used to compare differences between the groups. (p. 339)

Repeated Measures Designs With Counterbalancing □ In some studies, more than one treatment is administered to each subject. The treatments are provided sequentially, rather than concurrently. This is called a *repeated measures design*. Each subject is tested for response to each separate treatment. One difficulty encountered in this type of study is that exposure to one treatment may cause effects (called *carryover effects*) that persist and influence responses of the subject to later treatments. Subjects can improve as they become more familiar with the experimental protocol, which is called a *practice effect*. They may become tired or bored with the study, which is called a *fatigue effect*. The direct interaction of one treatment with another, such as the use of two drugs, can confound differences in the two treatments. Counterbalancing is a design strategy to guard against possible erroneous conclusions resulting from carryover effects in a repeated measures design. Using counterbalancing, subjects are randomly assigned to a specific sequencing of treatment conditions. This distributes the carryover effects equally across all the conditions of the study, thus canceling them out. The process of counterbalancing can become quite complicated when more than two treatments are involved. Counterbalancing is effective only if the carryover effect is essentially the same from treatment A to treatment B as it is from treatment B to treatment A. If one is more fatiguing than the other or more likely to modify response to the second treatment, counterbalancing will not be effective. An example of this design is Hasler and Cohen's (1982) study "The effect of oxygen administration on oral temperature assessment." The following is an excerpt from the abstract of that study:

> This study sought to determine if oxygen administration via aerosol mask, venti-mask, or nasal prongs altered oral temperature as assessed in the sublingual pockets of the mouth. The population included 40 healthy male and female volunteers. Oxygen was administered using a repeated measure design with the subjects serving as their own controls and the oxygen devices presented in a counterbalanced order. An electronic thermometer recorded the temperature at the end of each 15-minute treatment/control period. (p. 265)

The counterbalancing used in Hasler and Cohen's (1982, p. 266) study is illustrated in Table 10–1.

Randomized Clinical Trials □ These trials have been used in medicine since 1945. Tyzenhouse (1981) has proposed the utilization of the technique to examine areas of nursing practice, such as comparing traditional nursing care practices to newer.techniques. The design uses large numbers of subjects to test the effects of a treatment and compare the results with a control group who have not received the treatment (or who have received a more traditional treatment). Subjects are drawn from a reference population, using clearly defined criteria, and then randomly assigned to treatment or control groups. Baseline data and outcome data are collected in both groups; data are analysed and inferences are made from the findings. Because of the need for large samples, the study is carried out simultaneously in multiple geographic locations and coordinated by the primary researcher. Several problems must be confronted by the researcher using this technique. Coordination of a project of this type requires much time and effort. Keeping up with subjects is critical but may be difficult. Communication and cooperation of nurses assisting with the

TABLE 10–1
Sequence of Oxygen Device Presentation

Subject Order	Treatment Sequence
1	O-O-A-O-C-O-V-O-C-O-N-O
2	O-O-V-O-C-O-N-O-C-O-A-O
3	O-O-N-O-C-O-A-O-C-O-V-O
4	O-O-A-O-C-O-N-O-C-O-V-O
5	O-O-N-O-C-O-V-O-C-O-A-O
6	O-O-V-O-C-O-A-O-C-O-N-O

Note. These symbols are used to indicate: A = aerosol mask; V = venti-mask; N = nasal prongs; C = control period; O = temperature recording.

(Reprinted with permission from Hasler, M. E. & Cohen, J. A.: The effect of oxygen administration on oral temperature assessment. Nursing Research, 31(5):266, 1982. Copyright 1982 American Journal of Nursing Company.)

study in the various geographic locations is essential but sometimes difficult. Costs of conducting studies such as these can be higher than most nursing studies, and such studies usually require obtaining grant funding from outside sources. Nurses are often so convinced that current nursing practice is effective that they may resist following a protocol for care that does not coincide with their beliefs. Thus, the researcher may encounter attempts to ignore the protocol and provide traditional care. Utilization of this design could greatly improve the scientific base for nursing practice.

STUDIES THAT DO NOT USE TRADITIONAL RESEARCH DESIGNS

There are some approaches to research in which the research designs described in this chapter cannot be used. The purposes of these studies tends to be unlike those of other studies. These studies tend to be in highly specialized areas that require unique design strategies to accomplish their purposes. Designs for primary prevention and health promotion, secondary analysis, meta-analysis and methodological studies are described.

Primary Prevention and Health Promotion Studies

Studying primary prevention and health promotion involves applying a treatment of primary prevention (the cause) and then attempting to measure the effect (an event that does not occur if the treatment was effective). Primary prevention studies, then, attempt to measure things that do not happen. One cannot select a sample to study, apply a treatment and then measure an effect. The sample must be the community. The design involves examining changes in the community, and the variables are called *indicators*. A change in an identified indicator is inferred to be a consequence of the effectiveness of the prevention program (treatment). Specific indicators would depend on the focus of prevention. For example, the indicators identified by the National Institution on Drug Abuse include changes in drug-related perceptions, attitudes, knowledge and action; changes in prevalence and incidence of drug use, drug-related mortality/ morbidity; institutional policy/programs; youth/parent involvement in the community; and accident rates (French & Kaufman, 1981). Since one indicator alone would be insufficient to infer effect, multiple indicators and statistical analyses appropriate for these indicators must be used.

Secondary Analysis Designs

Secondary analysis involves studying data previously collected in another study. Data are reexamined using different organizations of the data and different statistical analyses than those previously used. The design involves analyzing data to validate the reported findings, examining dimensions previously unexamined or redirecting the focus of the data to allow comparison with data from other studies. An example of this design is Cox, Sullivan and Roghmann's (1984) study "A conceptual explanation of risk-reduction behavior and intervention development." An excerpt from the abstract of that study follows:

This study used a new conceptual model of health behavior to examine a specific risk-reducing response. Known to be at risk for fetal abnormalities because of maternal age, 203 women were examined for their acceptance or rejection of an amniocentesis test on the basis of individual characteristics and external significant factors. (p. 168)

Design: Since 1977, survey data have been collected to monitor the acceptance of prenatal screening by women at risk and by their care providers. Most of these data were collected through mail and telephone surveys; in addition, data from birth certificates, service logs, and census data from the Health Systems Areas were used. The study described here is a secondary data analysis of the original survey data. (p. 169)

Meta-analysis Designs

Meta-analysis involves merging findings from many studies that have examined the same phenomenon. The design incorporates specific statistical analyses. Specific statistical analyses are used to determine the overall findings from joint examination of reported statistical findings. Since studies seldom have exactly the same focus, conclusions are never absolute but do give some sense of unity to knowledge within that area (O'Flynn, 1982). An example of this design is Devine and Cook's (1983) study "A meta-analytic analysis of effects of psychoeducational interventions on length of postsurgical hospital stay." The following is an excerpt from the abstract of that study:

Forty-nine studies of the relationships between brief psychoeducational interventions and the length of postsurgical hospitalization are reviewed using meta-analysis. Results show that interventions reduce hospital stay by about 1 1/4 days and that reduction does not depend on whether the studies were published or not, whether the discharging physician was aware of the patient's experimental condition, or whether studies were lacking in internal validity. (p. 267)

Methodological Designs

Methodological studies are designed to develop the validity and reliability of instruments to measure constructs used as variables in research. The process is lengthy and complex. The average length of researcher time required to develop a research tool to the point appropriate to use in a study is 5 years. An example of this design is Brink's (1984) study "Value orientations as an assessment tool in cultural diversity." An excerpt from the abstract of that study follows:

Value Orientations is the term used for a theoretical construct and its cultural assessment tool that was developed by Florence Kluckhohn in the 1950s. The tool, tested in rural and urban areas, has been useful in identifying the dominant and variant values and beliefs that characterize groups. This paper describes the tool, its theoretical underpinning, and data analysis techniques with the Annang of Nigeria as an example of how the tool is used in context of a single culture. In addition, use of the tool with individual clients to establish possible areas of culture conflict in values is examined. (p. 198)

SUMMARY

Research design is a blueprint for the conduct of a study that maximizes control over factors that could interfere with the desired outcomes from studies. Selecting a design requires an understanding of certain concepts: causality, bias, manipulation, control and validity. In causality, there is an assumption that things have causes and that causes lead to effects. Nursing science must be built within a philosophical framework of multicausality and probability. Multicausality is the recognition that a number of interrelating variables can be involved in causing a particular effect. Probability deals with the likelihood that a specific effect will occur following a particular cause. Bias means to slant away from the true or expected. Manipulation means to move around or to control the movement, such as the manipulation of the independent variable. Control means having the power to direct or manipulate factors to achieve a desired outcome.

Validity is a measure of the truth or accuracy of a claim. When conducting a study, the researcher is confronted with major decisions regarding four types of validity: statistical conclusion validity, internal validity, construct validity and external validity. Statistical conclusion validity is concerned with whether the conclusions about relationships drawn from statistical analysis are an accurate reflection of the real world. However, there are reasons why false conclusions can be drawn about the presence or absence of a relationship; these are called threats to statistical conclusion validity. Internal validity is the extent to which the effects detected in the study are a true reflection of reality, rather than being a result of the effects of extraneous variables. Any study can have threats to internal validity, and these validity threats can lead to a false-positive or false-negative conclusion. Construct validity examines the fit between the conceptual definitions and operational definitions of variables. The threats to construct validity are related to both previous instrument development and the development of measurement techniques as part of the methodology of a particular study. External validity is concerned with the extent to which study findings can be generalized beyond the sample used in the study. The most serious threat would lead to the findings being meaningful only for the group being studied.

Designs have been developed by researchers to meet unique research needs as they emerge. At present, nursing research is using designs developed by other disciplines. These designs are a useful starting point but nurse scientists must go beyond these to develop designs that will more appropriately meet the needs of nursing's knowledge base. The chapter concludes with a discussion of designs for nursing research, including designs for exploratory (quantitative and qualitative), descriptive, correlational, quasi-experimental and experimental studies.

References

Abdellah, F. G. & Levine, E. (1979). *Better patient care through nursing research*. New York: Macmillan Publishing Company, Inc.

Brink, P. J. (1984). Value orientations as an assessment tool in cultural diversity. *Nursing Research*, 33(4), 198–203.

Campbell, D. T. & Stanley, J. C. (1963). *Experimental and quasi-experimental designs for research*. Chicago: Rand McNally College Publishing Company.

Carney, K. & Burns, N. (1985). Hospice care: some insights on nature, demand, and cost. In L.

F. Paradis (Ed.), *Hospice handbook: a guide for managers and planners* (pp. 281–300). Rockville, Maryland: An Aspen Publication.

Chen, S. C., Barkauskas, V. H. & Chen, E. J. (1984). Health problems encountered by nurse practitioners and physicians in general medicine clinics. *Research in Nursing and Health*, 7(2), 79–86.

Clinton, J., Beck, R., Radjenovic, D., Taylor, L., Westlake, S. & Wilson, S. E. (1986). Time-series designs in clinical nursing research: human issues. *Nursing Research*, 35(3), 188–191.

Cook, T. D. & Campbell, D. T. (1979). *Quasi-experimentation: design and analysis issues for field settings*. Chicago: Rand McNally College Publishing Company.

Cox, C. L., Sullivan, J. A. & Roghmann, K. J. (1984). A conceptual explanation of risk-reduction behavior and intervention development. *Nursing Research*, 33(3), 168–173.

Craig, J. R. & Metze, S. P. (1979). *Methods of psychological research*. Philadelphia: W. B. Saunders Company.

Davis, W. E. Jr. (1978). ODWIN expansion program: a study in success. *Nursing Research*, 27(4), 230–232.

Devine, E. C. & Cook, T. D. (1983). A meta-analytic analysis of effects of psychoeducational interventions on length of postsurgical hospital stay. *Nursing Research*, 32(5), 267–274.

Diers, D. (1979). *Research in nursing practice*. Philadelphia: J. B. Lippincott Company.

Dittmar, S. S. & Dulski, T. (1977). Early evening administration of sleep medication to the hospitalized aged: a consideration in rehabilitation. *Nursing Research*, 26(4), 299–303.

Durand, B. (1975). A clinical nursing study: failure to thrive in a child with Down's syndrome. *Nursing Research*, 24(4), 272–286.

Ellison, E. S. (1983). Parental support and school-aged children. *Western Journal of Nursing Research*, 5(2), 145–153.

Farr, L., Keene, A., Samson, D. & Michael, A. (1984). Alterations in circadian excretion of urinary variables and physiological indicators of stress following surgery. *Nursing Research*, 33(3), 140–146.

Fisher, Sir, R. A. (1935). *The designs of experiments*. New York: Hafner Publishing Company.

Flaskerud, J. H. (1984). A comparison of perceptions of problematic behavior by six minority groups and mental health professionals. *Nursing Research*, 33(4), 190–197.

French, J. F. & Kaufman, N. J. (1981). *Handbook for prevention evaluation: prevention evaluation guidelines*. Rockville, Maryland: National Institute on Drug Abuse.

Gill, N. E., White, M. A. & Anderson, G. C. (1984). Transitional newborn infants in a hospital nursery: from first oral cue to first sustained cry. *Nursing Research*, 33(4), 213–217.

Goldberg, W. G. & Fitzpatrick, J. J. (1980). Movement therapy with the aged. *Nursing Research*, 29(6), 339–346.

Goodwin, L. D. (1984). Increasing efficiency and precision of data analysis: multivariate vs. univariate statistical techniques. *Nursing Research*, 33(4), 247–249.

Greenleaf, N. P. (1983). Labor force participation among registered nurses and women in comparable occupations. *Nursing Research*, 32(5), 306–311.

Greer, D. S., Mor, V., Sherwood, S., Morris, J. M. & Birnbaum, H. (1983). National hospice study analysis plan. *Journal of Chronic Disease*, 36, 737–780.

Harris, R. B. & Hyman, R. B. (1984). Clean vs. sterile tracheotomy care and level of pulmonary infection. *Nursing Research*, 33(2), 80–85.

Hartfield, M. T., Cason, C. L. & Cason, G. J. (1982). Effects of information about a threatening procedure on patients' expectations and emotional distress. *Nursing Research*, 31(4), 202–206.

Hasler, M. E. & Cohen, J. A. (1982). The effect of oxygen administration on oral temperature assessment. *Nursing Research*, 31(5), 265–268.

Hinshaw. A. S. (1981). Problems in doing research: compromise? always!: where? how much? *Western Journal of Nursing Research*, 3(1), 109–113.

Isaac, S. & Michael, W. B. (1971). *Handbook in research and evaluation*. San Diego, California: EDITS Publishers.

Kerlinger, F. N. (1973). *Foundations of behavioral research* (2nd ed.). New York: Holt, Rinehart and Winston.

King, I. & Tarsitano, B. (1982). The effect of structured and unstructured pre-operative teaching: a replication. *Nursing Research*, 31(6), 324–329.

Lamb, K. (1979). Effect of positioning of postoperative fractured-hip patients as related to comfort. *Nursing Research*, 28(5), 291–294.

McCain, L. J. & McCleary, R. (1979). The statistical analysis of the simple interrupted time-series quasi-experiment. In T. D. Cook & D. T. Campbell (Eds.), *Quasi-experimentation: design and analysis issues for field settings* (pp. 233–293). Chicago: Rand McNally College Publishing Company.

Magilvy, J. K. (1985). Quality of life of hearing-impaired older women. *Nursing Research*, 34(3), 140–144.

Marut, J. S. & Mercer, R. T. (1979). Comparison of primiparas' perceptions of vaginal and cesarean births. *Nursing Research*, 28(5), 260–266.

Metzger, B. L. & Schultz, S. II. (1982). Time series analysis: an alternative for nursing. *Nursing Research*, 31(6), 375–378.

Neale, J. M. & Liebert, R. M. (1980). *Science and behavior: an introduction to methods of research* (2nd ed.). Englewood Cliffs, New Jersey: Prentice-Hall, Inc.

Newman, M. A. (1979). *Theory development in nursing*. Philadelphia: F. A. Davis Company.

Newman, M. A. & Gaudiano, J. K. (1984). Depression as an explanation for decreased subjective time in the elderly. *Nursing Research*, 33(3), 137–139.

Norris, S., Campbell, L. A. & Brenkert, S. (1982). Nursing procedures and alterations in transcutaneous oxygen tension in premature infants. *Nursing Research*, 31(6), 330–336.

O'Flynn, A. I. (1982). Meta-analysis. *Nursing Research*, 31(5),314–316.

Parsons, L. C. & Beek, D. V. (1982). Sleep-awake patterns following cerebral concussion. *Nursing Research*, 31(5), 260–264.

Parsons, L. C. & Wilson, M. M. (1984). Cerebrovascular status of severe closed head–injured patients following passive position changes. *Nursing Research*, 33(2), 68–75.

Penckofer, S. H. & Holm, K. (1984). Early appraisal of coronary revascularization on quality of life. *Nursing Research*, 33(2), 60–63.

Powers, M. J. & Wooldridge, P. J. (1982). Factors influencing knowledge, attitudes, and compliance of hypertensive patients. *Research in Nursing and Health*, 5(4), 171–182.

Reichardt, C. S. (1979). The statistical analysis of data from nonequivalent group designs. In T. D. Cook & D. T. Campbell (Eds.), *Quasi-experimentation: design and analysis issues for field settings* (pp. 147–206). Chicago: Rand McNally College Publishing Company.

Rice, V. H. & Johnson, J. E. (1984). Preadmission self-instruction booklets, postadmission exercise performance, and teaching time. *Nursing Research*, 33(3), 147–151.

Sandelowski, M. (1986). The problem of rigor in qualitative research. *Advances in Nursing Science*, 8(3), 27–37.

Selltiz, C., Wrightsman, L. S. & Cook, S. W. (1976). *Research methods in social relations* (3rd ed.). New York: Holt, Rinehart and Winston.

Spector, P. E. (1981). *Research designs*. Beverly Hills: Sage Publications.

Timm, M. M. (1979). Prenatal education evaluation. *Nursing Research*, 28(6), 338–342.

Tuckman, B. W. (1978). *Conducting educational research*. New York: Harcourt Brace Jovanovich, Inc.

Tyzenhouse, P. S. (1981). Technical notes: the nursing clinical trial. *Western Journal of Nursing Research*, 3(1), 102–109.

Ventura, M. R., Young, D. E., Feldman, M. J., Pastore, P., Pikula, S. & Yates, M. A. (1984). Effectiveness of health promotion interventions. *Nursing Research*, 33(3), 162–167.

Waltz, C. F. & Bausell, R. B. (1981). *Nursing research: design, statistics and computer analysis*. Philadelphia: F. A. Davis Company.

Wooldridge, P. J., Leonard, R. C. & Skipper, J. K. Jr. (1978). *Methods of clinical experimentation to improve patient care*. St. Louis: The C. V. Mosby Company.

Ziemer, M. M. (1983). Effects of information on postsurgical coping. *Nursing Research*, 32(5), 282–287.

11

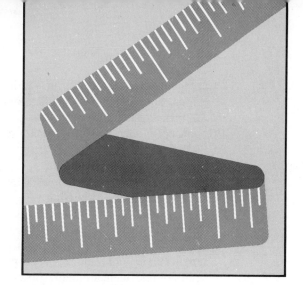

The Role of Measurement

Measurement is the process of assigning "numbers to objects (or events or situations) in accord with some rule" (Kaplan, 1963, p. 177). The numbers assigned can indicate numerical values or categories. The "rules" ensure that the assignment will be performed consistently from one subject (or event) to another and, eventually, if the measurement strategy is found to be meaningful, from one study to another. A component of measurement is instrumentation. Instrumentation is the application of specific rules to develop a measurement device (instrument). An instrument is used to examine a specific variable. The purpose of instrumentation is to produce trustworthy evidence that can be used in evaluating the outcomes of research.

The rules of measurement established for research are similar to those used in nursing practice. For example, when pouring a liquid medication, the measuring container is held at eye level. When taking a patient's temperature, we check to be sure that the patient has not recently drunk ice water or smoked a cigarette. When measuring the abdominal girth to detect increases in ascites, we mark the skin on the abdomen to be sure that the measure is always taken the same distance below the waist.

However, rules have not been established for measuring many concepts in nursing practice. For example, how can the effectiveness of preoperative teaching be measured? Can the length of hospitalization, number of complications, amount of pain medication, patient expressions of satisfaction be used to measure the effectiveness of preoperative teaching? There are many abstract concepts, such as compliance, stress, coping, pain management, anxiety or social support, that seem to influence health and recovery from illness. But measurement of these ideas is primarily intuitive and varies from nurse to nurse. Therefore, developing consistent measures of these abstract concepts is a major concern in nursing.

This chapter provides a beginning base of information about measurement in nursing research to guide the attitude development and decisions of beginning researchers and consumers of research. An introduction to measurement theory and major concepts is presented. Measurement strategies, including physiologic measurement, observational measurement, interviews, questionnaires and scales, and specific instruments used in nursing research are discussed.

Measurement Theory

Measurement theory and the rules within this theory have been developed to direct the measurement of abstract and concrete concepts. An understanding of the logic within measurement theory is important to the selection, utilization and development of measurement instruments. As with most theories, measurement theory uses terms that must be understood within the context of the theory. The following explanation of the logic of measurement theory includes definitions of directness of measurement, measurement error, levels of measurement, reference of measurement, reliability and validity.

DIRECTNESS OF MEASUREMENT

Measurement must begin by clarifying the object, characteristic or element to be measured. Only then can strategies or techniques be developed to measure it. In some cases, identification of the measurement object and measurement strategies can be quite simple and straightforward, as when we are measuring concrete factors such as a person's height or wrist circumference. This is referred to as *direct measurement*. The technology of health care has made direct measures of concrete elements such as height, weight, temperature, time, space, movement, heart rate and respiration very familiar to us. Technology is available to measure many bodily functions and biological and chemical characteristics. Nurses are also experienced in gathering direct measures of attribute variables such as age, gender, ethnic origin, diagnosis, marital status, income and education.

However, in many cases in nursing, the characteristic to be measured is an abstract idea such as stress, caring, compliance or pain. If the element to be measured is abstract, clarification is usually achieved through conceptual definition. The conceptual definition is then used to select or develop appropriate means of measuring the concept. The tool used in the study must match the conceptual definition. When abstract concepts are measured, the concept is not directly measured; instead, indicators or attributes of the concept are used to represent the abstraction. This is referred to as *indirect measurement*. For example, indicators of coping might be the frequency or accuracy of problem identification, the speed or effectiveness of problem resolution, level of optimism and self-actualization behaviors. Rarely, if ever, can a single measurement strategy completely measure all the aspects of an abstract concept.

MEASUREMENT ERROR

There is no perfect measure. Error is inherent in any measurement strategy. *Measurement error* is the difference between what exists in reality and what is measured by a research tool. Measurement error exists in both direct and indirect measures and can be random or systematic. Direct measures, which are considered to be highly accurate, are subject to error. For example, the scale may not be accurate, the machine may be precisely calibrated but it may change with use, the tape measure may not be held at exactly the same tightness.

There is also error in indirect measures. Efforts to measure concepts usually result in measuring only part of the concept or measures that identify an aspect of the concept but also include other elements that are not part of the concept. Figure 11–1 shows a Venn diagram of the concept A measured by instrument A-1. As can be seen, A-1 does not measure all of A. In addition, some of what A-1 measures is outside the concept of A. Both of these are examples of errors in measurement.

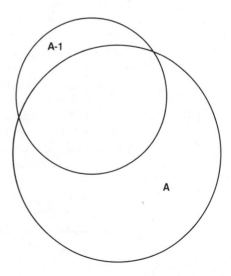

FIGURE 11–1. Measurement error when measuring a concept.

Types of Measurement Errors

There are two types of error that are of concern in measurement: random and systematic error. To understand these types of errors, we must first understand the elements of a score on an instrument or an observation. According to measurement theory, there are three components to a measurement score: the true score (T), the observed score (O) and the error score (E). The true score is what we would obtain if there were no error in measurement. Because there is *always* some measurement error, we *never* know the true score. We only know the observed score. The theoretical equation of these three measures is:

$$O = T + E$$

The error addressed by E is *random error*. The smaller the error term, the more closely O (observed score) reflects T (true score). Therefore, using measurement strategies that reduce the error term increases the accuracy of the measurement. This equation is a means of conceptualizing random error and not a basis for calculating it. Since the true score is never known, the random error is never known, only estimated.

There are a number of factors that can occur during the measurement process that can result in random error. These include (1) transient personal factors such as fatigue, hunger, attention span, health, mood, mental set and motivation; (2) situational factors such as a hot stuffy room, distractions, the presence of significant others, rapport with the researcher and playfulness or seriousness of the situation; (3) variations in the administration of the measurement such as interviews in which wording or sequence of questions is varied, questions are added or deleted or different coders code responses differently; and (4) processing of data such as errors in coding, a subject accidentally marking the wrong column, punching the wrong key while entering the data into the computer or totaling instrument scores incorrectly.

Random error causes individuals' observed scores to vary haphazardly around their true score. For example, with random error, one subject's observed score may be higher than his or her true score, whereas another subject's observed score may be lower than his or her true score. According to measurement theory, the sum of random errors is expected to be zero, and the random error term (E) is not expected to be correlated with the true score term (T). Thus, random error will not influence the direction of the mean but, rather, will increase the amount of unexplained variance around the mean. When this occurs, estimation of the true score is more diffuse.

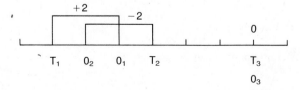

FIGURE 11-2. Conceptualization of random error.

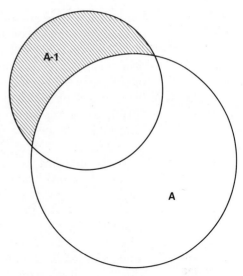

FIGURE 11–3. Conceptualization of systematic error.

If a variable were measured for three subjects and the random error was diagrammed, it might appear as demonstrated in Figure 11–2. The difference between the true score of subject one (T_1) and the observed score (O_1) is two positive measurement intervals. The difference between the true score (T_2) and observed score (O_2) for subject two is two negative measurement intervals. The difference between the true score (T_3) and observed score (O_3) for subject three is zero. The random error for these three subjects is zero ($+2 \ -2 \ +0 = 0$). In viewing this example, one must remember that this is only a means of conceptualizing random error.

In a study, the measurement error that is not random is systematic. A conceptualization of systematic error is presented in Figure 11–3. Systematic error (represented by diagonal lines in the figure) is due to the part of A-1 that is outside of A. This part of A-1 measures factors other than A and will bias scores in a particular direction.

Systematic error is considered part of T (true score) and reflects the true measure of A-1, not A. When the true score (with systematic error) is added to the random error (which is 0), it equals the observed score (Fig. 11–4). There will be some systematic error in almost any measure; however, a close link between the abstract theoretical concept and the development of the

$$T + E = O$$

T (True Score with Systematic Error) + E (Random Error of 0) = O (Observed Score)

FIGURE 11–4. Systematic error within the equation for measurement score.

instrument will greatly decrease systematic error. The refinement of an instrument is also a means of decreasing systematic error.

Another effective means of diminishing systematic error is to use more than one measure of a concept. Preferably a variety of data collection methods, such as interview and observation, are used. This technique is referred to as the *multimethod-multitrait technique* and was developed by Campbell and Fiske (1959). Using this technique, more dimensions of the abstract concept can be measured, and the effect of the systematic error on the composite observed score decreases. Figure 11–5 illustrates how more dimensions of concept A are measured by using instruments A-1, A-2, A-3 and A-4. The scores obtained from the four instruments are combined in such a way to give a single observed score for concept A.

For example, anxiety could be measured by: (1) administering Taylor's Manifest Anxiety Scale, (2) recording blood pressure readings, (3) asking the subject about anxious feelings and (4) observing the subject's behavior. The results of each of these measures would then be combined in some way to give a single observed score of anxiety for each subject.

In some studies, instruments are used to examine relationships. Consider a hypothesis in which the relationship between concept A and concept B is being tested. In Figure 11–6, the true relationship between concepts A and B is represented by the area enclosed in the dark lines.

If two instruments (A-1 and B-1) were used to examine the relationship

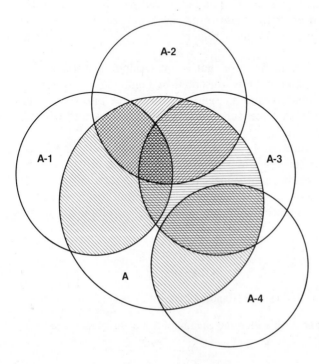

FIGURE 11–5. Multiple measures of an abstract concept.

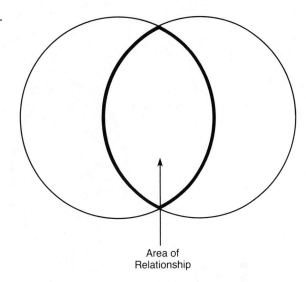

FIGURE 11–6. True relationship of concepts A and B.

Area of
Relationship

between concepts A and B, the part of the true relationship actually reflected by these measures is represented by diagonal lines in Figure 11–7. As the instruments (A-1 and B-1) provide a more accurate measure of concepts A and B, more of the true relationship between concepts A and B will be measured.

If additional instruments (A-2 and B-2) are used to measure concepts A and B, more of the true relationship might be reflected. Figure 11–8 demonstrates the parts of the true relationship that might be reflected using two instruments to measure concept A (A-1 and A-2) and two instruments to measure concept B (B-1 and B-2).

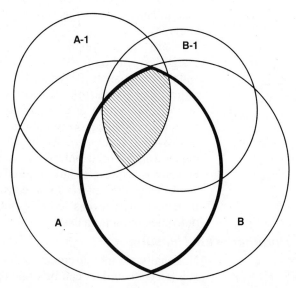

FIGURE 11–7. Examining a relationship using one measure of each concept.

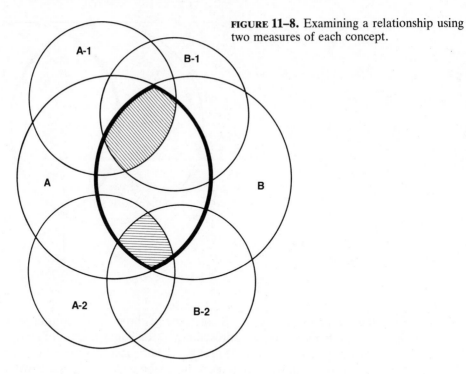

FIGURE 11–8. Examining a relationship using two measures of each concept.

LEVELS OF MEASUREMENT

The traditional levels of measurement have been used for so long that the categorization system has been considered absolute law and inviolate. The system was developed by Stevens in 1946. Stevens organized the rules for assigning numbers to objects so that a hierarchy in measurement was established. The levels of measurement from lower to higher are nominal, ordinal, interval and ratio.

In recent years, controversy has erupted over justification for the categories, leading to two factions in regard to the system: the fundamentalists and the pragmatists. Pragmatists consider measurement to occur on a continuum rather than by discrete categories, whereas fundamentalists adhere rigidly to the original system of categorization. The primary focus of the controversy is related to classification of data into the categories of ordinal and interval. The controversy developed because many of the current statistical analysis techniques can be used only with interval data. Many pragmatists believe that if Stevens' rules were rigidly adhered to, few if any measures in the social sciences would meet the criteria to be considered interval level data. They also believe that violating Stevens' criteria does not lead to serious consequences in the outcomes of data analysis.

Nominal-Scale Measurement

Nominal-scale measurement is the lowest of the four measurement categories. It is used when data can be organized into categories of a defined property but the categories cannot be compared. Thus, one cannot say that one category is higher than another or that category A is closer to category B than to category C. The categories differ in quality but not quantity. Therefore, one cannot say that subject A possesses "more" of the property being categorized than does subject B. (Rule: The categories must be unorderable.) Categories must be established in such a way that a datum will fit into only one of the categories. (Rule: The categories must be exclusive.) All the data must fit into the established categories. (Rule: The categories must be exhaustive.)

Data such as gender, race, marital status and diagnoses are examples of nominal data. When data are coded for entry into the computer, the categories are assigned numbers. For example, gender may be classified as 1 = male, 2 = female. The numbers assigned to categories in nominal measurement are used only as labels and cannot be used for mathematical calculations.

Ordinal-Scale Measurement

Data that can be measured at the ordinal-scale level can be assigned to categories of an attribute that can be ranked. There are rules for how one ranks data. As with nominal scale data, the categories must be exclusive and exhaustive. With ordinal-scale data, the quantity of the attribute possessed can be identified. However, it cannot be demonstrated that the intervals between the ranked categories are equal. Therefore, ordinal data are considered to have unequal intervals.

Level of education is frequently used as an ordinal scale measure. Many scales used in nursing research are ordinal levels of measure. For example, one could rank intensity of pain, degrees of coping, levels of mobility, ability to provide self-care or daily amount of exercise on an ordinal scale. Using daily exercise, the scale could be 0 = no exercise; 1 = moderate exercise, no sweating; 2 = exercise to the point of sweating; 3 = strenuous exercise with sweating for at least 30 minutes a day; 4 = strenuous exercise for at least 1 hour per day.

Interval-Scale Measurement

Interval scales have equal numerical distances between intervals of the scale in addition to following the rules of mutually exclusive categories, exhaustive categories and rank ordering. Interval scales are assumed to be a continuum of values. Thus, the magnitude of the attribute can be much more precisely defined. However, it is not possible to provide the absolute amount of the attribute because of the absence of a zero point on the interval scale.

Temperature is the most commonly used example of an interval scale. A difference between a temperature of 70° and 80° is the same as the difference between a temperature of 30° and one of 40°. Changes in temperature can be precisely measured. However, it is not possible to say that a temperature of 0° means the absence of temperature.

Ratio-Level Measurement

Ratio-level measures are the highest form of measure and meet all the rules of other forms of measures: mutually exclusive categories, exhaustive categories, rank ordering, equal spacing between intervals and a continuum of values. In addition, ratio-level measures have absolute zero points. Weight, length and volume are commonly used examples of ratio scales. All of these have absolute zero points at which a value of zero indicates the absence of the property being measured, such as zero weight means the absence of weight. In addition, because of the absolute zero point, one can justifiably say that object A weighs twice as much as object B, or that container A holds three times as much as container B.

Statistical Analyses and Levels of Measurement

The level of measurement is associated with the types of statistical analyses that can be performed on the data. Therefore, it is advisable to obtain the highest level of measurement possible. For example, age can be grouped into categories such as 20 to 29, 30 to 39 and so on. However, more sophisticated analyses can be performed if the actual age of each subject is obtained. Mathematical operations are limited in the lower levels of measurement. With nominal levels of measurement, it is only possible to use summary statistics such as frequencies, percentages and contingency correlation procedures. With ordinal level measurement, a mean cannot be obtained, which is necessary for most advanced statistical analyses. Although nonparametric analyses can be performed using the median, these approaches to analysis are not as powerful as parametric techniques.

The controversy over levels of measurement is related to the statistical operations that can justifiably be performed with scores from the various levels of measure. Fundamentalists believe that appropriate statistical analysis is contingent upon the level of measurement. They disagree with the contention that the scaling procedures used for most psychosocial instruments provide interval-level data. For example, the Likert Scale (discussed later in this chapter) uses a scale of strongly disagree, disagree, uncertain, agree and strongly agree. Fundamentalists claim that equal intervals do not exist between these categories. It is not possible to prove that there is the same magnitude of feeling between uncertain and agree as there is between agree and strongly agree. Therefore, parametric analyses cannot be used. Pragmatists believe that with many measures taken at the ordinal level, such as scaling procedures, an underlying interval continuum is present that justifies the use of parametric statistics. Our position is more like that of the pragmatists than of the fundamentalists. However, much data in nursing research are obtained using crude measurement methods that can only be classified into the lower levels of measurement. Therefore, we have included the nonparametric procedures needed for their analysis in Chapter 17.

REFERENCE OF MEASUREMENT

Referencing involves comparing a subject's score against a standard. There are two types of testing that involve referencing: norm-referenced testing and criterion-referenced testing. *Norm-referenced testing* involves the use of standardized tests that have been carefully developed over several years and have extensive reliability and validity data available. The best-known norm-referenced test is the MMPI (Minnesota Multiphasic Personality Inventory), which is commonly used in psychology and occasionally in nursing research. Many psychological tests are norm referenced and must be ordered from a psychological testing company and returned to it after data collection for analysis. Usually, this service is provided for a fee.

Criterion-referenced testing involves the comparison of a subject's score with a criterion of achievement that includes the definition of target behaviors. When these behaviors are mastered, the subject is considered proficient in the behavior. The criterion might be a level of knowledge or desirable patient outcome measures. Criterion measures are not as useful in research as they might be in evaluation studies. Norm referencing will generally lead to higher levels of measurement and greater variability than will criterion-referenced testing and, thus, to increased possibility of achieving statistical levels (0.05, 0.01, 0.001) of significance.

RELIABILITY

Reliability is concerned with how consistently the measurement technique measures the concept of interest. For example, if one were using a scale to obtain the weight of subjects, one would expect the scale to indicate the same weight if the subject stepped on and off the scale several times. A scale that did not show the same weight each time would be unreliable.

If two data collectors were observing the same event and recording their observations on a carefully designed data collection instrument, one would hope that the recordings would be comparable. The equivalence of their results would indicate the reliability of the measurement technique. In addition, if the same questionnaire is administered to the same individuals at two different times, one hopes that the individuals' responses to the items remain the same. If their responses vary each time the test is administered, there is a chance that the instrument is not reliable.

Reliability testing is considered a measure of the amount of random error in the measurement technique. It is concerned with such characteristics as dependability, consistency, accuracy and comparability. Since all measurement techniques contain some random error, reliability exists in degrees and is usually expressed as a form of correlation coefficient, with a 1.00 indicating perfect reliability and 0.00 indicating no reliability. A reliability of 0.80 is considered the lowest acceptable coefficient for a well-developed measurement tool. Reliability testing focuses on three aspects of reliability: stability, equivalence and homogeneity.

Stability

Stability is concerned with the consistency of repeated measures. This is usually referred to as *test-retest reliability*. This measure of reliability is generally used with physical measures, technological measures and paper-and-pencil scales.

Use of the technique requires an assumption that the factor to be measured remains the same at the two testing times and that any change in the value or score is a consequence of random error.

Retesting physical measures and equipment can be performed in a short period of time, or the equipment can be used for a period of time and then tested to determine the necessary frequency of recalibration. With paper-and-pencil measures, a period of 2 weeks to a month is recommended between the two testing times. After retesting, correlational analysis is performed on the scores from the two measures. A high correlation coefficient indicates high reliability.

Test-retest reliability has not proved to be as effective with paper-and-pencil measures as was originally anticipated. There are a number of problems with the procedure. Subjects may remember their responses at the first testing time, which will lead to overestimating the reliability. Subjects may actually be changed by the first testing and therefore respond to the second test differently, leading to underestimation. In tests that measure such factors as attitudes, the assumption that the attitude being measured does not change between the two measurement periods may not be justifiable. If the factor being measured does change, the test is not a measure of reliability. In fact, if the measures stay the same when the attitude has changed, it may be an indication of unreliability.

Equivalence

The focus of equivalence is on comparing two versions of the same paper-and-pencil instrument or two observers measuring the same event. When two observers are being compared, it is referred to as *interrater reliability*. When two paper-and-pencil instruments are being compared, it is referred to as *alternate forms*, or *parallel forms, reliability*. Alternate forms of instruments are of more concern in the development of normative knowledge testing. However, when repeated measures are part of the design, alternate forms of measurement, although not commonly used, would improve the design. Demonstrating that one is actually testing the same content in both tests is extremely complex and rarely used in clinical research.

Determining interrater reliability is a more immediate concern in research and is used in many observational studies. There are two techniques for determining interrater reliability. Both techniques require that two or more raters observe and record the same event or that the same rater observe and record an event on two occasions. The first procedure for calculating interrater reliability requires a simple computation involving a comparison of the agreements obtained between raters on the coding form with the number of possible agreements. This calculation is performed using the following equation:

$$\frac{\text{number of agreements}}{\text{number of possible agreements}}$$

This formula tends to overestimate reliability, and this is particularly a problem when the rating requires only a dichotomous alternative. In this case, there is a 50 per cent probability that the raters will agree on a particular item by chance alone. Appropriate correlational techniques can be used to provide a more accurate estimate of reliability. If more than two raters are involved, coefficient alpha may be used.

Homogeneity

Tests of instrument homogeneity are used primarily with paper-and-pencil tests and address the correlation of various items within the instrument. The original approach to determining homogeneity was *split-half reliability*. This strategy was a way of getting at test-retest reliability without administering the test twice. Rather, the instrument items were split in half, and a correlational procedure was performed between the two halves. The Spearman-Brown formula has generally been used for this procedure. One of the problems with the procedure was that although items were usually split into odd-even items, it was possible to split them in a variety of ways. Each approach to splitting the items would yield a different reliability coefficient. Therefore, the researcher could continue to split the items in various ways until a satisfactorily high coefficient was obtained.

More recently, testing the homogeneity of all the items in the instrument has been seen as a better approach to determining reliability. Although the mathematics of the procedure are complex, the logic is simple. One way to view it is as though one conducted split-half reliabilities in all the ways possible and then averaged the scores to obtain one reliability score. This procedure examines the extent to which all the items in the instrument measure the same construct. It is a test of *internal consistency*. The procedures used for this process are Cronbach's alpha coefficient and, when the data are dichotomous, K-R 20 (Kuder-Richardson formula).

If the coefficient value were 1.00, each item in the instrument would be measuring exactly the same thing. When this occurs, one might question the need for more than one item. A slightly lower coefficient (0.8 to 0.9) indicates an instrument that will reflect more richly the fine discriminations in levels of the construct. Magnitude can then be discerned more clearly.

Other approaches to testing internal consistency include correlating each item with the total score for the instrument. In this procedure, often used in instrument development, items that do not correlate highly may be deleted from the instrument. Factor analysis and analysis of variance may also be used to develop reliability of instruments.

VALIDITY

The validity of an instrument is a determination of the extent to which the instrument actually reflects the abstract concept being examined. In Figure 11–9, validity (the shaded area) is illustrated by the extent to which the instrument A-1 reflects the concept A. As measurement of the concept improves, validity improves. The extent to which the measurement tool measures items other than the concept is referred to as *systematic error* (also

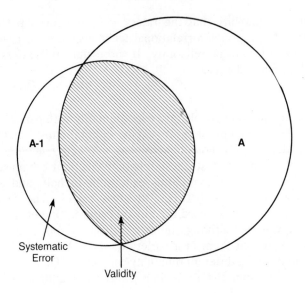

FIGURE 11–9. Representation of instrument validity.

identified in the figure). As systematic error decreases, validity increases. Validity will vary from one sample to another and from one situation to another; therefore, validity testing actually validates the use of an instrument for a specific group or purpose, rather than being directed toward the instrument itself.

Validity, as reliability, is not an all-or-nothing phenomenon but rather a matter of degree. No instrument is completely valid. Thus, we must determine the degree of validity of a measure rather than whether or not validity exists. Defining the validity of an instrument requires years of work. Many equate the validity of the instrument with the rigorousness of the researcher. The assumption is that since the researcher develops the instrument, the researcher must also "develop" the validity. However, this is to some degree an erroneous view. As Brinberg and McGrath (1985) so aptly say:

> Validity is not a commodity that can be purchased with techniques. Validity, as we will treat it, is a concept designating an ideal state—to be pursued, but not to be attained. As the roots of the word imply, validity has to do with truth, strength, and value. The discourse of our field has often been in tones that seem to imply that validity is a tangible "resource," and that if one can acquire a sufficient amount of it, by applying appropriate techniques, one has somehow "won" at the game called research. We reject this view. In our views, validity is not like money—to gain and lose, to count and display. Rather, validity is like integrity, character, or quality, to be assessed relative to purposes and circumstances. (p. 13)

One obtains validity, not for the instrument, but for the instrument in relation to a particular use (Carmines & Zeller, 1979). An instrument may be very valid in one situation but not valid in another. Therefore, validity must be reexamined in each study situation. For example, Beck, Weissman, Lester and Trexler (1974) developed a tool to measure hopelessness using hospitalized suicidal patients. Later, one of us (Burns, 1981) used the instrument in another study examining family members of cancer patients. One had to question whether a tool to measure hopelessness in the original population would be valid to measure hopelessness in family members of cancer patients. A computer search revealed that although the instrument had been used in 17 studies, none of the studies had reexamined the validity or reliability of the instrument. Further statistical analyses indicated that the instrument was indeed valid for both purposes.

There are three primary types of validity: content validity, predictive validity and construct validity. Within each of these types are subtypes, so the number of types of validity can seem very confusing to the beginning researcher. These types of validity are not discrete; each interrelates with the others to form a broad picture of the validity of the measurement.

Content Validity

Content validity verifies that the method of measurement actually measures the expected content. This type of validity is very important for knowledge testing but is less significant in clinical research. In education, blueprints of content are developed, and the test items are then developed from these blueprints in order to improve content validity.

One subtype of content validity is face validity. *Face validity* is a very primitive type of validity that verifies basically that the instrument "looks" like or gives the appearance of measuring the content. It is an intuitive type of validity in which subjects or colleagues are asked to read the instrument and evaluate the content. Using a similar type of validity, *expert validity*, the instrument may be sent to experts in a particular field of research across the country for their evaluation of the content. This step can be very useful for further development of the instrument (and thus content validity).

Predictive Validity

Predictive validity is sometimes referred to as *criterion validity*. Predictive validity determines the effectiveness of the instrument as a predictor of a future event. For example, we might determine the ability of a scale that measures health-related behaviors to predict the future health status of individuals. The future level of health of individuals might be predicted by examining reported stress levels of these individuals for the past 3 years. A tool that would be useful in gathering these data is the Holmes and Rahe Life Events Scale. Miller (1981) discussed the validity and reliability of the Holmes and Rahe Life Events Scale in measuring stress levels in a variety of populations. The accuracy of predictive validity is determined by correlational analysis. *Concurrent validity*, which is considered a type of predictive validity, is the ability to predict the current value of one measure based on the value obtained on the measure of another concept. For example, one might be able to predict the self-esteem score of an individual who had a high score on an instrument to measure coping.

Construct Validity

Construct validity is the degree to which a measurement strategy measures the construct it was designed to measure. Developing construct validity of an instrument is a process that requires many years of work by a number of scientists. As discussed in Chapter 7, constructs (or concepts) are the basic building blocks of a theory. Many of the measures used in nursing research are abstract constructs rather than concrete representations of the real world. One can easily see the connection between a tape measure as a measure of length and length as axiomatically associated with the theory of measurement. It is not easy to see the connection between Taylor's Manifest Anxiety Scale as a measure of anxiety and its association with related theory. However, this is the connection that must be made to demonstrate the validity of a specific measure of a construct.

Construct validity is now considered the most important type of validity to examine. Other types of validity alone cannot sufficiently demonstrate a valid measurement method. Thus, in critiquing studies and considering instruments for use in studies, one must look for evidence of construct validity. Therefore, being familiar with the process of examining construct validity is important in utilizing research findings, conducting research or developing new instruments.

There are a number of steps involved in developing construct validity, which occur over a period of many years. The identification and discussion of these steps in the literature varies with the author. The following discussion is designed to bring clarity and a sense of logical flow to the process of construct validity. The steps include concept analysis, factorial validity, contrasted groups approach, convergent validity, divergent validity, discriminant validity, nomological network validity and successive verification.

1. *Concept Analysis.* Concept analysis is the first step in theory development and is necessary to clarify the connotative meaning of an abstract term (Walker & Avant, 1983). One of the outcomes of concept analysis is identification of the domain of the construct. From this domain, methods can be developed to measure the construct.

2. *Factorial Validity.* After an instrument has been developed that measures the domain of the construct, data can be collected using the instrument. Factor analysis is performed on the data to examine relationships between the various items of the instrument. Items that do not fall into a factor (and thus do not correlate with other items) may be deleted. This analysis will also indicate whether the items in the instrument reflect a single construct or several constructs.

3. *Contrasted Groups Approach.* When the instrument is satisfactorily developed, hypotheses are generated about the expected response of various groups to the construct. Samples are selected from at least two groups that are expected to have opposing responses to the items

in the instrument. The instrument is administered, and the responses are analyzed using statistical procedures such as analysis of variance or t-test. If the groups' responses are significantly different in the expected directions, evidence has been added to the validity of the instrument.

4. *Convergent Validity.* A search is made for other measures of the construct. If possible, a variety of measurement strategies are included. This idea of using multiple measures to examine a construct is illustrated in Figure 11–5. Multiple measures of the construct are administered to the same subjects at the same time. Correlational analysis is performed. If the measures are positively correlated, the validity of each instrument is strengthened.

5. *Divergent Validity.* A search is made for instruments that measure the opposite of the construct. If possible, this instrument is administered at the same time as the instruments used to test convergent validity. Correlational procedures are performed with all the measures of the construct. If the divergent measure is negatively correlated with other measures, validity for each of the instruments is strengthened.

6. *Discriminant Validity.* A search is made for instruments that measure concepts related to but not the same as the construct of interest. It is important that the instrument be useful in finely discriminating between these related concepts. If possible, this instrument is administered simultaneously with other instruments during the studies described previously.

7. *Nomological Network Validity.* This approach to construct validity, although not named at the time, was originally described by Cronbach and Meehl (1955). The procedure tests propositions (predicted relationships between constructs) included within the theoretical framework. A tightly developed theory is not necessary for the procedure to be effective. The procedure requires a series of correlational studies and experimental studies. If the predicted relationships between concepts (propositions) are accurate, the relationships between propositions are tested. Although several statistical procedures will be used during the various studies, path analysis should be the eventual aim of the process. During this process, the construct validity of all the constructs within the theory will be tested.

8. *Successive Verification.* After initial validity and reliability studies are conducted on the instrument, the results of the studies are usually published. At that point, other researchers begin using the instrument in unrelated studies. As the results of these studies are published, with additional information on validity and reliability of various types of samples and mean scores on the instrument items, the validity of the instrument is further verified. Each time that an instrument is used in a study contributes to the construct validity information of the instrument.

OBTAINING VALIDITY IN QUALITATIVE RESEARCH

One of the most serious concerns related to qualitative research has been the lack of strategies to determine the validity of the measurements that led to the development of theory. Qualitative researchers tend to work alone. Biases in their work, which threaten validity, can easily go undetected. Miles and Huberman (1984) caution the qualitative researcher to be alert to the occurrence of the "holistic fallacy." This occurs as the researcher becomes more and more sure that his or her conclusions are correct and that his or her model does in fact explain the situation. This feeling should arouse suspicion and alert the researcher to take action to validate his or her findings. Recently, Miles and Huberman (1984) described 12 strategies for examining the validity of qualitative measures.

1. ***Checking for Representativeness.*** Qualitative measurement can be biased by either the attention of the researcher or a bias in the people from whom they obtain their measures. To ensure that measures are representative of the entire population, a search should be made for sources of data not easily accessible. The researcher assumes that observed actions are representative of actions that occur when the researcher is not present. However, efforts must be made to determine whether observed activities are representative of events occurring in the absence of the researcher.

2. ***Checking for Researcher Effects.*** In many cases, the researcher's presence can alter behavior, leading to invalid measures. The researcher must remain on the site long enough to become familiar, use unobtrusive measures and seek input from informants to avoid this effect.

3. ***Triangulating.*** The qualitative researcher must compare all the measures from different sources to determine the validity of the findings.

4. ***Weighting the Evidence.*** Qualitative research involves reducing large amounts of data during the process of coming to conclusions. In this process, some evidence is "captured" from this mass of data and is used in reaching those conclusions. The researcher must review the "strength" of the captured data to validate the conclusions. The researcher determines the strength of the evidence from the source, circumstances of data collection and researcher's efforts to validate the evidence. The researcher must actively search for reasons why the evidence should not be trusted.

5. ***Making Contrasts/Comparisons.*** Contrasts between subjects or events in relation to the study conclusions should be examined. For example, if nursing supervisors consider an action to be very important but staff nurses consider it simply another administrative activity, this is a contrast. The two extreme positions should be examined. Then a decision must be made about whether the difference is a significant one.

6. ***Checking the Meaning of Outliers.*** Exceptions to findings should be identified and examined. It is these exceptions that are referred to as outliers. The outliers provide a way to test the generality of the findings.

7. ***Using Extreme Cases.*** Certain types of outliers, referred to as extreme cases, can be useful in confirming conclusions. The researcher can compare the extreme case to the theoretical model that was developed and determine the key factor that causes the model not to fit the case.

8. ***Ruling Out Spurious Relations.*** This strategy requires the examination of relationships identified in the model in order to consider the possibility of a third variable influencing the situation.

9. ***Replicating a Finding.*** Documenting the findings from several independent sources increases the dependability of the findings and diminishes the risk of the "holistic fallacy." The findings can be tested with new data collected later in the study or data from another site or data set. The second option is more rigorous.

10. ***Checking Out Rival Explanations.*** The qualitative researcher is taught to keep several hypotheses in mind and to constantly compare the plausibility of each with the possibility of one of the others being more accurate. However, near the end of data analysis, when the researcher is more emotionally wedded to one idea, it is very useful to get someone not involved in the research to act as a devil's advocate. Questions should be directed toward "what could disprove the hypothesis?" or conversely "what does the present hypothesis disprove?" Evidence that does not fit the hypothesis should be carefully examined.

11. ***Looking for Negative Evidence.*** This action naturally flows from the search for outliers and the search for rival explanations. In this step, there is an active search for disconfirmation of what is believed to be true. The researcher goes back through the data, seeking evidence to disconfirm the conclusions. However, the inability to find disconfirming evidence never decisively confirms the conclusions reached by the researcher.

12. ***Obtaining Feedback from Informants.*** Conclusions should be given to the informants, and feedback should be sought from them about the accuracy of the causal network developed. Although researchers have been getting feedback from informants throughout the analysis period, feedback after completion of the model will provide a different type of verification of information.

Measurement Strategies in Nursing

Until recently, many nurse researchers have had limited understanding of measurement theory and rules. Because of this, some of the researchers' decisions regarding the selection of measurement strategies have threatened the quality and meaningfulness of the research. A decision often made by novice researchers is to find a measurement tool (any tool) and then design a study to fit the tool. Another poor measurement decision is to develop and use a tool in a study without examining the reliability and validity of the tool. Tool development, a sophisticated process, generally requires at least a year of work. Another ineffective measurement decision is to select instruments that have little or no connection with the framework or design of the study. This decision causes a serious threat to both measurement and design validity.

A concerted effort is being made within the nursing research community to modify the instrumentation problems just described. Tool development to measure nursing phenomena has increased strikingly in the last few years. Journals are requiring at least some documentation of validity and reliability of instruments if the study is to be published. However, to a great extent, broad modification of the prevalent attitudes toward measurement is dependent on the influence of those teaching nursing research and those supervising theses and dissertations.

Nursing, as a discipline, must consider what types of activities might improve measurement in research and can or should be undertaken by nurse researchers with various levels of preparation. Tool development requires a great deal of sophistication in research techniques and, in our judgment, should be performed primarily by those with doctoral preparation. Developing a tool and using it in a study without prior work to develop validity and reliability is not acceptable for any researcher. We would suggest that Master's level researchers place increasing emphasis on conducting studies that will add to the validity and reliability information available on existing tools and that these studies must be published.

There are a wide variety of strategies available from which to select measurement techniques for a nursing study. The design of studies is often limited by the researcher's unawareness of strategies that have been successfully used in the past. Additionally, an examination of possible techniques can often stimulate the creative thinking of the researcher and lead to the development of approaches not thought of previously. Many nursing phenomena have not been examined because no one has thought of a way to measure them. Common measurement approaches used in nursing research include physiologic measures, observations, interviews, content analyses, questionnaires and scales. Other methods of measurement discussed include the Q Sort, magnitude scaling, Delphi technique, projective techniques and diaries.

PHYSIOLOGIC MEASUREMENT

Much of nursing practice is oriented toward the physiologic dimensions of health. Therefore, many of our questions require the measurement of these dimensions. Initial interest in research related to clinical practice centered on examining the effects of physical care practices, studying such basic care activities as mouth care; decubitus care; the effect of preoperative teaching on postoperative recovery; and infection control related to urinary bladder catheterization, intravenous therapy and tracheostomy care. Unfortunately, studies in these areas declined long before sufficient information was available to form an adequate empirical base for nursing practice.

Even at this fairly simple level, finding valid ways to measure the variables of interest was difficult and required considerable time and expense to develop. For example, how does one measure changes in a decubitus ulcer? What criteria can be used to determine the effectiveness of a mouth care regimen? Creativity, imagination and attention to detail are needed to develop effective physiologic measurement strategies.

In recent years, there has been an upsurge of interest in studying physiologic factors. One element fostering this interest has been nurses who, during the 1970s, chose to obtain their doctoral preparation in the physiologic sciences. With a strong theoretical base for designing physiologic studies, these nurse scientists have begun adding to the empirical base of nursing. Lindsey (1982, 1983, 1984) has listed studies from 1970 to 1980 that measured physiologic variables. Lindsey (1982) used a classification schema developed by Barnard that provides a useful way of thinking about physiologic measures. The schema identifies phenomena related to "(1) the individual, (2) the individual's environment and (3) nursing therapeutics" (p. 345). The individual's environment is subdivided into "(a) the effect of manipulation of some environmental factor and (b) the effect of some naturally occurring environmental factor" (p. 345).

Lindsey (1983) listed physiologic variables used in the studies she reviewed:

Physiological variables used to quantify aspects of the phenomena studied by nurse investigators over this past decade have been numerous and have included the following list: tracheobronchial secretions, tracheal damage, arterial blood gases, nasopharyngeal O_2 concentration, transcutaneous O_2 tension, O_2 consumption, breathing patterns, pulmonary artery and pulmonary capillary wedge pressures, ventilatory function (volume and rate), temperature (in a variety of locations), blood pressure, heart rate, rhythm, and conduction, respiratory rate, premature ventricular contractions, cardiac muscle contractility, hot flash characteristics, internal jugular blood flow velocity, ventricular fluid drainage, healing, contamination/bacterial colonization, urine pH, urinary hemoglobin, urinary Na/K ratio, histological structure of several tissues, integrity of mucosal barrier, sodium reabsorption, blood glucose levels, plasma cortisol, plasma glycerol, secretory immunoglobulin A, 2,3-diphosphoglycerate, palmar sweat index, judgment of duration of a time interval, signs and symptoms and complications of a variety of clinical conditions, speech characteristics, noise, sleep-wake patterns, position, motor activity, limb activity, length and weight gain, development/maturation, caloric intake, feeding behavior, gastric motility, nausea/vomiting and even stool transit time. Identification of criterion measures for quantification remains a substantial problem and the extent to which an indirect measure is precisely reflective of the phenomenon under investigation is a significant question. (p. 56)

Measurements of physiologic variables can be either direct or indirect. These measures must be carefully linked conceptually with the framework of the study. The logic of operationalizing the concept in a particular way must be well thought out and made clear. Parsons and Wilson (1984) measured the cerebrovascular status of their subjects using indirect measures of the physiologic variables heart rate, mean arterial blood pressure, mean intracranial pressure and cerebral perfusion pressure. These physiological variables are clearly related to cerebrovascular status in the theoretical framework of this study.

Many measurement strategies require the use of instrumentation. If so, the researcher must determine where to obtain the equipment and must often seek funding for this purpose. The researcher must either learn to operate the equipment or make arrangements with someone who has these skills to participate in the study. Care must be taken that the equipment operate in an optimal fashion. In some cases, the equipment must be recalibrated regularly to ensure consistent readings. Recalibration means that the equipment is reset to ensure precise measurements. We recalibrate the bathroom scales periodically to make sure that the weight indicated is accurate.

Some procedures require laboratory analysis. If so, arrangements must be made with a laboratory to perform the needed analyses. In some cases, invasive procedures are involved. In these circumstances, great care must be taken to protect the subjects and to follow guidelines for informed consent and institutional approval.

In publishing the results of a physiologic study, the measurement technique must be described in great detail. This allows adequate critique of the study and facilitates replication of the study by others. At present, few replications of physiologic studies have been reported in the literature. The following section describes physiologic measurement strategies of two recently published studies.

Hilton (1985) studied the level of sound in intensive care areas. She describes her instrumentation in the following way:

Decibel levels of sound were measured using a microphone suspended on the end of a cable at the head of the patient's bed connected to a Type 1 Precision Integrating Sound Level Meter Type 2218 (Bruel & Kjaer) which in turn was wired to the Noise Level Recorder Type 2306 (Bruel & Kjaer). The range of sound was set at 40-90 dB(A) and the decibels calibrated by a Sound Level Calibrator Type 4230 (Bruel & Kjaer). Paper speed was 1 mm/sec when the observer was present and .3mm/sec otherwise.

To measure the LEQ, a small Integrating Sound Level Meter Type 2225 (Bruel & Kjaer), with Data Storer Type C101 (Bruel & Kjaer), was suspended near the headboard. Later this meter was connected to a Data Processor Type C102 (Bruel & Kjaer) which analyzed average sound levels in LEQs for selected time intervals. Printouts in graph and digital form were obtained of average sound levels in LEQs. (pp. 284–285)

Baun (1984) developed a study to determine physiological determinants of successful endotracheal suctioning. Instrumentation is described as follows:

Prior to and immediately following the suction sequence, the following variables were measured: functional residual capacity (FRC) determined by the helium dilution technique for mechanically ventilated patients (Sufer and Schlobohm 1974); long-thorax compliance calculated as the quotient of exhaled tidal volume recorded from the output of a Wedge Spirometer divided by the translungthorax (tracheal) pressures recorded from the output of a Harvard Apparatus pressure transducer connected through an adapter to the proximal end of the inflated endotracheal tube; carbon dioxide (CO_2) production obtained from mixed expired CO_2 obtained from the analysis of the contents of a Douglas Bag in which the expired gas has been collected for approximately 3 minutes through the use of a Sierra valve connected to the endotracheal tube; and simultaneous systemic arterial and mixed venous samples drawn over a period of 1 minute (Suter, Lindauer, Fairley, and Schlobohm 1975) and analyzed for pH, carbon dioxide tension (P_{CO_2}), oxygen tension (P_{O_2}), O_2 saturation, O_2 content, and bicarbonate according to standard laboratory techniques. All pH, P_{CO_2} and P_{O_2} values obtained for this study were corrected to the patient's body temperature. From the above measured variables, the following criterion variables were calculated: arterial-venous oxygen tension difference (a-vD_{O_2}), alveolar-arterial oxygen tension difference (A-aD_{O_2}), physiologic deadspace (V_D/V_T), shunt fraction (Q_{VA}/Q_T), and cardiac output (CO) by the Fick principle.
　　During the suction sequence, arterial samples were drawn into heparinized syringes (Adams, Morgan-Hughes and Sykes 1967) through a multistopcock manifold connected to the femoral arterial line and immediately placed on ice (Eldridge and Fretwell 1965). The distal end of the manifold was connected to a Harvard constant withdrawal pump so that a fresh supply of arterial blood was available for each sample. Since the arterial line did not contain more than 5 ml, the pump was turned on in advance of the sample time so that 5 ml would be cleared from the line. Arterial samples were drawn at baseline, at the end of 30 sec. of hyperinflation at 5 sec. intervals during the 20 sec. period of suction, at 10 sec. intervals during the 30 sec. period of hyperinflation after suction, at 30 sec. intervals for the next minute and then at one minute intervals for the next 3 minutes. During long pauses between samples, the Harvard pump was turned off to prevent the unnecessary withdrawal of blood but turned on long enough before the next sample to assure that fresh blood was withdrawn. There was a total blood loss of less than 50 ml to each patient studied. (p. 216)*

OBSERVATIONAL MEASUREMENT

Although measurement by observation is most commonly used in qualitative research, it is used to some extent in all types of studies. Measurement in qualitative research is not distinct from analysis; rather, the two occur simultaneously. For more detail on measurement and analysis in qualitative research, refer to Chapter 17. Measurement of observations is not quite as simple as it sounds. One must first decide what is to be observed and then determine how to ensure that every variable is observed in a similar manner in each instance. Observation tends to be more subjective than other types of measurement and, thus, is often seen as less credible. However, in many cases, this is the only possible approach to obtain important data for the body of knowledge. As with any means of measurement, consistency is very important. Therefore, much attention must be given to training data collectors. If the measurement technique is complex, written instructions should be provided. Opportunities for pilot testing of the technique should be used, and data on interrater reliability should be generated.

Unstructured Observations

In only a few types of qualitative studies does one simply spontaneously observe and record what is seen with no prior planning. This type of measurement is referred to as *unstructured observation*. Although unstructured observations give freedom to the observer, there is a risk of loss of objectivity and a possibility that the observer may not remember all the details of the observed event. The technique is very artistic in nature and requires someone with a very good memory and extremely effective interpersonal skills who is highly skilled in spontaneous reconceptualization.

Structured Observations

The first step in structured observational measurement is to carefully define what is to be observed. From that point, the concern is with how the observations are to be made, recorded and coded. In most cases, a category system is developed for organizing and sorting the behaviors or events being observed. The extent to which these categories are exhaustive varies with the study.

Category Systems □ The observational categories should be mutually exclusive. If the categories overlap, the observer will be faced with making judgments as to what category should contain each observed behavior, and data collection will not be consistent. In some category systems, all behavior is not recorded. Only that behavior that is of interest is recorded. Most category systems require some inference by the observer from the observed event to the category. The greater the degree of inference required, the more difficult the category system is to use. Some systems are developed to be used in a wide variety of studies, whereas others are specific to the study for which they were designed. The number of categories used varies considerably with the study. An optimal number for ease of use and therefore effectiveness of observation is 15 to 20 categories.

Checklists □ Checklists are techniques of indicating whether or not a behavior occurred. In this case, tally marks are generally placed on a data collection form each time the behavior is observed. Behaviors other than those on the checklist are ignored. In some studies, multiple tally marks may be placed in various categories while one is observing a particular event. However, in other studies, the observer must select a single category by which to place the tally mark.

Rating Scales □ Rating scales, which will be discussed in a later section, can be used for observation as well as for self-report. A rating scale allows the observer to rate the behavior or event on a scale. This provides more information for analysis than the dichotomous data, which indicates only that the behavior either occurred or did not occur.

Kerr (1985) used observational measurement in examining the variables space use, privacy and territoriality in a hospital environment. The data collection process is described below:

An observational study was conducted on two medical and two surgical wards of a recently constructed 832-bed research and teaching hospital... The four wards chosen were virtually identical in architectural design and space allocated to staff. For example, the places where the ward secretaries sat, their chairs, counter spaces, tables, and the chart racks they used were standardized. Similarly, the head nurse offices, doctors' offices, clinical nurse stations, nurse substations, and widths of counters and hallways were the same throughout the four wards. These standardized fixed and semifixed features of the environment allowed the data from all wards to be analyzed both in terms of the total sample of observations as well as in terms of the observations made on each ward. (pp. 203–204)

The instrument used in this study to measure the space occupied by a subject by his or her two nearest neighbors and their behavior over a working day was a modified form of the Behavior Sampling Instrument developed by Fairbanks et al. (1977). (p. 204)

Subjects were observed for one day, from the time each one entered the ward in the morning until they left for the day. When the second hand of the observer's watch reached zero seconds, the following variables were recorded: Time, space occupied by the focal subject, his or her nearest neighbor, space occupied by the neighbor, their behavior, age, sex, and role. The same data were obtained for the person second closest to the focal subject if applicable. (pp. 204–205)

Censullo, Lester and Hoffman (1985) conducted a study examining rhythmic patterning in mother–newborn interaction. They used the Dyadic Interaction Code (DIC) for their study. The code is based on Tronick's five dyadic phases of initiation, mutual orientation, greeting, play and disengagement. The code is used to score behaviors from a rank of 1, for disengagement, to a rank of 6, for highly engaged. As scores move toward level 6, "positive affect, level of arousal, and animation increase" (p. 344). The observation measurement was described as follows:

> Comforting procedures were first offered to enhance opportunity for social interaction, then each infant was placed in the mother's lap. The mother was seated on a chair with her back to the video monitor. She was asked to hold her baby upright at about a 30° angle, facing her. The specific instructions were, "Please hold the baby in front of you, like this (demonstrated), so that each of you has a full view of the other's face. Just play with your baby, doing whatever you normally do to keep your baby's attention. After 3 minutes we will tell you to stop." The interaction was filmed by placing a mirror at an angle in front of the mother, the camera held behind her shoulder, so that her face and the infant's were recorded on the videotape. The camera person was not in the mother's line of vision, decreasing further distractions during the interaction.
>
> The DIC was used to score the 3-minute mother-newborn interaction sequence from the videotapes, by recording the time and code level that corresponded to each change in dyadic behavior lasting at least 2 seconds. Each film was scored twice by the senior author by placing the tape on "pause" and writing the time and new behavioral level in a log. Interrater agreement was 90%. (p. 344)

INTERVIEWS

Interviews involve verbal communication between the researcher and the subject, during which information is provided to the researcher. Although this measurement strategy is most commonly used in exploratory studies (quantitative and qualitative) and descriptive studies, it can be used in other types of studies. This measurement approach is frequently used in survey designs. There are a variety of approaches to conducting an interview, ranging from a totally unstructured interview in which the content is completely controlled by the subject, to interviews in which the content is similar to a questionnaire, with the possible responses to questions carefully designed by the researcher.

Planning measurement by interview requires careful, detailed work and has almost become a science in itself. Many excellent books are available on the techniques of developing interview questions. Researchers planning to use this strategy should consult a text on interview methodology prior to designing their instrument. Because nurses frequently use interview techniques in nursing assessment, the dynamics of interviewing are familiar; however, using the technique for measurement in research requires greater sophistication.

Unstructured Interviews

Unstructured interviews are used primarily in exploratory studies. The researcher may be seeking to understand how the subject organizes ideas on a particular topic or to identify attitudes. In some cases, this type of interview may be used as a step in developing a more precise measurement tool in a particular area of study.

The interview may be initiated by asking a broad question such as "Describe for me your experience with..." After the interview is begun, the role of the interviewer is to encourage the subject to continue talking, using techniques such as nodding the head or making sounds that indicate interest. In some cases, the subject may be encouraged to further elaborate on a particular dimension of the topic of discussion.

Structured Interviews

Structured interviews include strategies that provide increasing amounts of control by the researcher over the content of the interview. Questions asked by the interviewer are designed by the researcher prior to the initiation of data collection, and the order of the questions is specified. In some cases, the interviewer is allowed to further explain the meaning of the question or modify the way in which the question is asked so that the subject can better understand the question. In more structured interviews, the interviewer must ask the question precisely as it has been designed. If the subject does not understand the question, the interviewer can only repeat the question. The subject may be limited to a range of responses previously developed by the researcher, similar to those in a questionnaire. If the possible responses are lengthy or complex, they may be printed on a card that is handed to the subject for selection of a response.

Designing Interview Questions

The development and sequencing of interview questions are similar to that used in questionnaires and will be elaborated on in the section entitled Questionnaires. Briefly, questions progress from broad and general to narrow and specific. Questions are grouped by topic, with fairly "safe" topics being addressed first, and sensitive topics reserved until late in the interview process. Less interesting data, such as age, educational level, income and other demographic information are usually collected last. These data should not be collected in an interview if they can be obtained from another source such as a patient record. The wording of questions in an interview is dependent on the education level of the subjects. The wording of certain questions may have a variety of interpretations by different subjects, and the researcher should anticipate this. After the interview protocol has been developed, feedback should be sought from an expert in interview technique and also from a content expert.

Pretesting the Interview Protocol

When the protocol has been satisfactorily developed, it should be pilot tested on subjects similar to those who will be used in the study. This allows the researcher to identify problems in the design of questions, sequencing of questions or procedure for recording responses. It also allows an assessment of the reliability and validity of the interview instrument.

Training Interviewers

Developing skills in interviewing requires practice. Interviewers should be very familiar with the content of the interview. They must anticipate situations that might occur during the interview and develop strategies for dealing with them. One of the most effective methods of developing a polished approach is role-playing. Playing the role of the subject can give the interviewer insight into the experience of a subject and thus facilitate an effective response to particular situations.

The interviewer must learn how to establish a permissive atmosphere in which the subject will be encouraged to respond to sensitive topics. Methods of maintaining an unbiased verbal and nonverbal manner must also be developed. The wording of a question, the tone of voice, raising an eyebrow or shifting body position can all communicate a positive or negative reaction of the interviewer to the subject's responses. Positive as well as negative verbal or nonverbal communications can alter the data.

Preparing For an Interview

If the interview is to be lengthy, an appointment should be made. The researcher should be nicely dressed but not overdressed and should be prompt for the appointment. The site selected for the interview should be quiet, allow privacy for the interaction and provide a pleasant environment. Instructions given to the subject about the interview should be carefully planned prior to the interview. For example, the interviewer might say "I am going to ask you a series of questions about.... Before you answer each question you need to.... Select your answer from the following... and then you may elaborate on your response. I will record your answer and then, if I am not clear, I may ask you to explain some aspect further."

Probing

Probing is used by the interviewer to obtain more information in a specific area of the interview. In some cases, the question may be repeated. If the subject has said "I don't know," the interviewer may press for a response. In other situations, the interviewer may further explain the question or ask the subject to explain statements that have been made. At a deeper level, the interviewer may pick up on a comment made by the subject and begin asking questions to obtain further meaning from the subject. Probes should be neutral to avoid biasing the subject's responses. Probing should be done within reasonable guidelines to prevent the subject from feeling that he or she is being "cross-examined" or "grilled" on a topic.

Recording Interview Data

Data obtained from interviews are recorded either during the interview or immediately following the interview. The recording may be in the form of handwritten notes or tape recordings. If notes are hand recorded, the interviewer might need instruction in the recording of concise, accurate information.

The interviewer must be able to identify key ideas (or capture essential data) in an interview and to concisely record this information. The recording of data must be done without distracting the interviewee. In fact, some interviewees will not respond if they notice that the researcher is taking notes or is taping their responses. In these situations, the interviewer must record essential information immediately after the interview. Tape recording requires the permission of the subject. These tapes must be transcribed prior to data analysis. In transcribing tapes, the interviewer will frequently capture and record essential data rather than extract the information verbatim from the tape. The data from unstructured interviews are the most difficult to capture and record. Content analysis is frequently used to capture the meaning within the data.

Advantages and Disadvantages of Interviews

Interviewing is a flexible technique that can allow the researcher to explore greater depth of meaning than can be obtained with other techniques. Interpersonal skills can be used to facilitate cooperation and elicit more information. There is a higher response rate to interviews than to questionnaires, leading to a more representative sample. Interviews allow collection of data from subjects unable or unlikely to complete questionnaires, such as the very ill or those whose reading, writing and ability to express themselves is marginal.

Interviews are a form of self-report, and the researcher must assume that the information provided is accurate. Interviewing requires much more time than questionnaires and scales and thus is more costly. Because of time and costs, sample size is usually limited. Subject bias is always a threat to the validity of the findings, as is inconsistency in data collection from one subject to another.

Gloeckner (1984) used an interview to measure subject perceptions of sexual attractiveness after ostomy surgery. The interview schedule was developed based on the researcher's experience, questions obtained from previous studies and tools available in the literature. "The interview consisted of 21 questions that addressed sexual information received, changes in sexual attractiveness, changes in sexual functioning, and reactions of a spouse or partner" (p. 89). Subjects rated each question on a scale from 1 to 5, with 1 being very low, and 5 being very high. The ratings were used for three points in time: "(1) within 1 year prior to ostomy surgery, (b) within the first year after surgery, and (c) now, at the time of interview" (p. 89). Interviewing took place in the subjects' homes and responses were tape recorded. Interviews required about 1 hour of time.

CONTENT ANALYSIS

Content analysis uses recorded words as the source of data. The technique provides a systematic means of measuring the frequency, order or intensity of occurrence of words, phrases or sentences. Categories are developed for the data, and/or statistical analyses are conducted. Initially, the specific characteristics of the content to be measured must be defined, then rules are developed by the researcher for identifying and recording these characteristics.

The researcher first selects a specific unit of analysis, which may be individual words, word combinations or themes. This unit of analysis is often an indicator of an abstract concept. Then, the data to be analyzed are identified. The data may be the universe (all written sources of the data), such as all articles or newspaper stories written on a particular topic, or the researcher may randomly select a portion of the universe (such as every fourth paragraph, every 10th word, a 3-minute segment from a tape recording) to analyze. Criteria are then developed for coding the data into categories. Data collectors are trained to classify the data into the categories, and levels of interrater reliability are identified.

The technique can be used on existing written data, which allows the study of individuals unobtrusively. These data sources are often available for long periods of time, which allows the researcher to examine changes over time. However, the process is time consuming. In addition, judgment is required in interpreting the meaning of the written communication of others, resulting in a risk of subjectivity (Waltz, Strickland & Lenz, 1984).

Burns and Carney (1985) used content analysis to collect data from the handwritten patient care notes of hospice care. The data were then used to describe the process of hospice care. The tool for the content analysis contained 75 care activities. The following is a list of some of the activities identified.

1. Rearrange environment for care
2. Discuss legal concerns or obtain legal assistance
3. Provide physical care
4. Provide spiritual support
5. Allow expression of feelings
6. Encourage family to take care of themselves
7. Teach hospice pain management
8. Discuss expected physical changes

Powers, Murphy and Wooldridge (1983) used content analysis to examine the recorded content of two experimental nursing approaches related to teaching in a hypertensive education program. Their procedures for content analysis are described below:

Two variations of content analysis were used in the present study. The first involved formulating content categories and then coding nurse-patient verbal behaviors using the entire statement by the nurse or patient as the unit of analysis. The second phase of analysis was concerned with developing a system of units for quantifying the relative amounts of time spent on the content categories. (p. 4)

The teaching checklist included the following: concept of blood pressure, measurement of blood pressure and blood pressure values, concept of hypertension as a lifelong disease, risk factors and complications, basic pathology of hypertension, rationale for treatment, medication schedules and side effects, dietary restrictions, weight control and exercise, smoking, and stress/life-style. The pilot categorization schema consisted of 32 categories; later, several were collapsed, leaving the final schema with 24 categories.

After the categories were identified, the unit of analysis was specified as a cycle of verbal exchange between nurse and patient, that is, one complete statement by the nurse followed by the patient's response... For ease of coding, each interaction unit from the typed transcripts was mounted on separate 5 × 8 cards. Each unit was then assigned a category based upon the predominant theme of the exchange... Ten interviews, five high indirect and five low indirect, were drawn randomly from the sample of 62 interviews for purposes of piloting the coding schema and assessing reliability. Two coders were trained and familiarized with categorizing schema. The ten pilot interviews comprising 756 interaction units were coded independently to determine reliability... To estimate the constancy of the two coders over time, a percentage agreement was calculated for each observer after the pilot interviews were coded a second time. (pp. 4–5)

Questionnaires

A questionnaire is a printed self-report form designed to elicit information that can be obtained through written responses of the subject. The information obtained through questionnaires is similar to that obtained by interview, but the questions tend to have less depth. The subject is unable to elaborate on responses or ask for clarification of questions, and the data collector cannot use probe strategies. However, questions are presented in a consistent manner, and there is less opportunity for bias than in the interview.

The primary measurement devices in survey designs are the interview and the questionnaire. Questionnaires can be designed to determine facts about the subject or persons known by the subject; facts about events or situations known by the subject; or beliefs, attitudes, opinions, levels of knowledge or intentions of the subject. They can be distributed to very large samples, either directly or through the mail. The development and administration of questionnaires has been the topic of many excellent books focusing on survey techniques that can be helpful in the process of designing a questionnaire. Two nursing methodology texts (Shelley, 1984; Waltz, Strickland & Lenz, 1984) provide detailed explanations of the questionnaire development procedure. Although questions on a questionnaire appear easy to design, the development of questions should be the result of careful planning.

Like interviews, questionnaires can have varying degrees of structure. Some questionnaires ask open-ended questions, which require written responses from the subject. Others ask closed-ended questions, which have options selected by the researcher. Data from open-ended questions are often difficult to interpret and require the use of content analysis to extract meaning. This form of questionnaire is not advised when data are obtained from large samples.

Development of Questionnaires

The first step in either selecting or developing a questionnaire is to identify the information desired. For this purpose, a blueprint or table of specifications is developed. The blueprint should identify the essential content to be covered by the questionnaire, and the content should be at the educational level of the potential subjects. It is difficult to stick to the blueprint in designing the questionnaire because it is tempting to add "just one more question" that seems a "neat idea" or a question that someone insists "really should be included." As the questionnaire becomes longer, fewer subjects will be willing to respond and more questions will be left blank.

The second step is to search the literature for questionnaires that match the developed blueprint. Questionnaires are compiled and published in instrument books such as the book by Ward and Lindeman (1979) entitled *Instruments for measuring nursing practice and other health care variables*. Sometimes published studies include questionnaires, but frequently you must contact the authors of a study in order to receive a copy of their questionnaire. Unlike scaling instruments, questionnaires are seldom copyrighted. Researchers are encouraged to use questions in exactly the same form as those in previous studies to facilitate comparing results between studies. However, questions that are poorly written should be modified, even if it interferes with comparison with previous results.

For some studies, the researcher can find a questionnaire in the literature that matches the questionnaire blueprint that has been developed for a study. However, frequently, the researcher must add items to or delete items from an existing questionnaire to accommodate the blueprint developed. In some situations, items from two or three questionnaires are combined to develop an appropriate questionnaire.

Sometimes the questionnaire blueprint requires the development of a few items or an entirely new questionnaire. An item on a questionnaire has two parts: a lead-in question and a response set. Each lead-in question must be carefully designed and clearly expressed to avoid influencing the response of the respondent. Because of this, "value laden words" and leading questions that indicate the bias of the researcher must be avoided. The degree of formality with which the question is expressed and the permissive tone of the question are, in many cases, important for obtaining a "true" measure. Each question should clearly instruct the subject as to how to respond (*i.e.*, choose one, mark all that apply), or instructions should be included at the beginning of the questionnaire. If a question includes a term with which the respondent may not be familiar or for which there are several meanings, the term must be defined. These skills in writing "good" questions can be acquired through books and formal coursework in questionnaire development.

Each item in a questionnaire has a *response set*, which provides the parameters within which the question is to be answered. This response set can be very open and flexible as it is with open-ended questions or very narrow and directive as it is with closed-ended questions. For example, an open-ended question might have a response set of three blank lines. With closed-ended questions, the response set includes a specific list of alternatives from which to select. The response sets for closed-ended questions must be carefully designed and clearly expressed. This set must include all possible responses to the question. If the information sought is factual, this can be accomplished by including "other" as one of the possible responses. However, it must be recognized that the item "other" is essentially lost data. Even if the response is followed by a statement such as "Please explain," it is rarely possible to analyze the data meaningfully. If a large number of subjects (greater than 10 per cent) select the alternative "other," the alternatives included in the response set might not be appropriate for the population studied.

After the questionnaire items have been developed, the ordering of these items should be carefully planned. Questions related to a specific topic should be grouped together. General items are included first, progressing to more specific items. More important items might be included first, progressing to items of lesser importance. Questions of a sensitive nature, or those that might be threatening should appear last on the questionnaire. In some cases, the response to one item may influence the response to another. If so, their order must be carefully considered. Any open-ended questions should be included last, because their responses will require more time than closed-ended questions. The general trend is to include demographic data about the subject at the end of the questionnaire.

Instructions on how to mark responses on the questionnaire should be included either on a cover page or at the beginning of the form. The subject should know whether to circle, underline or fill in a circle as he or she responds to items. In large studies, scantron sheets may be used to speed up data entry into the computer and to decrease errors. This decision should be carefully thought out, however, because subjects who are not familiar with these sheets may make errors in entering their responses (thus decreasing measurement validity), and fewer subjects may be willing to complete the questionnaire.

A cover letter should accompany the questionnaire, explaining the purpose of the study, the name of the researcher, the approximate amount of time required to complete the form and organizations or institutions supporting the study. Instructions should include an address to which the questionnaire can be returned. This address should be at the end of the questionnaire as well as on the cover letter and the envelope. Respondents will often discard both the envelope and the cover letter, and, after completion of the questionnaire, they will not know where to send it.

A pilot test of the questionnaire should be performed to determine the clarity of questions, effectiveness of instructions, completeness of response sets, time required to complete the questionnaire and successfulness of data collection techniques. As with any pilot test, the subjects and techniques should be as similar to those planned for the large study as possible. In some cases, some open-ended questions are included in a pilot test to obtain information for the development of closed-ended response sets for the large study.

Questionnaire Validity

One of the greatest risks in developing response sets is leaving out an important alternative or response. For example, if the questionnaire item addressed the job position of nurses working in a hospital and the sample included nursing students, a category must be included that indicates the student role. When seeking opinions, there is a risk of obtaining a response from an individual who actually has no opinion on the subject. When an item requests knowledge that the respondent does not possess, his or her guessing interferes with obtaining a "true" measure.

The response rate to questionnaires is generally lower than that with other forms of self-report, particularly if the questionnaires are mailed out. If the response rate is lower than 50 per cent, the representativeness of the sample is seriously in question. The response rate for mailed questionnaires is usually small (25 to 30 per cent), so the researcher is frequently unable to obtain a representative sample, even with randomization. Strategies that can increase the response rate include enclosing a stamped, addressed envelope and sending a postcard 2 weeks after the questionnaire was mailed to those who have not returned it. Sometimes a phone call follow-up is made to increase the return rate of questionnaires.

Commonly, respondents fail to mark responses to all the questions, which is especially a problem with long questionnaires. This can threaten the validity of the instrument. In some cases, responses will be written in if the respondent does not agree with the available choices, or comments may be written in the margin. Generally, these responses cannot be included in the analysis; however, a record should be kept of such responses. It is advisable to decide prior to distributing the questionnaires those questions that are critical to the research topic. If any of these questions is omitted in a questionnaire, it is not included in the analysis.

Consistency in the way that the questionnaire is administered is important to validity. For example, administering some questionnaires in a group setting and mailing out others is not wise. There should not be a mix of mailing to business addresses and home addresses. If questionnaires are administered in person, the administration should be consistent. Several problems in consistency can occur: (1) Some subjects may ask to take the form home to complete it and return it later, whereas others will complete it in the presence of the data collector; (2) some subjects may complete the form themselves, whereas others may ask a family member to write the responses that the respondent dictates; and (3) in some cases, the form may be completed by a secretary or colleague rather than by the individual. These situations lead to biases in responses that are unknown to the researcher and that alter the "true" measure of the variables.

Analysis of Questionnaire Data

The data from questionnaires are usually ordinal in nature, limiting analysis for the most part to summary statistics and nonparametric statistics. However, in some cases, t-tests or ANOVA are used to test for differences between responses of various subsets of the sample. Discriminant analysis may be used to determine the ability to predict membership in various groups from responses to particular questions. Burns (1986) used a questionnaire to examine smoking patterns of nurses in the state of Texas. Items from that questionnaire, which demonstrates a variety of response sets, are given in Figure 11–10.

SCALES

Scales, a form of self-report, are a more precise means of measuring phenomena than are questionnaires. The majority of scales have been developed to measure psychosocial variables. However, self-reports can be obtained on physiologic variables, such as pain, nausea or functional capacity, using scaling techniques. Scaling is based on mathematical theory, and there is a branch of science in

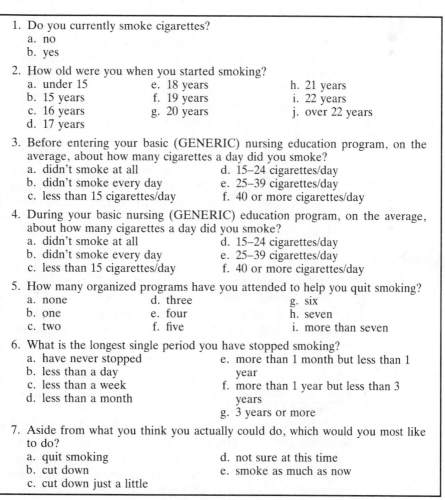

1. Do you currently smoke cigarettes?
   a. no
   b. yes

2. How old were you when you started smoking?
   a. under 15   e. 18 years   h. 21 years
   b. 15 years   f. 19 years   i. 22 years
   c. 16 years   g. 20 years   j. over 22 years
   d. 17 years

3. Before entering your basic (GENERIC) nursing education program, on the average, about how many cigarettes a day did you smoke?
   a. didn't smoke at all   d. 15–24 cigarettes/day
   b. didn't smoke every day   e. 25–39 cigarettes/day
   c. less than 15 cigarettes/day   f. 40 or more cigarettes/day

4. During your basic nursing (GENERIC) education program, on the average, about how many cigarettes a day did you smoke?
   a. didn't smoke at all   d. 15–24 cigarettes/day
   b. didn't smoke every day   e. 25–39 cigarettes/day
   c. less than 15 cigarettes/day   f. 40 or more cigarettes/day

5. How many organized programs have you attended to help you quit smoking?
   a. none   d. three   g. six
   b. one   e. four   h. seven
   c. two   f. five   i. more than seven

6. What is the longest single period you have stopped smoking?
   a. have never stopped   e. more than 1 month but less than 1
   b. less than a day   year
   c. less than a week   f. more than 1 year but less than 3
   d. less than a month   years
                              g. 3 years or more

7. Aside from what you think you actually could do, which would you most like to do?
   a. quit smoking   d. not sure at this time
   b. cut down   e. smoke as much as now
   c. cut down just a little

FIGURE 11–10. Smoking questionnaire.

which the primary concern is the development of measurement scales. From a point of view of scaling theory, there is expected to be considerable measurement error (random error) and systematic error in a single item. Therefore, in most scales, the various items on the scale are summed to obtain a single score. These are referred to as *summated scales*. There is less random and systematic error in using the total score of a scale. Using several items in a scale to measure a concept is comparable to using several instruments to measure a concept (see Fig. 11–5). The various items in a scale increase the dimensions of the concept that are reflected in the instrument. Each item in a scale is a variable. A scale with numerous items requires a large sample for adequate analysis. For example, if a scale had 30 items and 5 to 10 subjects were needed for each variable in a study for analysis, the sample must include 150 to 300 subjects. The types of scales described include rating scales, the Likert scale, the semantic differential and the Q sort.

Rating Scales

Rating scales are the most crude form of measure using scaling techniques. A rating scale lists an ordered series of categories of a variable, assumed to be based on an underlying continuum. A numerical value is assigned to each category. The fineness of the distinctions between categories varies with the scale. Rating scales are commonly used by the general public. In conversations, one can hear statements such as "on a scale of one to ten, I would rank that...." Rating scales are easy to develop; however, one must be careful to avoid end statements that are so extreme that no subject will select them. A rating scale could be used to rate the degree of cooperativeness of the patient or the value placed by the subject on the nurse–patient interactions. For example, Burns (1974) used the following rating scale (Fig. 11–11) to examine differences in nurse–patient communication of cancer patients and other medical-surgical patients.

Likert Scale

The Likert scale was developed by a social psychologist, Rensis Likert. The scale is designed to determine the opinion or attitude of a subject and contains a number of declarative statements with a scale after each statement. The Likert scale is the most commonly used of the scaling techniques. The original version of the scale consisted of five categories from which the subject could select: (1) strongly disagree, (2) disagree, (3) uncertain, (4) agree and (5) strongly agree. Values are placed on each response, with a value of 1 on the most negative response and a value of 5 on the most positive response (Nunnally, 1978).

There have been several modifications of the scale used in instruments. Sometimes seven options are given, sometimes only four. There has been controversy over the use of the uncertain or neutral category, which allows the subject to avoid making a clear choice of positive or negative statements. Thus, sometimes, only four or six options are offered, with the uncertain category omitted. This is referred to as a *forced choice* version. Sometimes, respondents

1. Nurses come into my room
   a. rarely
   b. sometimes
   c. whenever I call them
   d. frequently just to speak or check me
2. I would <u>like</u> nurses to come into my room
   a. rarely
   b. sometimes
   c. whenever I call them
   d. frequently just to speak or check me
3. When a nurse enters my room, she usually
   a. talks very little
   b. trys to talk about things I do not wish to discuss
   c. talks only about casual things
   d. is willing to listen or discuss what concerns me
4. When a nurse enters my room, I would <u>prefer</u> that she
   a. talk very little
   b. talk only when necessary
   c. talk only about casual things
   d. be willing to listen or discuss what concerns me
5. When a nurse talks with me she usually seems
   a. not interested
   b. in a hurry
   c. polite but distant
   d. caring for me as a person
6. When a nurse talks with me, I would <u>prefer</u> that she be
   a. not interested
   b. in a hurry
   c. polite but distant
   d. caring for me as a person
7. When a nurse talks with me she usually
   a. stands in the doorway
   b. stands at the foot of the bed
   c. stands at the side of the bed
   d. sits beside the bed
8. When a nurse talks with me I would <u>prefer</u> that she
   a. stand in the doorway
   b. stand at the foot of the bed
   c. stand at the side of the bed
   d. sit beside the bed
9. When a nurse talks with me, she is
   a. strictly business
   b. casual
   c. friendly but does not talk about feelings
   d. open to talking about things I worry or think about
10. When a nurse talks with me, I would <u>prefer</u> that she keep the conversation
    a. strictly business
    b. casual
    c. friendly but not talking about feelings
    d. open to talk about things I worry or think about

FIGURE 11–11. Communication rating scale.

Illustration continued on following page

11. Nurses talk with me about things important to me
    a. rarely
    b. sometimes
    c. frequently
    d. as often as I need to talk
12. I would like for the nurse to talk with me about things important to me
    a. rarely
    b. sometimes
    c. frequently
    d. as often as I need to talk
13. The nurse looks me in the eye when she talks with me
    a. rarely
    b. sometimes
    c. frequently
    d. very frequently
14. I would prefer that the nurse look me in the eye when she talks with me
    a. rarely
    b. sometimes
    c. frequently
    d. very frequently
15. When a nurse talks to me, she touches me
    a. rarely
    b. sometimes
    c. frequently
    d. very frequently
16. When a nurse talks with me, I would prefer that she touches me
    a. rarely
    b. occasionally
    c. frequently
    d. very frequently
17. My feelings about nurses talking to me are
    a. They should do their work well and otherwise leave me alone.
    b. They may talk if they need to; it does not bother me.
    c. I enjoy talking with the nurses.
    d. When the nurse lets me talk with her about things important to me, I feel that she cares for me as a person.
On question 18, please mark as many answers as you wish.
18. I would like to feel free to talk with the nurse about my
    a. illness
    b. future
    c. financial problems
    d. feelings about myself
    e. feelings about my family
    f. life up to this time

FIGURE 11–11 *Continued*

will become angry at forced choice items and refuse to complete the scale. Researchers who use the forced choice version consider an item that is left blank as a response of "uncertain." However, responses of "uncertain" are difficult to interpret, and, if a large number of respondents select that option or leave the question blank, the data may be useless.

An instrument using a Likert scale usually consists of 10 to 20 items addressing dimensions of a particular issue. Half of the statements should be expressed positively and half negatively to avoid inserting a bias in the responses. Scale values of negatively expressed items must be reversed prior to analysis. Usually, the values obtained from each item in the instrument are summed to obtain a single score for each subject. Although the values of each item are technically ordinal level data, the summed score is interval level data, thus allowing more sophisticated statistical analyses. The items (not actually part of a scale) in Figure 11–12 indicate the types of statements commonly used in Likert scales.

Semantic differentials

The semantic differential was developed by Osgood, Suci and Tannenbaum (1957) to measure attitudes or beliefs. A semantic differential scale consists of two opposite adjectives with a seven-point scale between them. The subject is to select one point on the scale that best describes his or her view of the concept being examined. The scale is designed to measure connotative meaning of the concept to the subject. Although the adjectives may not seem to be particularly related to the concept being examined, the technique can be used

	Strongly Disagree	Disagree	Uncertain	Agree	Strongly Agree
People with cancer almost always die					
Chemotherapy is very effective in treating cancer					
We are close to finding a cure for cancer					
I would work next to a person with cancer					
I could develop cancer					
Nurses take good care of patients with cancer					

FIGURE 11–12. Likert scale.

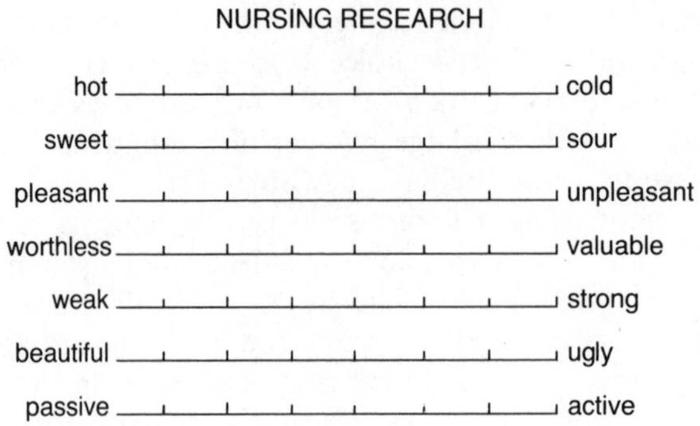

NURSING RESEARCH

FIGURE **11–13.** Semantic differential.

hot |_____| cold

sweet |_____| sour

pleasant |_____| unpleasant

worthless |_____| valuable

weak |_____| strong

beautiful |_____| ugly

passive |_____| active

to distinguish varying degrees of positive and negative attitudes toward a concept. Figure 11–13 illustrates the form used for this type of scale.

Some semantic differentials use descriptive phrases, rather than the original adjectives used by Osgood, Suci and Tannenbaum (1957) to develop the semantic differential instrument. Burns (1981, 1983) developed a semantic differential to measure beliefs about cancer that uses descriptive phrases. Figure 11–14 includes descriptive phrases from a 23-item scale.

In the semantic differential, values are assigned to each of the spaces, from 1 to 7, with 1 being the most negative response and 7, the most positive. The placement of negative responses to the left or right of the scale should be randomly varied to avoid global responses (in which the subject places checks in the same column of each scale. Each line is considered one scale. The values for the scales are summed to obtain one score for each subject. Factor analysis is used to determine the factor structure, which is expected to reflect three factors or dimensions: evaluation, potency and activity. The researcher must explain theoretically why particular items on the scale cluster together in the factor analysis. Thus, the development of the instrument contributes to theory development. Factor analysis is also used to evaluate the validity of the instrument. With some of these instruments, three factor scores, each representing one of the dimensions, are used to describe the subject's responses and are a basis for further analysis (Nunnally, 1978).

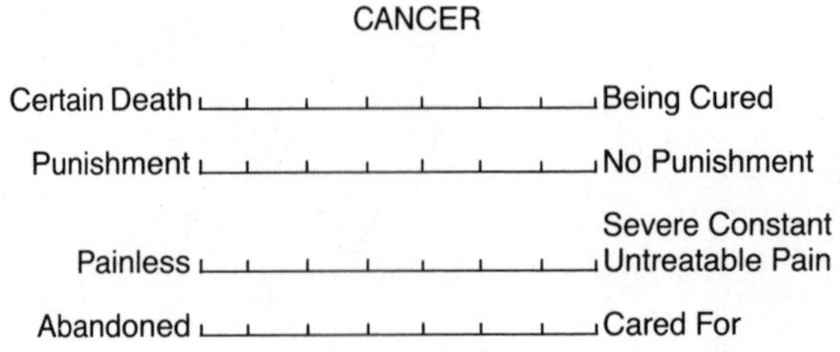

CANCER

Certain Death |_____| Being Cured

Punishment |_____| No Punishment

Painless |_____| Severe Constant Untreatable Pain

Abandoned |_____| Cared For

FIGURE **11–14.** Burns cancer beliefs scale.

Q SORT

The Q sort is a technique of comparative rating. It uses cards to categorize the importance placed on various words or phrases in relation to the other words or phrases in the list. Each phrase is placed on a separate card. The subject is instructed to place the cards in a designated number of piles, usually 7 to 10 piles. However, the subject is limited in the number of cards that may be placed in each pile. If the subject must sort 59 cards, category 1 may allow only 2 cards, category 2, 5 cards; category 3, 10 cards; category 4, 25 cards; category 5, 10 cards; category 6, 5 cards; category 7, 2 cards. Thus, the placing of the cards fits the patterns of a normal curve. The subject is usually advised to first select the cards that he or she wishes to place in the two extreme categories, then work toward the middle category, which contains the largest number of cards. Subjects are free to change the positions of cards until they are satisfied with the results. The Q sort method can also be used to determine the priority of or most important items to include in the development of a scale. In the previously mentioned example, the behaviors sorted into categories 5, 6 and 7 might be organized into a 17-item scale.

Wyers, Grove and Pastorino (1985) used the Q-sort technique to reduce 75 behaviors of the clinical nurse specialist (CNS) role to 40 essential behaviors. In a pilot study, these investigators identified 75 behaviors from the literature and from interviews with nursing administrators, nursing educators and CNSs. These 75 behaviors were sorted into 7 categories by 24 subjects (7 nursing administrators, 8 nursing educators and 9 CNSs) to identify 40 essential behaviors of the CNS role.

MAGNITUDE SCALING

One of the problems of concern in scaling procedures is the difficulty in obtaining fine discrimination of values. A recent effort to resolve this problem is magnitude scaling. This technique clearly provides interval-level data, and some researchers argue that it provides ratio-level data. It is particularly useful in scaling stimuli (Lodge, 1981). The scale is a line 100 mm in length. The extremes of the stimuli are placed at each end of the line. The subject is asked to place a mark through the line to indicate the intensity of the stimuli. A ruler is then used to measure the distance between the left end of the line and the mark placed by the subject. This measure is the value of the stimuli. The technique provides a way to use more complex statistical analyses on the data. An example of a magnitude scale is shown in Figure 11–15.

DELPHI TECHNIQUE

The Delphi technique is used to measure the judgments of a group of experts, assess priorities or make forecasts. It provides a means to obtain the opinion

FIGURE **11–15.** Magnitude scale.

No Pain _____ Extreme Pain

of a wide variety of experts across the country to provide feedback without the necessity of meeting together. Using the Delphi technique, the opinions of individuals cannot be altered by the persuasive behavior of a few people at a meeting.

To implement the technique, a panel of experts is identified. A questionnaire is developed that addresses the topics of concern. Although most responses are closed-ended questions, there are usually opportunities on the questionnaire for open-ended responses by the expert. The questionnaires are then returned to the researcher, and results are summarized. The outcome of the statistical analysis is returned to the panel of experts, along with a second questionnaire. Respondents with extreme responses to the first round of questions may be asked to justify their responses. The second round of questionnaires is returned to the researcher for analysis. This procedure is repeated until data reflect a consensus among the panel. A model of the Delphi technique was developed by Couper (1984) and is presented in Figure 11–16.

Lindeman (1975) conducted a Delphi survey to determine research priorities in clinical nursing research. She used a panel of 433 experts, both nurses and nonnurses with a wide range of interests. Four rounds of a 150-item questionnaire were sent to the panel. The report, published in *Nursing Research*, is frequently cited in discussing the directions for nursing research.

PROJECTIVE TECHNIQUES

Projective techniques are based on the assumption that the responses of individuals to unstructured or ambiguous situations reflect the attitudes, desires, personality characteristics and motives of the individual. The technique is most frequently used in psychology and includes such techniques as the Rorschach Inkblot Test, Machover's Draw-A-Person Test, word association, sentence completion, role-playing and play techniques. The technique is an indirect measure of data that is unlikely to be obtained directly. Analysis of the data requires that inferences be made as to the meaning and thus is subjective. Many of the tests require extensive training for administration and interpretation and thus have not been frequently used in nursing research. However, with the increased frequency of interdisciplinary research, their use in nursing studies may increase. At present, the technique is used in nursing primarily in studying children (Waltz, Strickland & Lenz, 1984).

DIARIES

A recent approach to obtaining information from subjects that must be collected over time is to ask the subjects to keep a record or diary of events. The data in this diary can then be collected and analyzed by researchers. A diary, which allows recording shortly after an event, is more accurate than obtaining the information through recall at an interview. A disadvantage is that keeping the diary may, in some cases, alter the behavior or events under study. For example, if a person were keeping a diary of the nursing care that he or she

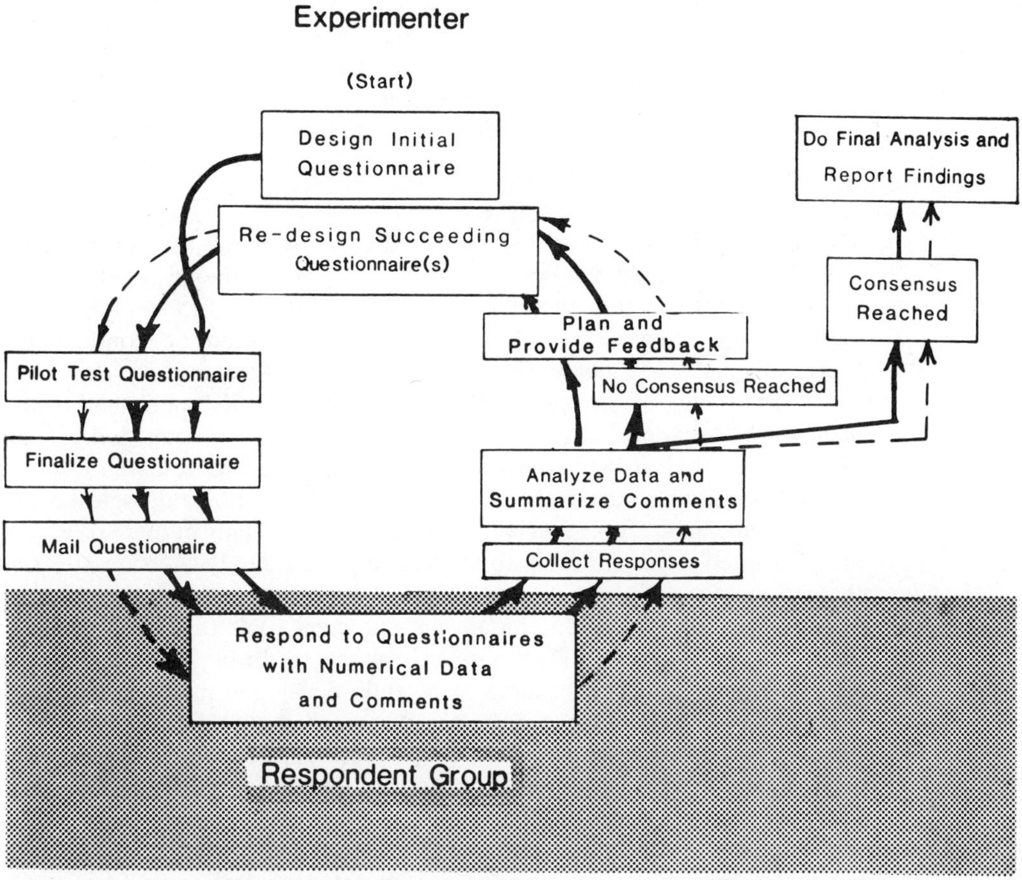

Experimenter

(Start)

FIGURE 11–16. Delphi technique sequence model. (From Couper, M. R.: The Delphi technique: Characteristics and sequence model. Advances in Nursing Science, 7(1):75, 1984. Copyright 1984. Reprinted with permission of Aspen Publishers, Inc.)

was providing to patients, that care might be changed based on the insights he or she gained from recording the information in the diary.

This technique provides a means to obtain data on topics of particular interest within nursing that have not been accessible by other means. Some potential topics for diary collection include expenses related to a health care event (particularly out-of-pocket expenses), self-care activities (frequency and time required), eating behaviors, exercise behaviors and care provided by family members in a home care situation.

Selection of an Existing Instrument

Selecting an instrument for measurement of the variables in a study is a critical process in research. The method of measurement must fit closely to the conceptual definition of the variable. The initial reaction of the beginning researcher is that no methods of measurement exist and a tool must be developed by the researcher. At the time, this seems to be the simplest solution, since the researcher has a clear idea of what needs to be measured. This solution, however, should not be used unless all else fails. The process of tool development is lengthy and requires considerable research sophistication.

Locating Existing Instruments

The first step should be an extensive search for existing measurement tools. The researcher should first determine measurement techniques used in previous related studies. If this search does not lead to satisfactory measurement methods, an extensive search of the literature should be conducted that specifically addresses measurement of the concept of interest.

There are many reference books that have compiled published measurement tools. An appendix is provided at the end of this chapter that lists many of the books that may be of interest in designing nursing research (Appendix 11–1). In addition, nurse researchers who specialize in methodological research are publishing many tools specific for nursing studies. Many of these publications are also listed in an attached appendix (Appendix 11–2). A computer search that specifically addresses measurement of the concept of interest can also be helpful. Dissertations often contain measurement tools that have never been published, so a review of Dissertation Abstracts might be helpful.

Another important source of recently developed measurement tools is word-of-mouth communication between researchers. Information on tools is often presented at research conferences years before publication. There are often networks of researchers working on similar topics. Thus, questioning available nurse researchers can lead to a previously unknown tool. These researchers are often easily contacted by telephone or letter and are usually willing to share their tools in return for access to the data to facilitate work on developing validity and reliability information.

Examining Existing Instruments

You must examine several instruments to find the one most appropriate for your study. The selection of an instrument for research requires careful consideration of how the instrument was developed, what the instrument measures and how to implement it. The following questions need to be addressed when examining an instrument.
1. Does this instrument measure what you want to measure?
2. Is the instrument reflective of the conceptual definition of the variable?
3. How does the population you are to administer the instrument to compare with the other populations that have been studied using this instrument?
4. What is the process for obtaining, administering and scoring the instrument?
5. How are the scores interpreted?

6. What is the time commitment for the subjects and researcher for administration of the instrument?
7. Does the instrument show evidence of reliability and validity testing?

Describing an Instrument in a Written Report

Information about the instrument must be included in the research proposal and final research report. When describing an instrument, you should identify the type of instrument, who developed the instrument, what information is measured by it and the population for whom it was designed. Other researchers who have used the instrument should be identified. The reliability and validity information should be reported from the initial testing of the instrument and from studies conducted by other researchers. A description of the administration and scoring of the instrument is necessary for critiquing the methodology of the study and for replication. Lamontagne, Mason and Hepworth (1985) studied the effects of relaxation on anxiety in children. They measured children's anxiety using the Gillis Child Anxiety scale. Their published study included the following description of the instrument:

The Gillis (1980) Child Anxiety Scale (CAS) is a 20-item instrument designed for children in kindergarten through fifth grade. Items are read aloud and subjects are asked to respond by circling the appropriate answers which are color-coded and presented in a picture-type format. In this study, items were recorded on an audiocassette tape provided by Gillis and administered by the teachers.

The instrument is scored by converting raw scores to stens and percentiles. Sten scores 4 through 7 indicate an average range of anxiety, whereas scores 8 through 10 reflect levels of anxiety higher than the norm and scores 1 through 3 lower than the norm.

Gillis and Cattell (1979) provided reliability data from a sample of first-, second-, and third-grade children. The reliability coefficient for the test-retest procedure was .85 for second-graders, and the overall coefficient for first through third grades was .81. Internal consistency was supported with a Kuder-Richardson 20 coefficient of .73. Using the CAS and the anxiety scale (IPAT) developed for children by Krug, Scheier, and Cattell (1976), construct validity was established at .81, $p < .01$, for one sample of 192 boys and girls, and .74, $p < .05$, for another 251 children. (p. 290)

Summary

Measurement is the process of assigning numbers to objects, events or situations in accord with some rule. The numbers assigned can indicate numerical values or categories. A component of measurement is instrumentation. Instrumentation is the application of specific rules to develop a measurement device or instrument. A variety of measurement strategies are necessary to examine the concrete and abstract concepts relevant to nursing.

Measurement theory and the rules within this theory have been developed to direct the measurement of abstract and concrete concepts. Measurement theory addresses the directness of measurement, measurement error, levels of measurement, reference of measurement, reliability and validity. There is direct and indirect measurement. The technology of health care has made direct measures of concrete elements such as height, weight, heart rate, temperature and blood pressure very familiar. Indirect measurement is used with abstract concepts, when the concepts are not measured directly, but when the indicators or attributes of the concepts are used to represent the abstraction. Measurement error is the difference between what exists in reality and what is measured by a research tool. Measurement exists in both direct and indirect measures and can be random or systematic. The levels of measurement from lower to higher are nominal, ordinal, interval and ratio. Referencing involves comparing a subject's score against a standard. There are two types of testing that involve referencing: norm-referenced testing and criterion-referenced testing.

Reliability in measurement is concerned with how consistently the measurement technique measures the concept of interest. Reliability testing is considered a measure of the amount of random error in the measurement technique. Reliability testing focuses on three aspects of reliability: stability, equivalence and homogeneity. The validity of an instrument is a determination of the extent to which the instrument actually reflects the abstract construct being examined. Validity, as reliability, is not an all-or-nothing phenomenon but rather a matter of degree. No instrument is completely valid. There are three primary types of validity: content validity, predictive validity and construct validity. Content validity verifies that the method of measurement actually measures the expected content. Predictive validity determines the effectiveness of the instrument as a predictor of a future event. Construct validity is the degree to which a measurement strategy measures the construct that it was designed to measure. Developing construct validity for an instrument is a process that requires many years of work by a number of scientists. The steps include concept analysis, factorial validity, contrasted groups approach, convergent validity, divergent validity, discriminant validity, nomological network validity and successive verification. Examining validity in qualitative research is also complex; 12 strategies for examining this validity were described.

Common measurement approaches that are used in nursing research include physiologic measures, observations, interviews, content analyses, questionnaires and scales. Other methods of measurement discussed include the Q sort, magnitude scaling, Delphi technique, projective techniques and diaries. These approaches were described and examples of each were given. The chapter concludes with a discussion of how to select a measurement strategy for studying a variable and how to describe this measurement technique in the research proposal or report.

Appendix 11-1: Sources of Instruments for Nursing Research

Anastasi, A. (1982). *Psychological testing* (5th Ed.). New York: Macmillan Publishing Co., Inc.

Andrulis, R. (1977). *A source book of tests and measures of human behavior*. Springfield, Illinois: Charles C. Thomas, Publisher.

Bauer, J. D. & Ackerman, P. G. (1982). *Clinical laboratory methods* (9th Ed.). St. Louis: The C. V. Mosby Company.

Beere, C. A. (1979). *Women and women's issues: a handbook of tests and measurements*. San Francisco: Jossey-Bass Publishing Co.

Bonjean, C. M., Hill, R. J. & McLemore, S. D. (1967). *Sociological measurement: an inventory of scales and indices*. San Francisco: Chandler Publishing Co.

Buros, O. K. (1970). *Personality tests and reviews*. Lincoln: University of Nebraska Press.

Buros, O. K. (1974). *Tests in print II*. Lincoln: University of Nebraska Press.

Buros, O. K. (1978). *The eighth mental measurements yearbook*. Lincoln: University of Nebraska Press.

Cattell, R. B. (1967). *Objective personality and motivation tests: a theoretical introduction and practical compendium*. Urbana: University of Illinois Press.

Chun, K-T, Cobb, S. & French, J. R. Jr. (1975). *Measurement for psychological assessment: a guide to 3000 original sources and their applications*. Ann Arbor, Michigan: Institute for Social Research, University of Michigan.

Ciminero, A. R., Calhoun, K. S. & Adams, J. E. (1977). *Handbook of behavioral assessment*. New York: John Wiley & Sons.

Comrey, A. L., Backer, T. E. & Glaser, E. M. (1973). *A sourcebook for mental health measures*. Los Angeles: Human Interaction Research Institute.

Cromwell, L., Weibell, F. J. & Pfeiffer, E. A. (1980). *Biomedical instrumentation and measurements* (2nd Ed.). Englewood Cliffs, New Jersey: Prentice-Hall, Inc.

Ferris, C. (1980). *A guide to medical laboratory instruments*. Boston: Little, Brown and Company.

Geddes, L. A. & Baker, L. E. (1975). *Principles of applied biomedical instrumentation* (2nd Ed.). Philadelphia: Chilton Book Co.

Goldman, B. A. & Busch, J. C. (1982). *Directory of unpublished experimental mental measures* (Vol. 3). New York: Human Sciences Press.

Haynes, S. N. (1978). *Principles of behavior assessment*. New York: Halstead Press.

Haynes, S. N. & Wilson, C. C. (1979). *Behavioral assessment*. San Francisco: Jossey-Bass.

Johnson, O. G. (1971, 1976). *Tests and measurements in child development: handbook I and handbook II* (Vols. 1 and 2). San Francisco: Jossey-Bass Publishing Co.

Lake, D. G., Miles, M. B. & Earle, R. B. Jr. (1973). *Measuring human behavior: tools for the assessment of social functioning*. New York: Teachers' College Press, Columbia University.

Lyerly, S. B. (1981). *Handbook of psychiatric rating scales* (2nd Ed.). New York: Research and Education Association.

Miller, D. C. (1983). *Handbook of research design and social measurement* (4th Ed.). New York: Longman.

Mitchell, J. V. Jr. (Ed.) (1983). *Tests in print III*. Lincoln: University of Nebraska Press.

Pfeiffer, J. W., Heslen, R. & Jones, J. E. (1976). *Instrumentation in human relations training* (2nd Ed.). La Jolla, California: University Associates, Inc.

Price, J. L. & Mueller, C. W. (1985). *Handbook of organizational measurement*. Massachusetts: Pitman Publishing Co.

Reeder, L. G., Ramacher, L. & Gorelnik, S. (1976). *Handbook of scales and indices of health behavior*. Pacific Palisades, California: Goodyear Publishing Co.

Robinson, J. P. et al. (1969). *Measurement of occupational attitudes and occupational characteristics*. Ann Arbor, Michigan: Survey Research Center Institute for Social Research.

Robinson, J. P. & Shaver, P. R. (1973). *Measures of social psychological attitudes* (revised edition). Ann Arbor, Michigan: Survey Research Center Institute for Social Research.

Shaw, M. E. & Wright, J. M. (1967). *Scales for the measurement of attitudes*. New York: McGraw-Hill Book Company.

Straus, M. A. & Brown, B. W. (1978). *Family measurements techniques: abstracts of published instruments (1935–1974)* (revised edition). Minneapolis: University of Minnesota Press.

Sweetland, R. C. & Keyser, D. J. (1983). *Tests: a comprehensive reference for assessments in psychology, education and business*. Kansas City, Mo.: Test Corporation of America.

Walker, D. K. (1973). *Socioemotional measures for preschool and kindergarten children*. San Francisco: Jossey-Bass Publishing Co.

Ward, M. J. & Fetler, M. E. (1979). *Instruments for use in nursing education research*. Boulder, Colorado: Western Interstate Commission for Higher Education.

Ward, M. J. & Lindeman, C. (1979). *Instruments for measuring nursing practice and other health care variables*. DHEW Publication No. HRA 78-53 (Vol. 1) and HRA 78-54 (Vol. 2). Hyattsville, Maryland.: U.S. Government Printing Office.

Weiss, M. (1973). *Biomedical instrumentation*. Philadelphia: Chilton Book Co.

Appendix 11–2: Publications From Recent Methodological Research in Nursing

Andersen, M. (1980). A psychosocial screening tool for ambulatory health care clients: a pilot study of validity. *Nursing Research*, 29(6), 347–351.

Atwood, J. R. & Gill-Rogers, B. P. (1984). Metatheory, methodology, and practicality: issues in research uses of Rogers's science of unitary man. *Nursing Research*, 33(2), 88–91.

Baker, C. M. (1985). Maximizing mailed questionnaire responses. *Image: The Journal of Nursing Scholarship*, 17(4), 118–121.

Ballard, S. & McNamara, R. (1983). Quantifying nursing needs in home health care. *Nursing Research*, 32(4), 236–241.

Benner, P. (1985). Quality of life: a phenomenological perspective on explanation, prediction, and understanding in nursing science. *Advances in Nursing Science*, 8(1), 1–14.

Blank, D. M. (1985). Development of the infant tenderness scale. *Nursing Research*, 34(4), 211–216.

Bowles, C. (1986). Measure of attitude toward menopause using the semantic differential model. *Nursing Research*, 35(2), 81–85.

Brandt, P. A. & Weinert, C. (1981). The PRQ—a social support system. *Nursing Research*, 30(5), 277–280.

Brink, P. J. (1984). Value orientations as an assessment tool in cultural diversity. *Nursing Research*, 33(4), 198–203.

Cox, C. L. (1985). The Health self-determinism index. *Nursing Research*, 34(3), 177–183.

Craig, H. M. (1985). Accuracy of indirect measures of medication compliance in hypertension. *Research in Nursing and Health*, 8(1), 61–66.

Cranley, M. S. (1981). Development of a tool for the measurement of maternal attachment during pregnancy. *Nursing Research*, 30(5), 281–284.

Crisham, P. (1981). Measuring moral judgment in nursing dilemmas. *Nursing Research*, 30(2), 104–110.

Dagenais, F. & Meleis, A. I. (1982). Professionalism, work ethic, and empathy in nursing: the nurse self-descriptive form. *Western Journal of Nursing Research*, 4(4), 407–422.

Dawson, C., Schirmer, M. & Beck, L. (1984). A patient self-disclosure instrument. *Research in Nursing and Health*, 7(2), 135–147.

Dennis, K. E. (1986). Q methodology: relevance and application to nursing research. *Advances in Nursing Science*, 8(3), 6–17.

Derdiarian, A. K. (1983). An instrument for theory and research development using the behavioral systems model for nursing: the cancer patient (part 1). *Nursing Research*, 32(4), 196–201.

Derdiarian, A. K. & Forsythe, A. B. (1983). An instrument for theory and research development using the behavioral systems model for nursing: the cancer patient (part II). *Nursing Research*, 32(5), 260–266.

Doerr, B. T. & Hutchins, E. B. (1981). Health risk appraisal: process, problems, and prospects for nursing practice and research. *Nursing Research*, 30(5), 299–306.

Duxbury, M. L., Henly, G. A. & Armstrong, G. D. (1982). Measurement of the nurse organizational climate of neonatal intensive care units. *Nursing Research*, 31(2), 83–88.

Ellison, E. S. (1985). A multidimensional, dual-perspective index of parental support. *Western Journal of Nursing Research*, 7(4), 401–424.

Fawcett, J. & Frye, S. (1980). An exploratory study of body image dimensionality. *Nursing Research*, 29(5), 324–327.

Felton, G., Reed, P. & Perla, S. (1981). Measurement of nursing students' and nurses' attitudes toward cancer. *Western Journal of Nursing Research*, 3(1), 62–75.

Ferrans, C. E. & Powers, M. J. (1985). Quality of life index: development and psychometric properties. *Advances in Nursing Science*, 8(1), 15–24.

Fleming, J. (1981). An evaluation of the use of the Denver developmental screening test. *Nursing Research*, 30(5), 290–293.

Fox, R. N. & Ventura, M. R. (1984). Internal psychometric characteristics of the quality patient care scale. *Nursing Research*, 33(2), 112–117.

Geden, E., Beck, N., Brouder, G. & O'Connell, E. (1983). Identifying procedural components for analogue research of labor pain. *Nursing Research*, 32(2), 80–83.

Goetz, A. A. & McTyre, R. B. (1981). Health risk appraisal: some methodologic considerations. *Nursing Research*, 30(5), 307–313.

Goldsmith, J. W. (1981). Methodological considerations in using videotape to establish rater reliability. *Nursing Research*, 30(2), 124–127.

Goodwin, L. D. & Prescott, P. A. (1981). Issues and approaches to estimating interrater reliability in nursing research. *Research in Nursing and Health*, 4(3), 323–337.

Goodwin, L., Prescott, P., Jacox, A. & Collar, M. (1981). The nurse practitioner rating form Part II: methodological development. *Nursing Research*, 30(5), 270–276.

Gortner, S. R., Hudes, M. & Zyzanski, S. J. (1984). Appraisal of values in the choice of treatment. *Nursing Research*, 33(6), 319–324.

Hageman, P. T. & Ventura, M. R. (1981). Utilizing patient outcome criteria to measure the effects of a medication teaching regimen. *Western Journal of Nursing Research*, 3(1), 25–36.

Haussmann, R. K. D., Hegyvery, S. T. & Newman, J. F. (1976). *Monitoring quality of nursing care, part II—assessment and study of correlates*. Department of Health, Education, and Welfare (DHEW) Publication No. HRA 76-7, Washington, D.C.: U.S. Government Printing Office.

Hilbert, G. A. (1985). Accuracy of self-reported measures of compliance. *Nursing Research*, 34(5), 319–320.

Hinshaw, A. S. & Atwood, J. R. (1982). A patient satisfaction instrument: precision by replication. *Nursing Research*, 31(3), 170–175.

Holm, K. & Kavanagh, J. (1985). An approach to modifying self-report instruments. *Research in Nursing and Health*, 8(1), 13–18.

Holzemer, W. L., Schleutermann, J. A., Farrand, L. L. & Miller, A. G. (1981). A validation study: simulations as a measure of nurse practitioners' problem-solving skills. *Nursing Research*, 30(3), 139–144.

Hoskins, C. N. (1983). Psychometrics in nursing research—further development of the interpersonal conflict scale. *Research in Nursing and Health*, 6(2), 75–83.

Hoskins, L. M., McFarlane, E. A., Rubenfeld, M. G., Walsh, M. B. & Schreier, A. M. (1986). Nursing diagnosis in the chronically ill: methodology for clinical validation. *Advances in Nursing Science*, 8(3), 80–89.

Hyman, R. B. & Woog, P. (1982). Stressful life events and illness onset: a review of crucial variables. *Research in Nursing and Health*, 5(3), 155–163.

Hymovich, D. P. (1981). Assessing the impact of chronic childhood illness on the family and parent coping. *Image*, 13(3), 71–74.

Hymovich, D. P. (1983). The chronicity impact and coping instrument: parent questionnaire. *Nursing Research*, 32(5), 275–281.

Hymovich, D. P. (1984). Development of the chronicity impact and coping instrument: parent questionnaire (CICI:PQ). *Nursing Research*, 33(4), 218–222.

Jacox, A. K., Prescott, P. A., Collar, M. K. & Goodwin, L. D. (1981). *The nurse practitioner rating form: a primary care process measure*. Wakefield, Mass.: Nursing Resources.

Jalowiec, A., Murphy, S. P. & Powers, M. J. (1984). Psychometric assessment of the Jalowiec coping scale. *Nursing Research*, 33(3), 157–161.

Jordan-Marsh, M. (1985). Development of a tool for diagnosing changes in concern about exercise: a means of enhancing compliance. *Nursing Research*, 34(2), 103–107.

Kerr, J. A. C. (1982). An overview of theory and research related to space use in hospitals. *Western Journal of Nursing Research*, 4(4), 395–405.

Laffrey, S. C. (1986). Development of a health conception scale. *Research in Nursing and Health*, 9(2), 107–113.

LaMonica, E. L. (1981). Construct validity of an empathy instrument. *Research in Nursing and Health*, 4(4), 389–400.

LaMonica, E. L., Oberst, M. T., Madea, A. R. & Wolf, R. M. (1986). Development of a patient satisfaction scale. *Research in Nursing and Health*, 9(1), 43–50.

Lasky, P., Buckwalter, K. C., Whall, A., Lederman, R., Speer, J., McLane, A., King, J. M. & White, M. A. (1985). Developing an instrument for the assessment of family dynamics. *Western Journal of Nursing Research*, 7(1), 40–57.

Leatt, P., Bay, K. S. & Stinson, S. M. (1981). An instrument for assessing and classifying patients by type of care. *Nursing Research*, 30(3), 145–150.

Lewis, F. M., Firsich, S. C. & Parsell, S. (1979). Clinical tool development for adult chemotherapy patients: process and content. *Cancer Nursing*, 2(2), 99–108.

Lowery, B. J. (1981). Misconceptions and limitations of locus of control and the I-E Scale. *Nursing Research*, 30(5), 294–298.

McCorkle, R. & Young, K. (1978). Development of a symptom distress scale. *Cancer Nursing*, 1(5), 373–378.

McGuire, D. B. (1984). The measurement of clinical pain. *Nursing Research*, 33(3), 152–156.

McLaughlin, F. E., Carr, J. W. & Delucchi, K. L. (1981). Measurement properties of clinical simulation tests: hypertension and chronic obstructive pulmonary disease. *Nursing Research*, 30(1), 5–9.

Majesky, S. J., Brester, M. H. & Nishio, K. T. (1978). Development of a research tool: patient indicators of nursing care. *Nursing Research*, 27(6), 365–371.

Miller, P., Wikoff, R., McMahon, M., Garrett, M. J. & Johnson, N. (1982). Development of a health attitude scale. *Nursing Research*, 31(3), 132–136.

Miller, T. W. (1981). Life events scaling: clinical methodological issues. *Nursing Research*, 30(5), 316–320A.

Minckley, B. B., Burrows, D., Ehrat, K., Harper, L., Jenkin, S. A., Minckley, W. F., Page, B., Schramm, D. E. & Wood, C. (1979). Myocardial infarct stress-of-transfer inventory: development of a research tool. *Nursing Research*, 28(1), 4–10.

Mishel, M. H. (1981). The measurement of uncertainty in illness. *Nursing Research*, 30(5), 258–263.

Mishel, M. H. (1983). Adjusting the fit: development of uncertainty scales for specific clinical populations. *Western Journal of Nursing Research*, 5(4), 355–370.

Mishel, M. H. (1983). Parents' perception of uncertainty concerning their hospitalized child. *Nursing Research*, 32(6), 324–330.

Mitchell, E. S. (1986). Multiple triangulation: a methodology for nursing science. *Advances in Nursing Science*, 8(3), 18–26.

Morgan, B. S. (1984). A semantic differential measure of attitudes toward black American patients. *Research in Nursing and Health*, 7(3), 155–162.

Munhall, P. L. (1986). Methodological issues in nursing research: beyond a wax apple. *Advances in Nursing Science*, 8(3), 1–5.

Murawski, B. J., Penman, D. & Schmitt, M. (1978). Social support in health and illness: the concept and its measurement. *Cancer Nursing*, 1(5), 365–371.

Murphy, S. P., Powers, M. J. & Jalowiec, A. (1985). Psychometric evaluation of the hemodialysis stressor scale. *Nursing Research*, 34(6), 368–371.

Norbeck, J. S. (1985). What constitutes a publishable report of instrument development? *Nursing Research*, 34(6), 380–382.

Norbeck, J. S., Lindsey, A. M. & Carrieri, V. L. (1981). The development of an instrument to measure social support. *Nursing Research*, 30(5), 264–269.

Norbeck, J. S., Lindsey, A. M. & Carrieri, V. L. (1983). Further development of the Norbeck social support questionnaire: normative data and validity testing. *Nursing Research*, 32(1), 4–9.

Olade, R. A. (1984). Evaluation of the Denver developmental screening test as applied to African children. *Nursing Research*, 33(4), 204–207.

Padilla, G. V. & Grant, M. M. (1985). Quality of life as a cancer nursing outcome variable. *Advances in Nursing Science*, 8(1), 45–60.

Palisin, J. (1981). The neonatal perception inventory: a review. *Nursing Research*, 30(5), 285–289.

Phaneuf, M. C. (1976). *The nursing audit: self-regulation of nursing practice*. Norwalk, Connecticut: Appleton-Century-Crofts.

Prescott, P. A., Jacox, A. K., Collar, M. & Goodwin, L. (1981). The nurse practitioner rating form part I: conceptual development and potential uses. *Nursing Research*, 30(4), 223–228.

Pridham, K. F. & Chang, A. S. (1985). Parents' beliefs about themselves as parents of a new infant: instrument development. *Research in Nursing and Health*, 8(1), 19–29.

Rhodes, V. A., Watson, P. M. & Johnson, M. H. (1984). Development of reliable and valid measures of nausea and vomiting. *Cancer Nursing*, 7(1), 33–41.

Roberts, C. S. & Feetham, S. L. (1982). Assessing family functioning across three areas of relationships. *Nursing Research*, 31(4), 231–235.

Rock, D. L., Green, K. E., Wise, B. K. & Rock, R. D. (1984). Social support and social network scales: a psychometric review. *Research in Nursing and Health*, 7(4), 325–332.

Ruffing-Rahal, M. A. (1986). Personal documents and nursing theory development. *Advances in Nursing Science*, 8(3), 50–57.

Sanders, S. A. (1986). Development of a tool to measure subjective time experience. *Nursing Research*, 35(3), 178–182.

Schwirian, P. M. (1978). Evaluating the performance of nurses: a multidimensional approach. *Nursing Research*, 27(6), 347–351.

Sexton, D. L. (1983). Some methodological issues in chronic illness research. *Nursing Research*, 32(6), 378–380.

Smyth, K., Sparacino, J., Hansell, S. & Call, J. (1980). Engagement-involvement and blood pressure change: a methodological inquiry. *Nursing Research*, 29(5), 270–275.

Stevenson, J. S. (1982). Construction of a scale to measure load, power, and margin in life. *Nursing Research*, 31(4), 222–225.

Stricklin, M. L. V. (1979). Mental health patient assessment record: interobserver reliability. *Nursing Research*, 28(1), 11–15.

Tilden, V. P. (1985). Issues of conceptualization and measurement of social support in the construction of nursing theory. *Research in Nursing and Health*, 8(2), 199–206.

Topf, M. (1986). Methodology corner: response sets in questionnaire research. *Nursing Research*, 35(2), 119–121.

Ulin, P. R. (1981). Measuring adjustment in chronically ill clients in community mental health care. *Nursing Research*, 30(4), 229–235.

Uphold, C. R. & Harper, D. C. (1986). Methodological issues in intergenerational family nursing research. *Advances in Nursing Science*, 8(3), 38–49.

Ventura, M. R., Fox, R. N., Corley, M. C. & Mercurio, S. M. (1982). A patient satisfaction measure as a criterion to evaluate primary nursing. *Nursing Research*, 31(4), 226–230.

Ventura, M. R., Young, D. E., Feldman, M. J., Pastore, P., Pikula, S. & Yates, M. A. (1985). Cost savings as an indicator of successful nursing intervention. *Nursing Research*, 34(1), 50–53.

Wandelt, M. A. & Ager, J. (1975). *Quality patient care scale*. Norwalk, Connecticut: Appleton-Century-Crofts.

Wandelt, M. A. & Stewart, D. S. (1975). *Slater nursing competencies rating scale*. Norwalk, Connecticut: Appleton-Century-Crofts.

Weiss, S. J. & Davis, H. P. (1985). Validity and reliability of the collaborative practice scales. *Nursing Research*, 34(5), 299–305.

Williams, P. D. (1984). The metro-Manilla developmental screening test: a normative study. *Nursing Research*, 33(4), 208–212.

Woods, N. F. (1981). The health diary as an instrument for nursing research: problems and promise. *Western Journal of Nursing Research*, 3(1), 76–92.

Worth, A. M., Dougherty, M. C. & McKey, P. L. (1986). Development and testing of the circumvaginal muscles rating scale. *Nursing Research*, 35(3), 166–168.

References

Baker, C. M. (1985). Maximizing mailed questionnaire responses. *Image: The Journal of Nursing Scholarship*, 17(4), 118–121.

Baun, M. M. (1984). Physiological determinants of a clinically successful method of endotracheal suction. *Western Journal of Nursing Research*, 6(2), 213–228.

Beck, A., Weissman, A., Lester, D. & Trexler, L. (1974). The measurement of pessimism; the hopelessness scale. *Journal of Consulting and Clinical Psychology*, 42(6), 861–865.

Blalock, H. M. Jr. (1982). *Conceptualization and measurement in the social sciences*. Beverly Hills: Sage Publications.

Brinberg, D. & McGrath, J. E. (1985). *Validity and the research process*. Beverly Hills: Sage Publications.

Burns, N. (1974). *Nurse-patient communication with the advanced cancer patient*. Unpublished master's thesis, Texas Woman's University, Dallas, Texas.

Burns, N. (1981). *Evaluation of a supportive-expressive group for families of cancer patients*. Unpublished doctoral dissertation, Texas Woman's University, Denton, Texas.

Burns, N. (1983). Development of the Burns cancer beliefs scale. *Proceedings of the American Cancer Society Third West Coast Cancer Nursing Research Conference*, 308–329.

Burns, N. (1986). Research in progress. American Cancer Society, Texas Division.

Burns, N. & Carney, K. (1985). The caring aspect of hospice: a study. In L. F. Paradis (Ed.), *Hospice handbook: a guide for managers and planners* (pp. 249–279). Rockville, Maryland: Aspen Systems Corporation.

Campbell, D. T. & Fiske, D. W. (1959). Convergent and discriminant validation by the multitrait-multimethod matrix. *Psychological Bulletin*, 56(2), 81–105.

Carmines, E. G. & Zeller, R. A. (1979). *Reliability and validity assessment.* Beverly Hills: Sage Publications.

Censullo, M., Lester, B. & Hoffman, J. (1985). Rhythmic patterning in mother–newborn interaction. *Nursing Research,* 34(6), 342–346.

Couper, M. R. (1984). The Delphi technique: characteristics and sequence model. *Advances in Nursing Science,* 7(1), 72–77.

Cronbach, L. J. & Meehl, P. E. (1955). Construct validity in psychological tests. *Psychological Bulletin,* 52(4), 281–302.

Ebener, M. K. (1985). Reliability and validity basics for evaluating classification systems. *Nursing Economics,* 3(6), 324–327.

Fox, R. N. & Ventura, M. R. (1983). Small-scale administration of instruments and procedures. *Nursing Research,* 32(2), 122–125.

Gloeckner, M. R. (1984). Perceptions of sexual attractiveness following ostomy surgery. *Research in Nursing and Health,* 7(2), 87–92.

Hilton, B. A. (1985). Noise in acute patient care areas. *Research in Nursing and Health,* 8(3), 283–291.

Kaplan, A. (1963). *The conduct of inquiry: methodology for behavioral science.* New York: Harper and Row Publishers. Inc.

Kerr, J. A. C. (1985). Space use, privacy, and territoriality. *Western Journal of Nursing Research,* 7(2), 199–219.

Kirk, J. & Miller, M. L. (1986). *Reliability and validity in qualitative research.* Beverly Hills: Sage Publications.

Knapp, T. R. (1985). Validity, reliability, and neither. *Nursing Research,* 34(3), 189–192.

Kruskal, J. B. & Wish, M. (1978). *Multidimensional scaling.* Beverly Hills: Sage Publications.

Lamontagne, L. L., Mason, K. R. & Hepworth, J. T. (1985). Effects of relaxation on anxiety in children: implications for coping with stress. *Nursing Research,* 34(5), 289–292.

Lindeman, C. A. (1975). Delphi survey of priorities in clinical nursing research. *Nursing Research,* 24(6), 434–441.

Lindsey, A. M. (1982). Phenomena and physiological variables of relevance to nursing, review of a decade of work: part I. *Western Journal of Nursing Research,* 4(4), 343–364.

Lindsey, A. M. (1983). Phenomena and physiological variables of relevance to nursing, review of a decade of work: part II. *Western Journal of Nursing Research,* 5(1), 41–63.

Lindsey, A. M. (1984). Research for clinical practice: physiological phenomena... research priorities for critical care nursing. *Heart and Lung,* 13(5), 496–507.

Lodge, M. (1981). *Magnitude scaling: quantitative measurement of opinions.* Beverly Hills: Sage Publications.

Lynn, M. R. (1985). Reliability estimates: use and disuse. *Nursing Research,* 34(4), 254–256.

McIver, J. P. & Carmines, E. G. (1981). *Unidimensional scaling.* Beverly Hills: Sage Publications.

Miles, M. B. & Huberman, A. M. (1984). *Qualitative data analysis: a sourcebook of new methods.* Beverly Hills: Sage Publications.

Miller, T. W. (1981). Life events scaling: clinical methodological issues. *Nursing Research,* 30(5), 316–320A.

Nunnally, J. C. (1978). *Psychometric theory* (2nd ed.). New York: McGraw-Hill Book Company.

Parsons, L. C. & Wilson, M. M. (1984). Cerebrovascular status of severe closed head–injured patients following passive position changes. *Nursing Research,* 33(2), 68–75.

Powers, M. J., Murphy, S. P. & Wooldridge, P. J. (1983). Validation of two experimental nursing approaches using content analysis. *Research in Nursing and Health,* 6(1), 3–9.

Osgood, C. E., Suci, G. J. & Tannenbaum, P. H. (1957). *The measurement of meaning.* Urbana: University of Illinois Press.

Romancyzk, R. G. et al. (1973). Measuring the reliability of observation data: a reactive process. *Journal of Applied Behavioral Analysis,* 6, 175.

Selltiz C., Wrightsman, L. S. & Cook, S. W. (1976). *Research methods in social relations* (3rd Ed.). New York: Holt, Rinehart and Winston.

Shelley, S. I. (1984). *Research methods in nursing and health.* Boston: Little, Brown and Company.

Sullivan, J. L. & Feldman, S. (1979). *Multiple indicators: an introduction.* Beverly Hills: Sage Publications.

Walker, L. O. & Avant, K. C. (1983). *Strategies for theory construction in nursing.* Norwalk, Connecticut: Appleton-Century-Crofts.

Waltz, C. F., Strickland, O. L. & Lenz, E. R. (1984). *Measurement in nursing research.* Philadelphia: F. A. Davis Company.

Ward, M. J. & Lindeman, C. (1979). *Instruments for measuring nursing practice and other health care variables.* DHEW Publication No. HRA 78–53 (Vol. 1) and HRA 78–54 (Vol. 2). Hyattsville, Maryland: U. S. Government Printing Office.

Wyers, M. E., Grove, S. K. & Pastorino, C. (1985). Clinical nurse specialist: in search of the right role. *Nursing Outlook,* 6(4), 202–207.

12

Conducting Research Ethically

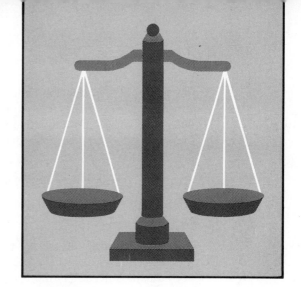

Nursing research must not only have the potential to generate and refine knowledge but also must be ethical in its development and implementation. Since the knowledge essential to the discipline of nursing requires studying human subjects, the protection of human subjects' rights will be an ethical consideration in many nursing studies. The ethical implications of using human subjects in research have been examined with increasing frequency during the last 40 years, primarily because of the Nazi medical experiments of World War II. Since the rights of human research subjects have not been protected by certain investigators, ethical codes and regulations have been developed to promote ethical conduct in research.

What does conducting research ethically involve? This is a question that has been debated without resolution for many years by researchers, politicians, philosophers, lawyers and even research subjects. The debate about ethics and research continues, probably because of the complexity of human rights issues, the abstractness of the ethical codes and regulations governing research and the variety of interpretations of these codes and regulations.

Even though the phenomenon of conducting research ethically defies clear delineation, there are certain ethical actions that investigators should take in conducting research. These actions include (1) protecting the human rights

335

of subjects, (2) balancing benefits and risks of a study, (3) securing informed consent and (4) submitting the research proposal for institutional review. This chapter focuses on the ethical codes and regulations and the actions of researchers that promote conducting research ethically.

Historical Events Affecting the Development of Ethical Codes and Regulations

Since the 1940s, the ethical conduct of researchers has received increasing attention because of the mistreatment of human research subjects. Three experimental projects have been highly publicized for their unethical treatment of human subjects: (1) the Nazi medical experiments, (2) the Jewish Chronic Disease Hospital Study and (3) the Tuskegee Syphilis Study. Although nurse researchers are unlikely to be involved in atrocities as extreme as these, knowledge of these unethical projects can serve as examples that can provide a basis for examining nursing studies. Some of the human rights violated in these studies could be violated in a subtle way in nursing studies. In addition, these experiments influenced the formulation of ethical codes and regulations that nurse researchers must follow in conducting research.

NAZI MEDICAL EXPERIMENTS

From 1933 to 1945, some of the most serious, unethical activities were conducted by the Third Reich in Europe. The programs of the Nazi regime included sterilization, euthanasia and numerous medical experiments. These programs were developed to produce a population of racially pure Germans or "Aryans" that were destined to rule the world. The Nazis encouraged population growth in the "Aryans" (good Nazis) and sterilized those regarded as racial enemies such as the Jews. They also practiced what they called "euthanasia", which involved killing various groups of people who were racially impure such as the insane, deformed or senile. In addition, numerous medical experiments were conducted on prisoners of war and racially "valueless" persons, such as the Jews, who had been confined to the concentration camps. The experiments involved exposing subjects to high altitudes, freezing temperatures, malaria, poisons, spotted fever (typhus) and untested drugs (Institute of Society, Ethics and the Life Sciences, 1976). These medical experiments were conducted not only to generate knowledge about humanity but also to destroy certain groups of people.

These studies violated numerous rights of human research subjects. The selection of subjects for these studies was unfair, because it was racially based. The subjects had no opportunity to refuse participation in these studies; they were prisoners who were coerced or forced to participate. As a result of these experiments, the subjects were frequently killed or sustained permanent physical, mental and social damage. These experiments were not conducted by a few isolated scientists and doctors; they were: "the product of coordinated policy-making and planning at high governmental, military, and Nazi Party levels, conducted as an integral part of the total war effort" (The Nuremberg Code, 1949, p. 285).

NUREMBERG CODE

Those involved in the Nazi experiments were brought to trial before the Nuremberg Tribunals, which made public their unethical research activities. The mistreatment of human subjects in these experiments led to the development of the Nuremberg Code in 1949. This ethical code of conduct contains rules, some general, others specific, that were developed to direct investigators in conducting research ethically. The code includes guidelines for voluntary consent; withdrawal of subjects from studies; protection of subjects from physical and mental suffering, injury, disability and/or death; and the balance of benefits and risks in a study (Table 12–1). This code was formulated mainly to direct the conduct of biomedical research; however, the rules in this code are essential to the conduct of research in other behavioral sciences, such as sociology, psychology and nursing.

DECLARATION OF HELSINKI

The Nuremberg Code provided the basis for the development of the Declaration of Helsinki, which was adopted in 1964 and revised in 1975 by the World

---

TABLE 12–1
The Nuremberg Code

1. The voluntary consent of the human subject is absolutely essential . . .
2. The experiment should be such as to yield fruitful results for the good of society, unprocurable by other methods or means of study, and not random and unnecessary in nature.
3. The experiment should be so designed and based on the results of animal experimentation and a knowledge of the natural history of the disease or other problem under study that the anticipated results will justify the performance of the experiment.
4. The experiment should be so conducted as to avoid all unnecessary physical and mental suffering and injury.
5. No experiment should be conducted where there is an *a priori* reason to believe that death or disabling injury will occur, except, perhaps, in those experiments where the experimental physicians also serve as subjects.
6. The degree of risk to be taken should never exceed that determined by the humanitarian importance of the problem to be solved by the experiment.
7. Proper preparations should be made and adequate facilities provided to protect the experimental subject against even remote possibilities of injury, disability, or death.
8. The experiment should be conducted only by scientifically qualified persons. The highest degree of skill and care should be required through all stages of the experiment of those who conduct or engage in the experiment.
9. During the course of the experiment the human subject should be at liberty to bring the experiment to an end if he has reached the physical or mental state where continuation of the experiment seems to him to be impossible.
10. During the course of the experiment the scientist in charge must be prepared to terminate the experiment at any stage, if he has probable cause to believe, in the exercise of the good faith, superior skill and careful judgment required of him that a continuation of the experiment is likely to result in injury, disability, or death to the experimental subject. . . .

(From The Nuremberg Code, 1949, pp. 285–286).

Medical Assembly. The Declaration of Helsinki differentiated therapeutic research from nontherapeutic research (Levine, 1979). Therapeutic research provides the patient an opportunity to receive an experimental treatment that might have beneficial results. Nontherapeutic research is conducted to generate knowledge for a discipline, and the results from the study might benefit future patients but will probably not benefit those acting as research subjects (Purtilo & Cassel, 1981). The type of research, therapeutic or nontherapeutic, is significant in explaining potential benefits and risks to prospective research subjects. The Declaration of Helsinki was adopted by most institutions that conduct clinical research; however, neither this document nor the Nuremberg Code has prevented some investigators from conducting unethical experiments.

JEWISH CHRONIC DISEASE HOSPITAL STUDY

Another highly publicized case of unethical experimentation was a study conducted at the Jewish Chronic Disease Hospital in the 1960s. The purpose of this study was to determine the patients' rejection responses to live cancer cells. Twenty-two patients were injected with a suspension containing live cancer cells that had been generated from human cancer tissue (Hershey & Miller, 1976).

The rights of these patients were not protected, because they were not informed that they were taking part in research and that the injections they received were live cancer cells. In addition, the study was never presented to the research committee of the Jewish Chronic Disease Hospital for review, and the physicians caring for the patients were unaware that the study was being conducted. The physician directing the research was an employee of the Sloan-Kettering Institute for Cancer Research, and there was no indication that this institution had conducted a review of the research project (Hershey & Miller, 1976). The research project was conducted without the informed consent of the research subjects and without institutional review and had the potential to cause the research subjects injury, disability or death. These actions violate both the Nuremberg Code and the Declaration of Helsinki.

TUSKEGEE SYPHILIS STUDY

In 1932, the United States Public Health Service (USPHS) initiated a study of syphilis in black males in the small, rural town of Tuskegee, Alabama. The study, which continued for 40 years, was conducted to determine the natural course of syphilis in the adult, black male. The research subjects were two groups of black males: one group included 400 males who had untreated syphilis, and the second group included 200 males who were found not to have syphilis, who served as a control group. The subjects, who consented to the study, were not informed about the purpose and procedures of the experiment and some were unaware that they were part of an experiment. The subjects were examined periodically, but none of them received treatment for syphilis, even when penicillin was determined to be an effective treatment for the disease in the 1950s. Information about an effective treatment for syphilis was withheld from the research subjects, and steps were taken to actually keep the subjects from receiving treatment (Brandt, 1978).

Published reports of the Tuskegee Syphilis Study first started appearing in 1936, and additional papers were published every 4 to 6 years. No effort was made to stop the study; in fact, in 1969, the Center for Disease Control decided that the study should continue. The study received public attention in 1972, and only then did the Department of Health, Education and Welfare stop the study. The study was investigated and found to be "ethically unjustified," but the racial implications of the study were never addressed (Brandt, 1978). There are still many unanswered questions related to this study, such as: Why was this study ever allowed to be conducted? Where were the checks and balances in the government system that should have stopped the study from continuing for 40 years? Why was public outrage the only effective means for halting the study?

DEPARTMENT OF HEALTH, EDUCATION AND WELFARE (DHEW) REGULATIONS

The continued conduct of harmful, illegal research made additional controls necessary. In 1973, the DHEW published its first set of proposed regulations on the protection of human research subjects. By May of 1974, clinical researchers were presented with very stiff regulations for research involving human subjects. By this time, the DHEW had already published additional regulations to protect persons having "limited capacities to consent," such as the ill, mental impaired and dying (Levine, 1981).

Researchers had gone from a few, vague regulations to almost overwhelming regulations that would legally control the research they conducted. Literally all research involving human subjects had to undergo institutional review. All nursing studies, which frequently involved minimal risks to human subjects, had to be reviewed. Institutional review did provide protection for human research subjects, but reviewing all studies, without regard for the degree of risk involved, overwhelmed the review process and greatly increased the time required for a study to be approved.

NATIONAL COMMISSION FOR THE PROTECTION OF HUMAN SUBJECTS OF BIOMEDICAL AND BEHAVIORAL RESEARCH

Since the issue of protecting human subjects in research was far from resolved by the DHEW regulations, the National Commission for the Protection of Human Subjects of Biomedical and Behavioral Research was formed. This commission was established by the National Research Act (Public Law 93-348) passed in 1974. Its goals were to identify the basic ethical principles that should underlie the conduct of biomedical and behavioral research involving human subjects and to develop guidelines based on these principles.

The Commission identified three *ethical principles* as relevant to the conduct of research involving human subjects: the principles of respect for persons, beneficence and justice. The principle of respect for persons states that persons have the right to self-determination and the freedom to participate or not participate in research. The principle of beneficence encourages the researcher to "above all, do no harm." The principle of justice indicates that human subjects should be treated fairly. The Commission developed guidelines based on these three ethical principles and made recommendations to the Department of Health and Human Services (DHHS). The Commission fulfilled its charges and was dissolved in 1978 (National Commission for the Protection of Human Subjects of Biomedical and Behavioral Research, 1978).

In 1980, the DHHS developed a set of regulations in response to the Commission's recommendations; these regulations were much more reasonable than those proposed in 1973–1974. The DHHS regulations include (1) general requirements for informed consent, (2) documentation of informed consent, (3) Institutional Review Board (IRB) review of research, (4) exempt and expedited review procedures for certain kinds of research and (5) criteria for IRB approval of research (Department of Health and Human Services, January 26, 1981). These regulations are discussed in this chapter.

Protection of Human Rights

Human rights are claims and demands that have been justified in the eyes of an individual or by the consensus of a group of individuals. Having rights is necessary for the self-respect, dignity and health of an individual (Sasson & Nelson, 1971). Conducting research ethically requires that researchers and reviewers of research recognize and protect the rights of human research subjects. The human rights that require protection in research are (1) the right to self-determination, (2) the right to privacy, (3) the right to anonymity and confidentiality, (4) the right to fair treatment and (5) the right to protection from discomfort and harm (American Nurses' Association, 1985; American Psychological Association, 1982).

RIGHT TO SELF-DETERMINATION

The right to *self-determination* is based on the ethical principle of respect for persons, which states that humans are capable of self-determination or controlling their own destiny. Therefore, humans should be treated as autonomous agents, who have the freedom to conduct their lives as they choose without external controls (Beauchamp & Walters, 1982). Prospective subjects are treated as *autonomous agents* by informing them about a proposed study and allowing them to voluntarily choose to participate or not participate. In addition, subjects have the right to terminate participation in a study at any time without penalty. These are elements of informed consent, which are described later in this chapter.

Violation of the Right to Self-Determination

A subject's right to self-determination is violated if he or she is coerced to participate in a study. *Coercion* occurs when an overt threat of harm or excessive reward is intentionally presented by one person to another in order to obtain compliance (National Commission for the Protection of Human Subjects of Biomedical and Behavioral Research, 1978). Some subjects are coerced to participate in research because they fear harm or discomfort if they do not participate. For example, some students feel forced to participate in research to protect their grades or prevent negative relationships with the faculty conducting the research. Other subjects are coerced to participate in studies because they believe that they cannot refuse the excessive rewards offered, such as large sums of money, special privileges and jobs.

An individual's right to self-determination is violated when he or she becomes a research subject without realizing it. Some researchers have exposed persons to experimental treatments without their knowledge, which is exemplified in the Jewish Chronic Disease Hospital study. Some researchers use covert methods of data collection, in which data are collected without subjects' knowledge. *Covert data collection* involves the "development of descriptions of natural phenomena using information that is provided as a matter of normal activity" (Reynolds, 1979, p. 76). Covert data collection frequently does not violate a subject's right to self-determination unless the research deals with sensitive aspects of a subject's behavior, such as illegal conduct, drug use, sexual behavior or use of alcohol (Department of Health and Human Services, January 26, 1981).

The use of deception in research can also violate a subject's right to self-determination. *Deception* is the actual misinforming of subjects for research purposes. An example of deception is the Milgram (1963) study, in which the subjects were to administer electric shocks to another person. The subjects thought that they were administering the shocks to another person, but the person was really a professional actor who pretended to receive the shocks. Some of the subjects experienced severe mental tension, almost to the point of collapse, related to their activities in this study.

The use of deception is not uncommon in social and psychological research, but it is a controversial research activity. Nurse researchers planning to use deception in their studies should examine the ethical and methodological implications of this activity as well as the implications that deception has for the future of nursing research (Kelman, 1967).

Persons with Diminished Autonomy

Some persons have *diminished autonomy* because of legal or mental incompetence, terminal illness or confinement to an institution. These persons require additional protection of their right to self-determination because they have a decreased ability or inability to give informed consent. In addition, these persons are vulnerable to coercion and deception. Many researchers believe that persons with diminished autonomy should not be used as research subjects if other subjects can be used (Hayter, 1979). In certain situations, these persons must be used as subjects, because the knowledge needed to provide their nursing care can be gained only by studying them.

Legally and Mentally Incompetent Subjects

Children (minors), the mentally ill and unconscious patients are legally and/or mentally incompetent to give informed consent. These individuals lack the ability to comprehend information about a study and to make decisions regarding participation in or withdrawal from the study. The use of these persons as research subjects is considered more ethical if the research is therapeutic, where the subjects have the potential to benefit from the experimental process (Watson, 1982).

Terminally Ill Subjects

In conducting research on terminally ill subjects, the investigator should determine (1) Who will benefit from the research? and (2) Is it ethical to conduct research on individuals who will probably not benefit from the study? Some researchers believe that these subjects' potential risks are increased and their potential benefits are minimal or none. In addition, the dying subject's condition could affect the study results and lead the researcher to misinterpret those results (Watson, 1982). Other investigators support conducting research on terminal subjects to generate necessary knowledge. Some terminally ill individuals are very willing subjects, because they believe that participating in research is a way for them to contribute to society before they die. Others want to take part in research because they believe that the experimental process will benefit them.

Subjects Confined to Institutions

Many nursing studies involve hospitalized patients who have some diminished autonomy. Their autonomy is diminished because they are confined to settings that are externally controlled by health care personnel and because their level of health is altered (Besch, 1979). Some hospitalized patients feel obligated to be research subjects, because they want to assist a particular nurse or physician with his or her research. Others feel coerced to participate, because they fear that their care will be adversely affected if they refuse. Nurses conducting research with hospitalized patients must make every effort to protect these subjects from feelings of coercion.

In the past, prisoners have experienced diminished autonomy in research projects because of their confinement. Prisoners can feel coerced to participate in research because they fear harm or desire the benefits of early release, special treatment or monetary gain. The researcher must evaluate the prospective subject's capability of self-determination and respect and protect subjects with diminished autonomy.

RIGHT TO PRIVACY

Privacy is the freedom an individual has to determine the time, extent and general circumstances under which private information will be shared with or withheld from others. Private information includes one's attitudes, beliefs, behaviors, opinions and records. The research subject's privacy is protected if the subject is informed and consents to participate in a study and voluntarily shares private information with a researcher (Hayter, 1979).

Invasion of Privacy

An *invasion of privacy* occurs when private information is shared without an individual's knowledge or against his or her will. Invading an individual's privacy might cause loss of dignity, friendships or employment. Other damaging consequences such as feelings of anxiety, guilt, embarrassment or shame might occur. Research subjects experience an invasion of privacy most frequently during the data collection process. Some researchers develop questionnaires that request very private information, such as (1) Are you an illegitimate child? (2) Were you an abused child? (3) What are your sexual activities? (4) Does your father or mother drink to excess? or (5) What is the intelligence of your mother and father? Other researchers have gathered data from subjects without their knowledge by taping conversations, observing through one-way mirrors and using hidden cameras and microphones. In these situations, the subjects have no knowledge that their words and actions were being shared with the researcher, which is an invasion of their privacy.

The invasion of subjects' right to privacy brought about the Privacy Act of 1974. This act caused the data collection methods to be scrutinized and stated that data cannot be gathered from subjects without their knowledge. This act also stated that individuals have the right to access their own records and the right to prevent access of others to their records (Hayter, 1979). One of the reasons for the Privacy Act was the increased technology that made it possible to collect and rapidly disseminate data without the knowledge or control of the subjects.

RIGHT TO ANONYMITY AND CONFIDENTIALITY

Based on the right to privacy, the research subject has the right to anonymity and the right to assume that the data collected will be kept confidential. *Anonymity* exists if the subject's identity cannot be linked, even by the researcher, with his or her individual responses. An investigator should design a study to achieve subject anonymity if possible (Sasson & Nelson, 1971). *Confidentiality* is the management of private information. This means that if a subject shares private information, the researcher must refrain from sharing that information without the authorization of the subject (Levine, 1981).

Breach of Confidentiality

A breach of confidentiality occurs when a researcher by accident or direct action allows an unauthorized person to gain access to raw data of a study. This breach of confidentiality could lead to the identification of the subject's identity, a violation of the right to anonymity. Breaches of confidentiality of data about religious preferences, sexual practices, income, racial prejudices, drug use, child abuse and personal attributes (such as intelligence, honesty and courage) are serious because of the possible social harm that the subject might experience. For example, sharing information about an employee's drug and alcohol abuse with his or her employer and fellow employees, who had no knowledge of the abuse, could cause the individual to be rejected by co-workers and/or to lose his or her job.

Protection of Anonymity and Confidentiality

Researchers have a responsibility to protect the anonymity of subjects and the confidentiality of the data collected during the study and after the study is completed. In data collection using questionnaires, the subject's identity frequently does not need to be known by the researcher. The questionnaires can have code numbers or letters on them rather than any information that will reveal the identity of the subject. When it is necessary for researchers to collect data from subjects more than one time, the subjects would have to be identified by name. However, the subjects' names should be kept separate from the data collection tools. If signed consent forms are used, these forms should not be stapled to the questionnaire or other data collection tools. This would make it easy for unauthorized persons to readily identify the subjects and their responses. If possible, the data collected should be immediately entered into the computer using code numbers or letters for identification. The original data collection questionnaires or tools should be locked in a secure place or destroyed.

In data analysis, the data should be group analyzed so that an individual cannot be identified by his or her responses. If the subjects are divided into groups for data analysis and there is only one subject in a group, that subject's data should be combined with another group or the data should be deleted. In writing the research report, the investigator should report the findings so that an individual cannot be identified by his or her responses.

Some nurse researchers have encountered health care professionals who believe that they should have access to information about the patients in the hospital and will request to see the data collected. Sometimes family members or close friends would like to see the data collected on specific subjects. The confidentiality of the data collected must be maintained. When requesting permission to conduct a study, it should be made clear to health care professionals, family members or others in the setting that the raw data will not be shared. Breaches of confidentiality can harm subjects psychologically and socially as well as destroy the trust that the subject had in the researcher.

RIGHT TO FAIR TREATMENT

The right to fair treatment is based on the ethical principle of justice. This principle states that each person should be treated fairly and that the person should receive what he or she is due or owed (Beauchamp & Walters, 1982). In research, the selection of subjects and their treatment during the course of a study should be fair.

Fair Selection of Subjects

In the past, injustice in subject selection resulted from social, cultural, racial and sexual biases in society. For many years, research was conducted on categories of individuals who were thought to be especially suitable as research subjects: the poor, charity patients, prisoners, slaves, peasants, dying persons and others who were considered "undesirable" (Reynolds, 1979). Researchers treated these subjects carelessly and had little regard for the harm and discomfort they experienced. The Nazi medical experiments, Tuskegee Syphilis Study and the Jewish Chronic Disease Hospital Study all exemplify unfair subject selection.

The selection of a population to study and the specific subjects to study should be fair, and the risks and benefits of a study should be fairly distributed based on the subject's efforts, needs and rights. Subjects should be selected for reasons directly related to the problem being studied and not for "their easy availability, their compromised position, or their manipulability" (National Commission for the Protection of Human Subjects of Biomedical and Behavioral Research, 1978, p. 10). Another concern with subject selection is that some researchers select subjects because they like them and want them to receive the specific benefits of a study. Other researchers have been swayed by power or money to make certain individuals subjects so that they can receive potentially beneficial treatments. Random selection of subjects can eliminate some of the researchers' biases that might influence subject selection.

Fair Treatment of Subjects During the Course of the Study

Researchers and subjects should have a specific agreement about what the subject's participation involves and what the role of the researcher will be (American Psychological Association, 1982). While conducting a study, the researcher should respect that agreement. If the data collection requires appointments with the subjects, the experimenter should be on time and should terminate the data collection process at an agreed upon time. The activities or procedures that the subject is to perform should not be changed without the subject's consent. The benefits promised the subjects should be provided. For example, if subjects are promised a copy of the study findings, they should receive those findings soon after the study is completed. In addition, subjects who participate in studies should receive equal benefits, regardless of age, race and socioeconomic level. Treating the subjects fairly will facilitate the data collection process and will probably decrease the withdrawal rate from the study.

RIGHT TO PROTECTION FROM DISCOMFORT AND HARM

The right to protection from discomfort and harm is based on the ethical principle of beneficence. This principle states "above all, do no harm" and indicates that members of society should take an active role in preventing discomfort and harm and promoting good in the world around them (Frankena,

1973). Therefore, researchers should conduct their studies to protect subjects from discomfort and harm and try to bring about the greatest possible balance of benefits over harm. Discomfort and harm can be physiological, emotional, social and economical in nature. Reynolds (1972) identified five categories of studies based on levels of discomfort and harm: (1) no anticipated effects, (2) temporary discomfort, (3) unusual levels of temporary discomfort, (4) risk of permanent damage and (5) certainty of permanent damage.

No Anticipated Effects

In some studies, there are no positive or negative effects that are expected for the subjects. For example, studies that involve reviewing patients' records, students' files, pathology reports or other documents have no anticipated effects on the subjects. In these types of studies, the researcher does not interact directly with the research subjects. However, even in these situations, there is a potential risk that the subject's right to privacy might not be protected.

Temporary Discomfort

Studies that cause temporary discomfort are described as minimal risk studies, in which the discomfort encountered is similar to what the subject would experience in his or her daily life and ceases with the termination of the experiment (DHHS, January 26, 1981). Many nursing studies require the completion of questionnaires or participation in interviews, which usually involves minimal risk(s) for the subjects. The physical discomforts might include fatigue, headache or muscle tension. The emotional and social risks might include anxiety, embarrassment or stress associated with responding to certain questions. The economic risks might include the time of being involved in the study or travel costs to the experimental site.

Some nurses conduct clinical studies that require the implementation of a treatment that may involve minimal risk. For example, a study might involve examining the effects of exercise on the glucose level of diabetics and the subjects would have to test their blood sugar two extra times per day. In this study, there is discomfort when the blood is drawn, and there is a potential risk of physical changes that might occur with exercise. The subjects might also experience anxiety and fear associated with the additional blood drawing, and the drawing of blood could be an added monetary expense. The diabetic subjects in this study would experience very similar discomforts in their daily lives, and the discomforts would cease with the study's termination.

Unusual Levels of Temporary Discomfort

In studies that have unusual levels of temporary discomfort, the subjects frequently experience discomfort during the study and after the study has been terminated. For example, subjects might experience muscle weakness, joint pain and dizziness after participating in a study that required them to be confined to bed for 7 days to determine the effects of immobility. In these types of studies, the physical discomforts experienced are more severe, such as the deep pain experienced with the drawing of blood gases. Studies that require subjects to experience failure, extreme fear or threats to their identity or to act in unnatural ways involve risks of unusual levels of temporary discomfort. For example, asking a subject to relive a rape experience could initiate severe feelings of fear and guilt. In these types of studies, the subjects should have an opportunity to receive postexperimental treatment, such as psychiatric counseling or follow-up care for physical discomfort.

Risk of Permanent Damage

Subjects participating in some studies have the potential to suffer permanent damage. The potential to suffer permanent damage is more of a risk in medical research than in nursing. For example, medical studies of new drugs and surgical procedures do have the potential to permanently damage the subjects. However, there are topics that nurses investigate that have the potential to permanently damage subjects emotionally and socially. Studies of sexual behavior, child abuse or drug use have significant risks for subjects. These types of studies have the potential to cause permanent damage to a subject's personality or reputation. There are also potential economic risks, such as less efficient job performance or loss of employment.

Certainty of Permanent Damage

In this type of research, the subjects will encounter permanent damage. Conducting research that will permanently damage subjects is highly questionable, regardless of the benefits that will be gained. The benefits gained frequently benefit other patients or clients but not the subjects.

Balancing benefits and risk in a study

Researchers and reviewers of research must balance the potential benefits and risks in a study to promote the conduct of research ethically. To balance benefits and risks, the researcher must project the outcome of a study and assess the potential benefits and risks based on this outcome (Fig. 12–1).

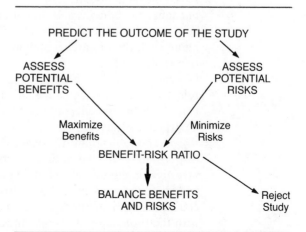

FIGURE 12–1. Balancing benefits and risks.

Assessment of Risk

Researchers must assess the type, degree and number of risks the subjects experience or might experience by participating in a study. The risks involved will depend on the problem studied and the procedures used to study the problem. Risks can be physical, emotional, social and economical in nature and can range from minimal discomfort to permanent damage. Studies can have actual and potential risks for the individual subjects and potential risks for the subjects' families and society. The researcher must try to determine whether or not the potential risk(s) are likely to occur. The risks of a study increase if the researcher fails to protect the rights of the subjects when implementing the research.

Assessment of Benefits

The benefit of knowledge to be gained from research can affect the individual subject, but, more importantly, this knowledge can have a forceful influence on a discipline and numerous members of society. The type of research conducted, therapeutic or nontherapeutic, affects the potential benefits for the subjects. In therapeutic nursing research, the individual subject has the potential to benefit from nursing care measures. The benefits might include improvement in the subject's physical condition, which could facilitate emotional and social benefits. In addition, the knowledge generated from the research might expand the subjects' and their families' understanding of their health.

The conduct of nontherapeutic nursing research is essential to generate and refine the knowledge base of nursing. The knowledge developed through research provides the basis for generating additional research and theory. A subject in any study has the potential to increase his or her understanding of the research process and an opportunity to know the findings from a particular study. Some subjects receive rewards, such as money or special privileges, for participating in research.

Maximizing Benefits and Minimizing Risks

After the benefits and risks have been assessed, the researcher attempts to maximize the benefits and minimize the risks by making changes in the purpose and/or procedures of the study. If the risks cannot be eliminated or further minimized, the researcher should be able to justify their existence. The benefit-risk ratio is developed from maximizing the benefits and minimizing the risks (Levine, 1981). If the risks highly outweigh the benefits, the study should be rejected and another study should be developed. If the benefits and risks balance or the benefits outweigh the risks, the researcher can justify conducting a particular study.

The obligation to balance the benefits and risks of studies is the responsibility of the individual researcher and of society. The individual investigator should balance the potential risks and benefits of a particular study and should protect the subjects from harm during the study. Society should be concerned with the benefits and risks of the entire enterprise of research and with the protection of all human research subjects from harm.

Obtaining Informed Consent

Obtaining informed consent from research subjects is an important aspect of conducting research ethically. Informing is the transmission of essential ideas and content from the investigator to the prospective subject. Consent is the prospective subject's agreement to participate in a study as a subject, which is reached after assimilation of essential information. Every prospective research subject, to the degree that they are capable, should have the opportunity to choose whether or not he or she will participate in research. The phenomenon of informed consent was formally defined in the first principle of the Nuremberg Code. This principle states that a person:

> ... should have legal capacity to give consent; should be so situated as to be able to exercise *free power of choice*, without the intervention of any element of force, fraud, deceit, duress, over-reaching or other ulterior form of constraint or coercion; and should have sufficient *knowledge* and *comprehension* of the elements of the subject matter involved as to enable him to make an understanding and enlightened decision... (Nuremberg Code, 1949, pp. 285–286).

This definition of informed consent has general acceptance in the research community and has been included in subsequent codes and regulations, but the interpretation of this definition continues to be controversial. Researchers vary in their opinions about what is essential information for informed consent and what is "sufficient knowledge and comprehension" of that information by a prospective subject. Researchers also vary in their methods of documenting informed consent. These controversial issues are addressed in a description of the three elements of informed consent: (1) essential information, (2) comprehension and (3) voluntarism.

ESSENTIAL INFORMATION FOR CONSENT

The information that investigators must provide prospective research subjects was identified by the DHHS (January 26, 1981). Informed consent involves the transmission of the following basic information to prospective subjects.

1. ***Introduction of Research Activities.*** The initial information presented to prospective subjects should clearly indicate that a study is to be conducted and that the individual is being asked to participate as a research subject. In clinical nursing research, the patient, serving as a research subject, should know which nursing activities are research activities and which are routine nursing interventions.

2. ***Statement of the Research Purpose.*** The researcher should state the immediate purpose of the research and any long-range goals related to the study. If the prospective subjects disagree with the researcher's goals or the intent of the study, they can immediately decline participation. Information regarding the duration of the study and the time commitment of the subjects should also be presented.

3. ***Selection of Research Subjects.*** The researcher must explain why these individuals were selected as possible subjects. For example,

the prospective subjects might have been selected because they were of a specific age group, belonged to a specific organization, had a specific disease or were hospitalized in a specific institution. At this time, investigators can determine whether the prospective subjects have the attributes that they are seeking.

4. *Explanation of Procedures.* The prospective subjects must receive a complete explanation of the procedures to be implemented in a study. The investigator should describe the research variables and the procedures or mechanisms that will be used to observe, examine, manipulate and/or measure these variables. In addition, the prospective subjects must know when the study procedures will be implemented, how many times and in what setting.

5. *Description of Potential Risks or Discomfort.* The prospective research subject must have information about the potential risks (physical, emotional, social and economical) that might result from the study. The investigator must indicate how the risks of the study have been and/or will be minimized.

   If the research involves more than minimal risks, an explanation as to whether any compensation is to be provided and whether any medical treatments are available if injury occurs should be given to the prospective subjects. If medical treatments are available, the type and extent of the treatments must be described. If appropriate, the prospective subject needs to know whether a procedure may involve risks to the subject (or the fetus, if the subject is or may become pregnant) that are not currently known or anticipated.

6. *Description of the Potential Benefits.* The investigator must explain the potential benefits of the research for the prospective subjects. Any financial advantages or other rewards for participating in the study should be described.

7. *Disclosure of Alternatives.* The investigator must disclose whether any appropriate, alternative procedures or courses of treatment exist that might benefit the subject. For example, the researchers of the Tuskegee Syphilis Study should have informed the research subjects with syphilis that penicillin was an effective treatment for the disease.

8. *Assurance of Confidentiality.* The prospective subjects require assurance that their responses will be kept confidential. In addition, the subjects need to know whether any of the data collected by the nurse researcher will become a part of their medical record. The subjects must be promised that their identity will remain anonymous in the research reports and publication of the study.

9. *Offer to Answer Questions.* The researcher must make an offer to answer any pertinent questions that are raised by the prospective subjects about the study and about their rights as subjects. The prospective subjects also need to know who to contact if they have further questions, want to withdraw from the study or are injured during the study; and they need a mechanism for contacting that person.

If the study involves greater than minimal risk, the researcher should encourage the prospective subjects to consult another person regarding their participation in the study. A trusted friend, family member or another nurse could consult with the prospective subject.

10. ***Noncoercive Disclaimer.*** A noncoercive disclaimer is a statement that participation in a study is voluntary and that refusal to participate will involve no penalty or loss of benefits for prospective subjects. This statement is very important in facilitating a relationship between prospective subjects and the investigator, especially if the relationship has a potential for coercion.

11. ***Option to Withdraw.*** Prospective subjects should know that they can withdraw from a study at any time without being penalized. However, researchers do have the right to ask subjects if they think that they will be able to complete the study, in order to decrease the number of subjects withdrawing early.

There may be circumstances where the "subject's participation may be terminated by the investigator without regard to the subject's consent" (DHHS, January 26, 1981). For example, if a particular treatment becomes potentially dangerous to a subject, the researcher has the responsibility to withdraw the subject from the study. Thus, prospective subjects should be told under what circumstances they might be withdrawn from a study. The researcher should also make a general statement about the circumstances that could lead to the termination of the entire project (Levine, 1981).

12. ***Consent to Incomplete Disclosure.*** Some studies require that the research subjects not be totally informed about the purpose of a study, because that knowledge will alter the subjects' actions. However, prospective subjects must know when they are not being completely informed about a study. The researcher must ensure that there are no undisclosed risks to the subjects that are more than minimal. The subjects' questions regarding the study should always be answered truthfully.

Subjects who are exposed to nondisclosure of information need to know when and how they will be debriefed about the study. The researcher *debriefs* the subjects by informing them of the actual purpose of the study and the results that were obtained. If the subjects experience adverse effects related to the study, the researcher should make every attempt to reconcile them (Jacobson, 1973).

COMPREHENSION OF CONSENT INFORMATION

Informed consent implies not only the imparting of information by the researcher but also the comprehension of that information by the subjects. Studies have been done to determine subjects' levels of comprehension after receiving the essential information for consent, and their comprehension was frequently low (Levine, 1981). The researcher must take the time to "teach" the prospective subjects about the study. The amount of information to be taught depends on the subjects' knowledge of research and the specific research topic. The risks and benefits of a study should be discussed in detail, using examples that are relevant to the prospective subject. The specific procedures to be used in the study and the subjects' rights should be outlined and described in depth to the subjects.

The consent information should be written and verbalized in lay terminology, not professional jargon. The terms used should be at the level of understanding of the prospective subjects. For example, a study designed for the general public should have consent information that is at an eighth grade level of education. The information for consent should be presented without loaded or biased terms that might coerce a subject into participating in a study.

The comprehension of subjects with diminished autonomy is a more complex phenomenon. The researcher should make every effort to present the information at the level at which these subjects can understand. In addition, the researcher must present the essential information for consent to the legally authorized representative of the prospective subject (Levine, 1981).

Assessing Subjects' Comprehension

The researcher can take steps to determine the prospective subject's level of comprehension. After receiving the information for consent, the subjects could be asked key questions: "(1) What is the purpose of this study? (2) What risks are involved in the study procedures? (3) What does your participation in this study involve? (4) Approximately how long will your participation in this study take? (5) When can you withdraw from this study? (6) How will your name be associated with the study data? (7) With whom will the study information be shared? and (8) What direct personal benefit will come to you as a result of participating in this study?" (Silva, 1985, p. 121). In some high-risk studies, the prospective subjects have been given tests about the consent information, and they did not become subjects unless they passed the tests (Hershey & Miller, 1976).

VOLUNTARY CONSENT

Consent to participate in a study is valid only if that consent is given voluntarily. Voluntary consent is obtained after the prospective subject has been given essential information about the study and has shown comprehension of this information. Voluntary consent means that the prospective subject has decided to take part in a study of his or her own volition without coercion or any undue influence (Levine, 1981). Some researchers, because of their authority, expertise or power, have the potential to coerce subjects into participating in research. Researchers should be cautious that their persuasion of prospective subjects does not become coercion. The rewards offered in a study should be congruent with the risks that the subjects must take.

DOCUMENTATION OF INFORMED CONSENT

Informed consent can be documented in different ways. The method of documentation used depends on the degree of risk involved in the study and the discretion of the researcher and those reviewing the study. DHHS (January 26, 1981) has developed rules and regulations to direct researchers in documenting informed consent. Most studies require a written consent form, but, in some studies, the consent form is waived.

Waived Consent

The requirements for written consent are usually waived in studies that present no more than minimal risk of harm to subjects and involve procedures that do not require written consent (DHHS, January 26, 1981). For example, researchers collecting relatively innocuous data using questionnaires would not need to obtain written consent from the subjects. The subject's completion of the questionnaire may serve as consent. The top of the questionnaire might contain a statement: "Your completion of this questionnaire indicates your consent to participate in this study." In addition, the subjects should receive a letter or verbal explanation that would provide the essential information for informed consent.

Written Consent Form

Written consent can be a short or long form. The short consent form includes the following statement: "The elements of informed consent required by law have been presented orally to the subject or the subject's legally authorized representative" (DHHS, January 26, 1981). The elements of informed consent are presented in this chapter under the heading "Essential Information for Consent." If the researcher uses this method, a witness must be present for the oral presentation. A written summary of the oral presentation must be provided to the subject, and the subject must sign the written summary and the short consent form. Copies of the summary and short consent form are given to the subject and the witness. The short form might be used in studies that present minimal or moderate risk to the subjects.

The long consent form includes all the essential information of informed consent. Reading the form should explain the proposed study to the prospective subjects; however, it is wise to also verbally explain the study to the subjects. The form is signed by the subject and is witnessed by the investigator or research assistant collecting the data. This type of consent is appropriate for studies of minimal and high risk. An example consent form is presented in Figure 12–2. All persons signing the consent form should receive a copy of it, which includes the subject, researcher and any other witnesses.

Studies that involve subjects with diminished autonomy need a written consent form. If these prospective subjects have some comprehension of the study and agree to participate as subjects, they should sign the consent form. However, the form should also be signed by their legally authorized representative. The representative should indicate his or her relationship to the subject under the representative's signature.

```
┌─────────────────────────────────────────────────────────────────┐
│                          CONSENT FORM                             │
│  Study Title: The Needs of Family Members of Critically Ill Adults│
│  Investigator: Linda S. Norris, R.N.                              │
│        Ms. Norris is a nurse studying the emotional and social    │
│  needs of family members of patients in the Intensive Care Units  │
│  (research purpose). She believes the study will provide          │
│  information that will enable nurses to identify family members'  │
│  needs and to assist family members with these needs (study       │
│  benefits). I understand that identifying my needs might cause     │
│  some anxiety and/or fatigue (study risks). I realize that the    │
│  study will take approximately 20 minutes of my time and will     │
│  involve filling out a questionnaire (research procedures).       │
│        I know that my participation in this study is strictly      │
│  voluntary (voluntary consent). I know that I have the right to    │
│  withdraw at any time and that the care of my family member        │
│  and my relationship with the health care team will not be         │
│  affected (option to withdraw).                                    │
│        If I have any questions about the study or about being a    │
│  subject, I know I can call Ms. Norris. I may reach her at         │
│  999–9999 (office) or 555–5555 (home) (opportunity to ask          │
│  questions).                                                        │
│        I agree to participate in this study, and I have received   │
│  a copy of this consent form. I have been assured that my         │
│  identity will not be revealed while the study is being conducted  │
│  or when the study is published (privacy and confidentiality).     │
│                                                                    │
│                                                                    │
│  ─────────────────────       ─────────────────────────────        │
│          Date                      Subject's Signature            │
│                                                                    │
│                                                                    │
│  ─────────────────────       ─────────────────────────────        │
│    Witness (If Appropriate)       Investigator's Signature        │
│                                                                    │
│                                                                    │
│  ─────────────────────                                            │
│  Relationship to Subject (if Appropriate)                         │
└─────────────────────────────────────────────────────────────────┘
```

FIGURE 12–2. Sample consent form.

The written consent form used in a high-risk study should include the signatures of two witnesses: (1) the researcher, and (2) an additional person. The additional person signing as a witness should actually observe the informed consent process and should not be otherwise connected with the study (Hershey & Miller, 1976). The witness could be a subject advocate or patient advocate who is employed in the institution. An advocate is important in the consent process if the prospective subject is in awe of the investigator and does not feel free to question the procedures of the study.

Tape Recording and Videotaping the Consent Process

Some researchers have chosen to tape record or videotape the consent process. This method documents what was said to prospective subjects and records the questions of the subjects and answers of the investigators. Tape recording and videotaping are time consuming and costly and are not really appropriate for studies of minimal or moderate risk. However, if a study has high risks, complete documentation of the consent process might be a wise precaution that could protect the subject and the researcher. Both the researcher and the subject would retain a copy of the tape recording or videotape.

Institutional Review

In institutional review, a study is examined for ethical concerns by a committee of peers. The first Federal policy statement on protection of human subjects

TABLE 12–2
Research Qualifying for Exemption From IRB Review

Exempt from coverage is most social, economic, and educational research in which the only involvement of human subjects will be in one or more of the following categories:

1. Research conducted in established or commonly accepted educational settings involving normal education practices.
2. Research involving the use of educational tests (cognitive, diagnostic, aptitude, achievement) if information taken from these sources is recorded in such a manner that subjects cannot be identified directly or through identifiers or code numbers linked to the subjects.
*3. Research involving survey or interview procedures or observations (including observation by participants) of public behavior, except where all of the following conditions exist:
   a. Responses and observations are recorded in such a manner that the human subject can be identified directly or through identifiers, or code numbers, linked to the subjects.
   b. The subject's responses or the observations recorded about an individual, if they became known outside the research, could reasonably place the subject at risk of criminal or civil liability or be damaging to the subject's financial standing or employability.
   c. The research deals with sensitive aspects of the subject's own behavior, such as illegal conduct, drug use, sexual behavior, or use of alcohol. All research involving survey or interview procedures is exempt, without exception, when the respondents are elected or appointed public officials or candidates for public office.
4. Research involving the collection or study of existing data, documents, records, pathological specimens, or diagnostic specimens, if these sources are publicly available or if the information is recorded by the investigator in such a manner that subjects cannot be identified, directly or through identifiers linked to subjects.
5. Unless specifically required by statute, research and demonstration projects which are conducted by or subject to the approval of the U.S. Department of Health and Human Services and which study, evaluate, or otherwise examine:
   a. programs under the Social Security Act or other public benefit or service programs,
   b. procedures for obtaining benefits or services under those programs,
   c. possible changes in or alternatives to those programs or procedures, or
   d. possible changes in methods or levels of payment for benefits or services under those programs.

*Not exempt when research subjects are children.
(Excerpted from the Federal Register of January 26, 1981)

by institutional review was issued by the United States Public Health Service (USPHS) in 1966. The USPHS indicated that research involving human subjects must be reviewed by a committee of peers or associates to determine:

> (1) the rights and welfare of the individual or individuals involved, (2) the appropriateness of the methods used to secure informed consent, and (3) the risks and potential medical benefits of the investigation. A description of the committee of the associates who will provide the review should be included (Levine, 1981, p. 209).

In 1974, DHEW passed the National Research Act, which required that all research involving human subjects undergo institutional review. The DHHS revised these guidelines in 1981. In this revision, there were certain studies identified that would qualify for exemption or expedited review by an institutional review board. Institutional Review Board (IRB) refers to a committee that reviews research to ensure that the investigator is conducting the research ethically. The IRB of the DHHS has two subcommittees: "the protocol review committee which approves or disapproves of requests for funds and the subject advisory committee which is responsible for protecting the rights of subjects of

TABLE 12-3
Research Qualifying for Expedited IBR Review

Expedited review (by committee chairpersons or designated members) for the following research involving no more than minimal risk is authorized:

1. Collection of: hair and nail clippings, in a nondisfiguring manner; deciduous teeth; and permanent teeth if patient care indicates a need for extraction.
2. Collection of excreta and external secretions including sweat, uncannulated saliva, placenta removed at delivery, and amniotic fluid at the time of rupture of the membrane prior to or during labor.
3. Recording of data from subjects 18 years of age or older using noninvasive procedures routinely employed in clinical practice. This includes the use of physical sensors that are applied either to the surface of the body or at a distance and do not involve input of matter or significant amounts of energy into the subject or an invasion of the subject's privacy. It also includes such procedures as weighing, testing sensory acuity, electrocardiography, electroencephalography, thermography, detection of naturally occurring radioactivity, diagnostic echography, and electroretinography. It does not include exposure to electromagnetic radiation outside the visible range (for example, x-rays, microwaves).
4. Collection of blood samples by venipuncture, in amounts not exceeding 450 milliliters in an eight-week period and no more often than two times per week, from subjects 18 years of age or older and who are in good health and not pregnant.
5. Collection of both supra- and subgingival dental plaque and calculus, provided the procedure is not more invasive than routine prophylactic scaling of the teeth and the process is accomplished in accordance with accepted prophylactic techniques.
6. Voice recordings made for research purposes such as investigations of speech defects.
7. Moderate exercise by healthy volunteers.
8. The study of existing data, documents, records, pathological specimens, or diagnostic specimens.
9. Research on individual or group behavior or characteristics of individual, such as studies of perception, cognition, game theory, or test development, where the investigator does not manipulate subjects' behavior and research will not involve stress to subjects.
10. Research on drugs or devices for which an investigational new drug exemption or an investigational device exemption is not required.

Excerpted from the Federal Register of January 26, 1981. Additional regulations that apply to research involving fetuses, pregnant women, human in vitro fertilization, and prisoners are available in the Federal Register, January 26, 1981, Subpart B and C.

biomedical or behavioral research" (Armiger, 1977, p. 334). Institutions, where most research is conducted, have IRBs to determine which studies will be conducted in that setting.

The DHHS rules and regulations state that studies are exempt from review if they have no apparent risks for the research subjects (Table 12-2). Studies that have some risks, but the risks are viewed as minimal, are expedited in the review process (Table 12-3). Minimal risk means "that the risks of harm anticipated in the proposed research are not greater, considering probability and magnitude, than those ordinarily encountered in daily life or during the performance of routine physical or psychological examinations or tests" (DHHS, January, 26, 1981).

Studies that have greater than minimal risks must receive a complete review by an IRB. A list of criteria must be followed in order to obtain IRB approval. These criteria include (1) risks to subjects are minimized, (2) risks to subjects are reasonable in relation to anticipated benefits, (3) selection of subjects is equitable, (4) informed consent will be sought and documented from each prospective subject or the subject's legally authorized representative, (5) the research plan makes adequate provision for monitoring the data collected to ensure the safety of subjects and (6) there are adequate provisions to protect the privacy of subjects and to maintain the confidentiality of data (DHHS, January 26, 1981). The process of seeking approval from a research review committee (IRB) to conduct a study is the focus of Chapter 13.

Summary

The ethical issues of conducting research have been debated without resolution for many years. The debate about ethics and research continues because of the complexity of human rights issues, the abstractness of the codes and regulations governing research and the variety of interpretations of these codes and regulations. Conducting research ethically requires that the investigator be knowledgeable of codes and regulations that govern research. Two historical codes that have a strong impact on the conduct of research are the Nuremberg Code and the Declaration of Helsinki. Recently, the Department of Health and Human Services (1981) has passed regulations that direct the ethical conduct of research. These regulations include (1) general requirements for informed consent, (2) documentation of informed consent, (3) Institutional Review Board (IRB) review of research, (4) exempt and expedited review procedures for certain kinds of research and (5) criteria for IRB approval of research.

Conducting research ethically requires protection of the human rights of subjects. Human rights are claims and demands that have been justified in the eyes of an individual or by the consensus of a group of individuals. The human rights that require protection in research are (1) the right to self-determination, (2) the right to privacy, (3) the right to anonymity and confidentiality, (4) the right to fair treatment and (5) the right to protection from discomfort and harm. The right to self-determination is based on the ethical principle of respect for persons, which states that humans are capable of determining and controlling their own destiny. Privacy is the freedom an individual has to determine the time, extent and general circumstances under which private information will be shared with or withheld from others. Based on the right to privacy, the research subject has the right to anonymity and the right to assume that the data collected will be kept confidential. Anonymity exists if the subject's identity cannot be linked, even by the researcher, with his or her responses. Confidentiality is the management of private information, which means that if a subject shares private information, the researcher must not share that information without the authorization of the subject. The right to fair treatment is based on the ethical principle of justice, which states that every person should be treated fairly and receive what he or she is due or owed. The right to protection from discomfort and harm is based on the ethical principle of beneficence, which states "above all, do no harm."

The rights of the research subjects can be protected by balancing benefits and risks of a study, securing informed consent and submitting the research for institutional review. To balance the benefits and risks of a study, the type, degree and number of risks are examined, and the potential benefits are identified. If possible, the risks should be minimized and the benefits maximized to achieve the best possible benefit-risk ratio. Informed consent involves the transmission of essential information, comprehension of that information and voluntary consent of the prospective subject. The guidelines for seeking consent from subjects and for institutional review were described. Researchers must be responsible for performing these ethical activities during the planning and implementation of research.

References

American Nurses' Association (1985). *Human rights guidelines for nurses in clinical and other research*. Kansas City, Missouri: American Nurses' Association (Document No. D–46 5M).

American Psychological Association (1982). *Ethical principles in the conduct of research with human participants*. Washington, D. C.: American Psychological Association, Inc.

Armiger, Sr. B. (1977). Ethics of nursing research: profile, principles, perspective. *Nursing Research*, 26(5), 330–336.

Beauchamp, T. L. & Walters, L. (1982). *Contemporary issues in bioethics* (2nd Ed.). Belmont, California: Wadsworth Publishing Company.

Besch, L. (1979). Informed consent: a patient's right. *Nursing Outlook*, 27(1), 32–35.

Brandt, A. M. (1978). Racism and research: the case of the Tuskegee syphilis study. *Hastings Center Report*, 8(6), 21–29.

Damrosch, S. P. (1986). Ensuring anonymity by use of subject-generated identification codes. *Research in Nursing and Health*, 9(1), 61–63.

Davis, A. (1985). Informed consent: how much information is enough? *Nursing Outlook*, 33(1), 40–42.

Department of Health and Human Services (DHHS) (January 26, 1981). Final regulations amending basic HHS policy for the protection of human research subjects. *Federal Regulations*, 46(16).

Frankena, W. K. (1973). *Ethics* (2nd Ed.). Englewood Cliffs, New Jersey: Prentice-Hall, Inc.

Hayter, J. (1979). Issues related to human subjects. In F. S. Downs & J. W. Fleming (Eds.), *Issues in nursing research*. Norwalk, Connecticut: Appleton-Century-Crofts.

Hershey, N. & Miller, R. D. (1976). *Human experimentation and the law*. Germantown, Maryland: Aspen Systems Corporation.

Institute of Society, Ethics and the Life Sciences (1976). Biomedical ethics and the shadow of Nazism. *Hastings Center Report*, 6(4), 1–20.

Jacobson, S. F. (1973). Ethical issues in experimentation with human subjects. *Nursing Forum*, 12(1), 59–71.

Kelman, H. C. (1967). Human use of human subjects: the problem of deception in social psychological experiments. *Psychological Bulletin*, 67(1), 1–11.

Levine, R. J. (1979). Clarifying the concepts of research ethics. *Hasting Center Report*, 9(3), 21–26.

Levine, R. J. (1981). *Ethics and regulation of clinical research*. Baltimore-Munich: Urban & Schwarzenberg, Inc.

Milgram, S. (1963). Behavioral study of obedience. *Journal of Abnormal and Social Psychology*, 67(4), 371–378.

National Commission for the Protection of Human Subjects of Biomedical and Behavioral Research (1978). *Belmont Report: ethical principles and guidelines for research involving human subjects*. Washington, D. C.: U. S. Government Printing Office, DHEW Publication No. (05) 78-0012.

Nuremberg Code (1949). In R. J. Levine (Ed.) (1981). *Ethics and regulation of clinical research* (pp. 285–286). Baltimore-Munich: Urban & Schwarzenberg, Inc.

Purtilo, R. B. & Cassel, C. K. (1981). *Ethical dimensions in the health professions*. Philadelphia: W. B. Saunders Company.

Reynolds, P. D. (1972). On the protection of human subjects and social science. *International Social Science Journal*, 24(4), 693–719.

Reynolds, P. D. (1979). *Ethical dilemmas and social science research*. San Francisco: Jossey-Bass Publishing Co.

Sasson, R. & Nelson, T. M. (1971). The human experimental subject in context. In J. Jung (Ed.), *The experimenter's dilemma*. New York: Harper & Row Publishers, Inc.

Silva, M. C. (1985). Comprehension of information for informed consent by spouses of surgical patients. *Research in Nursing and Health*, 8(2), 117–124.

Watson, A. B. (1982). Informed consent of special subjects. *Nursing Research*, 31(1), 43–47.

III

THE PRAGMATICS OF IMPLEMENTATION

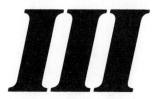
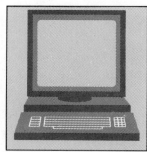
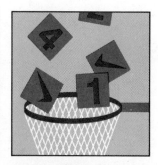
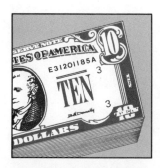
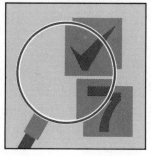
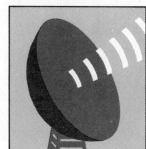
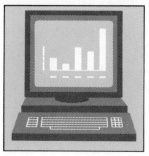

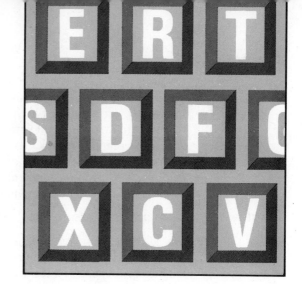

13

Proposal Writing for Research Approval

Most studies conceived are developed into a formal research proposal before the research project is initiated. A *research proposal* is a written plan that identifies the major elements of the study such as the research problem, subproblems and frame of reference, and outlines the methods and procedures to be used in studying the subproblems. The research proposal is a formal way to communicate ideas about a proposed study to obtain approval to conduct the study or to seek funding. *Seeking approval for the conduct and/or funding of a study* is a process that involves submission of a research proposal to a selected group for review and, in many situations, verbally defending that proposal. Seeking approval to conduct a study has become increasingly more complicated over the past few years because nurse researchers are conducting more complex studies using human subjects. This chapter focuses on developing a research proposal and seeking approval to conduct a study.

Writing a Research Proposal

A proposal should communicate a planned research project and demonstrate the qualifications of the researcher to conduct the study. Conducting research requires careful attention to details. Therefore, reviewers often judge a researcher's ability to attend to detail by the proposal presented for review. The skill with which the proposal is written influences whether a study is conducted in the real world and/or whether the study is funded. Proposal writing is a skill that is learned and refined with experience. A well-written proposal is concise, clear and complete (Cook, 1985; Shaw, 1963). Developing a proposal requires (1) the logical development of ideas, (2) the determination of the depth or detail of the proposal content, (3) the identification of critical points in a proposal and (4) the development of an aesthetically appealing copy.

Logical Development of Ideas

The ideas in a research proposal must logically build upon each other to justify or defend a study, just as a lawyer would logically organize information in the defense of a client in a legal case. The researcher should build a case for why a problem should be studied and propose an appropriate methodology for conducting the study. Each step in the research proposal builds on the problem statement to give a clear picture of the study to be conducted and its merit. *The Chicago manual of style* (1982) can be helpful in organizing the content of a proposal.

Determination of the Depth of a Proposal

Research proposals vary in length and depth. To some extent, the depth is determined by guidelines developed by schools, funding agencies and institutions where research is conducted. Guidelines provide specific directions for the development of a proposal and should be followed explicitly. Frequently, the omission and/or misinterpretation of a guideline is the basis for rejection of a proposal. In addition to following the guidelines, a researcher must determine the amount of information necessary to clearly describe each step of a study. The content in a proposal should be detailed enough to inform the reader, yet concise enough to be interesting and easily reviewed. Relevant content of a research proposal is discussed in the next section of this chapter.

Identification of Critical Points

In writing a proposal, the key or critical points must be clear to even the hasty reader. Critical points might be highlighted with bold type or underlined. Sometimes titles are created to highlight critical content, or the content is organized into tables or graphs. Critical content that should be identified in a proposal includes the research problem, significance of the problem, subproblems, framework, definitions of variables, assumptions, limitations, methodological procedures, budget and timetable.

Development of an Aesthetically Appealing Copy

The final copy of the proposal must be aesthetically appealing. Even a proposal with excellent content that is poorly typed or formatted will probably not receive full attention or respect and might offend the reviewer. An appealing copy is well typed on quality paper without spelling, punctuation or grammatical errors. The format used in typing the proposal should follow the format guidelines developed by the reviewer. If no particular format is requested, the American Psychological Association (APA) format is commonly used. An appealing copy is legible (print is dark enough to be read) and is neatly organized in a folder so that it can be easily examined by the reviewer.

Content of a Research Proposal

The content of a proposal should be written with the interest and expertise of the reviewers in mind. Proposals are frequently reviewed by faculty, agency members and representatives of funding institutions. Student researchers develop proposals to communicate their research projects to faculty and members of university human subjects review committees. Proposals are reviewed by individuals in agencies, such as agency officials or members of the research committee, who determine which studies will be conducted in an agency. Other researchers develop proposals in order to obtain funding for a research project (Chapter 14). The contents of a proposal vary depending on the reviewer and the guidelines developed for the review. However, the researcher would be wise to write the proposal in such a way that the material can easily be extracted for publication.

CONTENT OF A STUDENT PROPOSAL

Proposals written by students to satisfy requirements for a degree are usually developed according to specific guidelines outlined by faculty. Students should discuss these guidelines with the faculty member (usually the chair of their thesis or dissertation committee) who will be assisting them with their research project. Each faculty member has a unique way of interpreting and emphasizing aspects of the guidelines. In addition, a student should evaluate the faculty member's background regarding a research topic of interest and determine whether a productive working relationship can be developed. Faculty members who are actively involved in their own research have extensive knowledge and expertise that can be helpful to a novice researcher. A student's selection of a chair and members of a thesis or dissertation committee should be carefully thought out.

The content of a student proposal usually requires greater detail than the proposal developed for review by agency personnel or funding organizations. This proposal might be the first chapters of the student's thesis or dissertation. The content of the proposal is written in the future tense. A title page, which includes the title of the proposal, name of the investigator and the date the proposal was submitted, should precede the proposal. The first section of a proposal is an introduction to the research problem, the second section includes the review of relevant literature, the third section develops the frame of reference for the study and the fourth section describes the methods and procedures to be used in conducting the study. Some graduate schools require an in-depth development of these sections, whereas others require a condensed version of the same content. Another approach is that proposals for theses and dissertations be written in a form that can ultimately be submitted for publication. An example of research proposal guidelines that could be used in directing a student's development of a proposal for a quantitative or qualitative study is listed in Table 13–1.

Introduction

The introductory section identifies the research topic and problem and develops the background and significance for this problem. The background of a problem describes how the problem was identified and historically links the problem to nursing. The background information might include one or two major studies conducted to resolve the problem, some key theoretical ideas related to the problem and possible solutions to the problem. The significance of the problem addresses the importance of this problem in nursing practice and the expected generalizability of the findings. The interest of nurses, other health care professionals and health care consumers in the problem at the local, state, national or international level is part of determining the problem significance. This interest can usually be documented by citations from the literature. The background and significance of the problem is followed by a clear, concise statement of the research purpose. The purpose clarifies and narrows the focus of the study and identifies *why* the study is being conducted. The purpose might be to identify and describe variables and/or to examine relationships (associative and causal) of variables.

TABLE 13–1
Research Proposal Guidelines for Students

Research Proposal Guidelines

I. INTRODUCTION
   A. Statement of the Problem
   B. Background and Significance of the Problem
   C. Statement of the Purpose
II. REVIEW OF RELEVANT LITERATURE
   (Not part of the proposal in some qualitative studies)
   A. Review of Relevant Theoretical Literature
   B. Review of Relevant Research
   C. Summary
III. FRAME OF REFERENCE
   A. Development of the Conceptual or Theoretical Framework
   B. Formulation of Research Subproblems
   C. Definition of Major Variables
   D. Identification of Assumptions
IV. METHODS AND PROCEDURES
   A. Identification of the Research Design
   B. Identification of the Population and Sample
   C. Selection of a Setting
   D. Presentation of Ethical Considerations
   E. Planning Data Collection and Analysis
   F. Identification of Limitations
   G. Proposed Communication of Findings
   H. Presentation of the Study Budget and Timetable

Review of Relevant Literature

The review of relevant literature provides an overview of the essential information that will guide the development of a study. This section includes relevant theoretical information and studies. The theoretical information included is relevant to the proposed study but is not part of the study framework. The strengths and weaknesses of previous studies and studies currently being conducted are described. The recommendations, such as changing and/or expanding a study, made by other researchers are discussed related to the proposed study. The depth of the review of literature varies and might include only recent studies and theorists' works, or the review might include a number of past and current studies with a critique of these studies (Chapter 20) and an in-depth discussion of theorists' works. The review of literature should demonstrate that the researcher has command of the current empirical and theoretical knowledge regarding the proposed problem. Content from these sources should be related to the research problem and purpose. The sources cited in all sections of the proposal should be included in a reference list at the end of the proposal.

The review of relevant literature section concludes with a summary. The summary is a synthesis of the findings from previous research and theoretical information. In the summary, the current knowledge of a problem is described, and the gaps in the knowledge base are identified. Some qualitative approaches, such as phenomenology and grounded theory research, require that the major review of literature be conducted after the data are collected. Thus, the proposals for these types of study would not include the review of literature section.

Frame of Reference

A framework provides the basis for generating and refining a research problem and links that problem with the relevant theoretical knowledge in nursing or related fields. The framework includes concepts and relationships among concepts, which are sometimes represented in a model. The concepts to be studied are conceptually defined in the frame of reference. Depending on the type of research conducted, a conceptual framework or a theoretical framework is developed. A theoretical framework presents one theorist's work, whereas a conceptual framework includes ideas from one or more theorists.

In a proposal, the research subproblems are stated as objectives, questions or hypotheses, depending on the research purpose. Research subproblems identify the target population and the variables to be investigated. The subproblems must evolve from the study framework. A conceptual framework includes the concepts and/or relationships that are expressed in the subproblems. The theoretical framework identifies a proposition that provides the basis for the generation of an hypothesis. The variables and other key concepts identified in the subproblems are operationally defined in the proposal. The operational definitions of the variables should build upon the conceptual definitions and should indicate the procedures for measurement. Assumptions, statements that are taken for granted or are considered true, even though these statements have not been scientifically tested (Silva, 1981), should be stated in a proposal.

Methods and Procedures

The research approach, quantitative or qualitative, and specific type of study to be conducted are identified in the proposal. The design or general strategy for conducting the study is described, and sometimes a diagram of this strategy is included (see Chapter 10). The designs for exploratory studies (qualitative and quantitative) are flexible and sometimes unique to the study being conducted. Because of this uniqueness, the designs must be clearly described by the researcher. The designs of descriptive studies are more structured than exploratory studies but these designs are still quite flexible and require clear description. Presenting a design of correlational, quasi-experimental and experimental studies involves (1) describing how the research situation will be structured, (2) indicating the variables to be controlled and the methods of controlling them, (3) identifying uncontrolled extraneous variables and determining their impact on the findings and (4) describing the methods for assigning subjects to the treatment and control groups. The design should account for all the subproblems identified in the proposal. If a pilot study is planned, the design section of the proposal must describe the procedure for conducting the pilot and for incorporating the results into the proposed study.

The proposal describes the population to which the study findings are to be generalized. In addition, the target population from which the sample will be selected is identified. The criteria for selection of a subject and the rationale for these criteria are described. For example, a subject might be selected according to the following criteria: male, aged 20 to 50 years, hospitalized for 3 days and 2 days postoperative from abdominal surgery. The rationale for these criteria might be that the researcher wished to examine the effects of preoperative teaching about pain relief on adult males who recently had experienced hospitalization and abdominal surgery. The sampling method to be used and the approximate sample size are discussed in terms of their adequacy and limitations in investigating the research subproblems.

The selected setting for the study is described in the proposal. This description should include the name of the agency and the structure of the specific units where the study is to be conducted. The selected agency should have the potential for generating the type and size of sample required for the study. In addition, the structure and activities in the agency should be able to accommodate the proposed design of the study.

The ethical considerations that must be addressed in a proposal include the rights of the human subjects and the rights of the agency where the study is to be conducted. The protection of the subject's rights and the identification of the risks and potential benefits for the subject must be explained in detail. The proposal should address each risk and describe the actions that will be taken to reduce these risks for the subjects. A copy of the verbal explanation of the study and the proposed written consent form must be included in the appendix of the proposal. The researcher should also describe the risks and potential benefits for the institution where the study is to be conducted. If there are risks for the agency, the steps that will be taken to reduce or eliminate these risks should be outlined.

The data collection section of the proposal should address the kinds of information to be collected and clarify how this data will be collected. A copy of questionnaires, interview schedules, recording forms or other data collection tools should be included in the appendix of the proposal. Any special equipment that will be used or developed to collect data for the study should be discussed. The validity and reliability of the measurement tools must be addressed. If the tools or instruments have no reported validity and reliability, a pilot study is conducted by the researcher to test the instruments. If the intent of the proposed study is to develop an instrument, the process of instrument development must be described.

Data collection procedures and schedule should be described in the proposal. The investigator should identify who will collect the data. If more than one person will be involved in data collection, the proposal must describe the training of data collectors. The intent is to ensure that there is consistency among the data collectors (see Chapter 16). A method for recording data should be described, and an example data recording sheet should be included in the appendix. Data security should also be addressed, and the methods of data storage should be identified.

The methods proposed for analyzing the data are described in the proposal, and these data analysis techniques should be appropriate for the type of data collected. For example, if an associative hypothesis is developed, correlational analysis must be planned. If the researcher is using statistical tests to determine the differences among variables, a level of significance (0.01 or 0.05) must be identified in the proposal. The researcher should project the type of results that will be generated from the data analyses. Dummy tables, graphs and charts might be developed for the presentation of the results and included in the proposal appendix.

The investigator should project the possible findings for each subproblem and incorporate those projections in the proposal. The implications and meaning of possible findings should be examined in light of the study framework. For example, the researcher might consider what rejection or acceptance of a proposed hypothesis would mean in light of the study framework. Projecting a study's findings facilitates logical examination of possible findings, which is a necessary prerequisite for interpretation of research outcomes. Within the proposal, the researcher must indicate how the actual findings from the study will be communicated (Chapter 19). Communication of findings should include a written research report, verbal presentations and publication of the study.

The methods and procedures section of the proposal usually concludes with a discussion of study limitations. Limitations in research are methodological and theoretical. The methodological limitations might address areas of weakness in the design, sampling process, sample size, measurement tools or procedures and/or data analysis techniques. Theoretical limitations set boundaries for the generalization of study findings. For example, the accuracy of the theory and conceptual definitions in reflecting reality have a direct impact on the generalization of findings. Theory that has withstood frequent testing provides a stronger framework for the interpretation and generalization of findings.

Frequently, a budget and timetable are included in the appendix of a proposal. The budget projects the expenses for conducting the study. These expenses might include the costs for data collection tools and procedures; special equipment; consultants for data analysis; computer time; travel related to data collection and analysis; typing; copying; and developing, presenting and publishing the final report. Funded studies frequently include investigators' salaries and secretarial costs. The budget includes an estimated cost of each of these items. A timetable is needed to direct the steps of the research project and to facilitate the completion of the project on schedule. A timetable identifies the tasks to be done, who will accomplish these tasks and when they will be completed.

CONTENT OF A CONDENSED PROPOSAL

The content of proposals developed for review by agencies and funding institutions is usually a condensed version of the complete proposal. However, even though these proposals are condensed, the logical links between components of the study should be clearly demonstrated. The proposal should include the statement of problem, previous research that has been conducted in the area (usually limited to no more than three to five studies), research subproblems, framework, variables, design, sample, ethical considerations, plan for data collection and analysis and plans for dissemination of findings.

A proposal developed for a funding institution frequently includes a timetable, budget and description of the facilities. In addition, most of these proposals contain a one-page summary sheet or abstract at the beginning of the proposal, which summarizes steps of the study. The salient points of the study should be included on this page in simple, easy to read, nontechnical terminology. Most of the proposal reviewers for funding institutions are lay persons with no background in research or nursing. Inability to understand the terminology might put the reviewer on the defensive or create a negative reaction, which could lead to disapproval of the study. When multiple studies are examined by funding institutions, the summary sheet is often the basis for final decisions about the study. The summary should be concise, informative and designed to "sell" the study.

Frequently agency members who review research proposals examine the methods and procedures section closely. The proposal should clearly state the section of the institution to be used and the projected time span for the study. In addition, the data collection methods and any involvement of institutional personnel should be addressed. The proposal should identify any expected disruptions in institutional functioning and should indicate the mechanisms planned for preventing these disruptions. The researcher must recognize that anything that slows down or disrupts employee functioning costs the institution money and can interfere with the quality of patient care. Indications in the proposal that the researcher is aware of these concerns and has addressed ways to minimize their effect will increase the probability of obtaining approval to conduct the study.

Agency members are concerned with the feasibility of a research project and are very interested in the projected findings. They want to know how those findings might be used to impact patient care. Agencies have identified certain studies that are needed in their institution. Individuals who conduct studies in these areas are likely to receive not only approval but also support during the conduct of their study.

The proposal should document the researcher's credentials and a vitae may be requested. The committee will be interested in previous research, research publications and clinical expertise, especially if a clinical study is proposed. If the researcher is a graduate student, the committee may request the names of the university committee members and request verification that the proposal has been approved by the student's thesis or dissertation committee and the university human subjects review committee. Information should be provided on how the researcher can be reached, and the offer should be made to provide additional information if needed.

The researcher must determine the policy regarding the use of the facility's name in reporting findings. In many cases, using the facility's name can be done only with prior written administrative approval. The researcher may feel more free to report findings that could be interpreted negatively in terms of the institution if the agency is not identified. In some research institutions, a study cannot be submitted for publication by an employee without prior approval by the institution. Some institutions have rules about authorship of publications. Prior to conducting a study, researchers, especially employees of agencies, must clarify the rules and regulations of an agency regarding publication. In some cases, recognition of these rules must be included in the proposal if it is to be approved.

CONTENT OF A PREPROPOSAL

Sometimes a researcher will send a preproposal or query letter rather than a proposal to a funding institution. A *preproposal* is a short document of four to five pages plus appendix that is written to explore the funding possibilities for a research project. The parts of the preproposal are logically ordered as follows: "(1) letter of transmittal, (2) proposal for research, (3) personnel, (4) facilities and (5) budget" (Malasanos, 1976, p. 223). The preproposal provides a brief overview of the proposed project to determine whether the reader has an interest in funding the project. The proposal would include a statement of the problem, purpose of the research, identification of research subproblems, description of the methodology, methods for communicating the results and, most important, a statement of the significance of the work to knowledge in general and the funding institution in particular. The preproposal can save researchers a great deal of time and emotional energy in seeking funding, because they can focus the submission of their proposals for funding to only those institutions that indicate an interest in their projects. The development of preproposals and seeking funding for research are discussed in Chapter 14.

Seeking Approval for a Study

Initially, proposal reviews were limited to graduate students developing theses or dissertations and researchers seeking grant money. However, as a consequence of stricter rules related to the protection of human subjects, most nursing studies will be reviewed by at least one research committee. Seeking approval through these committees requires skills in writing and, in many cases, verbal defense of a research proposal. Little has been written providing guidance to the researcher who is going through the labyrinth of approval mechanisms. Information has been passed on verbally, or the researcher has had to depend on past experience or luck.

Seeking approval to conduct a study is an action that should be based on knowledge and guided by purpose. There are three purposes for approval mechanisms for studies: (1) to evaluate the quality of the study, (2) to ensure that adequate measures are being taken to protect human subjects and (3) to evaluate the impact of the conduct of the study on the reviewing institution. The desired outcome of the review may be to give approval to initiate data collection, to allow data collection at the reviewing institution or to provide grant funding.

APPROVAL MECHANISMS

An initial step in seeking approval is to determine exactly what committees in what agencies must grant approval before the study can be conducted. The researcher should take the initiative to determine the formal approval mechanisms rather than assume that they will be told if a formal review system exists. In determining the formal review system, the researcher needs to know the number and sequence of the committees that must review and approve a proposal. Sources of this information include administrative personnel, special projects officers or grant officers, clinicians who have previously conducted research or university faculty who are involved in research.

Graduate students usually require approval from their faculty committee, the university human subjects review committee and the committee in the institution where the data are to be collected. University faculty conducting research seek approval through the latter two committees. Nurses employed by an institution must seek approval only at the institution. If outside funding is sought, additional review committees are involved. Not all studies require review by the human subjects review committee; the types of studies that qualify for exempt or expedited review are discussed in Chapter 12.

In some cases, when multiple committees must review the study, an agreement has been made by the respective committees that review for the protection of human subjects will be done by only one of the committees, with the findings of that committee generally being accepted by other committees. For example, if the university human subjects review committee reviewed and approved a proposal for the protection of human subjects, the agency research committee might view that as a sufficient review. Review in other committees is then focused on approval to conduct the study within the institution or decisions to provide study funding.

PREPARING PROPOSALS FOR REVIEW COMMITTEES

The required proposal format and the guidelines for the content of the written proposal are usually available from the committee. Guidelines established by the committee should be followed carefully, particularly page limitations. Some committees refuse to review proposals that exceed these limitations. Reviewers in these committees are usually evaluating proposals in addition to other full-time responsibilities, and reading lengthy proposals utilizes the scarce time of the reviewer. The researcher must also determine if specific forms other than the research proposal must be completed by the review committee. Some additional information that the researcher should determine is when the committee meets, how long before the meeting the material should be submitted, the number of copies of the proposal required and what period of time is usually involved in committee review.

SOCIAL AND POLITICAL FACTORS

Social and political factors play an important role in obtaining approval to conduct a study. It behooves the researcher to treat these situations with as much care as the development of the study. The dynamics of the relationships among committee members is important to assess. This is especially important in the selection of a thesis or dissertation committee, so that the selected members are willing to work productively together.

A thorough assessment of the social and political situation in which the study will be reviewed and implemented may be crucial to the success of the study. The makeup of the committee is often a critical factor in obtaining approval. Committees may be made up of nurse clinicians who have never conducted research, nurse researchers or researchers in other disciplines. The reactions of each of these groups to a study could be very different. Sometimes the committees are made up primarily of physicians, which is often the case in health science centers. Physicians often are not oriented to nursing research methods. The lack of control in nursing studies concerns them, and some believe that the topics of these studies are not important. Sometimes they do not see the nurse researcher as credible because of educational differences, lack of previous experience in research and few published studies.

However, not all physicians hold this view. Many are strong supporters of nursing research, very helpful in suggesting changes in design to strengthen the study and willing to facilitate access to subjects. The researcher should anticipate potential responses of committee members, prepare the proposal to elicit a favorable response and consider means of minimizing negative responses. The researcher would be wise to meet with the chair of the agency research committee early in the development of the proposal. This meeting could facilitate (1) proposal development, (2) rapport of the researcher and agency personnel and (3) approval of the research proposal.

In addition to the formal committee approval mechanisms, the researcher will need the tacit approval of administrative personnel and staff who will be affected in some way by the study. In fact, these personnel can have a great influence on committee members reviewing the proposal. The researcher might seek out someone who is knowledgeable about the political systems of the institution and willing to share this information. There are multiple times and a myriad of ways in which support during data collection can make the difference between a successful and an unsuccessful study.

Obtaining informal approval and support often depends on the way in which a person is approached. The researcher should demonstrate interest in the institution and the personnel as well as interest in the research project. The relationships formed with agency personnel should be equal, sharing ones, because these people can often provide ideas and strategies for achieving success that might never occur to the researcher. These clinicians may be having their first close contact with a researcher, and interpretation of the researcher role and the study may be necessary. Clinicians tend to be more oriented in the present time than are researchers; they need to see the immediate impact of the study. They need to be able to see the possible effects that the study findings can have on nursing practice in their institution.

Conducting nursing research can provide benefits to the institution. Clinicians have an opportunity to see nursing research in action, which can influence their thinking and clinical practice if the relationship with the researcher is positive. Utilization of research findings may be enhanced, and clinicians may even become involved in research activities. All these activities can add prestige to an institution.

VERBAL DEFENSE OF A PROPOSAL

Graduate students conducting theses or dissertations will be expected to meet with their university committee members to verbally defend their proposal. Some institutions also require the researcher to meet with the research committee or a subcommittee to defend a proposal. In a verbal defense, the reviewers can evaluate the researcher as a person, the researcher's knowledge and understanding of the content of the proposal and his or her ability to reason and provide logical explanations related to the study. In a verbal defense of the proposal, the researcher might be able to persuade reluctant committee members to approve the study.

Appearance is important in a personal presentation, because it can give an impression of competence or incompetence. Since these presentations are businesslike, with logical and rational interactions, the researcher should dress in a businesslike manner. A researcher who is casually dressed might be perceived by the committee as not valuing the review process.

Nonverbal behavior of the researcher during the meeting is important. The researcher should appear calm, in control and confident. He or she should develop strategies to keep anxiety as low as possible, such as planning and organizing activities to prevent a time crunch just prior to the meeting. Knowledge of the personalities of committee members, their relationships with each other, vested interests of each member and their areas of expertise are important to know before the verbal defense. The researcher should arrive at the meeting early and assess the environment for the meeting. He or she should consider his or her seating position in relation to other committee members. The researcher should make an effort to place himself or herself so that all members of the committee can see him or her. The researcher should not be on one side of a table and all committee members on the other. This would feel uncomfortable to all those present and could stimulate an atmosphere similar to an interrogation rather than a scholarly interaction. Sitting at the side of a table rather than at the head of the table might be a strategic move to elicit support.

The verbal defense usually begins with a brief presentation of the study by the researcher. The presentation should be carefully planned, timed and rehearsed. Salient points should be highlighted, which can be accomplished by the use of audiovisuals. The presentation is followed by questions from the reviewers. The researcher should be prepared to defend or justify the methods and procedures of the study. Sometimes it is helpful to practice responding to questions related to the study with a friend as a means of determining the best ways to defend ideas without appearing defensive.

The reviewers will often suggest changes in the proposal that might make the study more acceptable. For the student, these suggested changes are part of the learning process in conducting research. The seasoned researcher can also benefit from reviewer suggestions. In institutional reviews, the researcher should attempt to gain a clear understanding of the reasons for the suggested changes and the impact of the changes on the proposed study. In some instances, the suggested changes may be of benefit to the institution but not to the study. If this situation occurs, the researcher must decide whether to accept the changes or approach other institutions. The researcher should remain receptive to suggestions, exploring with the committee the impact of the changes on the proposed study. The researcher should try to avoid taking criticisms of suggested changes personally. This is difficult to do, but it is important to maintaining an objective stance toward the study during the discussion. When the meeting has ended, the researcher should thank the members of the committee for their time. If a decision has not been made during the meeting, the researcher should ask when he or she will know the decision of the committee regarding the study.

CHANGING A PROPOSAL

In almost every proposal developed, some changes or adjustments are required before or during the implementation of the study. However, if the proposal has been approved by agency personnel or representatives of funding institutions, the proposal should not be radically changed. Before changing a proposal, researchers should ask themselves three questions: (1) What is to be changed? (2) Why is the change necessary? and (3) How will the change affect the implementation of the study and the study findings? (Diers, 1979). Students should seek advice from faculty members before making changes. Sometimes it is beneficial for seasoned researchers to discuss their proposed study changes with other researchers or agency personnel for suggestions and additional viewpoints. If a change is necessary, the researcher should revise the proposal and discuss the change with the members of the research committee in the agency where the study is being conducted. The committee members might indicate that the investigator can proceed with the study or that he or she will have to seek approval for the revised proposal. If a proposed study is funded, the necessary changes in the study must be discussed with the representatives of the funding agency. The funding agency has the power to approve or disapprove the changes. However, realistic changes that are clearly described and backed with a rationale will probably be approved.

Example Research Proposal

*Title: Proposed Investigation of Selected Psychosocial
Needs of Family Members of Critically Ill Adult Patients
(Investigator: Linda S. Norris, R.N.)*

BACKGROUND AND SIGNIFICANCE

One of the most important aspects of nursing is the interaction with the family, because the family is the critical intervening variable between society and the individual. Additionally, the quality of family life is closely related to the health of its members, which is particularly important for those who have a family member admitted to an intensive care unit. Traditionally, little attention has been given to the psychosocial needs of critically ill patients, and even less attention has been given to their families' psychosocial needs. Nurses are responsible for intervening with the psychosocial needs of critically ill patients and their families, often without adequate knowledge or background. Nurses' background for this is usually inadequate because of the lack of research regarding what constitutes the psychosocial needs of family members of critically ill adult patients (research problem). The purpose of this study is to describe the perceptions of selected family members and intensive care nurses concerning selected psychosocial needs of family members of critically ill adult patients hospitalized in intensive care.

REVIEW OF RELEVANT LITERATURE

Among the research conducted on the psychosocial needs of family members, Hampe (1975) attempted to determine whether spouses whose mates were terminally ill or had died could recognize their needs. Eight needs were subsequently identified: (1) to be with the dying person; (2) to be helpful to the dying person; (3) to be informed of the mate's condition; (4) to be assured of the comfort of the dying person; (5) to be informed of impending death; (6) to ventilate one's emotions; (7) for comfort and support from family members; and (8) for acceptance, support and comfort from health professionals. Ninety-three per cent of the spouses identified all eight needs. Building on Hampe's study, Breu and Dracup (1978) interviewed husbands and wives of coronary care unit patients. They found Hampe's needs were also experienced by these spouses and identified an additional need: the need for relief of initial anxiety.

A major study of family members' needs was conducted by Molter in 1976. Her research was done to identify what relatives of critically ill patients perceived as their needs, the importance of these needs, and whether or not they were being met. The study encompassed both a structured interview utilizing a list of 45 need statements to be rated on a scale of one to four, as well as personal interviews to check for other, uncovered needs. The universal need identified by Molter (1976) as very important was the need for hope; however, all the needs were considered very important by at least one relative.

The idea that needs are viewed differently by health care providers, patients, and families is supported in the literature in studies by Irwin and Meier (1973) and Carey (1973). During brief visiting periods, nurses often provide routine responses and generalized interventions to family members. These interventions are not adequate, because nursing care is frequently based on the needs as perceived by the staff. Nurses may be expending energy to cope with inaccurate or nonexistent needs. As a replication of Molter's work, this study will focus on selected psychosocial needs of family members of the critically ill adult patient. However, because additional studies have supported the idea of varying perceptions by health care providers and families, this study will also focus on the perception of family members' needs by intensive care nurses.

FRAME OF REFERENCE
Conceptual Framework

The conceptual framework for this study is the open system facet of Bertalanffy's General System Theory. The open system fosters a view of the family members as complex subsystems within the family system, separate from, yet open to, the environment. The health care system is also an open system, and nurses, as subsystems of the health care system, are key figures with whom critically ill adults and their family members interact. While in the health care system, family members experience psychosocial needs and the perceptions of these needs will affect nurses' interactions with family members of critically ill adults. This study will attempt to clarify and compare the perceptions of the subsystems of family members and intensive care nurses, regarding the psychosocial needs of family members of critically ill adults.

Research Subproblems

The specific research questions that will be investigated are (1) What selected psychosocial needs of family members are perceived as most and least important by selected family members of critically ill adult patients hospitalized in intensive care? (2) What selected psychosocial needs are most and least important for family members of critically ill adult patients as perceived by selected intensive care nurses? (3) Is there a difference between selected psychosocial needs of family members of critically ill adult patients as perceived by selected family members and intensive care nurses?

Definitions of Major Variables

1. *Psychosocial Needs*—Those requirements of a person having their origin in the mental apparatus, social actions, and/or the behavior of human beings. The selected psychosocial needs to be measured in this study are those identified in Molter's (1976) questionnaire, The Psychosocial Needs of Relatives of Critically Ill Patients.
2. *Family Member*—An adult (18 years or older) related to the patient by blood, marriage, or adoption who visits while the patient is in an intensive care unit.
3. *Critically Ill Adult*—Those patients (18 years or older) who have spent at least 48 hours in an intensive care unit.
4. *Intensive Care Nurses*—Registered nurses employed full-time in an intensive care unit for more than 6 months.
5. *Perception*—A mental image of a place, person, object, or event, interpreted in light of one's own life experiences (King, 1971).

Assumptions

The assumptions upon which this study will be based include (1) all individuals, therefore critically ill adults, are products of a family unit (Hymovich, 1974); (2) family members influence critically ill adults; (3) intensive care nurses are in a position to recognize the needs of family members; (4) family members will be able to recognize their needs; and (5) family members and intensive care nurses will respond to the research questionnaire truthfully and thoughtfully.

METHODS AND PROCEDURES

Study Design

The design of this study will be a descriptive survey that will be conducted at a major medical center in northeast Texas. Consent for this study will be obtained from the Institutional Review Board for Human Protection of the facility and from the attending physicians for each patient prior to contacting the family members. The study will include a pilot study that will be conducted to determine whether Molter's (1976) 45 need statements reflect the psycho-social needs of the family members of critically ill adult patients as perceived by intensive care nurses and family members. Molter's questionnaire has no recorded reliability and has only content validity, so further testing of the instrument is needed. In the pilot, these need statements will be given to a convenience sample composed of five graduate nursing students who are currently employed in intensive care units and five family members of critically ill adult patients, and a Q sort methodology will be used by the subjects to sort the needs. The data obtained from the Q sort will be used to generate median scores for each need statement. Each need statement with a median score lower than 2.00 will be evaluated for inclusion as is, inclusion with revision or removal from the questionnaire.

Sample and Setting

The setting for this study will be a medical center that houses six intensive care units, and all of these units will be utilized in the study. The sample of convenience will include 40 subjects, composed of 20 intensive care nurses and 20 family members of critically ill adult patients. A family member is defined as an adult who is related to the patient by blood, marriage or adoption who visited while the patient is in an intensive care unit. Only one relative per patient will be included in order to encompass the largest possible representation of patients' families. Intensive care nurses were defined as registered nurses employed full-time in an intensive care unit for more than 6 months.

Data Collection

In this study, the 20 family members will be contacted by the investigator during an ICU visit at least 48 hours after their family member is admitted to an intensive care unit. The 20 nurses will be contacted by the investigator individually in the intensive care unit or as a group following shift report. Each subject will receive the questionnaire as well as verbal and written instructions on how to complete the questionnaire and a demographic data form (Appendix). The verbal and written instructions will be the same for the family members and the intensive care nurses. The written instructions make up the consent form and include who the investigator is, the purpose of the study, and the potential benefits and risks to the subjects (Appendix). (The consent form for this study is included in Chapter 12.)

Data Analysis

A frequency analysis will be used to determine the means for each need statement for the family members and intensive care nurses. Means for the total questionnaire will also be calculated separately for the family members' and nurses' responses. A dummy table for presenting these results is included in this proposal (Table 13–2). An analysis of variance (ANOVA) will be used to determine whether a significant difference at the 0.05 level exists between

TABLE 13–2
Means for Psychosocial and Environmental Needs

Behavioral Needs	Family Members Group Mean	Nurses Group Mean	Difference
1. To feel accepted by hospital staff 2. To talk to the doctor every day 3. To know how the patient was being treated 4. To talk about feelings 5. To have directions as to what to do at bedside . . . . . . 30. To have explanations given in terms that are understandable			

the responses of the family members and the intensive care nurses on the questionnaire. In addition, a reliability alpha will be calculated for the questionnaire. The demographic data will be analyzed with descriptive statistics.

The results the investigator expects are that the need statements on the questionnaire will be marked highly or considered as very important by the family members as well as the nurses. However, the investigator believes that the responses of the family members and intensive care nurses will be significantly different.

Limitations

The findings from this study will have limited generalizability because the study will be conducted in one hospital in a specific geographic location with a limited number of subjects. The intent of this study is to investigate selected psychosocial needs of family members of critically ill adult patients; thus, the study will not provide a complete understanding of the psychosocial needs of family members whose significant others have been hospitalized.

TABLE 13–3
Study Timetable

Task to be Performed	Performer of Task	Completion of Task
1. Receive permission to use tool	Researcher	First month
2. Conduct pilot study	Researcher	First and second month
3. Develop form for demographic data	Researcher	Third month
4. Copy forms for data collection	Researcher	Third month
5. Develop rapport with agency personnel at data collection site	Researcher	Third month
6. Select sample	Researcher	Fourth month
7. Collect data	Researcher	Fourth and fifth month
8. Analyze data	Researcher	Sixth month
9. Interpret results	Researcher	Seventh month
10. Communicate findings	Researcher	1–2 yr

TABLE 13–4
Study Budget

Budget Items	Cost Per Item	Total Cost
1. Printing costs	2000 pages @ 0.05/page	$100.00
2. Consultant costs	4 hr @ 40/hr	$160.00
3. Computer time		$200.00
4. Supplies		$50.00
5. Travel costs		$100.00
6. Typing costs		$200.00
	TOTAL	$810.00

Communication of Findings

The investigator plans to communicate the findings from this study with the nurses in the agency where the study is to be conducted. The researcher also anticipates presenting the findings at research conferences, in particular, the local, yearly research conference. The study findings will also be developed into an article for submission for publication. A timetable (Table 13–3) and budget (Table 13–4) were developed for this study.

Summary

This chapter focused on developing a research proposal and seeking approval for the conduct or funding of a study. A research proposal is a written plan that identifies the major elements of the study such as the research problem, subproblems and frame of reference and outlines the methods and procedures to be used in studying the subproblems. A proposal should communicate a planned research project and demonstrate the qualifications of the researcher to conduct the study. There are usually four sections in a proposal: (1) introduction, (2) review of relevant literature, (3) frame of reference and (4) methods and procedures.

The content of a proposal should be developed with the interest and expertise of the reviewers in mind. Proposals are frequently reviewed by faculty, agency members and representatives of funding institutions. The contents of a proposal vary depending on the reviewer and the guidelines developed for review. The content of a student proposal usually requires greater detail than a proposal developed for review by agency personnel or funding organizations. Sometimes a researcher will send a preproposal or query letter to a funding institution rather than a proposal. A preproposal is a short document of four to five pages plus appendix that is written to explore the funding possibilities for a research project.

A research proposal is a formal way to communicate ideas about a proposed study to obtain approval to conduct the study or to seek funding. Seeking approval for the conduct or funding of a study is a process that involves submission of a proposal to a selected group for review and, in many situations, verbally defending that proposal. There are three purposes for approval mechanisms for studies: (1) to evaluate the quality of the study, (2) to ensure that adequate measures are being taken to protect human subjects and (3) to evaluate the impact of the conduct of the study on the reviewing institution. The researcher must determine exactly what committees in what agencies must give approval before the study can be conducted and/or funded. Then the formal review systems of these committees must be examined. Receiving approval to conduct a study and obtaining funding for a study require preparation of a scholarly proposal, examination of the social and political factors in the review committee and expert defense of the proposal to the review committee.

References

Cook, C. K. (1985). *Line by line: how to edit your own writing*. Boston: Houghton Mifflin Company.

Diers, D. (1979). *Research in nursing practice*. Philadelphia: J. B. Lippincott Company.

Geitgey, D. A. & Metz, E. A. (1969). A brief guide designing research proposals. *Nursing Research*, 18(4), 339–344.

Krathwohl, D. R. (1977). *How to prepare a research proposal* (2nd ed.). Syracuse: Syracuse University Bookstore.

Malasanos, L. J. (1976). What is the preproposal? What are its component parts? Is it an effective instrument in assessing funding potential of research ideas? *Nursing Research*, 25(3), 223–224.

Norris, L. S. (1984). *The psychosocial and environmental needs of family members of critically ill adult patients*. Unpublished master's thesis, University of Texas at Arlington, Arlington, Texas.

Norris, L. S. & Grove, S. K. (1986). Investigation of selected psychosocial needs of family members of critically ill adult patients. *Heart and Lung*, 15(2), 194–199.

Shaw, H. (1963). *Punctuate it right!* New York: Barnes & Noble Books.

Silva, M. C. (1981). Selection of a theoretical framework. In S. D. Krampitz & N. Pavlovich (Eds.), *Readings for nursing research* (pp. 17–28). St. Louis: The C. V. Mosby Company.

The University of Chicago Press (1982). *The Chicago manual of style* (13th ed.). Chicago: The University of Chicago Press.

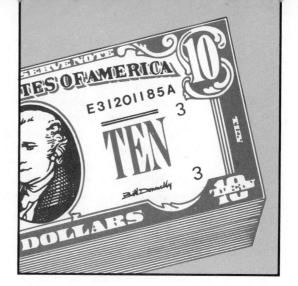

14

Seeking Funding for Research

Seeking funding for research is very important, both for the individual researcher and for the profession. Well-designed studies cost money. As the control of variance in and the complexity of the design increases, the cost of the study tends to increase. By obtaining funding, the researcher can conduct a complex, well-designed study. Funding indicates that the study has been reviewed by others who have recognized its scientific and social merit. In fact, the scientific credibility of the profession comes from the quality of studies conducted by its researchers. Thus, scientific credibility and funding for research are interrelated. Each incidence of funding enhances the status of the researcher and increases the possibilities of greater funding for later studies. In addition, funding provides some very practical advantages. Funding may reimburse part or all of the researcher's salary, releasing the researcher from other responsibilities to devote more time to conducting the study. The availability of research assistants allows the researcher to use time in more productive ways. Thus, skills in seeking funding for research are as important as skills in the conduct of research.

Purposes for Seeking Research Funding

There are two general types of grants sought in nursing: developmental grants and research grants. Developmental grant proposals are written to obtain

383

funding for the development of new programs in nursing such as a program designed to teach nurses to provide a new type of nursing care or a program to implement a new approach to patient care. Although these programs may involve evaluation, they seldom involve research. For example, the effectiveness of a new approach to patient care may be evaluated, but the findings can seldom be generalized beyond the unit or institution in which the patient care was provided. The emphasis is on implementing the new approach to care, not on research. Research grants provide funding specifically to conduct a study. Although there are some similarities between the two types of grant proposals, there are also important differences. The writing techniques and logical flow of ideas, as well as necessary content, differ. This chapter focuses on seeking funding for research.

The researcher may have one of two purposes for seeking research funding. First, the funding may allow the researcher to conduct a single study that is of immediate concern or interest. This is most common among nursing students who are conducting theses and dissertations. However, nurses in clinical practice may also develop an interest in a single study that has emerged from their clinical situation. Except in unusual circumstances, the person seeking funding for a single study, such as a master's thesis, must consider sources of small amounts of money. In most cases, this type of funding will not reimburse for salary and will pay only a portion of the costs of the study. Sources of funding are likely to be those described in the section entitled "Conducting Research On A Shoestring." These funds may pay for the costs of purchasing or printing instruments, postage, research assistants' salaries, travel to data collection sites, costs of computer analyses and/or the services of a statistician. If the researcher's experience is a positive one, further studies may be conducted later in his or her career. Thus, these small grants can be stepping stones to larger grants.

Another purpose for seeking funding is to initiate or maintain a career of conducting research. This is most common among nursing faculty and nurses employed in research positions in health care agencies. The individual planning to continue research activities throughout a career must plan a strategy for progressively more extensive funding of research activities. It is unrealistic, even in a university setting, to expect to be given the time and money needed to conduct full-time research without external funding. An aspiring career researcher must be willing to invest the time and energy into developing skills in grantsmanship. The researcher should develop a goal to obtain funding for that portion of time that it seems desirable to commit to research activities. This goal should be discussed with administrative personnel.

A specific area of study should be selected by the career researcher, and funding should be sought in this area. Funding agencies are usually more supportive of researchers who focus their research efforts in one specific area of study. Each study conducted within this area will increase the researcher's data base and familiarity with the area. Research designs can be built on previous studies. Publications of the studies will give increased credibility to the researcher's work. This base of previous research and knowledge greatly increases the probability of receiving further funding.

Ways to Learn Grantsmanship

Grantsmanship is not an innate skill; it must be learned. Learning the process requires a commitment of both time and energy. However, the payoff can be great. Strategies used to learn grantsmanship are described in the following section and are listed in order of increasing time commitment, involvement and level of expertise needed. The strategies are attending grantsmanship courses, developing a reference group, joining research organizations, participating on research committees or review panels, networking, assisting a researcher and obtaining a mentor.

ATTENDING GRANTSMANSHIP COURSES

Some universities offer elective courses on grantsmanship. Continuing education programs or sections of professional conferences sometimes offer topics related to grantsmanship. The content of these sessions may include the process of writing grants, techniques for obtaining grant funds and sources of grant funds. In some cases, representatives of funding agencies will be invited to explain funding procedures. This information is a useful beginning to developing skills in writing proposals.

DEVELOPING A REFERENCE GROUP

A reference group consists of individuals who share common values, ways of thinking and/or activities. They become a reference group to a particular individual when that person identifies with the group, takes on group values and behaviors and evaluates his or her own values and behaviors in relation to those of the group. For the new researcher moving into grantsmanship, this may mean switching from a reference group that views research and grant writing to be either "over their heads" or not worth their time, to a group for which it is an extremely valued activity. From this group will come the support and feedback necessary to develop grant-writing skills.

JOINING RESEARCH ORGANIZATIONS

Research organizations are another source of support and new information related to grant writing. Specifically in nursing, membership in the Council of Nurse Researchers, a component of the American Nurses Association, is an excellent source of information and support related to grant funding for research. To be a member, one must belong to the American Nurses Association and either be involved in nursing research or be supervising others who are conducting research. The Council is an important reference group for researchers. Communication is maintained through annual meetings and a newsletter.

The Council also provides opportunities for interaction with other nurse researchers on an international and national level and facilitates the development of networks of researchers conducting studies within the same area of interest.

SERVING ON RESEARCH COMMITTEES

Research committees exist in many work and professional organizations. Through membership on these committees, contacts with researchers can be made. Also, many research committees are involved in reviewing proposals for funding of small grants or granting approval to collect data in an institution. Reviewing proposals and making decisions about funding is an enlightening experience. Through these activities, researchers can become better able to critique their own proposals and revise them before submitting them for approval.

NETWORKING

Networking is a process of developing channels of communication between people with common interests in many parts of the country. Contacts may be by mail, telephone or arrangements to meet in groups. Through this process, nurses interested in a particular area of study can maintain contacts made at meetings by exchanging addresses and telephone numbers. These contacts provide opportunities for brainstorming, sharing ideas and problems and discussing grant-writing opportunities. In some cases, it is possible to write a grant to include members of a network in various parts of the country. When a proposal is being developed, the network, which may become a reference group, can provide feedback at various stages of the proposal development.

ASSISTING A RESEARCHER

Volunteering to assist with the activities of another researcher is an excellent way of learning research and grantsmanship. Graduate students can gain this experience by becoming a graduate research assistant. Assisting in the writing of a grant proposal can be particularly helpful. The assistant can read the researcher's proposals that have been funded. Examination of proposals that have been rejected can also be useful if the comments of the review committee are available. The criticisms of the review committee point out the weaknesses of the study and therefore clarify the reasons that the proposal was rejected. Examining these comments with the proposal can increase the insight of the new grant writer and also prepare him or her for similar experiences. However, some researchers are sensitive about these criticisms and may be reluctant to share them. If the experienced researcher is willing, it is enlightening to hear his or her perceptions and opinions about the criticisms.

OBTAINING A MENTOR

Learning effective means of acquiring funding is difficult. Much of the information needed is transmitted verbally, requires actual participation in grant-writing activities and is best learned in a mentor relationship. A mentor is a person who is more experienced professionally and who is willing to "teach the ropes" to a less-experienced professional. This type of relationship requires a great investment of time and energy on the part of both professionals. It has characteristics of both a teacher-learner relationship and a close friendship. Each must have an affinity for the other, from which a close working relationship can be developed. The relationship usually continues for a long period of time. Mentorship is not well developed in nursing. Nurses who have this opportunity should consider themselves fortunate.

Becoming a Funded Researcher

Many of us, as neophyte researchers, have had the fantasy of writing a grant proposal to the federal government or a large foundation for our first study and suddenly achieving "stardom" (100 per cent of our salary and everything needed to conduct the ultimate study, including a microcomputer, a secretary and multiple graduate research assistants). Unfortunately, in reality, this seldom occurs for an inexperienced researcher. The new researcher is usually caught in an interesting "Catch-22." One must be an experienced researcher in order to get funded; however, one needs funding in order to get release time to conduct research. The way out of this dilemma is to design initial studies that can realistically be done without release time and with little or no funding. This approach requires a commitment to putting in extra hours of work, which are often unrewarded, monetarily or socially. However, this type of study, well carried out and published, will provide the credibility one needs to begin the long road to major grant funding.

CONDUCTING RESEARCH ON A SHOESTRING

Ideas for studies often begin in grandiose ways. We envision the "ideal study." We follow all the "rules" in the textbooks and in research courses. When we begin to determine what is needed in time and money in order to conduct this wonderful study, we find our resources sadly lacking. This discovery should not lead us to give up the idea of conducting research. Rather, we should take stock of our resources and determine exactly what realistically can be done. Then we must modify our study to meet existing constraints. The modified study must remain "good research" but be scaled down to an achievable level. This might involve studying only one aspect of the original study, decreasing the number of variables examined, limiting the study to a single site or reducing the sample size. In many cases, only a minimum amount of money is needed to conduct small studies.

The next step is to determine potential sources for this small amount of money. In some cases, management in the employing institution can supply small amounts of money for research activities if a good case is presented for the usefulness of the study to the institution. In many universities, funds are available for intramural grants, which are obtained competitively by submitting a brief proposal to a university committee. Some nursing organizations also have money available for research activities. For example, Sigma Theta Tau, the honor society for nurses, provides small amounts of money for nursing research that can be obtained through submission to national, regional or local review committees. Another source is local volunteer agencies, such as the American Cancer Society and the American Heart Association. Although grants from the national offices of these organizations require greater sophistication in research, local or state levels of the organization may have small amounts of funds available for studies in the area of interest of the organization. Private individuals who are locally active in philanthropy may be willing to provide financial assistance for a small study in an area appealing to them. The trick is to know who to approach and how and when to approach them in order to increase the probability of success. Sometimes this requires knowing someone who knows someone who might be willing to provide financial support. It also requires more assertiveness than the other approaches to funding (Holmstrom & Burgess, 1982).

Requests for funding need not be limited to a single source. If a larger amount of money is needed than can be supplied by one source, funds can be sought from one source for a specific research need and from another source for another research need. Also, one source may be able to provide funds for a small segment of time, and another source can then be approached to provide funding to continue another phase of the study. A combination of these two strategies can also be used.

Seeking funding from local sources generally requires less skill in proposal writing than does other grants. Many times the process is very informal and may require only a two- or three-page description of the study. The important thing is knowing what funds are available and how to apply for them. Some of these funds go unused each year because nurses are not aware of their existence or think that they are unlikely to be successful in obtaining the money. This unused money leads granting agencies or potential granting agencies to the conclusion that nurses do not need more money for research.

Small grants are also available nationally. The American Nurses Foundation awards a number of $2100 grants on a yearly basis. The grants are competitive and are awarded to new investigators with promising ideas. Receiving funding from the American Nurses Foundation is held in high regard. Information is available on these grants from American Nurses Foundation, Inc., 2420 Pershing Road, Kansas City, Missouri 64108. Several of the federal granting agencies also provide New Investigator Awards through the Public Health Service. Information on New Investigator Awards can be obtained from the Federal Register, which is available in local libraries.

These grants do more than just provide necessary funds to conduct the research. They are the first step in being recognized as a credible researcher and in being considered for more substantial grants for later studies. Receipt of these small grants should be listed on vitae or biographical sketches as an indication of first level recognition as a researcher.

OBTAINING FOUNDATION GRANTS

Identifying Potentially Interested Foundations

There are multiple foundations in the United States that provide funding for research. The problem is to determine which foundations have interests in a particular field of study. When these foundations have been identified, the characteristics of the foundation must be determined, appropriate foundations selected, query letters sent, a proposal prepared and, if possible, a personal visit made to the foundation. Several publications list foundations and their interests. However, the most rapid means of determining this information is the Sponsored Programs Information Network (SPIN). This computerized information system assists researchers in locating the most appropriate funding sources to support their research interests. The data base contains approximately 2000 programs to provide information on federal agencies, private foundations and corporate foundations. Most universities and research institutions have access to SPIN.

Determining Foundation Characteristics

When these foundations have been identified, funding information should be gathered from each foundation. A foundation might fund only studies by female researchers or it may be interested only in studies of low-income groups. A foundation may fund only studies being conducted in a specific geographic region. The average amount of money awarded for a single grant and the ranges of awards should be determined for each foundation. If the average award of a particular foundation were $2500 and if $30,000 were needed, that foundation is not the most desirable source of funds. However, if the researcher has never been funded previously and the project could be conducted with less money, an application to that foundation could be combined with applications to other foundations to obtain needed funds. The book most useful in determining this information is *The Foundation Directory*, which is available from The Foundation Center, 888 Seventh Avenue, New York, New York 10106.

Verifying Institutional Support

Grant awards are most commonly made to institutions rather than to individuals. Therefore, it is important to determine the willingness of the institution to receive the grant and support the study. This willingness must be documented in the proposal. Supporting the study involves acceptableness of the study topic; adequacy of facilities and services; availability of space needed for the study; contributions that the institution is willing to make to the study such as staff time, equipment or data processing; and provision for overseeing the use of human subjects.

Sending Query Letters

The next step is to send a query letter to all foundations that might be interested in the planned study. The letter should be addressed to the name of the person who is director or head of the appropriate office rather than an impersonal title such as "Dear Director." Names of directors are available in a number of reference books or can be obtained by calling the organization's switchboard. The letter should reflect spontaneity and enthusiasm for the study. It should open by giving a reason why the letter is being sent to that particular foundation. The query letter should include a succinct description of the proposed study, an explanation of why the study is important, an indication of who will conduct the study, a description of what facilities are required and an expectation of the length and cost of the study. The qualifications of the researchers to conduct the study should be made clear. This is no time to be modest about credentials or past achievements. The letter should inquire about the foundation's interest in the topic and information on how to apply for funds. If a personal visit is possible, the letter should close with a request for an appointment.

Preparing Proposals

In preparing the proposal, guidelines for application should be followed carefully. In some cases, funding is sought from several sources. For example, funding requests may be submitted to an agency of the federal government, a nonprofit volunteer agency and several private foundations. The temptation is to send each source the same proposal, rather than retyping it to meet specific guidelines. This can be offensive and may lead to rejection of the proposal.

Making A Personal Visit

A personal visit to the foundation can be very helpful if this is feasible and permitted by the foundation. Some foundations wish to see only the written application, whereas others prefer personal contact. A visit should never be made without an appointment. Preparations should begin for the visit as soon as the appointment has been made. A fully developed proposal should be written before the visit. This allows the researcher to have carefully thought through the study and have ideas well developed and organized when he or she goes to the foundation. Friedman, speaking at a conference, suggested the following behaviors when visiting foundations: "One, be businesslike; two, be honest; three, know what you mean to do; four, ask questions; and finally, never, never argue with a foundation about the relevance of your proposed project to their program.... If they say it doesn't fit, it doesn't" (White, 1975, pp. 219–220). Although the visit may be informal in a social context, foundation representatives will tend to ask hard, searching questions about the study and the planned use of funding. In a way, it is similar to talking to a banker about a loan. Questions will be geared to help the foundation determine the following: Is the study feasible? Is the institution willing to provide sufficient support to permit the study to be completed? Is the researcher using all available resources? Have other sources of funding been sought? Has the researcher examined anticipated costs in detail and realistically? What are the benefits of conducting the study? Who will benefit, and how? Is the researcher likely to complete the study? Are the findings likely to be published? If the written proposal has not been submitted, the visit is an appropriate time to submit it. Additional information or notes prepared for the visit can be left with the foundation representatives for consideration as the decision is made.

OBTAINING FEDERAL GRANTS

The largest source of grant monies is the federal government—so much so that, in effect, the federal government influences what is studied and what is not. There are multiple divisions of the government through which funding can be requested. Information on funding agencies can be obtained from a document compiled by the federal government: *The Catalog of Federal Domestic Assistance*. This document is available from the U.S. Government Printing Office, Washington, D.C. 20402. Each agency has areas of focus and priorities for funding that change yearly. It is important to know these and prepare proposals within the areas in order to obtain funding. Therefore, calling or writing for the most recent list of priorities is essential. Most agencies funding nursing studies are within the Public Health Service. Therefore, the Public Health Service format for grant applications will be used to describe the process of preparing a grant application. Another important agency for nursing research, the Health Care Financing Administration (HCFA), is not within the Public Health Service and has a different format for grant applications.

Two approaches can be used to seek federal funding for research. The researcher can identify a significant problem, develop a study to examine it and submit a proposal for the study to an appropriate federal funding agency. Or, someone within the federal government can identify a significant problem, develop a plan through which the problem can be studied and publish a "Request For Proposals" (RFP) or a "Request For Applications" (RFA) from researchers.

Researcher-Initiated Proposals

If the study is researcher-initiated, it is useful for the researcher to contact an official within the government agency early in the planning process to inform the agency of the intent to submit a proposal. Each agency has established dates, usually twice a year, when proposals are reviewed. Preparation of the proposal should begin months ahead of this deadline. Agency officials are willing and even eager to provide assistance and feedback to the researcher during the development of the proposal. Proposals can be submitted prior to the deadline for comment and suggestions from agency staff, allowing modification of the proposal to more closely fit within agency guidelines, thus increasing the probability of funding. In many cases, proposals will fit within the interests of more than one government agency. It is permissible and perhaps desirable to request, at the time of submission, that the proposal be reviewed by two agencies within the Public Health Service.

Requests For Proposals (RFP)

An RFP is published in the Federal Register and usually has a deadline date that is only a few weeks after the publication. This means that the researcher must have a fairly good background in the field of study and be able to write a proposal quickly. Since a number of researchers will be responding to the same RFP and only one or a few proposals will be approved, these proposals are competitive. The agency staff will not be able to provide the same type of feedback as occurs in researcher-initiated proposals. The agency should be informed that a proposal is being submitted. Some questions that require clarification about elements of the RFP can be answered; however, other questions cannot be answered. The RFP allows a wide range of creativity in developing a study design to examine the problem of concern. After funding, the researcher has considerable freedom to conduct the study.

Requests For Applications

An RFA is similar to an RFP except that with an RFA, the government agency not only identifies the problem of concern but also describes the design of the study. The RFA is a contract for which researchers bid. A carefully written proposal is still required and must follow the RFA in detail. After funding, federal agency staff maintain much more control and supervision of the process of the study than is the case with an RFP.

Of the three types of proposals, the researcher-initiated proposal is the most important in achieving credibility as a researcher, because the identification of the problem and the design of the study originate with the researcher. However, at the present time, the government is funding fewer researcher initiated-studies and more RFAs. Receiving any federal funding for research is "a feather in the cap" of a researcher and warrants celebration.

Preparing a Grant Proposal

The Public Health Service (PHS) has established guidelines and forms (Form PHS 398) on which to write a proposal. These guidelines and forms are available from any of the PHS agencies and are usually kept in Special Projects Offices in universities and institutions involved in government-funded research. Forms for other agencies can be obtained by writing or calling the agency of interest. These guidelines list the sections to include in a proposal and page limitations for each section. These page limitations must be strictly adhered to. Some agencies will discard a proposal without review if one of the page limitations is not observed. The schedule for submission and review of a PHS proposal and beginning dates for the investigator's study are included in the PHS 398 form.

Proposals should be written with careful attention to detail, and instructions should be followed carefully. Every space on required forms should be completed. Reviewers seem to believe that if a researcher is careful about the details of a proposal, careful attention will also be given to details of the study.

Budget

The budget is one of the most difficult parts of a proposal to formulate and is usually one of the last to be completed. However, because of its importance and difficulty, development of the budget should be one of the first activities initiated. In a PHS grant, items in the budget must be categorized into personnel, consultants, equipment, supplies, travel, patient care, alterations and renovations, consortium/contractual costs and other expenses. These items are considered the *direct costs* of conducting the study. Most PHS grant proposals are for a 3-year period. A detailed budget is presented for the first year, and a less-specific budget is presented for the following years.

BUDGET FOR THE FIRST YEAR

Personnel

In most cases, salaries will be the largest item in the budget. Each individual whose salary will be completely or partially reimbursed by the grant must be identified. The principal investigator is listed first, followed by other professionals, staff personnel (such as secretaries) and students (research assistants).

Principal Investigator

The principal investigator (PI) is the individual who will have primary responsibility for administering the grant and will interact with the government during the period of the grant. The PI will have the responsibility for utilization of grant monies and submitting interim reports to the government on the progress of the study. Although some agencies will allow this responsibility to be shared between two individuals, the PHS will not. Therefore, if there are two or more investigators, one must be designated PI. There is increased status to being the PI, as well as increased responsibilities. If one has functioned as a PI and if the job was well done, that researcher's chances of obtaining funding for later studies are increased. During the funding period, there are opportunities for multiple interactions with agency staff. This provides an opportunity for further learning and developing contacts within the agency, which can be helpful when later grants are considered.

Co-Investigators

Co-investigators are professionals whose salaries are being paid partially or in full by the grant funding. Increasingly, the government is encouraging collaborative research, where the co-investigators may be in fields of study that are different from the PI. This is thought to allow the data to be examined from various perspectives, rather than being interpreted from the point of view of a single discipline. Problems that can occur with this approach include the increased difficulty in decision making and the interpersonal conflicts that can occur as the number of investigators increases.

The names of co-investigators should be included if the individuals are known. In some cases, such as secretary or research assistant, the individual must be hired after the grant is received. In this case, the personnel would be listed simply as secretary or research assistant.

The amount of involvement of each individual identified in the budget must be listed. The government assumes that an individual is committed to a 40-hour week; thus, 40 hours per week is considered 100 per cent time. However, if a person is working more than 40 hours, this is still seen as 100 per cent time. All of the commitments of a person can total only 100 per cent. If a person's salary is being reimbursed by several grants, the sum of committed time cannot be more than 100 per cent. If the proposal is funded, job-related activities must be decreased by the per cent of time committed to grant activities. Therefore, someone who is working 100 per cent of the time as a staff nurse and receives research funding for 50 per cent of salary must decrease staff nurse activities by 50 per cent. The proposal must show documentation that the employing institution will permit this decrease in job activities.

Salaries for each individual for the per cent of time involved in the study must be listed for the first year of the proposed study. In most cases, the salary remains consistent with salary levels of the supporting institution. The cost of fringe benefits paid by the employing institution must also be listed in a separate column. Fringe benefits include such items as workman's compensation, social security, retirement, unemployment insurance and health insurance.

Consultants

Consultants are individuals hired for a specific task during the study period. They may be paid by the hour or by the day. Although consultants are more likely to be used in a developmental grant, they are occasionally used in a research grant. For example, a computer programmer could be consulted to develop programs for data analysis, a statistician could be hired during the data analysis period or a psychologist could be employed to evaluate scores on psychosocial instruments.

Equipment

Each piece of equipment needed to conduct the study that must be purchased with grant money must be listed with the cost for purchase or leasing. These costs must be documented. This is often done by xeroxing the catalog page or other written documentation of the cost and including it in the appendices. However, catalog costs can be out of date. It is often safer to check with a vendor to determine current prices. Some researchers are inclined to include within the budget every item which can even loosely be connected with the study, such as microcomputers, typewriters and other office equipment. However, caution should be exercised. The supporting institution is expected to provide at least some resources for use with the study. If the equipment is available from the supporting institution, it will probably not be provided through the grant. If the proposal includes requests for unnecessary equipment, there is a greater likelihood of rejection. On the other hand, if necessary equipment is not requested, the study can be impaired.

Supplies

Supplies include all consumable goods needed during the study. This may include office supplies such as file folders, index cards and paper. It can also include such items as xeroxing, printing of instruments or clinical supplies unique to the conduct of the study. The cost for psychosocial instruments, which are ordered from a psychological testing company for the study, are listed under the supply section of the proposal.

Travel

Travel costs included are those required to conduct the study. For example, graduate research assistants may have to travel to a patient's home to collect data, or the investigator may have to travel to another city for some purpose directly related to the study. These costs should be documented to the extent possible. Travel costs for presenting the findings should be listed in this section.

Patient Care Costs

In some studies, patients are paid to participate in the study. In other situations, the care of patients is increased because they are participating in the study. For example, laboratory or x-ray studies that are beyond general patient care guidelines may be included. These costs are more common in medical research than in nursing research, but they can occur in clinical nursing studies.

Alterations and Renovations

In some cases, the facilities in which the study will be conducted must be modified for the purposes of the study. General remodeling is not allowed; however, a doorway may have to be moved or a partition installed or removed. The costs for these changes must be clearly identified.

Consortium/Contractual Costs

In some studies, agreements are made with other institutions or agencies to conduct portions of the study. In a consortium, professionals in several institutions are working jointly on the study. Because the study must be awarded to one specific institution (usually the institution employing the PI), the other institutions make up a consortium. Arrangements are made to pay portions of salaries or other costs incurred by each institution. A contract is made with another institution or agency that has agreed to take responsibility for a particular portion of the study. For example, a contract might be made with a psychological institution to score and analyze instruments used in a study. A contract would be drawn up with the institution agreeing to perform the desired activities for a specific fee. The contract would be included in the proposal.

Other Expenses

Miscellaneous expenses that do not pertain to other categories are included in this section. Items that might be listed include computer costs, library searches and expenses unique to a specific study.

BUDGET FOR THE ENTIRE PROJECT PERIOD

In most cases, federal grants are continued for more than 1 year. For each year of funding, a total amount needed for salaries is listed. This total amount should take into consideration such factors as promotions, salary increases and increases in fringe benefits that may occur. Many institutions will not pay the extra amount if it has not been provided for in the grant. Costs must be listed for each year for each budget item. The researcher must take into consideration potential increases as a result of economic inflation in areas such as travel. In some cases, researchers may use an inflation factor for each year for some items. For example, if a 5 per cent inflation factor were used, 5 per cent of the present cost of travel could be added to the budgeted amount requested for travel for the following year to cover increasing costs.

BUDGET JUSTIFICATION

After completing the budget, each item in the budget must be justified. This means that the researcher must explain, clearly and succinctly, how each person considered to be personnel will be used in the study, how his or her time will be used, why each item listed is necessary for the study, exactly how travel will be used and how the costs of computer time have been calculated. Some grant writers believe that the budget should be "padded," knowing that the reviewers will cut some items when the grant is reviewed. Other writers believe the reviewers are negatively influenced by "padding," which they readily recognize from their experience in reviewing grants, and may be more likely to reject the grant. A middle road between extreme austerity and heavy padding would seem advisable. If needed items are not included, reviewers may question the ability of the researcher to actually carry out the study. If the budget goes far beyond reasonable limits, the proposal may be rejected out of hand. It is difficult for the inexperienced grant writer to know reasonable limits. Consultation with an experienced grant writer can be helpful.

INDIRECT COSTS

Indirect costs are those costs incurred by the institution in administering the grant. These costs are, in a way, invisible; but if some effort is not made to reimburse for them, heavily funded institutions could experience severe difficulties. These costs include administrative costs, library costs, costs of secretarial time, costs for use of space and utilities, maintenance costs and cleaning costs. These indirect costs are negotiated between the institution and the agency. They are not included in the proposal, and the researcher is not usually responsible for negotiating them.

Biographical Sketches

A biographical sketch is included for each professional person included in the budget, starting with the PI. The sketch is limited to two pages and should include educational background, employment pattern, significant publications and papers presented at national meetings. Some researchers interpret "significant" to mean those publications and papers pertaining to the topic of the proposed study. It is through the biographical sketch that the reviewers judge the credibility of the researchers and their capacity to conduct the proposed study. They will be interested in publications because of the importance placed on publishing the findings from federally funded studies. Biographical sketches should be carefully developed and should describe the researchers in the most favorable way possible.

Resources and Facilities

In this section, the researcher should carefully describe the institution(s) in which the study will be conducted. Although these institutions may be familiar to the researcher, they are not usually known by the reviewers. This section is written assuming a total lack of familiarity with the institution. Size, numbers of people served, history of the institution, features that reflect quality, unique characteristics and values or philosophies that characterize the institution should be described. Details should be provided of the area in which the study will be conducted, describing, for example, the environment, the dimensions of space, anything that may be pertinent to the conduct of the study or the credibility of the institution.

Research Plan

This section of the proposal is similar to any other research proposal. Differences are the page limitations, the absence of a literature review as such and the necessity to document previous work of the researcher. The following format is not required but rather "suggested." Regardless of the format, the following questions should be answered: What do you intend to do? Why is the work important? What has already been done? How are you going to do the work? Because this section is likely to be extensive, a face page with a table of contents for the section is helpful to the reviewers.

AIMS

Aims are similar to purpose(s) of a study. Aims, as such, do not have to be listed in this section. This section is intended to provide a concise statement of what the study is intended to accomplish. Instead of aims, statements may be in the form of objectives, research questions or hypotheses. This section is limited to one page.

SIGNIFICANCE

The significance section combines the literature review and the significance components of a typical proposal. This section is limited to three pages and should (1) provide the background that led to the present proposal, (2) provide a critical evaluation of existing knowledge in the area and (3) identify gaps in the knowledge base that are expected to be filled by the present study. The importance of the study must be clearly explained. As part of indicating the importance, the aims, objectives, research questions or hypotheses must be linked to longer term objectives related to that field of knowledge.

PRELIMINARY STUDIES

This section can address two aspects of previous work related to the study: (1) previous studies conducted by the PI and co-investigators that document the credibility of the researchers and logically lead to the present study, and (2) preliminary or pilot studies conducted in preparation for the present study. The pilot studies may have been performed to establish validity and reliability of a measurement instrument, refine a data collection technique or conduct the entire study on a small sample. Diagrams, tables, graphs and charts related to the studies discussed may be included in this section or attached to the appendices. This section must sell the reviewers on the fact that the described investigators are well qualified to conduct the study and, in the case of RFPs and RFAs, are better qualified than other applicants.

EXPERIMENTAL DESIGN AND METHODS

The methodology of the study is discussed in detail in this section. Each portion of the methodology should easily relate to the aims, objectives, research questions or hypotheses. The methodology must be clear without being wordy. Reviewers have many studies to read in a short period of time. They often have a negative reaction to an unnecessarily long treatise on the topic.

Framework

The PHS does not require a framework for the study. However, when it is included, the beginning of the methodology section is an appropriate place to discuss it, since all other segments of the methodology should relate to it. The writer should keep in mind that reviewers will often be from other disciplines and may not be familiar with the theorists discussed. Therefore, the theoretical discussion should not assume any previous knowledge of the theories being explained. The framework section should be kept concise. The entire theoretical base does not need to be described, but the concepts used in the study should be defined. Relationships between concepts explained by the theory should be described. Propositions from the theory that are being tested in the study should be stated.

Sample

This section should include criteria for selection of subjects, strategies for obtaining subjects and the number of subjects anticipated to be included in the study. Researchers tend to expect to obtain more subjects than are actually included in the study. Granting agencies are particularly sensitive to decreases in sample size because of its effects on the generalizability of the findings. In some cases, funding may be withdrawn because sample size does not reach the numbers originally predicted. Therefore, the researchers should be particularly realistic in statements of sample size.

Instrumentation

Each tool used should relate back to the aims section. All measurement tools to be used in the study should be described in detail, with particular emphasis on validity and reliability. The length of time required for measurement with the tool should be discussed. Samples of questionnaires or scales should be included in the appendices. If mechanical equipment will be used for measurement, the equipment and the process of taking the measurement should be described in detail. If a tool is copyrighted, a permission letter from the copyright owner should also be included in the appendices.

Protocol for Data Collection

The proposal must give a step-by-step description of data collection techniques. If time permits, a pilot study should be conducted to test the data collection technique so that problems can be solved before submission of the proposal. Grant reviewers, who are experienced researchers, will usually recognize inherent problems with a data collection protocol before they occur. A pilot study is also useful for determining the length of time required for data collection. Frequently, the time required for data collection is underestimated by the researcher, as is the time required for completing data analysis and interpreting findings.

Data Analysis Techniques

Statistical techniques to be used in data analysis should be described, along with rationale for the selection of those particular statistics. This section should also describe the form in which results will be reported. If a statistical level of significance will be used, the level that will be considered significant must be stated in the proposal.

Sequence of Study Activities

A timetable showing the sequence of study activities must be developed and included in the proposal. It is helpful to make the timetable in the form of a table or graph. (See Table 13–3 in Chapter 13.) The timetable should show the activities of each investigator during the various stages of the study. It is important to allow sufficient time for the completion of written reports that must be made to the grantors. For a study lasting 3 or 4 years, it is reasonable to plan 6 months for analysis of data and completion of the final report.

New Methodologies

This section is usually brief but should address any new methods used in the course of the study. This might include new data collection techniques or new approaches to statistical analysis.

Potential Difficulties

The researcher should carefully think through difficulties that might occur in the course of the study. These difficulties should be pointed out and examined rather than glossed over. In most cases, the difficulties are obvious to the reviewers who are interested in whether the investigators are aware of them and prepared to deal with them. Difficulties might involve getting various agencies to work together or problems that might occur in attempting to gain access to specific data.

Limitations

Limitations to generalizing the study findings should be examined at the time of the proposal rather than on completion of the study. Therefore, limitations must be discussed in the proposal. Limitations in a grant proposal might be theoretical or methodological, as discussed in Chapters 3 and 13.

Alternative Approaches to Achieving Aims

Other strategies (alternative approaches) that could be used to conduct the study must be discussed. Potential difficulties and limitations for these alternative approaches should be identified. The selected design of the study should minimize both difficulties and limitations.

Human Subjects

Most nursing studies involve human subjects. This topic is discussed in Chapter 12. In order to protect human subjects, the proposal must describe the subject population, sample size and sample selection criteria such as age ranges, gender, ethnic background and health status. Rationale for the use of particular classes of subjects who are likely to be vulnerable, such as children or pregnant women, must be justified. Sources of data, recruitment of subjects and consent procedures must be described in detail. Potential risks to the subjects and the likelihood and the seriousness of each risk must be examined. Procedures for protecting the subjects against risks and their likely effectiveness must be explained. The researcher must discuss the risk-benefit ratio for the proposed study.

Literature Cited

References are listed only for material cited in the text of the proposal. Footnotes are not used. An exhaustive listing of all sources in which the topic of the study is discussed is not required. The major works in the area, primarily discussed in the "Significance" and "Preliminary Studies" sections, are listed in this section. Works reported should be relevant and current.

Appendices

Appendices should be listed alphabetically (for example, Appendix A). Each appendix should have a face page, with the appendix and contents listed.

Although pagination of the appendices is not required, it is very useful to the reviewers. Another helpful strategy is to include, at the beginning of the appendices, a table of contents of the appendices. The appendices should include letters in support of the study, instruments used in the study, tables or graphs referred to in the "Preliminary Studies" section, examples of relevant publications written by the investigators and other material specific to the study.

The Abstract

Although the abstract is one of the first pages of the proposal, it is usually completed last. In some cases, funding decisions are made based primarily on the abstract; therefore, the abstract should be carefully written to include pertinent information such as essential elements from each of the sections of the proposal previously described. Abstracts have space limitations and thus are difficult to write. Every word must be essential, which usually requires several revisions. An abstract should be written so that it is easily understandable by lay people and those in other professions.

The Federal Grant Review Process

After submission, grants are initially reviewed by staff members of the agency. These staff members then assign the proposal to a study section for scientific evaluation. The proposal is sent to two or more researchers considered qualified to evaluate the proposal. These scientists prepare a written critique of the study. The proposal is then sent to all the members of the study section. Each member may have 50 to 100 proposals to read in a 1- to 2-month period. Then, a meeting of the full study section is held. Each application is discussed by those who critiqued the proposal. Other members comment or ask questions. A majority vote determines whether the proposal is approved, disapproved or deferred. Approved proposals are assigned a numerical score used to develop a priority rating (White, 1975). A study that is approved is not necessarily funded. The PI will be notified at this point, whether or not the study was approved. At a later time, approved studies are further examined to determine actual funding. Funding begins with the proposal that has the highest rank order. Funding of proposals will continue until available funds are depleted. This process can take 6 months or longer. Because of this process, actual receipt of the money to initiate a grant may not occur for up to a year after submission of the proposal.

In many cases, researcher-initiated proposals are rejected after the first submission. The critique of the scientific committee is sent to the researcher on a "pink sheet." Often the agency staff will encourage the researcher to rewrite the proposal using the comments on the "pink sheet" and resubmit it to the same agency. The probability of funding is often greater the second time if suggestions are followed.

Review of RFPs or RFAs is slightly different. These applications first go through a technical (scientific) evaluation. Those proposals that pass the technical review are then evaluated from the standpoint of cost. After the financial review, the contracting officer may negotiate levels of funding with the proposal writers. Funding decisions are made based on identification of well-designed proposals that offer the best financial advantage to the government (White, 1975).

"Pink Sheets"

The reaction of a researcher to a pink sheet is usually anger and then depression. The proposal is rejected by the researcher, stuffed in a bottom drawer somewhere and forgotten. There really seems to be no way to avoid the anger and depression after a rejection because of the amount of emotional and time investment required to write a proposal. However, after a few weeks, it is advisable to examine the "pink sheet" again. The comments can be very useful in rewriting the proposal for resubmission. The learning experience of writing the proposal and evaluating the comments will also provide a background for seeking funding for another study.

A skilled grant writer will have approximately one proposal funded for every five submitted. The average is far less than this. Thus, the researcher must be committed to repeated efforts of proposal submission in order to achieve grant funding.

Receiving a Grant

Receiving notice that a grant proposal has been funded is one of the highlights in a researcher's career and warrants a celebration. However, when the euphoria begins to fade and reality sets in, careful plans must be made for implementing the study. To avoid problems, consideration should be given to managing the budget, hiring and training research personnel, maintaining the promised timetable and coordinating activities of the study.

MANAGING THE BUDGET

Although the supporting institution has ultimate responsibility for dispensing and controlling grant monies, the PI is also responsible for keeping track of budget expenditures and making decisions about how the money is to be spent. If this is the first grant received, the PI, who has no previous administrative experience, may need to seek some initial guidance in how to keep records and make reasonable budget decisions. If funding is through a federal agency, interim reports will include reports on the budget as well as the progress of the study.

TRAINING RESEARCH PERSONNEL

When a new grant is initiated, time must be set aside for interviewing, hiring and training grant personnel. Personnel who will be involved in data collection must learn the process, and then data collection must be refined to ensure that each data collector is consistent with other data collectors. This is referred to as *interrator reliability*. The PI must also set aside time to oversee the work of personnel hired for the grant.

MAINTAINING THE STUDY SCHEDULE

Plans must be made to initiate study activities on a time schedule in order to keep up with the planned timetable. If this is left to just happen, other work activities are likely to take precedence, delaying the grant work. Unexpected events do happen; however, careful planning can keep their impact to a minimum. The PI should constantly refer back to the timetable to evaluate progress. If the project falls behind schedule, actions must be taken to return to the original schedule or to readjust the timetable. Keeping on schedule will be a plus when it is time to apply for the next grant.

COORDINATING ACTIVITIES

During a large study, with several investigators and other grant personnel, coordinating activities can be a problem. It is useful to arrange meetings of all grant workers at intervals to facilitate sharing of ideas and problem solving. Records should be kept of discussions at these meetings. These actions can lead to a smoother functioning team.

Submitting Reports

Federal grants require the submission of interim reports. The federal agency involved will send written guidelines for the content of the reports, which will consist of a description of grant activities and expenditures of grant monies. There are usually set deadlines for the submission of these reports. It is important to set aside time for the preparation of the report, which usually requires compiling of figures and tables. In addition to the written reports, it is often useful to maintain contact by telephone with the appropriate staff at the federal agency.

Planning Your Next Grant

The researcher should not wait until funding from the first grant has ended to begin seeking funds for a second study because of the length of time required to obtain funding. In fact, it may be wise to have several studies in various stages of implementation ongoing. For example, one could be planning a study, collecting data on a second study, analyzing data on a third study and writing papers for publication on a fourth study. A full-time researcher could have completed one funded study, be in the last year of funding for a second study, be in the first year of funding for a third study and be seeking funding for a fourth study. This may sound unrealistic, but with planning, it is not. This strategy not only provides continuous funding for research activities but also facilitates a rhythm of research that prevents time pressures and makes use of lulls in activities in a particular study. To increase the ease in obtaining funding, the studies should be within the same area of research, each building on the previous studies.

Example Funding Proposal

An example proposal requesting funding for an exploratory survey follows. The proposal, as presented, is appropriate for submission to private funding agencies. A proposal to federal funding agencies is much more extensive.

NURSES AND SMOKING STUDY

Specific Aims

The aim of this study will be to examine patterns of smoking among nurses. Three populations will be examined: nurses who smoke, nurses who previously smoked and nurses who have never smoked. A randomly selected sample of nurses from across the United States will be surveyed to gather data on demographics, places of employment, attitudes about smoking, patterns of smoking, state of health and past efforts to stop smoking. The study will use an exploratory survey design. Findings will be used to develop specific strategies to help nurses stop smoking. The proposed budget for 3 years is $246,570.

Research Objectives

Three research objectives will be addressed: (1) to describe characteristics of the smoking nurse; (2) to examine differences among the smoking, exsmoking and nonsmoking nurses; and (3) to examine relationships among variables within the populations studied.

Significance and Literature Review

Smoking-related diseases among women are now of epidemic proportions. Although overall, smoking among health professionals has markedly decreased, smoking levels of nurses have remained high. In women, regular cigarette smoking usually begins between the ages of 12 and 25 years. Only a few published studies have examined smoking patterns among nurses. A study reported by the National Clearinghouse for Smoking and Health (USPHS, 1976) reported that the percentage of smokers among nurses had increased from 37 per cent in 1969 to 39 per cent in 1975. The percentage of smokers among physicians declined from 30 per cent in 1969 to 21 per cent in 1975. Smoking among dentists declined from 34 per cent in 1969 to 28 per cent in 1975. Smoking among pharmacists declined from 35 per cent in 1969 to 28 per cent in 1975. The percentage of nurses who smoked was greater than that of female adults in general and working female adults. Harvey (1983), reporting findings from the Harvard Nurses' Health Study (n = 121,964), reported that

34.5 per cent of nurses smoked. Dalton and Swenson (1983), surveying a random sample of registered nurses, found that nurses are not quitting smoking at the rate that occurs in other groups of smokers. Many nurses have made no attempt to stop smoking. Wagner (1985) reported a higher percentage of nurses who had never smoked (45 per cent compared with 40 per cent), a lower percentage of former smokers (27 per cent compared with 39 per cent) and a lower percentage of current smokers (28 per cent compared with 39 per cent) than the National Clearinghouse survey (USPHS, 1976).

Normally, women do not do more poorly than men in achieving initial cessation in treatment studies, but there is evidence to support the assumption that women are less successful in maintaining their abstinence (Gritz, 1978; Report of Surgeon General, 1981). A survey of young women (aged 18 to 35 years) revealed that light smokers had the greatest success rate in cessation (Yankelovich, Skelly & White, 1977). Present cessation programs do not seem to be effective with nurse populations. Factors that seem to influence the degree of recidivism among those who do attempt to stop smoking seem to be stress, weight control and self-esteem (Perri, Richards & Schultheis, 1977; Peterson, Lonergan, Hardinge & Teel, 1968; Russell, 1970; Rode, 1972).

Summary

Research is providing increasing bits of information in effective strategies to facilitate cessation of smoking. The major problems in motivating women to stop smoking appear to be psychosocial factors, the pharmacological effects of nicotine and physical dependency. Women seem to be less successful than men in maintaining their abstinence, and this appears to be due to psychosocial and demographic factors. Few studies have been conducted on the psychosocial and demographic factors specific to the nursing population. This information is needed to develop programs that are effective in motivating nurses to stop smoking and to help them remain nonsmokers for the remainder of their lives.

Framework

Studies now define four stages in a smoker's career: initiation, maintenance, cessation and resumption, or relapse (Lichtenstein & Brown, 1980). As one would speculate, psychosocial factors are the determinants of initiation. Together with cognitive factors and the pharmacological effects of nicotine, the psychosocial factors form the maintenance stage. Paradoxically, they are also responsible for the cessation stage, although the level of physical dependence plays a large role in success or failure. Relapse is an uncharted area and one that requires studying in greater depth. Psychosocial factors certainly play a large role, but so do social stress, withdrawal symptoms and other factors such as weight gain.

Data Collection Process

Subjects will be randomly selected for the study from the membership lists of the American Nurses Association. A questionnaire will be mailed to those selected. One month later, a second questionnaire will be mailed to those who failed to respond to the first questionnaire. A third abbreviated questionnaire will be mailed to those who failed to respond to the first two forms.

Instrument

The questionnaire will be a modified form of an instrument used in a study of smoking patterns of nurses in the state of Texas, conducted through the American Cancer Society. The instrument will be designed to allow scantron techniques to enter the data into the mainframe computer at the University of Texas at Arlington and yet allow the respondent to mark his or her answers on the same form on which the survey questions appear.

Analysis of Data

Data analysis will include descriptive statistics, Pearson's correlations, analysis of variance and regression analysis. Data will be interpreted within a motivation framework, and findings will be used to design strategies to assist nurses to stop smoking. The findings of the study will be submitted for publication in national journals.

Personnel

The study will require 50 per cent time from a nurse researcher, 100 per cent secretarial time, two graduate research assistants and consultant time from a SAS Programmer for data management.

Budget

	Year 1	Year 2	Year 3
Personnel	$ 50,000	$ 52,500	$ 55,125
PI	(22,000)	(23,100)	(24,255)
Secretary	(12,000)	(12,600)	(13,230)
Graduate Research Asst	(12,000)	(12,600)	(13,230)
Computer Programmer (12.00/Hr.)	(4,000)	(4,200)	(4,410)
Computer time	1,000	5,000	5,000
Printing	5,000	0	0
Postage	5,000	5,000	0
Travel	5,000	5,000	5,000
Consumables	1,000	1,000	1,000
Total	$ 67,000	$ 68,500	$ 66,125

TOTAL FOR 3 YEARS $201,625

SUMMARY

Seeking funding for research is very important, both for the individual researcher and for the profession. Researchers may have one of two purposes for seeking research funding. First, the funding may allow the researcher to conduct a single study that is of concern or interest. The second purpose is to initiate or maintain a career of conducting research. To receive funding, the skill of grantsmanship must be learned. Strategies used to learn grantsmanship are attending grantsmanship courses, developing a reference group, joining research organizations, participating on research committees or review panels, networking, assisting a researcher and obtaining a mentor.

Writing a grant proposal for funding requires a commitment to putting in extra hours of work, which are often unrewarded, monetarily and/or socially, at first. The first studies are usually conducted on a "shoestring" budget. A small amount of money might be obtained from a variety of sources such as management in employing institutions, universities (intramural grants) or nursing organizations. A study that is well carried out and published using limited funds will often give the credibility one needs to begin the long road to major grant funding.

Larger sums of money can be sought by writing foundation grants. The researcher must initially identify potentially interested foundations and determine the characteristics of those foundations. Foundation grant awards are most commonly made to institutions rather than to individuals. Therefore, it is important to determine the willingness of the institution to receive the grant and support the study. The institution's willingness must be documented in the proposal. Query letters are sent to all foundations that might be interested in the planned study. If a foundation is interested, a personal visit, if possible, should be made. The grant proposal must be developed according to the guidelines of the foundation.

The largest source of grant monies is the federal government. Two approaches can be used to seek federal funding for research. The researcher can identify a significant problem, develop a study to examine it and submit a proposal for the study to an appropriate federal funding agency. Or, someone within the federal government can identify a significant problem, develop a plan through which the problem can be studied and publish a "Request for Proposals" (RFP) or a "Request for Applications" (RFA) from researchers. The guidelines for preparing a grant proposal for the Public Health Service (PHS) were described in this chapter. The major sections of this grant proposal include budget (budget for the first year, budget for the entire project, budget justification and indirect costs), biographical sketches, resources and facilities, research plan, human subjects, literature cited, appendices and abstract.

After submission, grants are initially reviewed by staff members of the agency. Researchers who are writing their first federal grant frequently receive rejection notices. The critique of the scientific committee is sent to the researcher on a "pink sheet." Often the agency staff will encourage the researcher to rewrite and resubmit the proposal using the comments on the "pink sheet." When a grant proposal is funded, it is a time of celebration for the researcher. However, then the researcher must make careful plans for implementing the study. The principal investigator (PI) is responsible for keeping up with the budget, training research personnel, keeping up the schedule and coordinating activities. Federal grants require the submission of interim reports. A researcher should not wait until funding from the first grant has ended to begin seeking funds for a second study and then a third and then a fourth.

References

Abdellah, F. G. (1977). U.S. Public Health Service's contribution to nursing research—past, present, future. *Nursing Research*, 26(4), 244–249.

Fuller, E. O. (1982). The pink sheet syndrome. *Nursing Research*, 31(3), 185–186.

Gortner, S. R. (1981). Researchmanship: the politics of research revisited. *Western Journal of Nursing Research*, 3(3), 309–311.

Gortner, S. R. (1982a). Researchmanship: structures for research productivity. *Western Journal of Nursing Research*, 4(1), 119–124.

Gortner, S. R. (1982b). Researchmanship: research funding sources. *Western Journal of Nursing Research*, 4(2), 248–250.

Gortner, S. R. (1983). Researchmanship: maintaining the momentum. *Western Journal of Nursing Research*, 5(1), 104–106.

Holmstrom, L. L. & Burgess, A. W. (1982). Low-cost research: a project on a shoestring. *Nursing Research*, 31(2), 123–125.

Hyde, A. (1977). The American Nurses' Foundation's contributions to research in nursing. *Nursing Research*, 26(3), 225–227.

Meisenhelder, J. B. (1982). Networking and nursing. *Image*, 14(3), 77–80.

Oakley, D. (1981). A practical guide to political effectiveness: the case of federal funding for nursing research. *Nursing Research*, 30(6), 360–365.

Todd, A. H. & Gortner, S. R. (1982). Researchmanship: removing obstacles to research in the clinical setting. *Western Journal of Nursing Research*, 4(3), 329–333.

United States Department of Health and Human Services. (1982). *Application for public health service grant*. Instruction Sheet for PHS 398, Rev. 5/82 OMB No. 0925–0001.

White, V. P. (1975). *Grants: how to find out about them and what to do next*. New York: Plenum Press.

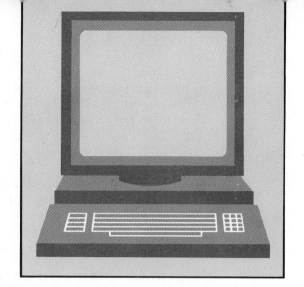

15

Using Computers for Research

The use of computers in society has soared in the last 10 years with the advancement of computer technology. Technological advances have increased the availability of computer equipment, while decreasing the equipment cost. An increasing number of health care systems are using computers, which has had an impact on nursing practice. In health care settings, computers are being used to calculate laboratory results; monitor patient responses (vital signs, fluid balance, cardiac arrhythmias, and so on); and store data such as patient records, nursing notes, and nursing care plans. In the near future, nurses will commonly use computers to generate nursing diagnoses and develop care plans based on these diagnoses. The data being computerized by health care systems hold many opportunities for clinical nursing research.

The use of computers by nurse researchers has increased at a rapid rate. Researchers are using computers to conduct literature searches; input, store and retrieve data; perform statistical analyses; and develop research reports. These activities can be performed by different types of computers: microcomputer, minicomputer and mainframe computer. Using a computer for research requires learning about the computer system, the process of computerizing data and the data analysis programs. The decision to use a computer in conducting a specific study must be made during the development of the proposal, because computer use requires planning. This chapter provides a background for determining when and how to use a computer in research by focusing on the computer system and computer-related research activities.

Computer System

Many nurses are intimidated by the complex computer equipment and overwhelmed by the computer's speed and multitude of functions. But those new to the computer should remember that it is merely an electronic device that requires human instructions in order to operate. With instructions from a computer user, the computer can load, process and store incoming data and report results. *Incoming data* are sets of facts that require processing, and *results* refer to data that have been processed to make them meaningful and useful to the user (Stern & Stern, 1983).

Computers, like any machine, require that the user take some time and effort to learn to operate them. Researchers, as computer users, should know the capabilities and limitations of the computer and the two basic parts of the computer, the hardware and software. In addition, they need some understanding of the different types of computers that are available.

COMPUTER CAPABILITIES

Computers have become invaluable to researchers because of their speed and accuracy. The computer has the capacity to process data in nanoseconds (billionths of a second) and picoseconds (trillionths of a second). Calculations that took humans weeks, months and even years to perform are performed by computers in seconds. With the advent of computers, researchers have been freed to perform more creative functions such as interpreting findings and generating additional problems for study.

In addition to speed, the computer is designed to virtually ensure the accuracy of the data that are processed. The statistical calculations conducted by the computer are frequently more accurate and reliable than those conducted by humans. This does not mean that the results produced by the computer are without errors; however, the errors that occur are almost always caused by humans rather than the computer. The two most frequent causes of errors in computer processing are inputting the data inaccurately (input errors) and providing inaccurate instructions (programming errors).

Computers are also capable of *iterative operations*, or the performance of a series of fixed functions numerous times without boredom or fatigue. For example, a computer could be programmed to calculate the mean and standard deviation for medication errors on every unit in the hospital for every week of the year. The computer's speed, accuracy and iterative ability frequently make the device cost-effective for the researcher. However, the cost saved with the computer is sometimes offset by the cost required to learn the computer system or to hire someone to operate the system.

Another valuable capability of the computer is the storage of data. The computer can store vast amounts of data in a small space and can rapidly make those data available to the user. For example, the results of the laboratory tests of every patient in the hospital could be stored by a computer, and the researcher could easily access the laboratory results of a specific sample of patients for a particular study. Before computers, researchers kept their raw data in boxes or files, which required a great deal of space and made it difficult to locate specific pieces of data. The storage of research data on computers requires less space, enables easy data retrieval and reduces the amount of data lost or misplaced.

The computer has facilitated communication by having the capacity to rapidly produce a printed copy of stored information. In addition, one computer terminal can be linked to another terminal, and information can be sent by various forms of telecommunication from one location to another. Information can be sent by telephone or microwave transmissions from one office to another within a building or from one country to another (Sweeney, 1985). A nurse researcher could send and receive data to or from researchers around the world in only seconds or minutes. With this capability, the computer can become a valuable source for communicating research findings.

COMPUTER LIMITATIONS

Computers do have limitations, and probably the greatest limitation is that computers cannot think. The computer is totally incapable of making even the slightest inference; only the computer user is capable of that higher mental function. Many users become very frustrated with a computer that will not operate because they have inadvertently omitted a step in providing instructions to the machine. The computer cannot provide that missing step; it can function only on the specific instructions provided.

Another limitation of the computer is that the instructions (programs) developed for the computer must be almost flawless in order for the machine to operate. For example, any misplaced period or comma in a computer program can interfere with the computer's processing. An even more serious problem is the inaccurate program that runs and produces inaccurate results. Researchers quickly learn to attend to details in writing programs and to evaluate the accuracy of the results received from the computer.

Since computers are mere machines, they do *crash* (lose power unexpectedly) and also break down at times. The time lost to repair the machine (*downtime*) and the cost of the repair are serious limitations. However, if the computer equipment is properly cared for, the need for repair is greatly reduced. Another problem that occurs when a computer either crashes or breaks down while one is using it is the loss of data. Data that have been entered in the system but have not been stored or saved may be lost when the computer crashes. This will frustrate even the most patient person. Researchers can reduce the probability of losing data by saving the data frequently and never leaving the computer system without saving the data entered. Many researchers have a back-up file for each set of data, and this file is updated frequently.

With the rapid expansion of computer usage, there is a growing concern about the individual's right to privacy. Many agencies, such as health care systems, banks and credit bureaus, keep extensive data banks of personal information. Many individuals are raising questions about what information should be computerized and who should have access to it. Another concern is that computers have become vulnerable to crime, and computerized information is being stolen. Many researchers take precautions to secure their computerized data so it will not be accessed without their permission, but these measures do not ensure data security. One way to secure data from all those but the most sophisticated of inquirers is the use of a software password. If the correct password is not entered, the computer will halt its function. The problems with privacy and computer crime will become more obvious as computer usage increases, and these problems will have to be addressed by society.

COMPUTER HARDWARE

Computer hardware is the machinery or physical equipment of the computer. The hardware consists of four main parts: (1) input device, (2) central processing unit (CPU), (3) output device and (4) external storage device. Figure 15–1 demonstrates that the instructions (program) and data are entered in the internal memory by the input device. From the memory, the instructions flow to the control unit. Based on these instructions, the control unit directs the

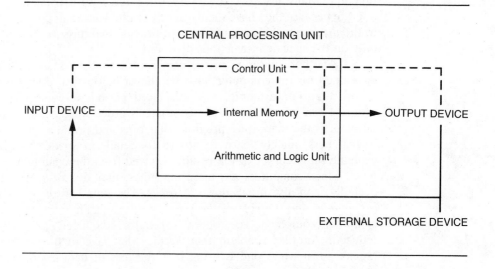

FIGURE 15–1. Computer hardware.

operations of the input device, internal memory, arithmetic and logic unit and output device. Figure 15–1 indicates the "flow of control" from the control unit to other parts of the computer system. Data entered in the internal memory can flow to the arithmetic and logic unit and be processed or flow to the output device. The information generated from the computer can be permanently stored in an external storage device, and the external storage devices can be used later as forms of input devices (Stern & Stern, 1983).

Input Devices

The input device enables the user to enter data and instructions in the computer system. There are a variety of input devices, but the most commonly used device is the keyboard with a display screen. The display screen or monitor is a cathode ray tube, which is commonly referred to as a *CRT* (Fig. 15–2).

Other input devices include card readers, magnetic tape drives, disk drives, optical scanners, touch- and light-sensitive monitor screens, and voice recognition devices (Ball & Hannah, 1984). The card reader inputs data from punched cards, which are prepared by a keypunch machine. This type of input device was frequently used a few years ago but is now almost obsolete. The use of the card reader has decreased because it is a slow method of inputting data and the cards are bulky and difficult to store. The keyboard, CRT and disk drive have replaced the card reader as an input device.

Magnetic tape drive and *disk drive* are frequently used input devices that input data from magnetic tapes (Fig. 15–3) and disks. The keyboard and CRT are used to control the recording of data on the magnetic tapes and disks, and

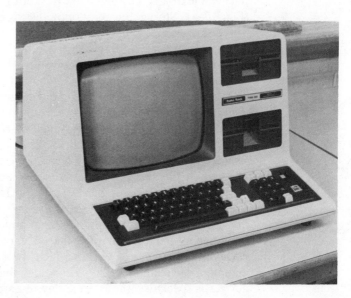

FIGURE 15–2. CRT and keyboard.

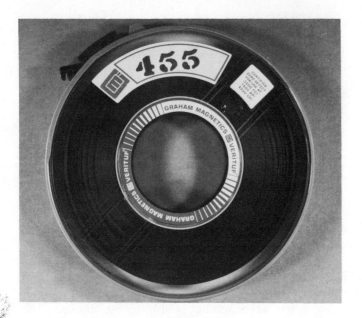

FIGURE 15–3. Magnetic tape.

these tapes and disks are used as external storage devices as well as forms of input devices.

Magnetic disks are of two basic types, flexible and rigid. An example of the flexible disk is the *floppy disk* (diskette), which is used in the microcomputer (Fig. 15–4). Storage on the floppy disk is either single-sided or double-sided. The disk can have double density, which increases the amount of information that can be recorded on the disk. The rigid magnetic disk is called a *hard disk* and looks like a large phonograph record. A number of these hard disks are stored in units called *disk packs*. The data from both the magnetic tapes and disks can rapidly be entered in the computer at a rate almost 100 times faster than a card reader can input data from punched cards (Grobe, 1984).

The *optical scanners* input data by reading specific marks, characters or bar codes. Scanners are used to input data from computerized answer sheets, such as those used for tests or certain questionnaires for research. The optical scanners in the supermarkets and other stores input data from the bar codes on products. Another input device that is similar in function to the optical scanner is the *touch- and light-sensitive screen*. The information is input through the use of touch or an optical scan wand (Ball & Hannah, 1984). This is a potential mechanism for inputting research data. Another input device is a *voice-activated input device*, in which the human voice is used to enter information in the computer. The technology that enables the use of voice-activated devices is speech synthesis. One day researchers may be able to verbally input

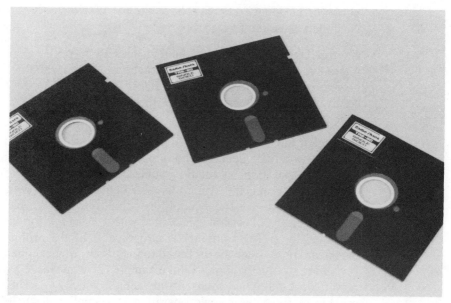

FIGURE 15–4. Floppy disks.

their data during the data collection process. The input device that is selected depends on the hardware available, the user's capabilities, the speed and accuracy of the data input device and the cost of the input device (Grobe, 1984). The researcher must evaluate these factors in determining a method for data input.

Central Processing Unit

The central processing unit (CPU) is the device that controls the computer operations and is considered the "brain" of the computer (Stern & Stern, 1983). The CPU includes the internal memory, the control unit and the arithmetic and logic unit. This unit is connected to the input and output devices by cables (Fig. 15–1).

Internal Memory □ The CPU includes the internal or primary memory that stores operating programs and monitors, tracks and temporarily stores data. The internal memory is not a permanent memory. If the computer system breaks down, the information in this memory would probably be lost if the user had not previously saved it. The internal memory consists of two types: random access memory (RAM), and read only memory (ROM). ROM is the permanent memory placed in the computer by the manufacturer, which usually cannot be changed by the user. RAM is accessible by the computer user, and data and programs can be entered and edited in this memory.

The capacity of the internal memory is measured in kilobytes (K) or megabytes. One *kilobyte* (1K) is approximately 1000 bytes, and a *megabyte* is a million bytes. A *byte* is a single character such as a number or letter in the alphabet. The size of the memory varies with the type of computer. Microcomputers or personal computers have the smallest memory, and the mainframe computers have the largest memory.

Control Unit □ The control unit in the CPU accesses instructions from the internal memory and uses these instructions to direct the functions of the input device, output device, internal memory and arithmetic and logic unit. The control unit also directs data from the internal memory to the arithmetic and logic unit and back (Fig. 15–1).

Arithmetic and Logic Unit □ The arithmetic and logic unit receives the data from the internal memory and processes the data. This unit conducts the arithmetic operations of addition, subtraction, multiplication and division. In a computer program, the symbol used to define addition is $+$, and the symbol for subtraction is $-$. The symbol for multiplication is $*$, which means that $2*3$ is 2 times 3, or 6. Division is indicated with a / symbol; for example, $6/2$ means 6 divided by 2. The computer is also capable of the arithmetic operation of exponentiation, which means raised to the power. The exponentiation operation is defined by the symbol $\wedge$; for example, $2\wedge3$ means 2 raised to the third power, or 2 multiplied by itself three times, which is 8. The computer is also capable of three basic logic operations of equal to $(=)$, less than $(<)$ and greater than $(>)$ (Peckham, 1978).

Output Devices

Output devices are used to display, print or store the information generated from the computer. The results could be displayed on a CRT, or a printer could be connected to the control unit to produce a printed copy. Floppy disks, hard disks and magnetic tapes are other forms of output that are used to store information from the computer.

The most frequently used output device is the *printer*, which is used to produce a *hard copy* (paper copy). The print on the hard copy can be either a solid character of letter quality or a dot-matrix character. The speed of the printer depends on whether the printer is a serial printer (prints one character at a time), a line printer (prints one line at a time) or a page printer (prints one page at a time). Page printers are faster but more expensive than the serial and line printers. The most commonly used printer is the line printer, which is moderate in price and speed (Stern & Stern, 1983).

Three other output devices that are used less frequently are the microfilm devices, plotters and voice output devices. The *microfilm recorder* enables computer output to be photographed so that it can be stored as microfilm. Some sources in the library are stored on microfilm, and some hospitals place patient records on microfilm. The *plotter* provides hard copy printouts of drawings and graphs, which are useful in developing research presentations and articles for publication. The *voice-activated output device* turns information from the computer into sounds comprehensible by humans.

External Storage Devices

The external storage device, or secondary memory, is a mechanism for permanently storing data and programs. The most common external storage devices are magnetic tapes and magnetic disks (floppy and hard disks) (Figs. 15–3 and 15–4). The data and programs stored on disks and tapes are organized into files, and each tape and disk must be clearly labeled so that the user knows what files are stored on each. Computer users should also have back-up copies of their disks and tapes to prevent loss of information if they become damaged, misplaced or stolen.

COMPUTER SOFTWARE

The computer software contains the instructions that direct the operations of the computer hardware. The instructions are called *programs*, which are written (programmed) by programmers. Researchers do not have to be programmers to use a computer, but they do need some knowledge of computer software. There are two types of software: the systems software, and the applications software. The *systems software* directs the operations of the computer system, input device, memory device, CPU and output device. An example of systems software used with the microcomputer or personal computer is the disk operating system (DOS).

Applications Software

The applications software is a program developed to solve a specific problem or perform a specific task. Developing applications software consists of the following steps: (1) define the problem or task, (2) design a solution, (3) write a program, (4) test the program and (5) document the program (Sweeney, 1985).

Programs can be written using a variety of computer languages. Some of the common computer languages are BASIC (**B**eginner's **A**ll-Purpose **S**ymbolic **I**nstruction **C**ode), FORTRAN (**For**mula **Tran**slator), PL~1 (**P**rogramming **L**anguage 1), PASCAL (named for Blaise Pascal) and COBOL (**CO**mmon **B**usiness-**O**riented **L**anguage). BASIC is the easiest language to learn and use in writing programs. This language encompasses both scientific and business applications. FORTRAN is one of the oldest languages developed for use by scientists, mathematicians and engineers. PL~1 is an all-purpose language designed for scientific and business applications. PASCAL is a relatively new language developed to teach programming concepts to students. This language has applications for science and business and has very good graphic capabilities. COBOL is the most frequently used language by business (Sweeney, 1985).

Some researchers develop programs for data collection. The software programs developed should be tested to determine whether or not the programs will work. If the program does not work, it must then be *debugged*, which means that the errors must be identified and replaced with accurate programming. The software developed should also be well documented. To document a program, the programmer should clearly and accurately (1) identify the language in which the program was written, (2) describe the capabilities and limitations of the program, (3) identify the equipment on which the program can be used, (4) describe how to use the program and (5) identify who to contact if the program fails to work.

There are a variety of software programs relevant to research that are available for purchase. Journals such as *Computers in Nursing*, *Softside Publications*, *Software Review* and *Softalk* are useful in keeping computer users current in software development. These journals advertise and critique the software programs that are available. Many publishers such as W. B. Saunders Company, J. B. Lippincott Company and the C. V. Mosby Company are involved in the development and distribution of software programs. Software should be purchased only after one has throughly examined the product. If software is not selected cautiously, users are frequently dissatisfied with the product or are even unable to use it. In selecting software for purchase, the user should (1) look for a well-tested program with good documentation, (2) ask for a list of current users and discuss the software with them, (3) participate in an in-depth demonstration, (4) inquire about vendor support for replacement and update of software and (5) check the vendor's financial status (Walker & Schwartz, 1984, p. 10).

TYPES OF COMPUTERS

There are three different types of computers: (1) microcomputer, (2) minicomputer and (3) mainframe computer. These computers vary in terms of their physical size, memory capabilities, processing speed and cost. With the rapid advancements in computer technology, these three types of computers are being constantly upgraded, which means that they are decreasing in size and cost and increasing in memory capabilities and processing speed.

Microcomputer

The microcomputer, which is frequently referred to as the personal computer, is a small device that fits on the desk-top. This computer has less memory (average 64K to 800K) and operates at a slower speed than the minicomputer or mainframe computer. However, the microcomputer is the least expensive of the three, ranging in cost from $600 to $10,000. Personal computers are used in hospitals, schools of nursing, small businesses and personal homes.

Minicomputer

The minicomputer is intermediate in memory size and speed. The memory capability of this computer is often greater than 50 megabytes. The minicomputer is about the size of a filing cabinet and costs $10,000 to $60,000 (Sweeney, 1985). Some hospitals use the minicomputer to run laboratory data, order supplies and determine patient bills.

Mainframe Computer

The mainframe computer has the largest memory (greater than 200 megabytes) and greatest speed of the three types of computers. These computers are sometimes as large as a room and can be used by a number of individuals from remote locations. Universities and large companies have mainframe computers because of the number of persons that must access the system and the amount of memory and speed needed to run programs and store data.

Computer Related Research Activities

Computers have become a vital part of nursing research, because a variety of research activities can be performed with the computer. Figure 15–5 identifies the types of computers (personal computer, minicomputer and mainframe computer) that are used in conducting research. The research activities that can be facilitated by the use of a computer include (1) literature review, (2) data input and storage, (3) statistical analysis, (4) model development and (5) word processing (Grobe, 1984; Schwirian, 1983). Each of these activities, except for the computerized literature searches which were described in Chapter 6, and the type of computer used to perform these activities is described.

DATA INPUT

The decision to input the data collected from a study in the computer should be made during the formulation of the research project. The researcher should identify what variables are to be studied, how these variables will be measured and whether the measurement of the variables produces quantitative (numerical) or qualitative (nonnumerical) data. Measurement of variables such as age, weight, height and vital signs produces quantitative data that can be easily entered in the computer.

Coding Data

Certain types of qualitative data can be coded for entry in the computer. *Coding* is the process of transforming qualitative data into numerical symbols that can be computerized. For example, the measurement of variables such as gender and race produces qualitative data that can be categorized and given numerical labels. Gender has two categories, female and male, and the female category could be identified by a 1, and the male category by a 2. The variable of race might include four categories: Caucasian, Black, Mexican-American and other. The Caucasian race could be represented by the numerical label of 1, Black race by 2, Mexican-American race by 3 and other by 4.

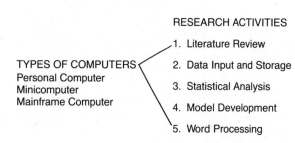

RESEARCH ACTIVITIES

TYPES OF COMPUTERS
Personal Computer
Minicomputer
Mainframe Computer

1. Literature Review
2. Data Input and Storage
3. Statistical Analysis
4. Model Development
5. Word Processing

FIGURE 15–5. Use of the computer in research.

Certain types of qualitative data do not lend to computerization, because the data are not easily coded. Data that are gathered using open-ended questions, where the subjects' responses are phrases, cannot be easily coded. Researchers' observations of human behaviors in complex, natural settings such as hospitals or places of employment produce data that are difficult to code. These are typical methods of data gathering for phenomenological, grounded theory and ethnographic research. Categorizing and putting a numerical label on certain types of qualitative data can distort the meaning of the data and/or can result in the loss of valuable responses. In addition, analysis of certain types of qualitative data requires frequent interpretations by the researcher that the computer is unable to perform.

Developing Data Collection Tools to Facilitate Coding

Questionnaires and other data collection tools may be developed so that the data collected can be easily coded and entered in the computer. The demographic sheet (Fig. 15–6) and questionnaire statements (Fig. 15–7) presented here were developed in a study of the essential behaviors of the Clinical Nurse Specialist Role (Wyers, Grove & Pastorino, 1985). The data generated with the demographic sheet and the questionnaire can be easily transformed into numerical symbols that can be computerized. To facilitate the transformation, the numerical symbols are included on the demographic sheet as well as on the questionnaire. The researcher could enter that data collected with this demographic sheet and questionnaire directly in the computer.

The coding categories developed for a study should be mutually exclu-

---

DEMOGRAPHIC SHEET
1. How many years have you been in a clinical nurse specialist role? _____
2. What is your clinical area of specialization?
   _____ (1) Medical/Surgical
   _____ (2) Pediatric
   _____ (3) Psychiatric
   _____ (4) Maternal/Child
   _____ (5) Other (please specify) _____
3. What is your position?
   _____ (1) Staff
   _____ (2) Line
4. To whom do you directly report?
   _____ (1) Director of Nursing
   _____ (2) Head Nurse
   _____ (3) Physician
   _____ (4) Inservice Director
   _____ (5) No one
   _____ (6) Other (please specify) _____
5. What is your salary range per year?
   _____ (1) $10,000–$15,000
   _____ (2) $15,001–$20,000
   _____ (3) $20,001–$25,000
   _____ (4) $25,001–$30,000
   _____ (5) over $30,000

FIGURE 15–6. Example demographic sheet.

CLINICAL NURSE SPECIALIST
COMPETENCY BEHAVIORS

Using the following six-point scale, please check the number that most accurately describes
your perception of the identified competency behaviors of the Clinical Nurse Specialist

BEHAVIOR	Least Essential Behavior					Most Essential Behavior
	1	2	3	4	5	6
1. Develops own framework for nursing practice						
2. Practices within the ANA ethical code						
3. Develops outcome criteria to evaluate patient care						
4. Initiates change in the health care delivery system						
5. Initiates collaborative relationships to improve health care delivery						

FIGURE 15–7. Example questionnaire.

sive, which means that the value for a specific variable should fit in only one category. For example, the salary ranges would not be mutually exclusive if they were categorized as (1) $10,000 to 15,000, (2) $15,000 to 20,000, (3) $20,000 to 25,000, (4) $25,000 to 30,000 and (5) $30,000 and over. These categories overlap, so a subject with a $25,000 income could mark category 3 or 4 or both. In this study, salary was put in ranges because subjects will usually mark a salary range but frequently will not list their specific salary. In addition, the single number representing each salary range is easier to computerize than is an actual salary.

The coding categories developed for a study should also exhaust the classification of all values that might appear in the study (Selltiz, Wrightsman & Cook, 1976). In question 2 of the demographic sheet, the categories of 1 to 4 do not exhaust the responses that subjects might make to this question, but category 5 does.

Developing a Codebook

After the development of the questionnaire or data collection tools and before data collection, the researcher should develop a plan for inputting the data in the computer. The plan for data input is developed in a codebook. A *codebook* documents the location and value of every variable entered in a computer file. In developing the codebook, the maximal value of each variable must be identified to determine how many columns will be needed to enter that variable in the computer. For example, if a study were to have more than 100 subjects but less than 1000, three columns would be needed for the respondents' identification numbers. In entering data in a computer, one must determine the number of columns per line for inputting data within a particular computer system.

If a codebook is developed, you will know what column(s) represent each variable and other information. Novice researchers mistakenly think that they can remember what data are in a file and how the data are sequenced in the file. However, with the passage of time or with the generation of additional projects, you will forget the data input format of each file. An example codebook is presented in Figure 15–8 for the demographic sheet and for the questionnaire in Figures 15–6 and 15–7.

Data Coding Sheet

Following the guidelines outlined by the codebook, the researcher develops a data coding sheet. The data coding sheet is a means of organizing the data so

FILE NAME—CNSDATA		
Data File Column	Variable Description and Other Codes	Question Number
1–3	Respondent Identification Number	
4	Blank Space	
DEMOGRAPHICS		
5–6	Years in CNS Role	1
7	Clinical Area of Specialization	2
	(1) Medical/Surgical	
	(2) Pediatric	
	(3) Psychiatric	
	(4) Maternal/Child	
	(5) Other	
8	Position	3
	(1) Staff	
	(2) Line	
9	Directly Report to:	4
	(1) Director of Nursing	
	(2) Head Nurse	
	(3) Physician	
	(4) Inservice Director	
	(5) No one	
	(6) Other	
10	Salary Range Per Year:	5
	(1) $10,000–$15,000	
	(2) $15,001–$20,000	
	(3) $20,001–$25,000	
	(4) $25,001–$30,000	
	(5) over $30,000	
11	Blank Space	
QUESTIONNAIRE		
12	Behavior 1	1
13	Behavior 2	2
14	Behavior 3	3
15	Behavior 4	4
16	Behavior 5	5

FIGURE 15–8. Codebook for clinical nurse specialist (CNS) study.

that it can be rapidly entered in the computer. Using the demographic sheet and questionnaire statements in Figures 15–6 and 15–7, the following data were collected on two subjects and placed on a coding sheet (Fig. 15–9).

Subject 1 has been a CNS for 10 years in medical-surgical nursing in a staff position, reports to the director of nursing and makes a salary in the $25,001 to $30,000 range. Subject 1 rated behavior 1 a **4**, behavior 2 a **6**, behavior 3 a **5**, behavior 4 a **5** and behavior 5 a **6**.

Subject 2 has been a CNS for 8 years in pediatric nursing in a staff position, reports to the director of nursing and makes a salary in the $20,001 to $25,000 range. Subject 2 rated behavior 1 a **5**, behavior 2 a **6**, behavior 3 a **6**, behavior 4 was left blank and behavior 5 a **6**.

When developing a coding sheet, the data must be *right-justified*, which means that the data must be entered in the column to the far right. On the example coding sheet in Figure 15–9, the 8 is right-justified by placing a 0 in column 5 and the 8 in column 6. If the 8 were placed in column 5, the computer would read the value as 80 rather than 8. The researcher must also determine the symbol to be used for missing data. In this example, the missing datum was identified by a blank space.

Cleaning Data

The data on the coding sheet should be cleaned, which involves checking the raw data on the demographic sheets, questionnaires or other data collection tools against the data on the coding sheet to determine any coding errors. The data entered in the computer are cleaned by scanning the data on the computer screen for errors and by checking the data printed out by the computer against the coding sheet. A computer program can be developed to clean the data. The program directs the computer to scan the data for numbers greater than or less than the possible values for a variable. In the example questionnaire provided in Figure 15–7, the behaviors are to be rated on a scale of 1 to 6. The computer could be programmed to scan the data entered from this questionnaire to identify any values greater than 6. Cleaning data to prevent errors is time consuming but essential to produce reliable findings.

Some researchers code the data they collect directly on coding sheets. Other researchers do not use code sheets but enter their data in the computer directly from their data collection tools. The most efficient method of entering data in the computer is to use the computer as a data collection tool; the data are entered in the computer as part of the data collection process. This method of inputting data requires less time because less coding and cleaning of data are necessary. In addition, the data are handled less, which decreases the chance for error.

Selection of Computers for Data Input

The computer selected for inputting the data depends on the amount of data to be analyzed and the type of analysis to be conducted. Large data files that require complex analyses are usually entered in the mainframe computer. Novice researchers frequently conduct studies that involve measurement of a

FIGURE 15-9. Data coding sheet.

limited number of variables and relatively simple statistical analyses. The data from these types of studies might be entered in the personal computer. Before selecting a type of computer, you should consult with an expert nurse researcher or computer expert about your data.

STORAGE OF DATA

The computer can be used to store data, which can be easily accessed for future work. You can add to, delete or reorganize the data in a computer file. The mainframe computer has the greatest capacity for storing research data, and these data can be easily accessed. When using the personal computer, the data must be stored on external storage devices such as floppy disks or hard disks.

Computerized Database

An increasing number of health care organizations are generating computerized databases (Bronzino, 1982). A *database* is a "structured compilation of information that can be scanned and retrieved by computer, that will provide comprehensive and detailed material, and that can be used for decisions, reports, and other purposes" like research (McElmurry & Newcomb, 1981). Computerized databases have the potential to reduce or even eliminate the data collection and data input steps for certain studies. However, not all data stored in computers are easy for researchers to access. Databases are organized by a database management system, and some of these systems are more useful for research than others. A useful database management system would enable the researcher to (1) create a database structure, (2) add new information, (3) sort the information, (4) search for the information, (5) report the data in the form you want, (6) correct or edit the data and (7) remove data when necessary (Sweeney, 1985).

MEDUS/A is an example of a database management system developed for medical research. This database includes the patient's profile (age, gender, medical diagnosis, previous medical diagnoses, previous surgeries, and so on) and patient care information (laboratory tests and results, doctor orders, medical treatments received, responses to treatments, and so on) (King, Strong & Goldstein, 1982). Researchers can search the database to find a list of cases (patients) that meet their specific criteria, and the data on these cases can be sorted separately, edited as needed and analyzed. MEDUS/A software can be used on the personal computer and minicomputer by novice programmers.

In nursing, there is a need for the development of computerized databases that will contain essential information for nursing research. The Midwest Alliance in Nursing (MAIN) has made an effort to identify the data elements that should constitute a comprehensive nursing information system.

Information Available on Computerized Databases

In hospital database management systems, there currently is a large amount of data available that could be used for clinical nursing research. Kathleen McCormick (1981) divided the data in the computer information systems into three categories: (1) Nursing Science in Patient Care, (2) Efficacy of Nursing Strategies in Solving Patient Problems and (3) Nursing Care Organization and Delivery. The Nursing Science in Patient Care data include "nursing diagnoses, signs and symptoms, physiological and psychological needs assessments, patient classifications, observations and procedures, medications administered, and communication with allied departments" (McCormick, 1981, p. 740). The Efficacy of Nursing Strategies in Solving Patient Problems category includes data on nursing actions and expected patient outcomes. The category of Nursing Care Organization and Delivery includes data on "error reporting, safety/ incidents, patient classifications, nursing computer time, nurse entry into computer, response time/down time/nurse time, unit transfers, community resources sought in discharge care planning, admissions, communication of nurses with other allied health professionals, discharges, deaths, transfers, and assignment of primary nurses" (McCormick, 1981, p. 741). Research conducted using information in computerized databases is critical to the advancement of nursing practice.

Long (1982) conducted a study of medication errors in 40 hospitals during a 1-year period. The data for this study were obtained from a computerized information system called the Variance Reporting System (VRS). Long found that 94.8 per cent of the medication errors occurred on the nursing unit, and 5.2 per cent took place in ancillary departments. The most frequently reported error was omission of the medication (28.4 per cent), wrong dosage was second (17.4 per cent) and wrong medication was third (14.9 per cent). The findings from this study identified the types of medication errors and the source of these errors, which could be useful in reducing these errors. The computerized database made it possible for the researcher to easily collect and analyze the data on medication errors from a large number of hospitals for a 1-year period.

In the near future, the amount and type of information stored by the computer will greatly increase, and the retrieval of this information will become easier. One must determine the availability of computerized databases and the usefulness of these databases for conducting nursing research. The increased availability of databases that are useful in research could greatly expand the nursing research conducted in clinical practice.

STATISTICAL ANALYSIS

Using the computer to conduct statistical analyses on data has greatly increased the accuracy of data analysis and decreased the time required to complete the analysis. However, not every research project requires a computer for data analysis. If you are conducting relatively simple analyses on a small amount of data, a handheld calculator is probably the best tool for conducting the analyses. You need to use the most economical and reasonable method for conducting data analyses, which sometimes involves the use of a calculator and other times a computer. If the computer is used, researchers can write their own statistical analysis programs or use preprogrammed statistical packages.

Writing a Data Analysis Program

Researchers with some programming experience can write their own programs for data analysis. The capabilities of the program depend on the skills of the programmer and the type of computer used. Simple analysis programs can be written for the personal computer using the BASIC programming language. The program presented in Figure 15–10 was developed to calculate the mean and standard deviation for any group of data collected.

The first line and line 150 of this program form a "do loop." The "do loop" is used to enter and analyze data for a sample size from 1 to 1000. The calculations performed in the "do loop" are identified in line 130, which instructs the computer to sum each datum point or piece of datum, and line 140, which directs the computer to sum the squares of the data points. Line 120 is a convention for exiting the data input mode, which indicates that when $X = 0$, the computer will exit the data input mode and proceed to line 160 to calculate the number of data points (pieces of data) entered (N). Line 170 of the program directs the computer to calculate the mean; and line 180, to calculate the standard deviation. The print lines 200 and 220 limit the expression of the mean and standard deviation to two places right of the decimal point.

This BASIC program could be used to calculate the mean and standard deviation for any group of data points, providing that the number of data points is not greater than 1000. A researcher could calculate the mean and standard deviation for variables such as pulse, respiration, temperature, blood pressure, height and weight that have been recorded on a group of subjects. For example, a researcher might record the pulses of 50 subjects before and after 30 minutes of exercise to determine the effect of exercise on heart rate. The pulses obtained from the 50 subjects before exercise could be entered in the computer using the basic program in Figure 15–10, and the mean and standard deviation could be calculated on these data. The pulses obtained from the 50 subjects after exercise could also be entered and analyzed with this basic program.

```
100    FOR N = 1 TO 1000
110    INPUT "ENTER DATA POINT ";X
120    IF X = 0 THEN 160
130    SUMX = SUMX + X
140    SUMX2 = SUMX2 + X∧2
150    NEXT N
160    N = N − 1
170    MEAN = SUMX/N
180    SX = SQR [(SUMX2 − SUMX∧2/N)/(N − 1)]
190    PRINT
200    PRINTING USING "THE MEAN IS ####.##";MEAN
210    PRINT
220    PRINT USING "THE STANDARD DEVIATION IS ####.##";SX
230    END
```

FIGURE 15–10. Statistical program in BASIC language.

Using Existing Analysis Programs

An increasing number of programs are being developed to analyze data on the personal computer. ABSTAT and MINISTAT are examples of such programs. MINISTAT was developed to store, organize and analyze clinical psychiatric data (Grobe, 1984). ABSTAT contains a variety of parametric and nonparametric statistical analyses. If you are planning to purchase a statistical software package for a personal computer, you should determine what packages are available, determine the capabilities of each package and use the software on your computer system. The personal computer is limited in the complexity of calculations that can be performed and the amount of data that can be analyzed.

Preprogrammed statistical packages (canned programs) are available for use on the mainframe computer, minicomputer and microcomputer. The common software packages include SPSS (Statistical Package for the Social Sciences), BMDP (Biomedical Computer Program—P-Series), SAS (Statistical Analysis System), ABSTAT and AIDA (Table 15–1). If you are considering using these preprogrammed software packages, you should consult an expert who will guide you in the selection of a manual, development of programs and evaluation of the computer printouts. Many universities provide special classes to assist individuals in using these software packages. The most frequently used preprogrammed software is SPSS, which is now entitled SPSS[x]. The SPSS[x] programs can be used to conduct numerous parametric and nonparametric

TABLE 15–1
Manuals for Software Packages

Program	Manual Title	Availability	Type of Computer
SPSS[x]	SPSS[x] User's Guide (1983) SPSS[x] Introductory Statistical Guide SPSS[x] Advanced Statistical Guide SPSS[x] Data Management	Publisher McGraw-Hill SPSS Inc. Suite 3000 444 North Michigan Avenue Chicago, Illinois 60611 (312) 329-2400	Mainframe
SAS	SAS User's Guide: Basic (1985) SAS User's Guide: Statistics (1985) SAS/ETS User's Guide (1984) SAS/GRAPHIC	SAS Institute Inc. Box 8000 Cary, North Carolina 27511	Mainframe
BMDP	Biomedical Computer Programs P-Series (1983)	University of California Press 2223 Fulton Street Berkeley, California 94720	Mainframe
ABSTAT	ABSTAT	Anderson-Bell POB 191 Canon City, Colorado 81212 (303) 275–1661	Microcomputer
AIDA	AIDA	Dr. David Lingwood Action-Research Northwest 11442 Marine View Dr., SW Seattle, Washington 98146 (206) 241-1645	Microcomputer

RUN NAME	BEHAVIORS
INPUT MEDIUM	CARD
N OF CASES	133
VARIABLE LIST	BEHAVIOR1 TO BEHAVIOR5
INPUT FORMAT	FIXED (11X,5F1.0)
FREQUENCIES	GENERAL = BEHAVIOR1 TO BEHAVIOR5
STATISTICS	ALL

FIGURE 15–11. Frequency program for SPSS[x].

analyses and to generate a multitude of tables, charts and graphs. The SPSS[x] programs are well documented in the user manuals (Table 15–1).

An example of a frequency program is listed in Figure 15–11, which was developed to calculate the frequencies on the behaviors listed in the questionnaire in Figure 15–7. A frequency program is used to calculate means, medians, modes, standard deviations and ranges for different variables. In this example, there are 133 subjects, and the program developed will direct the computer in running a frequency analysis on the first five behaviors of the questionnaire. A printout of the frequency information for Behavior 1 is presented in Figure 15–12.

The prepackaged programs have some limitations, because the user must know something about the programming language to input the data and the

CNS

FILE   NONAME   (CREATION DATE = 05/17/83)

V1

CATEGORY LABEL	CODE	ABSOLUTE FREQ	RELATIVE FREQ (PCT)	ADJUSTED FREQ (PCT)	CUM FREQ (PCT)
	1.	1	0.8	0.8	0.8
	2.	5	3.8	3.8	4.5
	3.	19	14.3	14.3	18.8
	4.	28	21.1	21.1	39.8
	5.	45	33.8	33.8	73.7
	6.	35	26.3	26.3	100.0
		------	------	------	
	TOTAL	133	100.0	100.0	

MEAN	4.624	STD ERR	0.102	MEDIAN	4.800
MODE	5.000	STD DEV	1.172	VARIANCE	1.373
KURTOSIS	-0.241	SKEWNESS	-0.634	RANGE	5.000
MINIMUM	1.000	MAXIMUM	6.000		

VALID CASES   133   MISSING CASES   0

FIGURE 15–12. Printout of frequency information.

program and something about the analysis to be performed. QUESTOR is a conversational statistical package that has been developed to deal with these problems. The user of QUESTOR is prompted by the program for all the information required for the analysis, then the machine transforms this information into the control language instructions for BMDP (Grobe, 1984).

MODEL DEVELOPMENT

Computers have the capacity to generate models of various cognitive activities such as decision making. These models can be used to direct research activities. An example is a computerized model developed by Lagina to diagnosis anxiety levels. The "computer diagnostic system was designed to help distinguish mild, moderate, and severe levels of anxiety among hospitalized patients" (Lagina, 1971, p. 484). Medicine has developed extensive computerized modeling systems for the diagnosis of diseases, such as HEME2 for diagnosing hematologic disorders (Grobe, 1984). As researchers become more familiar with computers, they can use them to develop models and to test the theories underlying these models.

WORD PROCESSING

Computers have provided researchers with word processing capabilities that are very useful in the development of the research report. One can use word processors to develop research articles for publications and speeches for presentations. The word processor enables one to easily reorganize content and rewrite sections. Spelling can be checked in research reports, and indexes can be generated for articles and books using word processor programs. If an article is rejected by a journal, the word processor makes it easy to rewrite the article to fit the style of another journal. Computers also have the capacity to produce black and white and color graphs and diagrams for presentations and articles.

Most journals require that typed copies of articles be submitted; these copies are easily produced by a letter quality printer. In the near future, journals will probably be accepting manuscripts on floppy disks. *Computers in Nursing* and *Western Journal of Nursing Research* are currently examining this prospect.

In the future, researchers will probably be sending articles by way of telecommunication from their computers directly to publishers' computers. The revisions required by the publisher could be transmitted by computer to the researcher, and the researcher could transmit back the revisions. The time required for this type of computer transmission would be much less than the time required to mail the information.

Summary

The use of computers by nurse researchers has increased at a rapid rate. Researchers are using microcomputers, minicomputers and mainframe computers to perform a variety of activities. Using a computer for research requires learning about the computer system. The computer has many capabilities: it is fast, accurate, capable of interactive operations and cost-effective. In addition, the computer can be used to store data and can facilitate communication. Computers do have limitations; for instance, they cannot think and require instructions (programs) to work. The system does break down at times and is vulnerable to crime.

There are two basic parts of the computer: the hardware and the software. Hardware is the machinery or physical equipment of the computer and consists of four main parts: input device, central processing unit, output device and external storage device. Computer software contains the instructions that direct the operations of the computer hardware, which are called programs. There are two types of software: the systems software and the applications software. The hardware and software are constantly being upgraded for the microcomputer (personal computer), minicomputer and mainframe computer.

The research activities that can be facilitated by the use of a computer include literature review, data input and storage, statistical analysis, model development and word processing. The decision to input data collected from a study in the computer should be made during the formulation of the research project. Instruments can be developed to facilitate coding. The plan for data input is developed in a codebook. A codebook documents the location and value of every variable entered in a computer file. Following the guidelines outlined by the codebook, the researcher develops a data coding sheet. The data coding sheet is a means of organizing the data so that they can be rapidly entered in the computer. The data entered in the computer should be cleaned to detect errors in coding and input.

The computer can be used to store data, which can be easily accessed for future work. An increasing number of health care organizations are generating computerized databases. A database is a structured compilation of information that can be scanned and retrieved by computer. Researchers should determine the availability of computerized databases and the usefulness of these systems for conducting nursing research. Computers are useful in conducting statistical analyses. One can write one's own statistical analysis program or use preprogrammed statistical packages. Computers have the capacity to generate models of various cognitive activities such as decision making. In addition, computers have provided researchers with word processing capabilities that are very useful in the development of the research report.

There are numerous opportunities for the use of computers in nursing research, and these opportunities are expanding every day. Nurse researchers should become aware of the types of computers available at their local university, and they might investigate the availability of computer hardware and software for purchase. One can take courses and/or consult with experts to expand one's knowledge of the computer system. In the future, the computer will be extremely useful in conducting many research activities.

References

Ball, M. J. & Hannah, K. J. (1984). *Using computers in nursing*. Reston: Reston Publishing Company, Inc.

Bronzino, J. D. (1982). *Computer applications for patient care*. Menlo Park: Addison-Wesley Publishing Company.

Grobe, S. J. (1984). *Computer primer & resource guide for nurses*. Philadelphia: J. B. Lippincott Company.

King, C., Strong, R. M., & Goldstein, L. (1982). MEDUS/A: distributing database management for research and patient care. In B. I. Blum (Ed.), *Proceedings of the sixth annual symposium on computer applications in medical care*. Los Angeles: Institute of Electrical and Electronics Engineers Computer Society, 818–826.

Lagina, S. M. (1971). A computer program to diagnose anxiety levels. *Nursing Research*, 20(6), 484–492.

Long, G. (1982). The effect of medication distribution systems on medication errors. *Nursing Research*, 31(3), 182–184, 191.

McCormick, K. A. (1981). Nursing research using computerized data bases. In H. G. Heffernan (Ed.), *Proceedings of the fifth annual symposium of computer applications in medical care*. Los Angeles: Institute of Electrical and Electronics Engineers Computer Society, 738–743.

McElmurry, B. J. & Newcomb, B. J. (1981). Clarification of the database concept. *Nursing Research*, 30(3), 155, 161, 176.

Murphy, J. R. (1979). Preparing research data for computerization. *American Journal of Nursing*, 79(5), 954–956.

Peckham, H. D. (1978). *Basic: a hands-on method*. New York: McGraw-Hill Book Company.

Saba, V. K. & McCormick, K. A. (1986). *Essentials of computers for nurses*. Philadelphia: J. B. Lippincott Company.

Schwirian, P. (1983). Schwirian's cube: the research dimension. *Computers in Nursing*, 1(1), 5.

Selltiz, C., Wrightsman, L. S. & Cook, S.W. (1976). *Research methods in social relations*. New York: Holt, Rinehart and Winston.

Stern, N. & Stern, R. A. (1983). *Computers in society*. Englewood Cliffs, New Jersey: Prentice-Hall, Inc.

Sweeney, M. A. (1985). *The nurse's guide to computers*. New York: Macmillan Publishing Company.

Walker, M. B. & Schwartz, C. M. (1984). *What every nurse should know about computers*. Philadelphia: J. B. Lippincott Company.

Wyers, M. E., Grove, S. K. & Pastorino, C. (1985). Clinical nurse specialist: in search of the right role. *Nursing and Health Care*, 6(4), 202–207.

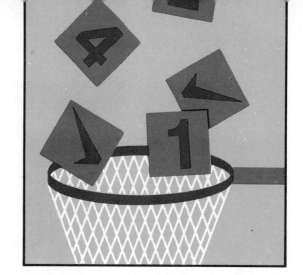

16

Planning and Implementing Data Collection

This chapter combines ideas related to both the thinking and the doing of research. Planning is the cognitive activity that moves the researcher from a broad image of a problem situation in nursing practice to a sophisticated investigation. Data collection is a pragmatic activity that propels the planned study from an idea to an actuality. The intent of this chapter is to generate a questioning attitude during the planning of the study and the data collection process.

Planning Throughout the Research Process

Planning research starts long before the research problem has been clearly formulated. Planning often starts in discussions with friends and colleagues when the idea of actually conducting a study is just beginning to nudge the surface of consciousness. Planning begins with an idea that catches the imagination. From this idea emerges consideration of the feasibility and importance of the idea. The rising sense of enthusiasm that begins to emerge provides the energy to begin the planning process.

Throughout the planning process, which continues until data collection begins, ideas should be written down as they occur. Idea people learn to keep paper and writing implements handy. Keeping a note pad at the bedside for the "two o'clocker" is good planning. As the elements of the study described in the earlier chapters of the text begin to develop, a plan for implementing the study logically emerges. Ideas may come from various sources. For example, developing the literature review reveals strategies other researchers have used in the same field of study. Sharing plans with colleagues can generate thoughts in new directions. Ideas often emerge during sleep. Often our unconscious continues to work while we sleep.

Problem solving, which includes considering alternatives, is as important as gathering ideas. Problematic reasoning is occurring while the basic elements of the study are being developed and again prior to finalizing the plan. The basic elements, including the research problem, frame of reference, research subproblems, variables and design must be examined in relation to each other. How can these components be put together in a way that is most likely to provide valid answers to the research problem? Do the components logically fit together? What changes could be made in the design to strengthen the study? Have all of the important variables related to the phenomenon under study been considered? Are there additional ways of measuring the dependent variables? This type of thinking must continue throughout the planning process.

In addition to these concerns, plans must be developed to implement the study. Beginning data collection is not as simple as it may seem. Careful thought must go into the process of implementing the proposed study. The setting for the study must be chosen, and plans must be made for acquiring a sample of subjects. The social environment in which the study will be conducted must be prepared and nurtured. The mechanics of conducting the study, such as time and costs, must be considered, data collection forms must be prepared and careful plans must be made for the actual collection of data. Plans must be made for how the data will be organized and analyzed. At this point, consideration should also be given to how the study findings will be examined or interpreted and disseminated. This extensive planning provides the groundwork for the implementation of the data collection process.

SELECTING A SETTING

The selection of an appropriate setting for conducting the study is crucial to its successful completion. The setting, of course, depends on the research problem. Experimental studies, which require very tight control over the environment and the manipulation of a treatment, may be set up in a laboratory. Some attempt may be made to have the best of both worlds—the control of the laboratory with the reality of a normal practice situation. For example, a small nursing unit could be set up within a hospital for the care of patients participating in a research project. However, most nursing studies will be conducted in field settings such as nursing units in hospitals, clinics or client homes rather than in a laboratory.

One must then determine the adequacy of the field setting as it is. Will the setting need to be modified in order to conduct the study? Are the modifications in terms of physical changes, work patterns or social interactions? The fewer changes in the setting required, the greater the generalizability of the study findings. And yet, in many cases, minimal disruption can lead to loss of researcher control, a concern in quasi-experimental and experimental studies. Will the conduct of the study disrupt the care of other patients? How will the presence and activities of the data collector affect the operations of the setting? The less disruption involved, the more receptive the institution will be to allowing the study to be done.

Some facilities are much more supportive of research endeavors than are others. However, an institution can be very supportive of medical research but not particularly supportive of nursing research. In institutions in which much research is being conducted, personnel within the institution may tend to be protective of patients who they may wish to use for their own studies. They may resist "outsiders" coming in and using "their" patients. Some facilities will claim to encourage research, but upon closer examination, one learns that approval of a study takes 3 to 6 months and that few studies have actually been conducted at the institution. It may be very helpful to talk with other nurses who have conducted research in that setting to determine institutional attitudes toward nursing research.

In selecting a setting, it is important to examine both administrative support and support from personnel who will be more directly related to the conduct of the study. Is research perceived as a valued activity? How will the staff react to having a researcher in the area? Have the personnel who will be directly involved previously worked with researchers? Can they accept, for example, not knowing the hypotheses of the study during the data collection period? Will they be cooperative or disruptive to the research effort? Will the researcher be allowed the freedom necessary to collect data?

In seeking sites for clinical studies, the authors have found a history of clinical practice in the community and clinical competence to be of great value. We have established working relationships with many administrative level personnel and clinicians. We have also developed good working relationships with physicians in the area. Our previous experience in conducting clinical nursing studies has increased the confidence of management level people that our work will not be disruptive and will be a positive experience for the setting.

Of course, an overriding concern in the selection of a setting is the availability of adequate numbers of subjects who meet criteria for inclusion in the study. The actual numbers of available subjects in the setting should be determined. In some cases, it may be possible to obtain this information from patient records. Other sources include nurses working with the type of patient needed or a frequency count of the number of observed instances of the phenomenon to be studied that occur over a given period of time.

Students sometimes have little option about selecting a setting (Diers, 1979). The setting may be the facility closest to the school. Individuals employed in a health care institution may be in similar circumstances and be limited to the employing institution as a research site. Even when students have no option in selecting a setting, they may be able to select from a variety of units within a facility. Some units may be more desirable than others for the implementing of a study. Strategies for seeking institutional approval for the conduct of a study are discussed in Chapter 13.

SELECTING A SAMPLE

A sample usually means people, but it may also be an instance of nurse-patient interaction, episodes of care or particular types of incidents such as being transferred from intensive care to a general unit (Diers, 1979). If the sample is people, the first step in selecting a sample is developing criteria that must be met for a person to be included as part of the sample. This is the "sampling frame." The criteria are developed from the research problem, the variables and their operational definitions. In a quasi-experimental or experimental study, the primary purpose of sampling criteria is to limit the effect of extraneous variables on the particular interaction between the dependent and independent variables. Subjects should be selected in order to maximize the effects of the independent variable and minimize the effects of variation in other variables.

Suppose that the researcher was studying the effects of a specific nursing intervention on postchemotherapy nausea in patients experiencing cancer. The subject would be a cancer patient receiving chemotherapy who is experiencing nausea. This is fairly obvious from the study as it is developed; however, at this point, it must be even more carefully thought out. Would the nausea experienced by all cancer patients receiving chemotherapy be the same, or could some cases of nausea be due primarily to the chemotherapy, whereas others are due primarily to disease processes and, in others, there is a combination of disease and chemotherapy? Would treatments for nausea due to all these factors be the same? Would responses to treatment be the same or differ in some important ways? Would the type of chemotherapy affect the severity and length of nausea experienced by the patient? Is severity of nausea related to response to the proposed treatment? Would the extent of nausea and the response to the planned nursing intervention vary depending on whether the patient received the chemotherapy at the hospital, the physician's office, an outpatient clinic or at his or her home? Would it be important whether the patient were receiving the first dose of chemotherapy or had been receiving it for a year? Is it important to include in the criteria the medications for nausea administered to the patient during and after chemotherapy? Generating answers to these questions will clarify the sampling frame for the proposed study.

Sampling criteria can become so restrictive that an adequate number of subjects cannot be found. To some extent, the number of restrictions that can safely be made will depend on the typical patient load in the selected setting. If the sample is limited to patients experiencing multiple myeloma, the researcher might have trouble finding enough subjects to justify conducting the study.

Perhaps the sampling frame for a study could be patients experiencing breast cancer who had not previously received chemotherapy; who were presently receiving a specific protocol of chemotherapy, including specific antiemetics; and who were receiving treatment in an outpatient clinic. Patients who were receiving their first treatment could be included in the sample. They could then be followed for a 6-month period and be given the treatment each time they received chemotherapy. Those selected as subjects could be randomly assigned to treatment and control groups. If the number of breast cancer patients being treated at the outpatient clinic were large enough, the sample itself could be randomly selected.

Sampling criteria may also include such characteristics as the ability to read, the ability to write responses on the data collection form and the ability to comprehend and communicate using the English language. Age limitations are often included. Subjects may be limited to those not participating in any other study. Subjects should be able to participate fully in the procedure for obtaining informed consent; this requirement may exclude those who are retarded, blind, deaf or mentally ill.

When criteria for subject selection have been established, sample size must be determined. The research design and the statistics to be used will influence this decision. If quasi-experimental or experimental designs are being used, the power of the study to detect causality will be determined in part by sample size. Case studies and qualitative studies may require limiting sample size to allow more intensive examination of the sample selected. There are practical factors that must also be instrumental in this decision, including the availability of subjects, limits on length of time for data collection and the complexity of data collection with a single subject. Many of the issues related to sampling are discussed in greater detail in Chapter 9.

Another matter related to sample that must be decided is the actual process of acquiring a sample for the study. If persons experiencing breast cancer are the subjects, a mechanism must be developed to determine when a person who meets the criteria is being admitted to the outpatient clinic. Should the clinic nurse call the researcher, or can the researcher be given a list of clinic appointments several days in advance? Will every person who meets the criteria be included in the study? How much prior notice will the researcher need to be able to get to the clinic, approach the patient about participating in the study and provide the treatment? How much time will the treatment require? What will the researcher do if several new patients are to be seen in the clinic within a short period of time? Will data be collected every day, or will specific days be designated for data collection? Is it possible that the day of the week or the time of day could be related to the severity of nausea after chemotherapy? This could influence findings if severity of nausea is related to the effectiveness of the intervention. Could limitations on data collecting times confound the findings? If data are collected on each patient for 6 months, the period during which new subjects will be enrolled must be decided upon.

As can be seen, much detailed planning must occur related to acquiring a sample before data collection can begin. Making decisions from these and other similar questions will affect the extent of control that the researcher will have over threats to the validity of the study findings.

DEVELOPING RELATIONSHIPS

After a decision has been made about the setting of the study, it is wise to begin establishing good working relationships with the personnel who will be involved in the study. In most institutions, the study proposal must be approved by a research review committee. However, in addition to this formal approval of the study, approval must occur at other levels within the social networks of the institution. In addition to approval, the researcher must have cooperation and support. In order to acquire these, the researcher must exhibit skills in public relations and salesmanship.

Meeting persons within the institution who will be involved in the study is essential. If the study is to be conducted in a hospital, this contact will involve those in administrative positions and those at the unit level. (See Germain's description of this process in her ethnographic study, described in Chapter 4.) The study should be explained to these individuals to the extent possible without interfering with the study. The impact of the study on work patterns within the institution must be explored with personnel. For example, in a study of nausea in breast cancer patients receiving chemotherapy, the clinic nurse may need to call the researcher or in some way keep track of breast cancer patients being scheduled to start chemotherapy. If patients are being followed for 6 months, the researcher must know the dates that patients are scheduled to return to the clinic and changes in appointment dates. Sometimes the times of appointments may have to be adjusted to allow time for data collection. The data collection process may mean that another nurse is in the room with the patient at a time when the clinic nurse usually performs other necessary tasks.

Staff nurses may also be concerned about how the researcher views them and their nursing care. Often, they believe that their nursing practice is being judged, which increases anxiety and can interfere with good working relationships. The staff response could alter care that might have an impact on the data being collected. Acceptance of the nursing staff and the patterns of care on the unit should be communicated both verbally and nonverbally. This does not mean that the researcher must approve of suboptimal care because acceptance and approval are different. Often, acceptance is a necessary precursor to facilitating positive change. Opportunities of the staff to establish a positive relationship with a nurse researcher can lead to changes in clinical practice and changes in administrative decision making. These changes are not necessarily immediate and may occur long after the study has been completed.

It is crucial that there be opportunities to get acquainted and share ideas and concerns before data collection begins. The need to maximize researcher control of the study situation can be worked out in these meetings. Joint planning of the data collection process and resolution of potential problems can make data collection a more pleasant experience. Nurses in clinical practice often do not place a high value on nursing research. The staff's values might be changed through discussions of the study's potential impact on patient care. In the study of effective nursing interventions for nausea after chemotherapy, for example, the researcher could offer to teach the treatment technique to the nurses when the study was complete.

Clinical nursing research should be a reciprocal activity. The institution has provided a facility and allowed some degree of disruption of staff activities. In return, the researcher can offer support and sometimes assistance to the institution. For example, the researcher can offer to present the study findings to group meetings after completion of the study. A copy of the study report can be provided for use by the institution. If the researcher is considered an expert in areas of interest to the institution, brief free consultative services may be highly valued by the institution. These kinds of activities pave the way for the next researcher seeking to conduct a study in that institution and also facilitate further studies by the same researcher.

CONSIDERING TIME AND COST FACTORS

Time is a factor that is often inadequately considered in conducting a study. Inexperienced researchers tend to underestimate the amount of time required for each activity of the study. Therefore, it is advisable to write out a time plan for completion of the study that indicates expected dates of completion. This time plan should include five dimensions: (1) developing the study, including the literature review; (2) obtaining approval to conduct the study; (3) collecting data; (4) analyzing data; and (5) writing the study report. From these dimensions, the researcher can develop a reasonable time frame within which to operate.

There are three factors that tend to disrupt time plans. First, there are some aspects, such as obtaining approval, over which the researcher has no control. The researcher may expect approval to be easy and require, at the most, 2 weeks, when, in fact, it is likely to be 2 months. Research committees tend to meet monthly, and sometimes these meetings are canceled. There may be deadlines for getting material to the committee for consideration each month. If there is a backlog of studies to consider, most recently submitted studies may be reviewed later.

Second, a researcher initially believes that data collection will require only a short period of time. But it usually requires two to three times longer than anticipated. Events during the data collection period are sometimes not under the control of the researcher. A sudden heavy workload of staff may make data collection temporarily difficult or impossible. The number of potential subjects might be reduced for a period of time. In some situations, approval for data collection stipulates that the physician's approval must be obtained for each subject prior to collecting data on that subject. Activities required to meet this stipulation such as contacting physicians, explaining the study and obtaining approval require extensive amounts of time. In some cases, many potential subjects are lost before the approval can be obtained, thus extending the time required to obtain additional subjects.

Third, research activities, by their nature, are self-initiated and self-paced. Procrastination is not uncommon. The two aspects of the study that seem to be most affected by procrastination are the literature review and writing the research report. Writing research reports is not like writing term papers in college courses. They are much more formal and rigid in content and format and usually require rewriting *many times*.

Cost is another factor that must be considered in planning a study. Measurement tools may cost money to rent or purchase. If questionnaires or scales are ordered from another source, there may be a fee for the scale and a fee for analyzing the data. Data collection forms must be typed and duplicated. In some cases, there are printing costs related to materials that are to be distributed during data collection such as teaching materials. In some studies, there are postage costs. If computer analyses are used, there may be costs involved in coding the data into the computer and conducting the analyses. If a statistician is employed, a fee must be paid to him or her. Sometimes it is necessary to hire a typist for the final report.

In addition to these direct costs, there are indirect costs. The researcher's time is a cost, and there are costs for traveling to and from the study site and for meals eaten out while working on the study. The cost of travel to communicate findings must also be anticipated and estimated in a budget. To prevent unexpected costs from being a surprise and perhaps delaying the study, costs should be examined in an organized manner during the planning phase of the study. We suggest developing a budget early in the planning process and revising it as plans are modified (Chapter 13). Seeking funding for at least part of the study costs can greatly facilitate the conduct of a study (Chapter 14).

Many researchers have difficulty making reasonable estimates of time and costs related to a study. We advise validating the time and cost estimates with an experienced researcher when possible. If time or cost estimates go beyond expectations, the time schedules and budget must be reformulated with a new projection for completion time and costs.

DEVELOPING DATA COLLECTION FORMS

Before data collection begins, the researcher must develop forms on which to record data. Before this process can occur, decisions must be made about what data will be collected. In addition to data related to the major variables identified in the study, data must also be collected on attribute variables. The researcher gathers these data to describe the sample. If a control group is used, the researcher must compare the experimental group and the control group to determine how comparable they are. How are these subjects different and how are they alike? Are there some key characteristics of subjects that might have influenced the study findings? In addition, these characteristics can be used for secondary analysis (Chapter 10). Secondary analysis may be conducted for the purpose of examining possible alternative hypotheses to the suggested findings of the study. For example, if the study findings indicated that the length of hospital stay was related to early ambulation, secondary analysis might examine whether length of hospital stay was related more to the age of the patients in that sample than to the variables initially studied.

We suggest that data be collected on such attribute variables as subject's age, gender, race, education, income or socioeconomic status, diagnosis and marital status if these seem in any way related to the study. Other variables that may be either extraneous or confounding should be collected, including subject's physician, length of illness or hospitalization, complications, date of data collection, time of day and day of week of data collection and any untoward events that occur during the data collection period. In some cases, the length of time required for data collection on individual subjects may be a confounding variable and should be recorded. If it is necessary to contact the subject at a later time, his or her address and telephone number should be obtained, but only with the subject's awareness and permission. Names of available family members may also be useful.

It is a frustrating experience in research to get to the analysis phase of the study and think "If only I had collected this little bit of data." However, the data collection process, which might include the completion of data collection forms, requires the subject's time. Subjects sometimes become impatient if too much data are sought; subjects can also be lost to the study. If the data can be obtained from patient records or any other written sources available, the subject should not be asked to provide this information.

Data collection forms should be developed for easy recording during data collection. A decision must be made about whether data are collected in "raw" form or coded at the time of collection. Coding will reduce the time required for data collection and analysis. For example, gender can be recorded as male or female or coded as 0 = male and 1 = female (Fig. 16–1). The codes developed should be indicated on the collection forms. For many items, the code for "other" should be included for unexpected classifications. If data are

__ __ __ 1 2 3	Subject Number
__ __ 4 5	Subject Age
__ 6	Subject Sex 0 = Male 1 = Female
__ 7	Marital Status 0 = Married 1 = Divorced 2 = Widowed 3 = Single 4 = Other

FIGURE 16–1. Data collection form for computer use.

to be coded into a computer, this should be considered in designing the forms. For computer use, forms must have one space for each column in the computer that that datum will use. For example, age would use two columns (unless someone were 100 years old). The subject number columns in Figure 16–1 would allow sufficient space for 999 subjects. Chapter 15 explains the development of data collection forms for the computerization of data.

Subjects' names should not be on coding forms—only the subject's number. A master list of subjects and associated coding numbers can be kept and secured by the researcher. The subjects' privacy and, in some cases, anonymity must be preserved. Decisions related to who, if anyone, other than the researcher will have access to subjects' names should be made early in the study. This information is part of informed consent, which is described in Chapter 12.

Qualitative studies often use note cards for data collection. In some cases, interviews are recorded verbatim, requiring note paper and perhaps carbons. Carbons are used to cross-file data and to provide the researcher with a copy while data are being typed. Giving the typist the only copy of data is taking a risk. Sometimes, interviews are recorded using tape recorders and videotapes. Plans must be made for acquiring this needed equipment, learning how to use it and determining whether it is in working order. Tapes should be checked soon after recording to ensure that the data were actually recorded. Duplicates of tapes should be made and kept in separate places.

Sometimes data may be recorded on scantron sheets, which can be directly entered into the computer by optic scanner. This greatly speeds up the process of entering data. There is a cost, in most cases, for this service. Subjects may be reluctant to use the scantron sheets, and some inaccuracies in the data may occur because of subject error in completing these sheets. However, errors also occur when data are manually entered in the computer or are transferred from a data collection form to a coding sheet.

With the advent of microcomputers, data collectors can code data directly into a microcomputer at the data collection site. A computer program must be written for entering the data. If a computer programmer is hired for this purpose, there is, of course, a fee involved. A microcomputer enables collection of much larger amounts of data with less error. Questionnaires might be placed within the microcomputer so that the subject could enter responses directly.

Very small data collection machines are available to allow the researcher to code data into the machine from observations as they occur. Gill, White and Anderson (1984) used this approach in their study of the first sustained cry of newborn infants. A variety of data collection machines are being developed, and many facilities are currently recording large amounts of data for use in research. These newer strategies are likely to revolutionize data collection techniques in the years to come.

PLANNING THE DATA COLLECTION PROCESS

Much thought should go into the process of data collection before it is actually initiated. Two dimensions of consistency must be addressed. The researcher must consider both consistency between subjects and consistency between data collectors if more than one data collector is used. Thus, one must consider how data will be collected and who will collect it.

Consistency in data collection between subjects is critical. The specific days and hours of data collection may influence the consistency of the data collected and thus should be carefully considered. For example, the state of mind of subjects from whom data are gathered in the morning may differ from that of subjects from whom data are gathered in the evening. Visitors are more likely to be present at certain times of day. Patient care routines vary with time of day. Subjects who are approached on Saturday may differ from subjects approached on weekday mornings. Subjects attending clinics on Saturday may have a full-time job, whereas those attending clinics on weekday mornings may be either unemployed or too ill to work.

Many variations can occur during the actual data collection phase that can alter the data obtained. The researcher should think through as many of these situations as possible prior to data collection to improve consistency. Questions with which the data collector may be confronted include the following: If interviews are being used, will the data collector take notes during the interview or wait until the interview is over and jot down notes from memory? If subjects are to complete forms or scales, is this to be done in the presence of the researcher or can the forms be picked up later? Can the subject take the forms home and bring them back later or mail them in? If the subject cannot fill out forms because of an intravenous infusion, no reading glasses or weakness, can a family member, the nurse or a data collector read the questions and record the subject's responses?

Decisions related to who collects the data must be made. Will the data all be collected by the researcher or will data collectors be used? Can data collectors be nurses working in the area? If data collectors are used, plans must be made for these individuals to receive equivalent training. In addition to training, written guidelines should be developed for the data collectors. Following training, data collectors must be evaluated to determine their consistency in the data collection process. The researcher should make as many decisions as possible before being confronted with these questions in the data collection situation.

PLANNING THE ORGANIZATION OF DATA

When data collection begins, the researcher will be confronted with much paper handling. The situation can quickly grow to a state of total confusion unless careful plans are made before data collection begins. Plans should be made to keep all data from a single subject together until analysis is begun. The subject code number should be written on each form, and one should check to ensure that all forms are present for each subject. Researchers have been known to sort their data by form, such as putting all the scales of one kind together, only to realize afterward that they had failed to code the forms with subject numbers first. They then had no idea which questionnaire belonged to which subject, and valuable data were lost.

Space should be allotted for storing forms. File folders should be purchased, and a labeling method should be designed to allow easy access to data. Color coding can sometimes be very useful. For example, if multiple forms are being used, the subject data form can be one color, the anxiety scale another color, the interview notes a third color. Envelopes can be used to hold small pieces of paper or note cards that might fall out of a file folder. Plans should be made to code data and enter it into the computer as soon as possible after data collection to help reduce the loss or disorganization of data.

PLANNING DATA ANALYSIS

In planning data analysis, the researcher considers a number of important questions. What statistical analyses are appropriate for the data? Of the analyses selected, which analyses are critical and which are off target for the identified subproblems? Will the data analyses be conducted manually or by computer? Should a consultant be sought for data analysis? What is the best way of presenting the results from data analyses: tables, graphs or narrative description?

PLANNING INTERPRETATION AND DISSEMINATION OF FINDINGS

Before the study is initiated, the researcher should predict possible findings and the meanings of these findings. What findings are anticipated for each subproblem? Are these findings consistent with previous research? What is the meaning of these findings in light of the framework? What is the usefulness of these findings? Questions addressed related to interpretation continue to emerge during data collection. When the researcher is in contact with subjects, ideas related to data analysis and interpretation are stimulated.

Identifying methods of disseminating findings is part of planning research. In planning the dissemination of findings, certain questions should be addressed. How much time will be needed to develop the research report? To whom should the research report be distributed? What other audiences should be informed of the study findings? What presentations should be planned to reach appropriate audiences? Where should the findings be published to reach those interested? The researcher should begin gathering information on calls for abstracts and author information in nursing journals during the planning stage. The journals should be perused to determine typical content. Query letters can be sent to journals that seem appropriate for publication of the findings (Chapter 19).

EVALUATING THE PLAN

After planning has been completed, the researcher should review the plan and evaluate it. The entire plan should be examined for the threats to validity discussed in Chapter 10. What threats are not controlled by the plan? Which of these threats could be of concern in this study? In what ways could the plan be modified to lessen these threats? After thorough review by the researcher, a trusted colleague should be sought to critique the proposed study. At this point, researchers often think that their study is the most wonderful plan ever developed. They have so much invested in the plan that they cannot examine it objectively. The objective critique of a trusted friend can sometimes save much frustration later.

The Process of Data Collection

The initiation of data collection is an exciting part of research. After all the planning, writing and negotiating, you are getting to the "real" part of research—the "doing" part. There is a sense of euphoria and excitement—an eagerness to get on with it. For a neophyte researcher, there is a sense of venturing into the unknown. And for all researchers, it really is the unknown. This section addresses the questions often asked by researchers entering new research ventures. Suggestions are provided for planning and problem solving to facilitate effective data collection.

Data collection is the process of acquiring subjects and collecting the data needed for the study. Depending on the study design, data may be collected on subjects by observing, measuring, testing, questioning, recording and/or gathering. The researcher is actively involved in this process either by collecting data or overseeing data collectors.

Data collection implements the plan previously discussed. Implementing the research plan, in effect, tests the expectations of the researcher (which are built into the plan) against reality. The researcher expects data collection to proceed at a specific pace and to be completed within a given period of time. Potential subjects and health professionals are expected to react to the study in anticipated ways. The environment in which the study is conducted is expected to remain somewhat consistent. The extent to which these expectations are upheld reflects to some degree the previous experience of the researcher. To the extent that events are consistent with the plan, the data collection process is somewhat routine and develops its own rhythm of activity.

The actual steps of collecting the data are specific to each study and are dependent on the research design (Chapter 10) and measurement techniques (Chapter 11). Data collection techniques for qualitative studies will differ from most quantitative designs. In qualitative research, data collection, measurement and analysis are not clearly differentiated. Qualitative data collection techniques are described in Chapters 4, 11 and 17. Many studies will include elements of both quantitative and qualitative data collection techniques.

Personal characteristics of the researcher are as important to the success of the study during data collection as is the concrete implementation of the research steps. Being knowledgeable about research is not a sufficient criterion for achieving success in data collection. Both knowledge and personal characteristics are essential. The pragmatics of data collection require personal discipline, alertness, quick thinking, interpersonal skills and flexibility. Effective people management and problem-solving skills are as important to data collection in research as they are in any other area of nursing practice.

DATA COLLECTION TASKS

The researcher performs five tasks during the process of data collection. These tasks are interrelated and occur concurrently rather than in sequence. The tasks include obtaining subjects, collecting data in a consistent way, maintaining research controls, protecting the integrity (or validity) of the study and solving problems that threaten to disrupt the study.

Obtaining Subjects

Subjects may be obtained only at the initiation of data collection or throughout the data collection period. The design of the study determines the method of selecting subjects. The method of acquiring subjects should be as consistent as possible with the research plan. Obtaining the number of subjects originally planned is critical, since data analysis and interpretation of findings may hinge on this achievement. Factors related to subject selection should be continually examined to determine possible biases in the sample actually obtained.

Maintaining Consistency

The key to data collection in any study is consistency. Consistency involves maintaining the data collection pattern for each collection event as it was developed in the plan. A good plan will facilitate consistency. However, developing a consistent plan is easier than implementing it. Consistency in the collection of data is critical to the validity of the study. Deviations, even though minor, should be noted and evaluated for their impact on interpreting the findings.

Maintaining Controls

Research controls were built into the plan to minimize the influence of intervening forces on study findings. Maintenance of these controls is essential. These controls are not "natural" in a field setting and letting them slip is easy. In some cases, these controls slip without the researcher realizing it. Maintaining control is more difficult than designing controls. In addition to maintaining controls included in the plan, the researcher should continually watch for previously unidentified extraneous variables that could be having an impact on the data being collected. These factors are often specific to a particular study and tend to become apparent during the data collection period. Extraneous variables identified during data collection must be considered during data analysis and interpretation of findings. These variables must also be included in the research report to allow other researchers to examine these variables in future designs.

Protecting Study Integrity

Protecting the integrity or validity of the study involves the first three tasks listed, but it must also be considered in a broad context. To accomplish this, the researcher will have to move away from the point of view of examining elements of data collection to viewing the process of data collecting as an entirety. Changes in one small component of data collection can modify other elements and thus alter the whole process in ways that threaten the validity of the outcomes.

Problem Solving

Skills in problem solving, usually related to the first four tasks identified, are often the key to successful data collection. Problems can be perceived either as a frustration or as a challenge. The fact that the problem occurred is not as important as the success of problem resolution. Therefore, the final and perhaps most important task of the data collection period may be problem resolution.

Little has been written about the problems encountered by nurse researchers. The research reports read as though everything went smoothly. The implication is that if you are a good researcher, you will have no problems. This is emphatically not true. Research journals generally will not provide sufficient space to allow description of problems encountered, and this gives a false impression to the inexperienced reader. A more realistic picture can be obtained by personal discussions with researchers about the process of data collection.

KINKS IN THE RESEARCH PLAN

Murphy's Law (If anything can go wrong, it will, and at the worst possible time) seems to prevail in studies as in other dimensions of life. For example, data collection almost always requires more time than was anticipated, and collecting the data is usually more difficult than was expected. Sometimes changes must be made in the way that the data are collected, in the specific data collected or in the timing of data collection. People react to the study in unpredicted ways. Institutional changes may force modifications in the research plan, or unusual or unexpected events may occur.

The researcher must be as consistent as possible in data collection but must also be flexible in dealing with unforeseen problems. Sometimes, sticking with the original plan at all costs is a mistake. Skills in finding ways to resolve problems that will protect the integrity of the study can be critical.

In preparation for data collection, possible problems should be anticipated, and possible solutions for these problems should be explored. In the remainder of this chapter, some of the common problems and concerns are described, and possible solutions are discussed. Problems that tend to occur with some regularity in studies have been categorized as people problems, researcher problems, institutional problems and event problems.

People Problems

Unfortunately, nurses cannot place a subject in a test tube in an experimental laboratory, instill one drop of the independent variable, and then measure the effect. Our studies are conducted by examining the subjects in interaction with their environments. When research involves people, nothing is completely predictable. People, in all their complexity and wholeness, have an impact on all aspects of nursing studies. And in some cases, this impact causes problems.

People react with people throughout several dimensions of the study. There will be researchers, potential subjects, family members of subjects, health professionals, institutional staff, and others ("innocent bystanders") interacting within the study situation. These interactions should be closely observed and evaluated by the researcher for their impact on the study.

Obtaining a Sample □ The first step in initiating data collection, obtaining a sample, may be the beginning of people problems. The researcher may find that few available people fit the sampling criteria or that many of those approached refuse to participate in the study, even though the requests seem reasonable. Appropriate subjects, who were numerous a month previously, seem to have disappeared. Institutional procedures may change, which might result in many potential subjects becoming ineligible for participation in the study. Subject criteria may have to be reevaluated, or additional sources for potential subjects sought. In research institutions that provide care for the indigent, patients tend to be reluctant to participate in research. This lack of participation might be due to exposure to frequent studies, a feeling of being manipulated and/or a misunderstanding of research in general or of a particular study. Patients may feel that they are being used or are afraid that they will be harmed.

Subject Mortality □ After a sample has been obtained, other problems can occur. Some subjects may agree to participate but then fail to follow through. Some may not complete needed forms and questionnaires or may fill them out incorrectly. Some subjects may not return for a second interview or not be home for an arranged visit. Although time has been invested in data collection with these people, data from them may have to be excluded from the study because of incompleteness.

Sometimes subjects must be dropped from the study because of changes in health status. For example, the patient may be transferred out of intensive care where the study is being conducted; the patient's condition may worsen, requiring different care; or the patient may die. Clinic patients may be transferred to another clinic or discharged from the service. In the community, subjects may choose to discontinue services, or limits of third-party reimbursement may force discontinuation of services that are being studied.

Subject mortality occurs in all studies to some extent. One way to deal with this is to anticipate the mortality rate and increase the planned number of subjects to ensure a minimally desired number of subjects who will complete the study. If subject mortality is higher than expected, the researcher may consider continuing data collection for a longer period of time to achieve the originally planned sample size. Completing the study with a smaller than expected sample size may become necessary. If so, the effect of a smaller sample on the power of planned statistical analyses should be considered; however, the smaller sample may not be adequate to test the hypotheses. Subject mortality is discussed in more detail in Chapter 9. The effect of sample size on statistical power is discussed in Chapter 17.

Subject As An Object □ The quality of interactions between the researcher and the subjects during the study is a critical dimension to maintaining subject participation in the study. When there is pressure in completing a study, people can be treated as objects rather than as subjects. In addition to being unethical, this also alters interactions, diminishes the subjects' satisfactions in serving as a subject and increases subject mortality. Subjects are scarce resources and should be treated with great care. Treatment of the subject as an object by the researcher can lead to similar patient treatment by other health care providers, which leads to poor quality of care. In this case, participation in the study is to the subject's detriment.

External Influences on Subject Responses □ People interacting with the subject or with the researcher or both can also have an important impact on the data collection process. Family members may not agree with the subject's participation in the study or may not understand the study process. These people will, in most cases, influence the subject's decisions related to the study. In many studies, time should be invested in explaining the study to and seeking the cooperation of family members.

Family members or other patients may also influence the subject's responses to questionnaires or interview questions. In some cases, the subject may ask the family member, a friend or another patient to complete study forms for him or her, or questions asked on the forms may be discussed with whomever happens to be in the room. When this occurs, the subject's real feelings may not be those recorded on the questionnaire. If interviews are conducted with other persons in the room, the subject's responses may be dependent on his or her need to respond in ways expected by the other persons. Sometimes, questions addressed verbally to the patient may be answered by a family member. Thus, the location in which a questionnaire or interview is completed may determine the extent to which it is a true reflection of the subject's feelings. If the location is varied in the degree of privacy from one subject to another, the subjects' responses may also vary. In most cases, the most desirable setting is one of a private area away from the distractions of others. If this is not possible, the presence of the researcher at the time that the questionnaire is completed may decrease the influence of others. If the questionnaire is to be completed later or taken home and returned at a later time, the probability of influence by others increases and the return of questionnaires greatly decreases. The seriousness of this to the integrity of the study depends on the nature of the questionnaire.

Passive Resistance □ Other health professionals and institutional staff working with the subject also have an effect on the data collection process. Some professionals will outwardly verbalize strong support for the study and yet passively interfere with the data collection process. For example, nurses providing care may fail to follow guidelines agreed upon for providing specific care activities being studied. Information needed for the study may be left off patient records. The researcher may not be informed of the admission of a new potential subject. A physician who has agreed to the utilization of his or her patients as subjects for the study may decide as each patient is admitted that this one is not quite right for the study or may be unusually unavailable to the researcher.

Nonprofessional staff may not realize the impact of the data collection process on their work patterns until data collection has been initiated. Their beliefs about how care should be provided (and has been provided for the last 20 years) may be violated by the data collection process. If ignored, their resistance can be the complete undoing of a carefully designed study. For example, a nursing aide's bathing routine may be disrupted by the study treatment; yet he or she may continue with his or her normal routine regardless of the study protocol.

Because of the potential impact of these problems, the researcher would be advised to carefully maintain communication and positive relationships with other professionals and staff during data collection. Problems that are recognized early and dealt with promptly have fewer serious consequences for the study than those that are ignored. However, not all problems can be resolved. Sometimes it is necessary to find effective ways to work around an individual or to counter the harmful consequences of passive resistance. These actions may require some creative solutions.

Researcher Problems

Some problems are a consequence of the interaction of the researcher with the study situation or lack of skill in data collection techniques. These problems are often difficult to identify because of the personal involvement of the researcher. However, their effect on the study can be serious.

Researcher Interactions □ The researcher can get so caught up in interactions with all the people involved in the study that adequate data collection on the subject under study is not completed. This is particularly likely to occur in qualitative studies in which some form of participant observation is being used. Researcher interactions can also interfere with data collection in interview situations. If the researcher is collecting data while surrounded by familiar professionals with whom he or she typically interacts socially and professionally, it is sometimes difficult to completely focus one's attention on the study situation. This lack of attention usually leads to loss of data.

Lack of Skill in Data Collection Technique □ The researcher's skill in using a particular data collection technique can affect the quality of data collected. The researcher who is unskilled at the beginning of data collection might practice the data collection technique planned for the study with the assistance of an experienced researcher. A pilot study to test the data collection techniques can be helpful. If data collectors are being used, they should also have opportunities to practice data collection techniques before the study is initiated. If skill is developed in the study itself, as skill increases the data being collected may change, confounding the study findings and threatening the validity of the study. If more than one data collector is used, changes in skill can occur more frequently than if the researcher is the data collector. The skills of data collectors should be evaluated during the study to detect any changes in their data collection techniques.

Researcher Role Conflict □ The professional nurse conducting clinical research often experiences a conflict between the role of researcher and that of clinician during the data collection period. As a researcher, one is observing and recording events. In some cases, involvement of the researcher in the event could alter the event and thus bias the results. It would be difficult to generalize the findings to other situations in which the researcher was not present to intervene. However, in some situations, the needs of patients must take precedence over the needs of the study. The dilemma is to determine when the needs of patients are great enough to warrant researcher intervention.

Some interventions are life threatening, such as respiratory distress and changes in cardiac function, and require immediate action by anyone present. Others are simple, are expected of any nurse available and are not likely to alter the results of the study. Examples of these interventions include giving the patient a bedpan, informing the nurse of the patient's need for pain medication or assisting the patient in opening food containers. These situations seldom cause a dilemma. Other situations, however, do not have as easy a solution.

Suppose, for example, that the study involved examining emotional responses of family members during and immediately after surgery. The study was designed to examine emotional responses within existing care situations using these subjects as a control group and then providing an experimental treatment consisting of a support system for families before and during surgery. Both sets of families are to be followed for 1 week after the surgery, measuring levels of anxiety, coping, amount of pain medication given to the patient and length of hospital stay. The researcher is currently collecting data on the control group. The data consist of demographic information and scales measuring anxiety and coping. One of the family members is in great distress. After completing the demographic information, she verbally expresses her fears and the lack of support she has received from the nursing staff. Two other subjects from different families hear the expressed distress and concur, moving closer to the conversation and looking to the researcher. Supportive responses from the researcher are likely to modify the results of the study, because these responses are part of the treatment to be provided to the experimental group. This is likely to narrow the difference between the two groups and thus decrease the possibility of showing a significant difference between the two groups. How should the researcher respond? Is there an obligation to provide support? To some extent almost any response by the researcher will be supportive. One alternative is to provide the needed support and not include these family members in the control group. Another alternative is to recruit the help of a nonprofessional to collect the data from the control group. However, one must recognize that most people will provide some degree of support in the described situation, even though their skills in supportive techniques may vary.

These dilemmas should be anticipated prior to data collection whenever possible. Pilot studies can be helpful in identifying dilemmas likely to occur in a particular study. Strategies can be built into the design to minimize or avoid dilemmas. Other dilemmas cannot be anticipated easily and must be responded to spontaneously. After the event, it is wise to reexamine the situation for its effect on study results and to consider options in case the situation arises again.

Maintaining Perspective □ From the previous discussion, one can see that there are both joys and frustrations in the process of data collection. The researcher must be able to maintain some degree of objective perspective during the situation and yet not take oneself too seriously. A sense of humor is invaluable. It is helpful to be able to allow oneself to feel the emotions experienced and then move to being the rational problem solver. Obviously, management skills and good mental health are very helpful to the serious researcher.

Institutional Problems

Institutions are in a constant state of change (even though they sometimes seem not to have changed for 20 years). They will not stop changing for the period of a study, and these changes often affect data collection. The nurse who has been most helpful in the study may be promoted or transferred. The unit on which the study is conducted may be reorganized, moved or closed during the course of the study. An area used for subjects' interviews may be transformed into an office or a store room or may be torn down for a new remodeling project. Patient record forms may be revised, omitting data that were being collected. The record room personnel may be reorganizing their files and be temporarily unable to provide needed charts.

These problems are, for the most part, completely outside the control of the researcher. It is helpful to keep an ear to the internal communication network of the institution for advance warning of impending changes. Contacts within the administrative decision-making system of the institution can allow a word to be put in about the impact of specific changes on an ongoing study. However, in many cases, data collection strategies might have to be modified to meet the newly emerging situation. Again, flexibility while maintaining the integrity of the study may be the key to continuing successful data collection.

Event Problems

Unpredictable events can be a source of great frustration during a study. Research tools ordered from a testing company may be lost in the mail. The duplicating machine may break down just before five hundred data collection forms were to be copied. A machine to be used in data collection may break down and require 6 weeks for repair. A computer ordered for data collection may not arrive when promised. A tape recorder may become jammed in the middle of an interview. After an interview, the data collector may discover that the play button rather than the record button on the recorder had been pushed, leaving no record of the interview. Data collection forms may be misplaced, misfiled or lost.

World events and nature can also play dirty tricks on researchers. Sometimes worldwide or national events influence subjects' responses to a study. For example, one of our graduate students was examining patients' attitudes related to renal dialysis. She planned to collect data for 6 months. Three months into data collection, three patients died as a result of the malfunction of a dialysis machine in the city where the study was being conducted. The event made national headlines. Obviously, this event could be expected to modify subjects' responses.

In attempting to deal with the impact of the event on the study, the graduate student could have modified the study and continued collecting data to examine the impact of news such as this on attitudes. However, the emotional climate of the clinics participating in the study was not conducive to this option. She chose to wait 3 months before collecting additional data, examining the data before and after the event for statistically significant differences in responses. Since there were none, she could justify using all the data for her planned study.

Other less dramatic events can also have an impact on data collection. If data collection for the entire sample is planned for a single time, a snow storm or a flood may require canceling the meeting or clinic. Weather may decrease attendance far below that expected at a support group or series of teaching sessions. A bus strike can disrupt transportation systems to such an extent that subjects can no longer get to the source of data collection. A new health care service may open in the city, which may decrease demand for the care activities being studied. On the other hand, an external event can also increase attendance at clinics to such an extent that existing resources are stretched and data collection is no longer possible.

These events are completely outside the control of the researcher and are impossible to anticipate. In most cases, however, restructuring the data collection period can salvage the study. In order to do this, it is necessary to examine all the possible alternatives by which one might collect the necessary data. In some cases, data collection can simply be rescheduled; in other situations, the changes needed may be more complex.

SERENDIPITY

Serendipity is the accidental discovery of something useful or valuable. During the data collection phase of studies, researchers often become aware of elements or relationships not previously identified. These aspects may be closely related to the study being conducted or have little connection with it. They come from the increased awareness of close observation. Because the researcher is focused on close observation, other elements in the situation can come into clearer focus and take on new meaning. This is similar to the open context discussed in Chapter 4. The researcher's perspective shifts, and new gestalts are formed.

Serendipitous findings are important to the development of new insights in nursing theory. They can be very important in terms of understanding the totality of the phenomenon being examined. Additionally, they lead to new areas of research that generate new knowledge. Therefore, it is essential to capture these insights as they occur. These events should be carefully recorded, even if their impact or meaning is not understood at the time. Sometimes, when notes are reexamined at a later time, patterns begin to emerge.

Serendipitous findings can also lead the unsuspecting researcher astray. It is possible to forget the original research plan and move right into examining the newly discovered dimensions. Although modifying data collection to include data related to the new discovery may be valid, the researcher must remember that there has not been time to carefully plan a study related to the new findings. Examination of the new data should only be an offshoot of the initial study. Data collected as a result of serendipitous findings can provide additional information to allow a carefully planned study to be designed at a later time. Serendipitous findings should be included in presentations and publications related to the study. Although the meaning of the discovery may not be understood, sharing the information may lead to insights by researchers studying related phenomena.

ACCESSING SUPPORT SYSTEMS

The researcher must have access to individuals or groups who can provide support and consultation during the data collection period. Support systems themselves have been the subject of much study in recent years. In some cases, support systems can be the source of both stress and support. However, more recent theorists propose that to be classified as support, the individual or group must enhance the ego strength of the individual. Three dimensions of support have been identified: (1) physical assistance; (2) provision of money or other concrete needs, such as information; and (3) emotional support. The researcher can readily use all these dimensions of support.

Academic Committees

In spite of the fact that theses and dissertation committees are basically seen as stern keepers of the sanctity of the research process, they also serve as support systems for neophyte researchers. In fact, committee members should be selected from faculty who are willing and able to provide the needed support. Experienced researchers among faculty are usually more knowledgeable about the types of support needed. Because they are directly involved in research, they tend to be more sensitive to the needs of neophyte researchers.

Institutional Supports

A support system within the institution in which the study is being conducted is also very important. These people have the knowledge of how the institution functions and their closeness to the study can increase their understanding of the problems experienced by the researcher and subjects. Their ability to provide useful suggestions and assistance should not be overlooked. Resolution of some of the problems encountered during data collection may be dependent on having someone within the power structure of the institution who can intervene. Also, because of their physical closeness to the data collection arena, they are often accessible when there is a need for support.

Personal Supports

In addition to professional supports, it is helpful to have at least one significant other with whom one can share the joys, frustrations and current problems of data collection. These people can often serve as mirrors to allow you to see the situation more clearly—and perhaps more objectively. Through personal support, feelings can be shared and released, allowing the researcher to achieve distance from the data collection situation. Discussions of alternatives to problem resolution can then occur.

Summary

Planning is the cognitive activity that moves the researcher from a broad image of a problem situation to a sophisticated investigation. Data collection is a pragmatic activity that propels the planned study from an idea to an actuality. Planning research starts long before the research problem has been clearly formulated. During planning, the researcher must continually question the rationale for each decision in developing the methodology of the study. The adequacy of the field setting and of sampling techniques should be questioned. After a decision has been made about the setting of the study, the researcher should begin establishing good working relationships with institutional personnel.

A time plan for completion of the study should be developed. Three factors tend to disrupt time plans: (1) factors over which the researcher has no control, such as obtaining approval; (2) changes in institutional functioning; and (3) procrastination. Direct and indirect costs related to the time plan should be identified.

Before data collection begins, the researcher must develop forms on which to record data and determine methods of coding the data. Methods of storing and organizing data should be thought through, and strategies of data analysis should be questioned. Before the study is initiated, the researcher should predict possible findings and the meanings of these findings. Identifying methods of disseminating findings is part of planning research. After the planning has been completed, the researcher should review the plan and evaluate it for threats to validity.

The plan previously discussed is implemented during the data collection process. Data may be collected on subjects by observing, measuring, testing, questioning, recording and/or gathering information. The actual steps in collecting the data are specific to each study and are dependent on research design and measurement techniques. Personal characteristics of the researcher are as important to the success of the study during data collection as is the concrete implementation of research steps.

The researcher performs five tasks during the process of data collection: (1) obtaining subjects, (2) collecting data in a consistent way, (3) maintaining research controls, (4) protecting the integrity (or validity) of the study and (5) solving problems that threaten to disrupt the study. Many problems can occur during the data collection phase. Problems that tend to occur with some regularity in studies have been categorized as people problems, researcher problems, institutional problems and event problems.

Two concerns of the data collection process are the handling of serendipitous findings and the researcher's access to support systems. Serendipity is the accidental discovery of something useful or valuable. During the data collection phase of studies, researchers often become aware of elements or relationships not previously identified. Serendipitous findings are important to the development of new insights in nursing theory. In addition, the researcher must have access to individuals or groups who can provide support and consultation during the data collection period. Support can be obtained from faculty serving on theses and dissertation committees, supports within the study setting and personal supports.

References

Diers, D. (1979). *Research in nursing practice*. Philadelphia: J. B. Lippincott Company.

Gill, N. E., White, M. A. & Anderson, G. C. (1984). Transitional newborn infants in a hospital nursery: from first oral cue to first sustained cry. *Nursing Research*, 33(4), 213–217.

Wooldridge, P. J., Leonard, R. C. & Skipper, J. K. Jr. (1978). *Methods of clinical experimentation to improve patient care*. St. Louis: The C. V. Mosby Company.

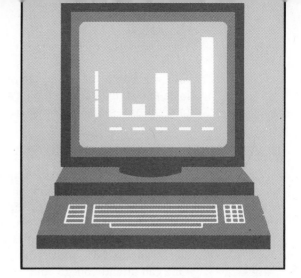

17

DATA ANALYSIS

Introduction

During data analysis, the data are gathered, summarized in various ways and carefully examined, often using a variety of analytical techniques. The period of data analysis is probably the most exciting part of research. In this period, one finally gets answers to the questions that initially generated the research activity. However, this enthusiasm can be clouded by fears and uncertainties, particularly if the researcher has an inadequate knowledge of analytical techniques.

MATHEMATICAL KNOWLEDGE NEEDED FOR RESEARCH

Mathematical reasoning is used throughout the research process; it is not confined to data analysis. A solid background in mathematical logic and statistical techniques is essential for conducting quality research. Analysis is not disconnected from the rest of the research process; it is an integral part. The approach to analysis is inextricably intertwined with the design of the study. Interpretation of the results of analysis must be made with a clear understanding of both the conduct of the study and the process of analysis.

The clinical nurse must have both mathematical logic and statistical reasoning to intelligently critique and utilize research findings. We suggest that the lack of both is a primary reason for the current lack of utilization of nursing research findings. Because the reader is unable to comprehend the mathematical logic and statistical terminology in the research approach, the entire report (in fact, all of research) is often rejected.

DEVELOPING MATHEMATICAL AND STATISTICAL SKILLS

Currently, more nurses are acquiring a sound knowledge base in mathematics and statistical reasoning than in the past. Students who enjoy mathematics tend to seek out faculty who are sophisticated in their use of statistical techniques. We encourage nurses who are interested in increasing skills in mathematical logic to seek out opportunities for additional coursework in mathematics and statistical analysis, both during and after formal nursing education programs. One can attend college courses without pursuing a degree. In addition, for the nurse researcher who is aware of a knowledge deficit related to statistics, we encourage searching the literature related to the specific statistical analyses being used in a particular study. In this way, knowledge can gradually be accumulated by the researcher as it is needed. Seeking out the mentorship, advice and guidance of researchers with a more comprehensive knowledge of the analyses being used is also very helpful.

USING COMPUTERS FOR ANALYSIS

Some beginning researchers may believe that they will not need mathematical and statistical knowledge because they plan to use computer analysis. They do not believe that they need to know mathematical formulas and statistical theory, because the computer "handles all of that." All they want to know is the *answer*. There is an enormous amount of information, however, provided in the computer printout. If the researcher finds the *answer* in the mass of computer output, its meaning can easily be misinterpreted. Computers conduct analysis on whatever data are provided. If the data entered into the computer are garbage (*e.g.*, numbers from the data are typed in incorrectly or data are typed into the wrong columns), the computer output will be garbage. If the data are inappropriate for the particular type of analysis selected, the computer program is often unable to detect that error, and the researcher's conclusions may be completely in error. Knowledge of the use of computers is important to the analytic process. However, it is important that computers be used wisely. The use of computers in research is discussed in more detail in Chapter 15.

USING "PACKAGED" COMPUTER PROGRAMS

"Packaged" computer analyses, such as SPSS^x (Statistical Packages for the Social Sciences), SAS (Statistical Analysis System) and BMDP (Biomedical Computer Programs) have been developed to make computer analysis simpler. Some of these analytic packages have been developed for the microcomputer (personal computer) as well as for the mainframe. The mathematical formulas are built into the program. When these programs are used, the manuals available demonstrate how to write the program and also provide a detailed discussion of the mathematical logic inherent within each type of analysis. The references at the end of each section in the manual suggest up-to-date and comprehensive sources related to each specific type of analysis. Even when packaged programs are being used, it is essential that the researcher understand the mathematical processes in the selected analytic technique. In this chapter, the computer programs to be used on the mainframe from SAS (1984; 1985a; 1985b), BMDP (1983) and SPSS^x (1983) are identified for specific statistical analysis techniques. In addition, programs from ABSTAT (1986), which was developed for the IBM personal computer, are provided for certain analysis techniques. The programs and the manual page numbers of these programs are presented in table form for each statistical analysis for easy reference.

USING PROGRAMMERS

In some cases, the researcher may employ a programmer to assist in writing the programs that give commands to the computer to implement the mathematical processes selected. Programmers are not statisticians; thus, they do not interpret the outcomes of analyses but are skilled in the use of computer languages. Computer languages are the techniques used to give detailed commands to the computer. Even when packaged programs are being used, a programmer, skilled in the use of common software packages, can be of great help in selecting the appropriate programs, writing them according to guidelines and speeding up the "debugging" process. In universities, computer science students are often available for programming services.

USING STATISTICIANS

Some researchers attempt to avoid the experience of data analysis altogether by taking their data to a statistician with an explanation of the questions to be answered or the specific analyses desired. The researcher can then return later to obtain the results, with an explanation by the statistician of the meaning of the findings.

This approach may seem the most desirable and simplest solution to data analysis, with the costs being the primary reason for choosing an alternative. However, in addition to relative costs, we believe that use of this approach does a serious injustice both to the researcher and to nursing. This strategy leaves the researcher in the same state of ignorance when the study is complete as when it started, thus inhibiting personal growth and the growth of nursing. There are approaches to utilizing the knowledge and skills of statisticians that can provide assistance without abdicating the total responsibility for data analysis to them.

One way to utilize the services of a statistician is to ask him or her to serve as an advisor during the analysis process. The statistician's knowledge can be sought to verify the researcher's approach to analysis. In this way, the statistician can be a source of additional information and thus assist in building the researcher's skills in statistical analysis. If the researcher experiences difficulties, the statistician can be available to assist in problem solving and critical examination of the analytic process.

Another approach to utilizing the knowledge of a statistician is to seek his or her counsel in order to crosscheck the work of the researcher. After the analysis is complete and conclusions have been reached by the researcher, a statistician can evaluate the work for accuracy and search out potential biases in the interpretation. This adds validity to the work and further strengthens the skills of the researcher.

Purposes of Statistical Analysis

Statistics can be used for a variety of purposes, including (1) to summarize, (2) to compare or contrast descriptively, (3) to test the proposed relationships in a theoretical model, (4) to infer that the findings from the sample are indicative of the entire population, (5) to examine causality, (6) to predict or (7) to infer from the sample to a theoretical model. The design selected for a study determines the purposes of the statistics used to analyze the data. To accomplish these purposes, a variety of statistical techniques have been developed.

Many research textbooks divide the statistical techniques into two sections, descriptive statistics and inferential statistics. This division has led to some erroneous thinking by beginning researchers. First, there may be the belief that descriptive statistics are to be used only in exploratory (qualitative and quantitative), descriptive and correlational studies and that inferential statistics are limited to use in quasi-experimental or experimental studies. Descriptive statistics are used in most quasi-experimental and experimental studies, as well as in studies in which the results will be limited to the sample under study. For example, description of the sample or samples used in the study requires the use of descriptive statistics.

The assumption is often made that if one uses *inferential statistics*, one is inferring from the sample to the population. Inferential statistics, although designed to allow inference from a sample statistic to a population parameter, are also commonly used to test hypotheses of similarities and differences in subsets of the sample under study, not a population. Inferences take place in the thinking of the researcher, not in the specific statistical analyses used. Inferences do not necessarily address causality in a population. Inferential thinking may be used to evaluate the probability of the existence of relationships in a population or to predict the probability of an event in the population. Causality, at best only an assumption, cannot be proved by any analysis. The mathematical theory concept of inference is discussed in more detail later in this chapter.

Organization of Chapter Content

Based on the aforementioned statements about statistical analysis and the development of the researcher, this chapter is designed to facilitate the researcher's performance of analysis, manually and/or by computer. The chapter also provides the statistical analysis information needed to conduct critiques of published research. It is assumed that the reader has had a prior course in statistics. For refreshing the memory of basic statistical concepts, we suggest referral to a basic statistics textbook.

In this text, two broad divisions of data analysis are made: *quantitative* techniques and *qualitative* techniques. Quantitative analysis techniques use numerical data, whereas qualitative techniques tend to use data in the form of words as the basis for the analysis. In the quantitative section, statistical techniques used primarily to summarize the data, or summary statistics, are described first. Then, quantitative analysis techniques are classified into two categories: *bivariate* or *multivariate*. Within the bivariate category, statistical analyses are further subdivided by the type of group (independent or dependent), by the number of groups (one, two or three or more) and by the type of data (nominal, ordinal, interval or ratio), for which these analyses are appropriate. Both parametric and nonparametric procedures are described. The analysis techniques in the multivariate category are organized according to increasing complexity. In addition to these traditional analysis techniques, some new approaches, such as time-series analysis and meta-analysis, are briefly discussed. In each section, the terms commonly used in discussing the analyses are defined. The qualitative analysis section includes descriptions of the techniques of analysis that are particularly relevant to this research approach.

Summary Statistics

Data analysis begins with summary statistics in any study in which the data are numerical. Summary statistics allow the researcher to organize the data in ways that give meaning and facilitate insight. It is like examining a phenomenon from a variety of angles in order to understand more clearly what is being seen. The angles from which the data can be examined will be limited to some extent by the level of measurement (nominal, ordinal, interval or ratio). These levels are described in Chapter 11. For some exploratory and descriptive studies, summary statistics will be the only approach to analysis of the data. Summary statistics also provide a means for describing the characteristics of the sample from which the data were collected.

FREQUENCY DISTRIBUTIONS

Frequency distributions are usually the first strategy used to organize the data for examination. In addition, frequency distributions are used to check for errors in coding and computer programming. There are two types of frequency distributions: ungrouped frequency distributions and grouped frequency distributions. In addition to providing a means to display the data, these distributions may be used for further analysis of the data.

Ungrouped Frequency Distribution

Most studies have some categorical data that are presented in the form of ungrouped frequency distributions. An ungrouped frequency distribution involves listing all possible measures of that variable and tallying each datum on the listing. The tally marks are then counted, and a table is developed to display the results. This approach is generally used on discrete rather than continuous data. Examples of data commonly organized in this manner include gender, race, marital status and diagnostic category of study subjects. Continuous data, such as test grades or scores on a data collection instrument, could be organized in this manner; however, if the number of possible scores is large, it is difficult to extract meaning from examination of the distribution.

Grouped Frequency Distribution

Some method of grouping is generally necessary when continuous variables are being examined. Age, for example, is a continuous variable. Many measures taken during data collection are continuous, including temperature, vital lung capacity, weight, scale scores and time. Grouping requires that the researcher make a number of decisions that will be important to the meaning derived from the data.

Any method of grouping results in loss of information. For example, if age is being grouped, a breakdown of under 65–over 65 will provide considerably less information than grouping by 10-year spans. The grouping should be made to provide the greatest possible meaning in terms of the purpose of the study. If the data are to be compared to data in other studies, groupings should be similar to those of other studies in that field of research to allow comparisons between studies.

The first step in developing a grouped frequency distribution is to establish a method of classifying the data. Although any number of classifications is possible, the general rule is that there should be at least 6 but not more than 20 groups. The classes that are developed must be exhaustive; each datum must fit into one of the identified classes. The classes must be exclusive; each datum can fit into only one of the established classes. A common mistake is to list ranges that contain overlaps. The range of each category must be equivalent. In the case of age, for example, if 10 years is the range, each category must include 10 years of ages. This rule is violated in some cases to allow the first and last categories to be open-ended and worded to include all scores above or below a specified point.

The precision with which the data will be reported is an important consideration. Will data be listed only in whole numbers, or will decimals be used? At how many decimal places will rounding off be performed? Data should not be reported with more precision on the tables and graphs than was actually obtained during data collection.

Percentage Distributions

Percentage distributions indicate the per cent of the sample whose scores fall in a specific group as well as the number of scores in that group. Percentage

TABLE 17–1
Example of a Cumulative Frequency Table

Score	Frequency	Per Cent	Cumulative Frequency (f)	Cumulative Per Cent
1	4	8	4	8
3	6	12	10	20
4	8	16	18	36
5	14	28	32	64
7	8	16	40	80
8	6	12	46	92
9	4	8	N = 50	100

distributions are particularly useful in comparing the present data with findings from other studies that have varying sample sizes. A cumulative distribution is a type of percentage distribution in which the percentages and frequencies of scores are summed as one moves from the top of the table to the bottom. Thus, the bottom category would have a cumulative frequency equivalent to the sample size and a cumulative percentage of 100 (Table 17–1). Frequency analysis can be conducted using the computer. Information about the programs used to conduct these calculations is presented in Table 17–2.

Displaying Frequency Distributions

Frequency distributions can be displayed using tables or graphs. Four types of graphs are commonly used: pie charts, bar charts, histograms and frequency polygons. Selection of an effective method of communicating the meaning found in the data is very important. Strategies for developing tables and graphs are described in Chapter 19.

MEASURES OF CENTRAL TENDENCY

A measure of central tendency is frequently referred to as an *average*. The term *average* is a lay term not commonly used in statistics because of its

TABLE 17–2
Computer Program Information
for Frequency Analysis

Computer Software	Computer Program Information
SAS	PROC FREQ; page 405
BMDP	P2D page 80
SPSS^x	FREQUENCIES page 265
ABSTAT	FREQ and ZSCOR page 75

vagueness. The measures of central tendency are the most concise statement of the nature of the data. The three measures of central tendency commonly used in statistical analyses are the mode, the median and the mean.

Mode

One of the simplest measures of central tendency is the mode. The mode can be determined by examination of an ungrouped frequency distribution of the data. The *mode* is the numerical value or score that occurs with greatest frequency. In Table 17–1, the mode of that data set is the score of 5, which occurred 14 times in the data set. The mode is the appropriate measure of central tendency for nominal data and is used in the calculation of some nonparametric statistics. A data set can have more than one mode. If two modes exist, the data set is referred to as bimodal. The mode does not necessarily indicate the center of the data set.

Median

The *median* is the score at the exact center of the ungrouped frequency distribution. The median is obtained by rank ordering the scores. If there are an uneven number of scores, exactly 50 per cent of the scores are above the median, and 50 per cent are below the median. If there are an even number of scores, the median is the average of the two middle scores. Thus, the median may not be an actual score in the data set.

Sometimes subjects have the same or tied scores. These tied scores have tied ranks. Under these circumstances, calculation of the median is more complex (Waltz, Strickland & Lenz, 1984). A frequency tabulation is necessary. Table 17–3 provides the raw scores, frequencies of these scores and the cumulative frequencies of these scores. (This is the same data set presented in Table 17–1). The median was calculated using these values. The steps for calculating the median for the data in the table follow:

1. The median score is the $N/2 = 50/2 = $ 25th score from the bottom.
2. Identify the score corresponding to the 25th score. The 25th score is located between the score interval of 4 and 5. These limits are identified in Table 17–3.

TABLE 17–3
Example Data Set for Calculation of the Median

	Score	Frequency (f)	Cumulative Frequency
	9	4	50
	8	6	46
	7	8	40
Upper Median Limit	**5**	**14**	**32**
Lower Median Limit	**4**	**8**	**18**
	3	6	10
	1	4	4
	N = 50		

3. The cumulative frequency in the lower limit of this interval is 18. Thus, 25 − 18 = 7 or 7 more scores are required to reach the 25th score.
4. The cumulative frequency in the upper limit of this interval is 32. The number of frequencies in the interval containing the 25th score is 32 − 18 = 14 frequencies.
5. The number of scores needed to reach the 25th score is 7 in this example. The 7 is divided by the number of frequencies in the interval containing the 25th score, which is 14. The fraction of 7/14, or 1/2, is multiplied by the width of the interval containing the 25th score. This interval is calculated by subtracting 5 − 4 = 1. Thus, 1/2 (1) = 1/2, or 0.5.
6. The 0.5 is added to the lower limit score of the median interval, which is 4. In the example, the median equals 0.5 + 4 = 4.5.

The median is not considered as useful statistically as the mean. However, it is not affected by extreme scores in the data (outlyers) as is the mean and thus may, in some cases, more accurately reflect the central tendency of the data. The median is the most appropriate measure of central tendency for ordinal data and is frequently used in nonparametric analyses.

The Mean

The most commonly used measure of central tendency is the mean. The *mean* is the sum of the scores divided by the number of scores being summed. The formula for calculating the mean is listed below.

$$\overline{X} = \frac{\Sigma X}{N}$$

where:
$\overline{X}$ = the mean
Σ = sigma (the statistical symbol for the process of summation)
X = a single raw score
N = number of scores being entered in the calculation

The mean was calculated for the data provided in Table 17–4.

$$\overline{X} = \frac{4 + 18 + 32 + 70 + 56 + 48 + 36}{50} = \frac{264}{50} = 5.28$$

The mean is the appropriate measure of central tendency for interval and ratio level data. This formula will be found repeatedly within more complex formulas of statistical analyses.

MEASURES OF DISPERSION

Measures of dispersion, or variability, give some indication of how scores in a sample are dispersed around the mean. These measures provide information

TABLE 17–4
Data for Calculation of Mean and Standard Deviation

Score X	Frequency (f)	fX	fX²
1	4	4	4 (1) = 4
3	6	18	6 (9) = 54
4	8	32	8 (16) = 128
5	14	70	14 (25) = 350
7	8	56	8 (49) = 392
8	6	48	6 (64) = 384
9	4	36	4 (81) = 324
	N = 50	ΣX = 264	ΣX² = 1636

about the data not available from measures of central tendency. They indicate how different the scores are—the extent to which individual scores deviate from one another. If the individual scores are similar, measures of variability are small and the sample is relatively *homogeneous* in terms of those scores. *Heterogeneity* (wide variation in scores) is important to obtain in order to conduct meaningful data analyses with parametric statistics. Heterogeneity is determined by measures of variability. The measures most commonly used are modal percentage, range, deviation scores, sum of squares, variance and the standard deviation.

Modal Percentage

The modal percentage is the only measure of variability appropriate for use with nominal data. The modal percentage indicates the relationship of the number of data scores represented by the mode to the total number of data scores. To determine the modal percentage, the frequency of the modal scores is divided by the total number of scores. For example, in Table 17–4, the mode is 5, 14 of the subjects scored 5, and the sample size is 50; thus, $14/50 = 0.28$. The result of that operation is then multiplied by 100 to convert it to a percentage. In the example given, the modal percentage would be 28 per cent, which means that 28 per cent of the sample is represented by the mode. The complete calculation would be $14/50(100) = 28$ per cent. This strategy allows comparison of the present data with other data sets.

Range

The simplest measure of dispersion is the range. The range is obtained by subtracting the lowest score from the highest score. The range for the scores in Table 17–4 is calculated as follows: $9 - 1 = 8$. The range is a difference score, which uses only the two extreme scores for the comparison. It is a very crude measure and is sensitive to outlyers. The range is generally reported but is not used in further analyses. It is not a very useful method of comparing the present data with that from other studies.

Difference Scores

Difference scores are obtained by subtracting each score from the mean. A difference score is sometimes referred to as a deviation score since it indicates the extent to which a score deviates from the mean. The difference score will be positive when the score is above the mean and negative when the score is below the mean. Difference scores are the basis for many statistical analyses and can be found within many statistical equations. The sum of difference scores is zero, making the sum a useless measure. The formula for difference scores is:

$$X - \overline{X}$$

The Sum of Squares

A common strategy used to allow meaningful mathematical manipulation of difference scores is to square them. These squared scores are then summed. When negative scores are squared, they become positive. Because of this, the sum will no longer equal zero. This mathematical maneuver is referred to as the *sum of squares* (SS). In this case, the SS is actually the sum of squared deviations. The equation for SS is:

$$SS = \Sigma (X - \overline{X})^2$$

The larger the value of SS, the greater the variance. Because the value of SS is dependent on the measurement scale used to obtain the original scores, comparison of SS with other studies is limited to studies using similar data. The sum of squares is a very valuable measure of variance and is used in many complex statistical equations. The SS importance is due to the fact that when deviations from the mean are squared, the sum is smaller than the sum of squared deviations from any other value from a sample distribution. This is referred to as the *least-squares principle* and is important in mathematical manipulations.

Variance

The variance is another measure commonly used in statistical analyses. The equation for variance (V) is:

$$V = \frac{\Sigma (X - \overline{X})^2}{N}$$

As can be seen, the variance is the mean or average of the sum of squares. Again, because the result is dependent upon the measurement scale used, it has no absolute value and can be compared only to data obtained using similar measures. However, generally, the larger the variance, the larger the dispersion of scores (Shelley, 1984).

Standard Deviation

The standard deviation is simply the square root of the variance. This is an important step mathematically because squaring mathematical terms changes them in some important ways. Obtaining the square root reverses this change. The equation for obtaining standard deviation (SD) is:

$$SD = \sqrt{\frac{\Sigma \, (X - \overline{X})^2}{N}}$$

Although this equation clarifies the relationships between difference scores, sum of squares and variance, using it requires that all these measures in turn be calculated. If the SD is being calculated directly by hand (or with the use of a calculator), the following computational equation is easier to use. The data from Table 17–4 were used to calculate the SD.

$$SD = \sqrt{\frac{\Sigma \, X^2 - (1/N) \, (\Sigma \, X)^2}{N - 1}}$$

$$SD = \sqrt{\frac{1636 - (1/50) \, (264)^2}{50 - 1}} = \sqrt{\frac{1636 - 1393.92}{49}} = \sqrt{4.94} = 2.22$$

Just as the mean is the "average" score, the standard deviation is the "average" difference (deviation) score. The standard deviation provides a measure of the average deviation of a score from the mean in that particular sample. It indicates the degree of error that would be made if the mean alone were used to interpret the data. Standard deviation is an important measure, both in understanding dispersion within a distribution and in interpreting the relationship of a particular score to the distribution. Descriptive statistics (mean, median, mode and standard deviation) can be calculated using the computer. The programs used to conduct these calculations are presented in Table 17–5.

THE SHAPES OF DISTRIBUTIONS

The shape of the distribution provides important information about the data being studied. The outline of the distribution shape is obtained using the frequency polygon. Then, within this outline, the mean, median, mode and standard deviation can be graphically illustrated. This visual presentation of combined summary statistics provides increased insight into the nature of the distribution. As the sample size becomes larger, the shape of the distribution will more accurately reflect the shape of the population from which the sample was taken.

TABLE 17–5
Computer Program Information
for Descriptive Statistics

Computer Software	Computer Program Information
SAS	PROC FREQ page 405
BMDP	P4D page 86
SPSS[x]	FREQUENCIES page 265
ABSTAT	DESC page 74

Symmetry

Several terms are used to describe the shape of the curve (and thus the nature of a particular distribution). A symmetrical curve is one in which the left side of the curve is a mirror image of the right side. In these curves, the mean, median and mode are equal and are the dividing point between the left and right side of the curve (Fig. 17–1).

Skewness

Any curve that is not symmetrical is referred to as skewed or asymmetrical. Skewness may be exhibited in the curve in a variety of ways (Fig. 17–2). A curve may be positively skewed, which means that the largest portion of data is below the mean. For example, the data on length of enrollment in hospice are positively skewed. Thus, the majority of the people die within the first 3 weeks of enrollment, with increasingly smaller numbers surviving over a period of months. The curve can also be negatively skewed, which means that the largest portion of data is above the mean. For example, the data on the

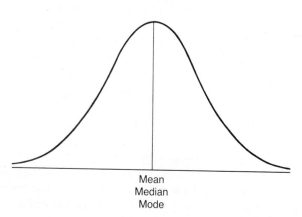

FIGURE 17–1. The normal curve.

Mean
Median
Mode

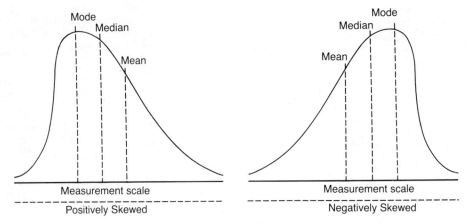

FIGURE 17–2. Skewness.

occurrence of chronic illness in a population are negatively skewed, with the majority of chronic illnesses occurring in older age groups.

In a skewed distribution, the mean, median and mode are not equal. Skewness interferes with the accuracy of many statistical analyses; therefore, mathematical equations have been developed to test for the skewness of the distribution of the sample being studied. Very few samples will be perfectly symmetrical; however, as the deviation from symmetry increases, the seriousness of the impact on statistical analyses increases. The test for skewness is expressed in the following equation:

$$\text{skewness} = \frac{\Sigma\,(X - \overline{X})^3}{N\,(SD^3)}$$

Using the equation, a result of zero indicates a completely symmetrical distribution; a positive number indicates a positively skewed distribution; and a negative number indicates a negatively skewed distribution. Statistical analyses conducted by computer will often automatically test for skewness, which is then indicated in the computer printout. Strongly skewed distributions must often be tested using nonparametric techniques, which make no assumptions of normally distributed samples. In a positively skewed distribution, the mean will be greater than the median, which will be greater than the mode. In a negatively skewed distribution, the mean will be less than the median, which will be less than the mode.

Modality

Another characteristic of distributions is their modality. Most curves are unimodal, which means that there is one mode and frequencies progressively decline as they move away from the mode. Symmetrical distributions are usually unimodal. However, curves can also be bimodal (Fig. 17–3) or trimodal.

FIGURE 17–3. Bimodal distribution.

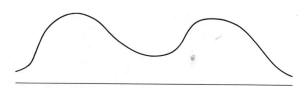

Kurtosis

Another term used to describe the shape of the distribution curve is *kurtosis*. Kurtosis explains the degree of peakedness of the curve, which is related to the spread of variance of scores. A relatively flat curve is referred to as *platykurtic*; an intermediate degree of kurtosis as *mesokurtic*; and an extremely peaked curve is termed *leptokurtic* (Fig. 17–4). Extreme kurtosis can also affect the accuracy of statistical analyses and is mathematically tested for in computer analyses. A common equation used to test for kurtosis is:

$$\text{kurtosis} = \frac{(X - \overline{X})^4}{N(SD^4)} - 3$$

Standardized Scores

Because of differences in the characteristics of various distributions, comparing a score in one distribution with a score in another distribution is difficult. To facilitate this comparison, a mechanism has been developed to transform raw scores into standard scores. Numbers that make sense only within the framework of measurements used within a specific study are transformed to numbers (*standard scores*) that have a more general meaning. Transformation to standard scores allows an easy conceptual grasp of the meaning of the score. A common standardized score is called a *Z score*. It expresses deviations from the mean (difference scores) in terms of standard deviation units. The equation for a Z score is as follows:

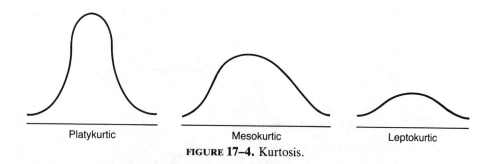

Platykurtic   Mesokurtic   Leptokurtic

FIGURE 17–4. Kurtosis.

$$Z = \frac{X - \overline{X}}{SD}$$

A score that falls above the mean will have a positive Z score, whereas a score that falls below the mean will have a negative Z score. The mean expressed as a Z score is zero. The standard deviation expressed as a Z score is 1. Thus, a Z score of 2 indicates that the score from which it was obtained is two standard deviations above the mean. A Z score of -0.5 indicates that the score was 0.5 standard deviations below the mean. The distribution of Z scores is included in Appendix B.

The Normal Curve

When data have been measured repeatedly in many samples using scales based on an underlying continuum, all the scores can be combined into one large sample. From this very large sample, one can develop a more accurate representation of the pattern of the curve in that population. In most cases, the curve is similar, regardless of the specific data that have been examined. This fact was discovered by an 18-year-old mathematician (Gauss) in 1795. Using this discovery, he developed a theoretical frequency distribution of all *possible* scores, which is referred to as the normal curve. No *real* distribution exactly fits the distribution. It is an expression of mathematical theory. The normal curve is symmetrical and unimodal and has continuous values. The mean, median and mode are equal. The values from the kurtosis and skewness equations are zero. The distribution is completely defined by the mean and standard deviation. The measures in the theoretical distribution have been standardized using Z scores. The proportion of scores that may be found in a particular area of the normal curve have been identified (Fig. 17–5).

As can be seen, 68 per cent of the scores will be within 1 standard

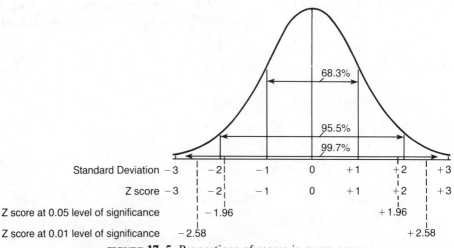

FIGURE 17–5. Proportions of scores in curve areas.

deviation above or below the mean, 95 per cent will be within 2 standard deviations above or below the mean and 99 per cent will be within 3 standard deviations above or below the mean. Even when a statistic, such as a mean, comes from a population with a skewed distribution, the sampling distribution developed from multiple means obtained from that skewed population will tend to fit the pattern of the normal curve. This phenomenon is referred to as the *Central Limit Theorem* and lends some justification to the argument for using parametric statistical analyses, even with data from skewed samples (Volicer, 1984).

THE SAMPLING DISTRIBUTION

The sampling distribution is developed from statistical values from many samples obtained from the same population. The purpose of the sampling distribution is to more precisely define the population. For example, the means from many samples in the population are often used to develop a sampling distribution. The mean of this distribution is referred to as the *mean of means*. A related distribution can be developed from the standard deviations of each sample. The mean of the standard deviation distribution is referred to as the *standard error*. Other values, such as correlations between variables, scores obtained from specific measures and differences between groups within the population can yield values that are then used to develop the sampling distribution. The sampling distribution provides information on all the possible values of identified dimensions of the population that can occur within that distribution. It contains multiple "normal curves" describing various dimensions of that specific population. We can then compare the mean or standard deviation of our sample with that of the sampling distribution. The mean of the sample then becomes an "estimate" of the mean of the sampling distribution. And the mean of the sampling distribution is an even more accurate "estimate" of the mean of the population.

In most cases, the actual population values are not known. (If they were, why would we be conducting the research?) Therefore, these values are "estimated." We "infer" from a sample value to an estimated population value. Although one might envision a scientist laboriously collecting data on large numbers of samples of varying sizes that were randomly selected from the population of interest, this is not the case. In fact, the distribution is developed mathematically and is thus an expression of mathematical theory.

SAMPLING DISTRIBUTION OF A STATISTIC

Just as it is possible to develop distributions of summary statistics within a population, it is possible to develop distributions of inferential statistical outcomes with varying sample sizes. These distributions involve the outcome of comparison of two or more samples. For example, if one repeatedly obtained two samples of the same size from the same population and tested for differences in the means using a t-test, a distribution could be developed from the resulting t values. Using this t distribution, one could determine the probability of obtaining a specific t value if two samples being studied were really from the same population. Using this approach, a distribution could be developed for samples of many varying sizes. Figure 17–6 illustrates the normal distribution for t values, which has a mean of 50 and a standard deviation of 10.

Such a distribution is based on probability and addresses the likelihood of obtaining a specific statistical outcome considering the sizes of the two samples tested. Statistical analysis makes an inference that the samples being tested can be considered part of the population from which the distribution was developed. The population addressed in these distributions is again a theoretical one of "all possible samples that could be tested with the statistic in question." It is then necessary to infer from this population to the population being considered in the study.

One of the important outcomes of this work is tables that have been developed that organize the statistical outcomes from various sample sizes that would have a low probability of occurring in the present theoretical population. This probability is expressed as *alpha*, commonly referred to as the *level of significance*. An explanation of level of significance is provided later in this chapter.

Parameters

In data analysis and in the interpretation of that analysis, reference is often made to the "population" with which the sample is being compared. Actually, there are *two* populations to which the sample is being compared; yet these two populations are not usually clearly differentiated in statistical discussions. The first population is the one discussed in Chapter 9. This population is in one sense "real" (concrete) and in another sense abstract. For example, if you are studying the effect of teaching on the behavior of new diabetics, you are generalizing to the behavior of all new diabetics who have been taught (concrete) and/or, theoretically, to the expected behavior of all new diabetics if they were taught (abstract).

In order to determine whether your sample is like all those in the "real"

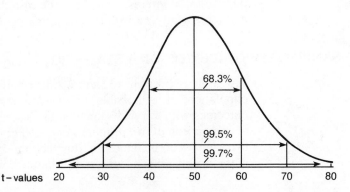

FIGURE 17–6. t Distribution.   t–values 20   30   40   50   60   70   80

population, you must compare them by some measures. For example, one strategy would be to compare the mean of your sample to the mean of the entire population. Unfortunately, it is highly unlikely that you *know* the mean of the entire population. Therefore, you must make an estimate of the mean of that population. You must know how good your sample is as an estimator of the parameters of that population.

First, you make some assumptions. You assume that the mean scores from multiple randomly selected samples of this diabetic population would be normally distributed. Emerging from this assumption is another assumption—that the behavior of the diabetic population will be distributed according to the theoretical normal curve—that difference scores and standard deviations can be equated to those in the normal curve.

This is where the second population comes in. If you assume that the "real" population in your study is normally distributed, you can also assume that this "real" population is comparable to the sampling distribution of the statistical analyses that you plan to use. Thus, you infer from your sample to the sampling distribution, the mathematically developed theoretical population made up of parameters such as the mean of means and the standard error. The parameters of this theoretical population are those measures of the dimensions identified in the sampling distribution. The *statistic* (X) is the numerical figure obtained from the sample. The *parameter* (μ) is the mean of that value within the sampling distribution. For example, the mean of the sample is a statistic; the mean of means (or the population mean) is a parameter (Barnett, 1982).

Perhaps you want to know whether certain behaviors of new diabetics who are provided specific information differ significantly from the same behaviors of new diabetics who are not given this information. If you tested the means from these two groups, would the means be so different that you could justify saying that they were from different populations because the means were statistically significantly different? To determine this, you would use a statistical analysis and compare the resulting value of the test statistic with the table value. This table value would indicate the population parameters for that statistic.

Parametric and Nonparametric Statistical Analyses

Both parametric and nonparametric techniques are valuable methods to analyze data. The choice of technique is, to some extent, determined by the type of data available for analysis. The most commonly used statistical analyses are parametric statistics. These approaches to analysis emerged from the work of Fisher and required meeting the following three assumptions before they could justifiably be used: (1) The sample was drawn from a normal distribution, (2) random sampling techniques were used to obtain the sample and (3) the data were measured at least at the interval level. The analyses were referred to as parametric because the findings were being inferred to the parameters of a normally distributed population.

These criteria greatly limited the situations and variables that could be studied. Therefore, a small group of mathematicians began to develop techniques that were nonparametric, or distribution free. These techniques could be used in studies that did not meet the assumptions just listed. These nonparametric techniques were gathered together by Siegel in a book published in 1956, which has remained the primary source for nonparametric analyses since that time.

Nonparametric techniques are not as powerful as parametric techniques; in other words, they are less able to detect differences. However, the techniques can be used with cruder forms of measurement that yield nominal or ordinal data. The techniques have continued to be considered inferior to parametric approaches by those who hold a very conservative point of view.

In recent years, there has been a greater tolerance to using parametric techniques when some of the assumptions were not met, recognizing that the analyses were robust to violation of assumptions. *Robust* means that the analysis will yield accurate results even if some of the assumptions are violated by the data used for the analysis. The criteria for classifying data as "interval" have been relaxed. The Central Limit Theorem has demonstrated that even when the population from which the sample was taken is not normally distributed, the means from multiple samples taken from it will be normally distributed. Therefore, there has been somewhat of a move back to the use of parametric techniques.

Estimation of Parameters

In most studies, there is interest in inferring the findings from the study sample to a population. To do this, one needs to know the parameters of that population. Unfortunately, one seldom knows the parameters of the population to which one wishes to infer; therefore, the parameters may have to be estimated. There are two approaches to estimating the parameters of a population: point estimation and interval estimation.

Point Estimation

A statistic that produces a value as a function of the scores in a sample is called an *estimator*. Much of inferential statistical analysis involves the use of point estimation to evaluate the fit between the estimator (a statistic) and the population parameter. A *point estimate* is a single figure that estimates a related figure in the population of interest. The best point estimator is the mean of the sample being examined. However, the mean of the sample rarely equals the mean of the population. In addition to the mean, other estimators used include the median, variance, standard deviation and the correlation coefficient.

The selection of an estimator is based on previous experience with the accuracy of that estimator in approximating the parameter. Three characteristics of the estimator are considered important: (1) unbiasedness, (2) consistency and (3) relative efficiency. An estimator is considered unbiased if the mean of the sampling distribution for the estimator is equal to the value of the parameter. The mean of the sample is the most unbiased estimator. The standard deviation is more biased than the mean. Consistency is also a concern. Even if an estimator is biased, if it is consistently biased in the same direction, it will tend to more closely estimate the population parameter as the sample size becomes larger. Relative efficiency refers to the precision or accuracy with which the estimation is made. The difference between the estimator and the parameter is referred to as the *variance error*. The variance error of the median is much greater than the variance error of the mean. In fact, the sample mean has less variance error than any other estimator. Therefore, the mean is commonly used in statistical analyses.

Interval Estimation

An interval estimate is a segment of a number line where the value of the parameter is thought to be. For example, using a sample with a mean of 40 and a standard deviation of 5, one might use the range of scores between two standard deviations below the mean to two standard deviations above the mean, (30,50) as the interval estimation. This provides a set of scores rather than a single score. The population mean is *probably* in this set of scores; however, there is no absolute certainty that the mean of the population lies within that range. Therefore, it is necessary to determine the probability that this interval estimate contains the population mean.

This need to determine probability brings us back to the sampling distribution. We know that 95 per cent of the means in the sampling distribution lie within two standard deviations of the mean of means (the population mean). If these scores are converted to Z scores, the unit normal distribution table can be used to determine how many standard deviations out from the mean of means one must go to establish an interval estimate that includes 70 per cent, 95 per cent or 99 per cent of the means in the distribution.

Examining the normal distribution, one finds that 2.5 per cent of the area under the normal curve lies below a Z score of -1.96, or $\mu - (1.96SD/\sqrt{N})$, and 2.5 per cent of the area lies above a Z score of 1.96, or $\mu + (1.96SD/\sqrt{N})$, where μ is the mean of means, SD is the standard deviation and N is the sample size. The probability is 0.95 that a randomly selected sample would have a mean within this range.

Confidence Intervals

When the probability of including the value of the parameter within the interval estimate is known (using the formula above), it is referred to as a *confidence interval*. In the previous example, the results would be expressed in the following format: "a 95 per cent confidence interval was constructed." In this case, the confidence coefficient is 0.95. The confidence interval does *not* imply that 95 per cent of the means in the sampling distribution will fall within this interval of values but that there is a 95 per cent probability that the population mean will fall within the interval.

Calculating the confidence interval involves using two formulas to identify the upper and lower ends of the interval. The formula for a confidence interval for a sample is presented below:

$$\overline{X} - 1.96SD/\sqrt{N} \qquad \overline{X} + 1.96SD/\sqrt{N}$$

If one had a sample with a mean of 40, a standard deviation of 5 and an N of 50, a confidence interval could be calculated.

$$40 - 1.96\left(\frac{5}{\sqrt{50}}\right) = 40 - 1.386 = 38.6$$

$$40 + 1.96\left(\frac{5}{\sqrt{50}}\right) = 40 + 1.386 = 41.4$$

These confidence intervals are usually expressed as (38.6,41.4). Confidence intervals can also be developed around correlation coefficients (Glass & Stanley, 1970, pp. 264–268).

Hypothesis Testing

Estimation compares a sample statistic to a population parameter. In hypothesis testing, one compares a sample statistic (such as a mean) with the same statistic from a second sample (or perhaps several other samples). This comparison is done through statistical analysis, which results in a statistical value. The statistical value is then compared to the mean value for that statistic listed in the sampling distribution for the statistic. The purpose is to determine whether the statistics from the different samples are similar enough to suggest that the samples probably came from the same population.

The approach to hypothesis testing emerges from a different tradition of mathematical theory than does estimation—that of decision theory. Based on the statistical analyses, the researcher must make a decision about whether the hypothesis is to be accepted or rejected. Using decision theory, a null hypothesis is developed that states that there is no difference between the samples. In other words, the samples are assumed to be from the same population. Then, if a difference is found according to the statistical analysis, the null hypothesis is rejected. If no difference is found, the null hypothesis is "accepted" or "retained." The existence of a difference is determined by using the sampling distribution of the statistical test. Therefore, one can determine the probability that a statistical value obtained is likely to occur in two samples selected from the same population. This probability is expressed as the level of significance.

Level of Significance

The level of significance, developed from decision theory, is the cutoff point used to determine whether the samples being tested are members of the same population or from different populations. This decision is based on the theoretical normal curve. As mentioned previously, 68 per cent of the means from samples in a population will fall within one standard deviation from the mean of means (μ), 95 per cent will fall within two standard deviations, 99 per cent within three standard deviations and 99.9 per cent within four standard deviations. This decision theory explanation of the expected distribution of means is equivalent to the confidence interval explanation described previously.

It is simply expressed differently. In keeping with decision theory, the level of significance sought in a statistical test must be *established prior to conducting the test*. In fact, the significance level should be established prior to collecting the data. In nursing studies, the level of significance is usually set at 0.05 or 0.01.

If one wishes to predict with a 95 per cent probability of accuracy, the level of significance would be $p \leq 1 - 0.95$ or $p \leq 0.05$. The statistical symbol ($\leq$) means "less than or equal to." Thus, $p \leq 0.05$ means there is a probability less than or equal to 5 per cent of making a decision error in the determination of significant differences between groups. The level of significance is often referred to as *alpha* or the Greek letter (α).

In computer analysis, the actual level of significance obtained from the data is frequently provided on the printout. For example, the actual level of significance might be $p \leq 0.03$ or $p \leq 0.07$. This level of significance should be provided in the research report as well as the level of significance set prior to the analysis.

Tailedness

On the normal curve, extremes of statistical values can occur at either end of the curve. Because this is true, the 5 per cent of statistical values that are considered statistically significant must be distributed between the two extremes of the curve. The extremes of the curve are referred to as *tails*. If the hypothesis is nondirectional and assumes that an extreme score can occur in either tail, the analysis is referred to as a *two-tailed test of significance* (Fig. 17–7).

In a *one-tailed test of significance*, the hypothesis is "directional," and extreme statistical values that occur on a single tail of the curve are of interest.

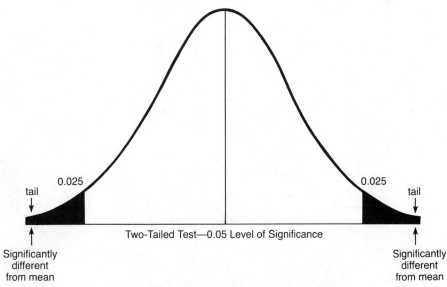

FIGURE 17–7. Two-tailed level of significance.

In this case, extreme statistical values occurring on the other tail of the curve are not considered significantly different. In Figure 17–8, which is a one-tailed figure, the portion of the curve in which statistical values will be considered significant are in the right tail of the curve.

Two cautions must be considered in using directional hypotheses. First, it is easier to obtain significance with a one-tailed statistical test and thus the risk of a Type I error (discussed below) is greater. Second, if the theory from which the hypothesis was developed is in error, extreme statistical values in the other tail of the curve will be overlooked and information needed to modify the existing theory will not be obtained.

Type I and Type II Errors

Two types of error can occur in making decisions about the meaning of a value obtained from a statistical test: Type I errors and Type II errors. A Type I error occurs when the researcher concludes that the samples tested are from different populations (there is a significant difference between groups) when, in fact, the samples are from the same population (there is no significant difference between groups). This error is possible because even though statistical values in the extreme ends of the tail of the curve are rare, they do occur within the population. In viewing Table 17–6, remember that the null hypothesis states that "there is no difference between groups."

There is a greater risk of a Type I error with a 0.05 level of significance than with a 0.01 level of significance. As the level of significance becomes more extreme, the risk of a Type I error decreases, as illustrated in Figure 17–9.

A type II error occurs when the researcher concludes that there is no

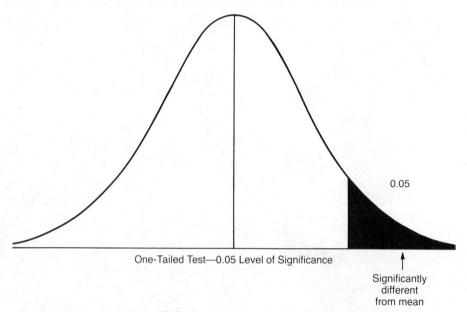

0.05

One-Tailed Test—0.05 Level of Significance

Significantly
different
from mean

FIGURE 17–8. One-tailed level of significance.

TABLE 17–6
Occurrence of Type I and Type II Errors

Data Analysis Indicates:	In Reality The Null Hypothesis Is:	
	True	False
results significant null rejected	Type I Error	correct decision (power)
results not significant null accepted	correct decision	Type II Error

significant difference between the samples examined when, in fact, a difference exists. This type of error occurs because in some cases there is some degree of overlap between the values of different populations, so that a value with a greater than 5 per cent probability of being within one population may in fact be within the dimensions of another population (Fig. 17–10).

As the risk of a Type I error decreases (by setting a more extreme level of significance), the risk of a Type II error increases. When the risk of a Type II error is decreased (by setting a less extreme level of significance), the risk of a Type I error increases. It is not possible to decrease both types of error simultaneously. Therefore, the researcher must decide which risk poses the greatest threat within a specific study. In fields such as medical research, for example, the effectiveness of one drug to treat cancer might be compared with the effectiveness of another drug. The risk of committing a Type I error (saying that one drug is more effective in treating cancer than another drug when it is not) is more serious than committing a Type II error (saying that one drug is no more effective in treating cancer than the other when one drug is more effective). Therefore, medical scientists would tend to set an extreme level of significance, such as 0.001. In nursing research, many studies are conducted with small samples and instruments that are not precise measures of the variables under study. In many nursing situations, multiple variables interact to lead to differences within populations. However, when one is examining

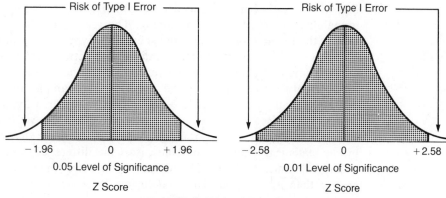

FIGURE 17–9. Risk of Type I error.

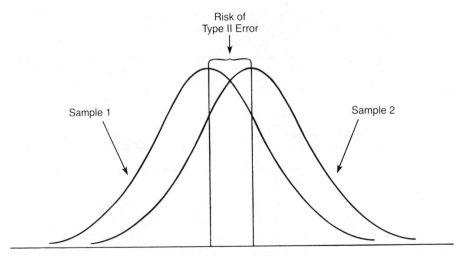

FIGURE 17–10. Risk of Type II error.

only a few of the interacting variables, small differences can be overlooked, leading to a false conclusion of no differences between the samples. In this case, the risk of a Type II error is a greater concern, and a more lenient level of significance is in order. Most nursing studies set the level of significance at 0.05.

Power Analysis

Until recently, the researcher's primary interest was in preventing a Type I error. Therefore, great emphasis was placed on the selection of a level of significance. Interpretation of the level of significance was so rigid that an alpha of 0.06 was treated the same as an alpha of 0.60. In both cases, the null hypothesis was accepted, the research hypothesis was rejected, and the findings were so reported in publications. This strategy is in keeping with the tenets of decision theory. Currently, using decision theory criteria, researchers are criticized for making statements such as "the findings approach significance at the 0.06 level." Support for decision theory is decreasing as support for probability theory increases in nursing. The reason for this changing point of view is the recognition of the seriousness of a Type II error in nursing studies.

A null hypothesis assumes no difference between the groups. Therefore, under the null hypothesis, the difference score in the measure of the dependent variable between groups would be zero. In a two-sample study, this would be expressed mathematically as $A - B = 0$. The research hypothesis would be stated as $A - B \neq 0$ where ($\neq$) means "not equal to." A Type II error occurs when the difference score is not zero but is small enough that it is not detected by the statistical analyses. In some cases, the difference is negligible and not of interest clinically. However, in many other cases, the difference in reality is greater than is indicated. This undetected difference is often due to research methodology problems.

Type II errors can occur for three reasons: (1) a stringent level of significance, (2) a small sample size and (3) a small difference in measured effect between the groups. Difference in measured effect is due to a number of factors, including a large variance in scores on the dependent variable within groups, crude instrumentation that does not measure with precision and/or confounding variables that mask the effects of the variables under study. The level of significance and the sample size are known prior to data collection. Strategies have been developed to calculate the expected size of the effect; therefore, it is possible to determine the risk of a Type II error and modify the study to decrease the risk if necessary.

The strategy used to determine the Type II error risk is *power analysis*. Power analysis is used to determine the power of the study to detect a significant difference that actually exists. Power analysis techniques have been presented in detail by Cohen (1977) in his book *Statistical Power Analysis for the Behavioral Sciences*. Power analysis is most commonly used to determine the sample size necessary for a particular study; however, it is also used to determine the level of power to detect differences in research reports that support the null hypotheses. *Power* is the probability that a statistical test will detect a significant difference that exists. Often, reported studies supporting the null hypothesis (in which power is unlikely to have been examined) will have only a 10 per cent power level to detect a difference if one exists. An 80 per cent power level is minimally acceptable. The technique of power analysis is important in planning and critiquing studies and in meta-analysis (described later in this chapter).

If the researcher conducts a power analysis and finds it unacceptably low and the power of the study cannot be increased, the risk of a Type II error may be so great that it is useless to conduct the study. In this type of study, statistical tests will not detect differences that exist. Deciding to conduct a study in these circumstances is costly in time and money, cannot add to the body of nursing knowledge and can actually lead to false conclusions.

Cohen (1977) has identified four parameters that must be included in a power analysis: (1) significance level, (2) sample size, (3) effect size (ES) and (4) power. If three of the four are known, the fourth can be calculated using power analysis formulas. Significance level and sample size are fairly straightforward. *Effect size* is "the degree to which the phenomenon is present in the population, or the degree to which the null hypothesis is false" (Cohen, 1977, pp. 9–10). For example, if one were measuring changes in anxiety levels, measured first when the patient is at home and then just prior to surgery, effect size would be large if a great change in anxiety was expected. Effect size must be calculated, and the calculations differ with the statistical test being used. These calculations will be described for some statistical tests later in the chapter. Power must also be calculated. However, Cohen has developed tables indicating the power level if the sample size, alpha level and effect size are given. The available power in a proposed study is relatively easy to determine using these tables. The power analysis should be reported in studies that support the null hypothesis. If power is high, it strengthens the meaning of the findings. If power is low, the researcher should address this in the discussion of implications. The modifications in the research methodology that resulted from the use of power analysis should also be reported.

Magnitude Estimation

When a statistical test determines that there are significant differences between groups (as in a t-test), the researcher has no information on the magnitude of the difference. Some researchers mistakenly assume that the extent of the level of significance provides this information; however, this is not the case. Magnitude estimation is a strategy to estimate the degree of difference between groups. Magnitude estimation of differences between groups when the dependent variable is continuous is commonly obtained using Pearson's Product-Moment Correlation Coefficient (discussed later in this chapter). Squaring the statistic r will indicate the amount of variance in the variable scores explained by group membership. If the amount of variance (r^2) is low, as frequently occurs in psychosocial variables, further studies should be conducted to identify other variables interacting in the situation, which together will explain a greater amount of the variance.

Degrees of Freedom

The concept of degrees of freedom (df) is a product of mathematical theory and is easier to calculate than it is to explain because of the complex mathematics involved in demonstrating the justification for the concept. Degrees of freedom involves the freedom of a score's value to vary given the other existing scores' values and the established sum of these scores. A simple example may provide beginning insight into the concept. Suppose difference scores are obtained from a sample of 4 and the mean is 4. The difference scores are -2, -1, $+1$ and $+2$. As with all difference scores, the sum of these scores is 0. As a result, if any three of the difference scores are calculated, the value of the fourth score is not free to vary. Its value will depend on the values of the other three in order to maintain a mean of 4 and a sum of 0. The degrees of freedom (df) in this example is three, since only three scores are free to vary. In this case and in many other analyses, degrees of freedom (df) is the sample size (N) minus one (N $-$ 1).

$$df = N - 1$$

In this example, df $= 4 - 1 = 3$ (Roscoe, 1969, p. 162). In some analyses, determination of levels of significance on tables of statistical sampling distributions requires knowledge of the degrees of freedom.

Bivariate Data Analysis

Bivariate analysis involves the comparison of summary values from two groups on the same variable or of two variables within a group. Selection of the statistical analysis will depend on the level of measurement (nominal, ordinal, interval or ratio) of the data and the subproblems (hypotheses, questions or objectives) posed by the study. Analyses could be conducted that are appropriate for the type of data but do not answer the questions within the study design. Bivariate analyses for both independent and dependent groups are discussed in this section. In *independent groups*, the selection of one subject is totally unrelated to the selection of other subjects. Therefore, the selection of each subject does not bias the selection of other subjects. In *dependent groups*, subjects or observations selected for data collection are, in some way, related to the selection of other subjects or observations. For example, if subjects serve as their own control by using the pretest as a control, the observations (and therefore the groups) are dependent. If matched pairs of subjects are used for control or treatment groups, the observations are dependent. The approaches to analysis for independent and dependent groups are discussed in this section.

INDEPENDENT GROUPS—NOMINAL DATA

The common tests used to analyze nominal data for independent groups are presented in Table 17–7. These are nonparametric tests. Nominal data are frequently organized using contingency tables. *Contingency tables*, or cross-tabulation, allows visual comparison of summary data output related to two variables within the sample. This is a useful preliminary strategy for examining large amounts of data. In most cases, the data are in the form of frequencies or percentages. Using this strategy, one can compare two or more categories of one variable to two or more categories of a second variable. The simplest version is referred to as a 2 × 2 table (two categories of two variables). Table 17–8 shows an example of a 2 × 2 contingency table from Knafl's (1985) study of how families manage a pediatric hospitalization.

The data are generally referenced in terms of rows and columns. The intersection between the row and column in which a specific numerical value is inserted is referred to as a *cell*. The upper left cell would be row 1, column 1. In the example in Table 17–8, the cell of row 1, column 1 has the value of 18, and the cell of row 1, column 2 has the value of 7 and so on. The output from each row and each column is summed, and the sum is placed at the end of the row or column. In the example, the sum of row 1 is 25; the sum of row 2, 37; the sum of column 1, 34 and the sum of column 2, 28. The per cent of the sample represented by that sum can also be placed at the end of the row or

TABLE 17-7
Independent Groups—
Nominal Data

Chi Square
Fisher's Exact Probability
Phi
Cramer's V
Contingency Coefficient C
Lambda

TABLE 17–8
The Relationship Between Parents' Reports of Impact on
Family Life and Outside Help

	Parents' Reports		
Outside Help	Neutral	Negative	Total
No*	18	7	25
Yes†	16	21	37
Total	34	28	62

*Includes cases from "Alone" category.
†Combines cases from "Some Help" and "Delegation" categories.
$p < 0.05$ $\chi^2 = 4.98$ $df = 1$
Modified from Knafl, 1985, p. 163.

column. The row sums and the column sums total to the same value, which is 62 in the example.

Although contingency tables are most commonly used to examine nominal or ordinal data, they can be used with grouped frequencies of interval data. However, one must recognize that information about the data will be lost when this is done with interval data. Therefore, it is not generally the technique of choice. A contingency table is sometimes useful when an interval level measure is being compared to a nominal or ordinal level measure.

In some cases, the contingency table is presented and no further analysis is conducted. The table is presented as a form of summary statistics. However, in many cases, statistical analysis of the relationships or differences between the cell values is performed. The most familiar analysis of cross-tabulated data is the use of the chi-square statistic. Chi-square (χ^2) is designed to test for significant differences between cells and is considered by some to imply causal inference. Some statisticians prefer to examine the data from a probability framework, using nonparametric correlational techniques to detect possible relationships (Goodman & Kruskal, 1954, 1959, 1963, 1972). Many correlational techniques can be used to analyze nominal data, and the techniques discussed include Phi, Cramer's V, Contingency Coefficient and Lambda. There are computer programs available to analyze data from cross-tabulation tables (contingency tables). These programs can generate output from chi-square and many correlational techniques and indicate the level of significance for each technique. The basic programs used to conduct analyses of cross-tabulated data are presented in Table 17–9. One should know which statistics are appropriate for one's data and how to interpret the outcomes from these multiple analyses. The information presented on each of these tests provides guidance in the selection of a test and interpretation of the findings.

Chi-Square Analysis

Chi-square tests for significant differences between observed frequencies within the data and frequencies that were expected. There are two chi-square tests: the chi-square test of independence and the chi-square "goodness of fit" test. The more commonly used χ^2 test is the test of independence, which follows.

TABLE 17–9
Computer Program Information
for Analyzing Cross-Tabulated
Data

Computer Software	Computer Program Information
SAS	PROC FREQ; TABLES A*B/ALL page 405
BMDP	P4F page 143
SPSS^x	CROSSTABS page 287
ABSTAT	XTAB page 93

Chi-Square Test of Independence

The chi-square test of independence tests whether the two variables being examined are independent or related. Chi-square is designed to test for differences in frequencies of observed data and compare them with the frequencies that could be expected to occur if the data categories were actually independent of each other. If differences are indicated, the analysis will not indicate where within the data the significant differences exist.

Assumptions. One assumption of the test is that there is only one entry of data for each subject in the sample. Therefore, if repeated measures from the same subject are being used for analysis, such as pretests and post-tests, chi-square is not an appropriate test. Another assumption is that there are data categorized in every cell in the contingency table. Therefore, no cells may have a frequency of zero. Until recently, each cell was expected to have a frequency of at least 5, but this requirement has been mathematically demonstrated not to be necessary. The test is distribution-free, or nonparametric, which means that there is no assumption of a normal distribution of values in the population from which the sample was taken.

Calculation. The formula is relatively easy to calculate manually and can be used with small samples, making it a popular approach to data analysis. The first step in the calculation of chi-square is to categorize the data, record the observed values in a contingency table and sum the rows and columns. Next, the expected frequencies are calculated for each cell. The expected frequencies are those frequencies that would occur if there were no group differences and are calculated from the row and column sums using the following formula:

$$E = \frac{(Tr)\,(Tc)}{N}$$

where:

E = expected cell frequency
Tr = row total for that cell
Tc = column total for that cell
N = total number of subjects in the sample

Thus, the expected frequency for a particular cell is obtained by multiplying the row total by the column total and dividing by the sample size. When the expected frequencies have been calculated for all the cells, the sum should be equivalent to the total sample size. The calculations of the expected frequencies for the four cells in Table 17–8 follow; they total 62 (sample size).

Cell 1,1

$$E = \frac{(25)\,(34)}{62} = 13.71$$

Cell 1,2

$$E = \frac{(25)\,(28)}{62} = 11.29$$

Cell 2,1

$$E = \frac{(37)\,(34)}{62} = 20.29$$

Cell 2,2

$$E = \frac{(37)\,(28)}{62} = 16.71$$

Using this same example, a contingency table could be constructed of the observed and expected frequencies (Table 17–10). The chi-square statistic is then calculated using the following formula:

$$\chi^2 = \Sigma \frac{(O - E)^2}{E}$$

where:

O = observed frequency
E = expected frequency

Note that the formula includes difference scores between the observed frequency for each cell and the expected frequency for that cell. These difference scores are squared, divided by the expected frequency and summed for each

TABLE 17–10
Contingency Table of Observed and Expected Frequencies

	Parents' Reports	
Outside Help	*Neutral*	*Negative*
No	O = 18 E = 13.71	O = 7 E = 11.29
Yes	O = 16 E = 20.29	O = 21 E = 16.71

O = observed frequencies
E = expected frequencies

TABLE 17–11
Framework for Developing a 2 × 2 Contingency Table

	Variable X		
Variable Y	*0*	*1*	*Totals*
0	A	B	A + B
1	C	D	C + D
Totals	A + C	B + D	N

cell. The chi-square value was calculated using the observed and expected frequencies in Table 17–10.

$$\chi^2 = \frac{(18 - 13.71)^2}{13.71} + \frac{(7 - 11.29)^2}{11.29} + \frac{(16 - 20.29)^2}{20.29}$$

$$+ \frac{(21 - 16.71)^2}{16.71} = 4.98$$

$$df = 1; \, p < 0.05$$

If the sample is smaller than 40 or if there are expected values less than 10, a correction factor (Yates correction factor) is included in the formula. In this case, 0.5 is subtracted from the difference score between observed and expected frequencies in each of the cells. This strategy prevents an inflated chi-square statistic from small cell frequencies, which could result in a Type I error.

A special chi-square formula is generally used with 2 × 2 tables that have samples of less than 40 or samples with categories of less than 10. In a 2 × 2 table, all cell frequencies must be at least 5. (If not, the Fisher's exact test should be used for the analysis.) The 2 × 2 chi-square formula, which contains the correction factor, is as follows:

$$\chi^2 = \frac{(n \mid AD - BC \mid - n/2)^2}{(A + B)(C + D)(A + C)(B + D)}$$

A, B, C and D are the observed frequencies in the 2 × 2 contingency table illustrated in Table 17–11. Bars in the formula ($\parallel$) indicate that absolute values are used for mathematical calculations. Absolute values ignore plus (+) and minus (−) signs. Although the formula appears more ominous than the original formula, it is somewhat easier to use for manual calculation.

With any chi-square analysis, to determine the significance of the value of the statistic, the degrees of freedom (df) must be calculated. The following formula is used for this calculation:

$$df = (R - 1)(C - 1)$$

where:

R = number of rows in the contingency table

C = number of columns in the contingency table

In the example presented previously, the chi-square value was 4.98, and the df was 1, which was calculated as follows: df = $(2 - 1)(2 - 1) = 1$. The computer programs that are useful in generating chi-square statistics are presented in Table 17–12.

Interpretation of Results. The chi-square statistic is compared to the chi-square values in the table in Appendix E. The table identifies the critical values of chi-square for specific degrees of freedom at selected levels of significance (usually 0.05 or 0.01). If the value of the statistic is equal to or greater than the value identified in the chi-square table, there is a significant difference between the two variables. If the statistic remains significant at more extreme probability levels, the largest p value at which significance is achieved is reported. The analysis indicates that there are group differences in the categories of the variable and that those differences are related to changes in the other variable. Although a significant chi-square indicates difference, the magnitude of the difference is not revealed by the analysis. If the statistic is *not* significant, there is no difference in the distribution of the two variables, and they are considered independent (Siegel, 1956).

Interpretation of the results is dependent on the design of the study. If the design were experimental, causality can be considered and the results can be inferred to the associated population. If the design were descriptive, differences identified are associated only with the sample under study. In either case, the differences found are related to differences among all the categories of the first variable and all the categories of the second variable. The specific differences among variables and categories of variables cannot be identified with this analysis. Often, in reported research, the researcher will visually examine the data and discuss differences in the categories of data as if they had been demonstrated to be statistically significantly different. These reports must be viewed with caution by the reader. Partitioning, the contingency

TABLE 17–12
Computer Program Information
for Chi-Square

Computer Software	Computer Program Information
SAS	PROC FREQ; TABLES A* (B, C)/CHISQ page 405
BMDP	P4F page 143
SPSS[x]	NPAR TESTS CHISQUARE page 673
ABSTAT	CHIFIT page 72

coefficient, the phi coefficient or Cramer's phi can be used to statistically examine the data to determine in exactly which categories the differences lie. The last three strategies can also shed some light on the magnitude of the relationship between the variables. These strategies are discussed later in this chapter.

In reporting the results, contingency tables are generally presented only for significant chi-square analyses (refer to Table 17–8). The value of the statistic is given, including the degrees of freedom and the p value. Data in the contingency table are sufficient to allow other researchers to repeat the chi-square analyses and thus check the accuracy of the analyses.

Partitioning of Chi-Square

Partitioning involves breaking up the contingency table into several 2×2 tables and conducting chi-square analyses on each table separately. Partitioning can be performed on any contingency table greater than a 2×2 with more than one degree of freedom. The number of partitions that can be conducted is equivalent to the degrees of freedom. The sum of the chi-square values obtained by partitioning is equal to the original chi-square value. There are some rules that must be followed during partitioning to prevent inflating the value of chi-square. The initial partition can include any four cells as long as two values from each variable are used. The next 2×2 must compress the first four cells into two cells and include two new cells. This process can continue until no new cells are available. The chi-square formula for 2×2 tables that includes the correction factor is used to calculate chi-square. The computer programs used to determine the chi-square values in the test of independent groups are the same for the partitioning of chi-square (Table 17–12). Using this process, it is possible to determine which cells have contributed to the significant differences found.

Fisher's Exact Probability Test

Fisher's exact probability test is particularly useful with nominal data and with small samples. It can be used in situations that do not meet the criteria for chi-square. Cells with a value of zero are allowed. The sample size should not exceed 30. The data must fit into a 2×2 contingency table. Neither row total can exceed 15. The procedure can be used with larger samples, with modifications in the analytic procedure (Siegel, 1956, pp. 96–104). The computer programs presented in Table 17–12 are used to generate the Fisher's exact probability test.

Phi

The phi (ϕ) coefficient is used to describe relationships in dichotomous, nominal data. It is also used with the chi-square test to detect exact difference(s) between categories. Phi is used only with 2×2 tables (Table 17–11).

Calculation □ If chi-square (χ^2) has been calculated, the following formula can be used to calculate phi. Using the data presented in Table 17–8, the following phi coefficient was calculated. The chi-square analysis indicated a significant difference, and the phi coefficient indicated the magnitude of effect.

$$\text{Phi} = \sqrt{\frac{\chi^2}{N}} \quad \text{Phi } (\phi) = \sqrt{\frac{4.98}{62}} = \sqrt{0.0803} = 0.283$$

where:

N = the total frequency of all cells

Alternatively, phi can be calculated directly from the 2 × 2 table, using the following formula (Siegel, 1956). Again the data from Table 17–8 are used to calculate the phi coefficient. The computer programs presented in Table 17–9 can be used to generate this statistic.

$$\text{Phi} = \frac{AD - BC}{\sqrt{(A + C)(B + D)(A + B)(C + D)}}$$

$$= \frac{(18)(21) - (7)(16)}{\sqrt{(34)(28)(25)(37)}} = 0.283$$

Interpretation of Results □ The phi coefficient can be compared to Pearson's product-moment correlation coefficient (r) except that two dichotomous variables are involved. Phi values range from -1 to $+1$, with the magnitude of the relationship decreasing as the coefficient nears zero.

Cramer's V

Cramer's V is a modification of phi used for contingency tables larger than 2 × 2. It is designed for use with nominal data. As with phi, the value of the statistic ranges from zero to one.

Calculation □ The formula can be calculated from the chi-square statistic. Using the data presented in Table 17–8, Cramer's V was calculated. The computer programs presented in Table 17–9 can be used to generate this statistic.

$$V = \sqrt{\frac{\chi^2}{N(L - 1)}} \quad V = \sqrt{\frac{4.98}{62(7 - 1)}} = \sqrt{0.01334} = 0.115$$

L = the smaller of either the number of columns or rows

N = total frequency of all cells

The Contingency Coefficient

The contingency coefficient (C) is used with two nominal variables and is the most commonly used of the three chi-square based measures of association.

Calculation □ The contingency coefficient can be obtained with the following formula. Using the data presented in Table 17–8, this statistic was calculated. The computer programs identified in Table 17–9 can also be used to generate this statistic.

$$C = \sqrt{\frac{\chi^2}{\chi^2 + N}} \quad C = \sqrt{\frac{4.98}{4.98 + 62}} = \sqrt{0.07435} = 0.273$$

The relationship demonstrated by C cannot be interpreted on the same scale as Pearson's r, phi or V because it does not reach an upper limit of one. The formula does not consider the number of cells, and the upper limit varies with the size of the contingency table. With a 2×2 table, the upper limit is 0.71; with a 3×3 table, the upper limit is 0.82; and with a 4×4 table, the upper limit is 0.87. Contingency coefficients from separate analyses can be compared only if the table sizes are the same.

Lambda

Lambda measures the degree of association (or relationship) between two nominal level variables. The value of lambda can range from zero to one. Two approaches to analysis are possible: asymmetric and symmetric. The asymmetric approach indicates the capacity to predict the value of the dependent variable given the value of the independent variable. Thus, when asymmetric lambda is used, it is necessary to specify a dependent and independent variable. Symmetric lambda measures the degree of overlap (or association) between the two variables and makes no assumptions regarding which variable is dependent and which is independent (Waltz & Bausell, 1981). The computer programs identified in Table 17–9 can be used to generate the asymmetric and symmetric lambda statistics. The computer printout will indicate the significance of these statistics.

INDEPENDENT GROUPS—ORDINAL DATA

The statistical tests commonly used to analyze ordinal data are presented in Table 17–13.

Median Test

The median test is a nonparametric test for differences in central tendency that uses the median rather than the mean as the sample value. It is less powerful

---

TABLE 17–13
Tests for Independent Groups—
Ordinal Data

Median Test
Mann-Whitney U
Kolmogorov-Smirnov Two-Sample Test
Wald-Wolfowitz Runs Test
Spearman Rank-Order Correlation
Kendall's Tau

than the Mann-Whitney U test (description follows) except with extremely small samples.

Calculation □ To begin calculations, a median is calculated for the combined scores. (The process for calculating the median was described earlier in this chapter.) Then the scores for each group are dichotomized (separated into scores above the median and scores on or below the median) based on the calculated median. These scores are then placed in a 2 × 2 contingency table (see Table 17–11). Cell A could include the number of scores in Group I that is above the median, while Cell B includes the number of scores in Group II above the median. Cell C could include the number of scores below the median for Group I, while Cell D includes the number of scores below the median for Group II. The median test is calculated using the chi-square formula. The chi-square distribution is given in Appendix E. The median test can be calculated using the programming information provided in Table 17–14.

Mann-Whitney U Test

The Mann-Whitney U test is the most powerful of the nonparametric tests, with 95 per cent of the power of the t-test to detect differences between groups. If the assumptions of the t-test are violated, the Mann-Whitney U test is more powerful. It can be used with samples as small as 6. Although ranks are used for the analysis, ties in ranks have little effect on the outcome of the analysis.

Calculation □ Prior to calculation, the scores from the two samples must be combined and ranked, with the lowest score assigned the rank of 1. Each score should also be identified as to group membership. If one had two groups (males and females) and the males scored 50, 55, 62 and 70 on an anxiety tool and the females scored 45, 58, 75, 76 and 77 on the same tool, these scores could be combined and ranked. The groups, scores and ranks of these scores are presented in Table 17–15. The formula for calculating the Mann-Whitney U test follows. The U statistic was calculated using the data presented in Table 17–15.

TABLE 17–14
Computer Program Information for Median Test

Computer Software	Computer Program Information
SAS	PROC FREQ; TABLES A*B/CHISQ page 405
SPSS[x]	NPAR TESTS MEDIAN page 685
ABSTAT	CHIFIT page 72

TABLE 17–15
Ranked Scores From Two Groups

Group	F	M	M	F	M	M	F	F	F
Score	45	50	55	58	62	70	75	76	77
Rank	1	2	3	4	5	6	7	8	9

$$\hat{U} = n_1 n_2 + \frac{n_1(n_1 + 1)}{2} - R_1$$

$$U' = n_1 n_2 - \hat{U}$$

where:

n_1 = number of observations in the smallest group
n_2 = number of observations in the largest group
R_1 = sum of ranks assigned to n_1
U = the smaller value of $\hat{U}$ or U'

$$\hat{U} = (4)(5) + \frac{4(4 + 1)}{2} - (2 + 3 + 5 + 6) = 20 + 10 - 16 = 14$$

$$U' = (4)(5) - 14 = 20 - 14 = 6$$

Interpretation of Results □ The equations for both $\hat{U}$ and U' must be calculated. If there are a number of ties in the sample that include four or more scores, a correction factor must be included to decrease the risk of a Type I error. (Siegel, 1956, p. 124 describes this correction factor.) Two tables are available to determine the significance of U. If n_2 is less than or equal to 8, the tables in Appendix F are used. If n_2 is between 9 and 20, the table in Appendix G is used. In the example, $U = 6$ and $n_1 = 4$ and $n_2 = 5$. The probability listed in the table in Appendix F is 0.206, which is not significant. If n_2 is greater than 20, the Z statistic is calculated using the following equation. The normal distribution (Appendix B) is used to determine the level of significance.

$$Z = \frac{U - n_1 n_2 / 2}{\sqrt{\frac{(n_1 n_2)(n_1 + n_2 + 1)}{12}}}$$

The Mann-Whitney U test can be calculated using the computer programs identified in Table 17–16. Computer programs select the appropriate equation based on the sample size and include the correction factor when necessary.

TABLE 17–16
Computer Program Information
for Mann-Whitney U Test

Computer Software	Computer Program Information
BMDP	P3S page 442
SPSS^x	NPAR TESTS M-W page 685
ABSTAT	MANN page 79

Kolmogorov-Smirnov Two-Sample Test

The Kolmogorov-Smirnov test is a nonparametric test used to determine whether two independent samples have been drawn from the same population. This test uses the cumulative frequency from two samples for analysis. Either grouped or ungrouped frequencies can be used. If groupings are used, the same intervals must be used for developing the distribution of each sample. Larger numbers of groups lead to a more meaningful analysis. For example, if age were being used, 5-year age spans would provide more meaningful analysis than 20-year spans. The test is sensitive to any differences in the distributions of the two samples, including differences in measures of central tendency, dispersion or skewness. There is less of a risk of a Type II error with this test than with chi-square when small samples are being examined.

Calculation ☐ The scores within two groups are ranked separately. The cumulative relative frequency is calculated for each rank by dividing the ranking by the number in the sample. In Table 17–17, a score of 2 is ranked 1 in a sample of 9; therefore, the relative frequency would be $1/9 = 0.11$. A difference score is obtained for each point on the distribution by subtracting the smaller relative frequency from the larger relative frequency. For the score of 2, sample one had no scores that low, so the cumulative probability was 0.00 and the difference score was $0.11 - 0.00 = 0.11$. The largest difference score in the example is indicated with an * in Table 17–17.

Interpretation of Results ☐ One difficulty with the Kolmogorov-Smirnov two-sample test is that one cannot determine whether the difference is in central tendency, dispersion or skewness; therefore, conclusions must be broad. The test compares the cumulative distributions of the two samples with the assumption that if they are from the same population, differences in the distribution will be only random deviations. If the deviation is large enough, it is considered evidence for rejecting the null hypothesis.

The largest difference score is identified and used to compare with the tabled values in Appendix H. If the difference score is equal to or greater than the table value, the test indicates a significant difference. In the example in Table 17–17, the largest difference score, 0.67, compared with the table value

TABLE 17–17
Ranking of Scores for the Kolmogorov-Smirnov Two-Sample Test

Sample 1 (n = 10)		Sample 2 (n = 9)		
Scores	Cumulative Probability	Scores	Cumulative Probability	Absolute Value of the Difference
	0.00	2	1/9 = 0.11	0.11
	0.00	3	2/9 = 0.22	0.22
	0.00	5	3/9 = 0.33	0.33
	0.00	6	4/9 = 0.44	0.44
	0.00	9	5/9 = 0.56	0.56
	0.00	10	6/9 = 0.67	0.67
11	1/10 = 0.10		0.67	0.57
12	2/10 = 0.20	12	7/9 = 0.78	0.58
13	3/10 = 0.30		0.78	0.48
14	4/10 = 0.40		0.78	0.38
15	5/10 = 0.50	15	8/9 = 0.89	0.39
18	6/10 = 0.60	18	9/9 = 1.00	0.40
19	7/10 = 0.70		1.00	0.30
21	8/10 = 0.80		1.00	0.20
23	9/10 = 0.90		1.00	0.10
25	10/10 = 1.00		1.00	0.00

of 0.578 at the 0.05 level for a two-sided test indicates that the samples are significantly different at the 0.05 level. Computer programs have been developed to compute the Kolmogorov-Smirnov two-sample test. These programs are identified in Table 17–18.

Wald-Wolfowitz Runs Test

The Wald-Wolfowitz runs test, a nonparametric test, is used to determine differences between two samples. It will reject the null hypothesis if the two samples differ in any way, including central tendency, variability or skewness.

Calculation □ The scores from the two samples are merged and ranked. The group membership of each score is recorded with the rank. Then the number of runs in the ranked series of scores is determined. A run is any sequence of scores from the same sample. In the example given, sample 1 is coded as A, and sample 2 is coded as B. The merged scores from samples A and B are presented below. Using this example, 6 runs were identified.

TABLE 17–18
Computer Program Information for Kolmogorov-Smirnov Two-Sample Test

Computer Software	Computer Program Information
SPSS[x]	NPAR TESTS K-S page 685
ABSTAT	KS2 page 77

2 3 5 6	9 10	11 11	12 13	14 15	16 17	18 19 21 23 25
B B B B	B B	A A	B B	A A	B B	A A A A A
1		2	3	4	5	6

Interpretation of Results □ The runs test assumes that if the samples are from the same population, the scores will be well mixed. Therefore, r, the number of runs, will be large. When the null hypothesis is false, r is small. The table for the runs test is found in Appendix I. For the samples in the example, the table value of r is 5, which means that the number of runs must be equal to or less than 5 to be significant. Since there are 6 runs in the example, the null hypothesis is accepted. This test can also be calculated using an SPSS^x program and the programming statement NPAR TESTS W-W. This program is discussed on page 685 of the SPSS^x user's guide.

The Spearman Rank-Order Correlation Coefficient (Rho)

The Spearman rho, a nonparametric test, is an adaptation of Pearson's product-moment correlation. This test is used when the assumptions of Pearson's analysis cannot be met. For example, the data may be ordinal, or the scores may be skewed.

Calculation □ The data must be ranked in order to conduct the analysis. Therefore, if scores from measurement scales are used to perform the analysis, the scores must be converted to ranks. As with all correlational analyses, there must be a score (or value) on each of two variables (variable X and variable Y) for each subject in the analysis. The scores on each variable are independently ranked. Rho is calculated based on difference scores between a subject's ranking on the first set of scores and their ranking on the second set of scores. The formula for this calculation is:

$$D = X - Y$$

As in most statistical analyses, difference scores are difficult to use directly in equations because negative scores tend to cancel out positive scores; therefore, the scores are squared for use in the analysis. The formula is as follows:

$$rho = 1 - \frac{6 \, \Sigma \, D^2}{N^3 - N}$$

where:

rho = Spearman correlation coefficient (derived from Pearson's r)

D = difference score between the ranking of a score on variable X and the ranking of a score on variable Y

N = number of paired ranked scores

Interpretation of Results □ When the equation is used on data that meet the assumptions of Pearson's correlational analysis, the results are equivalent or slightly lower than Pearson's r. If the data are skewed, rho has an efficiency of 91 per cent in detecting an existing relationship. One of the difficulties encountered in the use of rho occurs when there are ties in the rankings. Tied ranks occur when the scores or values on one variable obtained from two or more subjects are equivalent. In this case, each of the scores is assigned the same rank. If the tie involves two subjects and the untied ranks that would have been assigned are 3 and 4, the tied rank assigned to both subjects will be 3.5. A few ties will cause little problem, but if the number of ties is large, the tied ranks reduce the sum of squares and, thus, the ability to detect an existing correlation. In this case, a correction factor must be included in the sum of squares to adjust for the ties (Siegel, 1956, p. 207). The significance of rho must be tested as with any correlation; the formula used is presented below. The t distribution is presented in Appendix C, and the df = N − 2.

$$t = \text{rho} \sqrt{\frac{n-2}{1-\text{rho}^2}}$$

Computer programs have been developed for generating the Spearman correlation coefficient (rho) and for testing the significance of rho (Table 17–19). These programs will include the correction factor when appropriate.

Kendall's Tau

Kendall's tau is a nonparametric measure of correlation used when both variables have been measured at the ordinal level. It is considered the analysis of choice when large numbers of tied ranks occur within the data. It can be used with very small samples. The statistic tau reflects a ratio of the actual concordance obtained between rankings with the maximal concordance possible. Typically, the approach used by Siegel (1956) is used to calculate tau. However, more recently, Marascuilo and McSweeney (1977) have described the analysis in a way that lends itself to a briefer explanation of the process and is used in this text.

TABLE 17–19
Computer Program Information
for Spearman's Rho

Computer Software	Computer Program Information
BMDP	P3S page 444
SPSS[x]	NONPAR CORR page 665
ABSTAT	SRANK page 88

TABLE 17–20
Ranking of Scores for Calculation of Kendall's Tau

Subject	A	B	C	D	E
Scores on variable X:	3	5	6	9	12
Scores on variable Y:	4	2	6	8	7
Subject	**A**	**B**	**C**	**D**	**E**
Ranking on variable X:	1	2	3	4	5
Ranking on variable Y:	2	1	3	5	4

Calculation □ To calculate tau, rank the scores on each of the two variables independently. Arrange the paired scores by subject, with the lowest ranking score on variable X listed on the left and the ranking score on variable Y for the same subject in the column below. Subjects must be arranged in order of rank from left to right across the page. An example of the ranking of scores for 5 subjects on variables X and Y is presented in Table 17–20.

Next, comparisons are made of the relative ranking position between subjects on variable Y. (It is not necessary to compare rankings on variable X, because the data have been arranged in order by rank.) If the comparison is *concordant*, the ranking of the score on the right will be higher than the ranking of the score on the left and is assigned a value of +1. If the comparison is *discordant*, the ranking of the score on the right will be lower than the ranking of the score on the left and is assigned a value of −1. In Table 17–21, the comparisons are identified as concordant (+1) or discordant (−1) for the ranked scores identified in Table 17–20. In this example, the number of discordant pairs is 2; the number of concordant pairs is 8. The statistic S is then calculated using the following equation.

$$S = N_c - N_d \quad \text{Example: } S = 8 - 2 = 6$$

where:

N_c = number of concordant pairs
N_d = number of discordant pairs

TABLE 17–21
Calculation of Concordant–Discordant States in Kendall's Tau

Comparison Subjects	Value for X	Value for Y	State
A B	+ 1	− 1	Discordant
A C	+ 1	+ 1	Concordant
A D	+ 1	+ 1	Concordant
A E	+ 1	+ 1	Concordant
B C	+ 1	+ 1	Concordant
B D	+ 1	+ 1	Concordant
B E	+ 1	+ 1	Concordant
C D	+ 1	+ 1	Concordant
C E	+ 1	+ 1	Concordant
D E	+ 1	− 1	Discordant

At this point, tau is calculated using the following equation:

$$\text{Tau} = \frac{2\,S}{n(n-1)} \qquad \text{Example: Tau} = \frac{(2)\,(6)}{5(5-1)} = 0.6$$

where:

n = number of paired scores

When tied scores occur in the data, a correction must be made in the equation, and, in large samples, this is almost inevitable. In this case, when the ranking of two subjects is equal during the comparison process, a value of zero is recorded. Since equal rankings can also occur in the X variable, these must also be recorded. S is calculated directly rather than calculating concordant and discordant values separately. The Y column is summed excluding pairs in which the X variable was tied. Tau is then calculated using the following equation:

$$\text{tau} = \frac{S}{\sqrt{1/2\ n(n-1) - T_x}\ \ \sqrt{1/2\ n(n-1) - T_y}}$$

where:

S = sum of values of y

n = number of paired scores

T_x = number of tied observations in X variable

T_y = number of tied observations in Y variable

There are computer programs for calculating Kendall's Tau, and they are identified in Table 17–22.

Interpretation of Results □ If the ranking of values of X is not related to the ranking of values of Y, any particular rank ordering of Y is just as likely to occur as any other. Tau tests the probability that the two rankings are correlated. The significance of tau can be tested using the following equation for the Z statistic. The Z statistic was calculated using the previous example.

TABLE 17–22
Computer Program Information
for Kendall's Tau

Computer Software	Computer Program Information
SAS	PROC FREQ; TABLES A*B/ALL page 414
BMDP	P3S page 444
SPSS[x]	NONPAR CORR page 665

$$Z = \frac{tau - mean}{SD_{tau}} \quad Z = \frac{0.6 - 0}{\sqrt{\dfrac{2(10 + 5)}{(9)\,(5)\,(5 - 1)}}} = \frac{0.6}{0.408} = 1.47$$

where:

$$Mean = \mu_{Tau} = 0$$

$$SD_{tau} = \sqrt{\frac{2(2n + 5)}{9n\,(n - 1)}}$$

Table values of Z scores are available in Appendix B. The Z score for the example was 1.47, which is nonsignificant at the 0.05 level.

INDEPENDENT GROUPS—INTERVAL DATA

The common parametric tests used to analyze interval data for independent groups are presented in Table 17–23.

t-Test For Independent Samples

One of the most common parametric analyses used to test for significant differences between statistical measures of two samples is the t-test. The t-test uses the standard deviation of the sample to estimate the standard error of the sampling distribution. The ease in calculating the formula is attractive to researchers who wish to conduct their analyses "by hand." It is particularly useful when only small samples are available for analysis.

The t-test is frequently misused by beginning researchers who use multiple t-tests to examine differences in various aspects of data collected in a study. When this is done, there is an escalation of significance that results in a greatly increased risk of a Type I error. The t-test can be used only one time during analysis to examine data from the two samples in a study. A specialized version of the t-test, Hotelling's t, which controls for the escalation of significance, can be used if various t-tests must be performed on different aspects of the same data. Hotelling's t must be performed through computer analysis; programs for generating this t value are identified in Table 17–24. Analysis of variance is always a viable alternative to the t-test and is preferred by many researchers who have become wary of the t-test because of its frequent misuse.

| TABLE 17–23 |
| Tests for Independent Groups— |
| Interval Data |

| t-test—Independent Group |
| Pearson's Correlation |
| Cross-Lagged Panel Correlation |
| Analysis of Variance |
| Simple Regression |

TABLE 17–24
Computer Program Information
for t-Test

Computer Software	Computer Program Information
SAS	T TEST page 795
BMDP	P3D page 94
SPSS[x]	T-TEST page 431
ABSTAT	TIND page 90

Mathematically, the two approaches are basically the same when only two samples are being examined. Use of the t-test involves the following assumptions:

1. Sample means from the population are normally distributed.
2. The dependent variable is measured at the interval level.
3. There is equal variance in the two samples.

The t-test is robust to violation of its assumptions. *Robustness* means that the results of analysis can still be relied upon to be accurate when one of the assumptions has been violated. Sample groups do not have to be equal for this analysis—the concern is, rather, for equal variance. There are a variety of t-tests that have been developed for various types of samples. Independent samples means that the two sets of data were *not* taken from the same subjects and that the scores in the two groups are not related.

Calculation □ The t statistic is relatively easy to calculate. The numerator is the difference scores of the means of the two samples. The test uses the pooled standard deviation of the two samples as the denominator of the formula, which gives a rather forbidding appearance to the formula. The computational formula follows:

$$t = \frac{\overline{X}_a - \overline{X}_b}{\sqrt{\frac{\Sigma X_a^2 - \frac{(\Sigma X_a)^2}{n_a} + \Sigma X_b^2 - \frac{(\Sigma X_b)^2}{n_b}}{(n_a + n_b - 2)}} \left(\frac{1}{n_a} + \frac{1}{n_b} \right)}$$

where:

$\overline{X}_a$ = mean of sample 1
$\overline{X}_b$ = mean of sample 2
n_a = number of subjects in sample 1

n_b = number of subjects in sample 2

df = n_a + n_b − 2

In the following example, the t-test was used to examine the difference between a control group and an experimental group. The independent variable administered to the experimental group was a form of relaxation therapy. The dependent variable was pulse rate. The pulse rates for the experimental and control groups are presented in Table 17–25 with the calculations for the t-test.

$$t = \frac{77-70}{\dfrac{\sqrt{71376 - \dfrac{(924)^2}{12} + 58944 - \dfrac{(840)^2}{12}\left(\dfrac{1}{12} + \dfrac{1}{12}\right)}}{12 + 12 - 2}} =$$

$$\frac{7}{\dfrac{\sqrt{(71376 - 71148 + 58944 - 58800)\,(.1667)}}{22}} = \frac{7}{0.358} = 19.55$$

df = 12 + 12 − 2 = 22

There are a variety of computer programs available to generate the t value. These programs are identified in Table 17–24.

TABLE 17–25
Data and Computations for the t-Test

	Pulse Rate (Control Group)			
X_a	*Frequency (f)*	fX_a	X_a^2	fX_a^2
70	1	70	4900	4900
72	2	144	5184	10368
76	5	380	5776	28880
82	3	246	6724	20172
84	1	84	7056	7056
n_a = 12	$\overline{X}_a$ = 77	ΣX_a = 924		ΣX_a^2 = 71376

	Pulse Rate (Experimental Group)			
X_b	*Frequency (f)*	fX_b	X_b^2	fx_b^2
64	1	64	4096	4096
66	2	132	4356	8712
70	5	350	4900	24500
72	3	216	5184	15552
78	1	78	6084	6084
n_b = 12	$\overline{X}_b$ = 70	ΣX_b = 840		ΣX_b^2 = 58944

Power Analysis ☐ If the t statistic fails to reject the null hypothesis, power analysis should be performed. The effect size (ES) is calculated using the following formula:

$$ ES = \frac{|\overline{X}_a - \overline{X}_b|}{SD} $$

where:

    | | indicates the use of absolute scores that disregard negative symbols

    $\overline{X}_a$ = mean of sample 1

    $\overline{X}_b$ = mean of sample 2

    SD = standard deviation

Since the level of significance and the sample size are known and ES can be calculated, the power table for t-tests can be consulted to determine the power of the test to reject the null hypothesis. If the power is lower than 80, careful consideration should be given to the possibility of a Type II error. The power tables can be found in Appendix M.

Interpretation of Results ☐ To determine the significance of the t statistic, the degrees of freedom must be calculated. The value of the t statistic is then found on the table for the sampling distribution. If the sample size is 30 or less, the t distribution is used; a table of this distribution can be found in Appendix C. For larger sample sizes, the normal distribution may be used; a table of this distribution can be found in Appendix B. The level of significance and the degrees of freedom are used to identify the critical value of t. If the computed statistic is equal to or greater than the critical value, the groups are significantly different. Traditionally, one reports the smallest level of significance at which the computed t is greater than the critical value. Thus, if 0.05 had been selected as a cutoff point but the computed t remained significant at the 0.01 level, the 0.01 level would be reported. In the example presented in Table 17–25, the calculated t = 19.55, and the df = 22. This t value was significant at the 0.001 level.

    If the result indicates a significant difference between the samples, magnitude testing must be done to determine the amount of variance explained. This is performed using the Pearson's product-moment correlation procedure. Magnitude testing can be performed by the computer programs identified in Table 17–24. If the result indicates no significant difference, power analysis must be performed.

Bivariate Correlation

Bivariate correlation measures the extent of relationship between two variables. Multiple correlation, a more complex analysis technique, which examines relationships among three or more variables, will be discussed later in this chapter. Bivariate correlational analysis requires that data be collected from a single sample. Measures of the two variables to be examined must be available for each subject in the data set. Less commonly, data are obtained from two related subjects, such as blood lipid levels in father and son. Correlational analysis provides two pieces of information about the data: the nature of a relationship (positive or negative) between the two variables, and the magnitude (or strength) of the relationship. The outcomes of correlational analyses are symmetrical rather than asymmetrical. Symmetrical means that there is no indication from the analysis of the direction of the relationship. One cannot say from the analysis that variable A "leads to" or causes variable B.

Correlational studies examine the sample as it is; no experimental treatment is involved. In addition, most correlational studies do not have randomly selected samples. There has been a negative mindset among some researchers toward correlational studies because of these "weaknesses" in design and the fear of associating relationship with causation. Because of this concern, the use of correlational analysis has fallen into some degree of disrepute. However, correlational analysis provides important information about samples and populations. In any situation involving causality, a relationship will exist between the factors involved in the causal process. Therefore, the first clue to the possibility of a causal link is the existence of a relationship. As the strength of a relationship increases, the possibility of a causal link increases. The absence of a relationship precludes the possibility of a causal connection between the two variables being examined, given adequate measurement of the variables and the absence of other variables that might mask the relationship. Thus, a correlational study can be the first step in determining the dynamics important to nursing practice within a particular population. Determining these dynamics can allow us to increase our ability to predict and control the situation studied, whether or not we can ever clearly prove definite causal links. Earlier, we expressed concern over attempts to extract causation (perhaps artificially) between two variables in the complex situations that occur in nursing (even when using experimental designs). Determining causality is difficult because of the complexity of nursing situations. The point of view of probability is a more reasonable way of perceiving nursing situations than is causality.

Scatter Diagram

Developing a visual image of the raw data (values obtained on variables) is very useful before conducting correlational analyses. Thus, the first step in the examination of bivariate relationships is to display the data graphically. Scatter diagrams are a means for displaying this data. Some possible scatter diagrams are shown in Figure 17–11.

Perfect positive and perfect negative linear relationships are represented by all the dots forming a straight line (Fig. 17–11). The line representing the negative relationship is sometimes referred to as an *inverse relationship* because the scores being correlated vary inversely (in opposite directions). Thus, in a negative relationship, when one score is high, the other score is low. In a positive relationship, the scores being correlated vary together (in the same direction). Therefore, in a positive relationship, the scores being correlated will both be high or both be low. Perfect positive and negative relationships rarely,

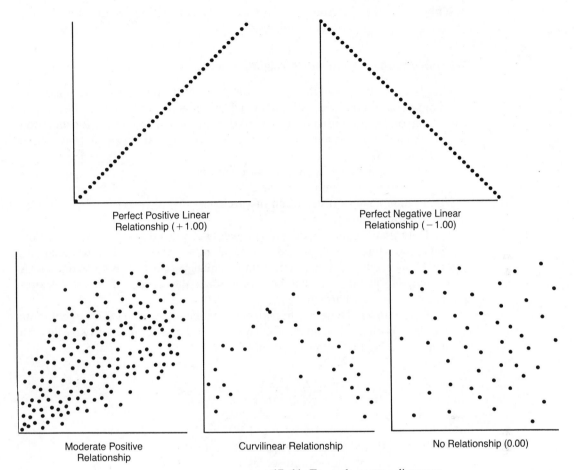

Perfect Positive Linear
Relationship (+1.00)

Perfect Negative Linear
Relationship (−1.00)

Moderate Positive
Relationship

Curvilinear Relationship

No Relationship (0.00)

FIGURE 17–11. Example scatter diagrams.

if ever, occur. Often, the diagram of a positive linear relationship in a study will be similar to the moderate relationship in Figure 17–11. When there is *no* correlation (relationship), the dots are scattered at random over the diagram. In some cases, the outcome is not a straight line but is curved, indicating a *curvilinear relationship*. In this case, analysis designed to test for linear relationships will not show a strong correlation.

After a scatter diagram has been developed, statistical analyses using the numerical values are necessary to obtain a more precise description of the relationship. The statistical analysis techniques used will depend on the type of data available. Correlational techniques are available for nominal, ordinal or interval types of data. Many of the correlational techniques (gamma, Somers' D, Kendall's tau, contingency coefficient, phi and Cramer's V) are used in conjunction with contingency tables. Many of these techniques were discussed previously in this chapter. Correlational techniques for interval data that are described are the Pearson's product-moment correlation coefficient and the cross-lagged panel correlation analysis.

Pearson's Product-Moment Correlation Coefficient

Pearson's correlation was the first of the correlation measures developed and is the most commonly used. All other correlation measures have been developed from Pearson's equation and are adaptations designed to control for violation of the assumptions that must be met in order to use Pearson's equation. These assumptions are:

1. Interval measurement of both variables
2. Normal distribution of variables
3. Independent distribution of variables
4. Homoscedasticity

Data that are *homoscedastic* are evenly dispersed both above and below the regression line, which indicates a linear relationship on a scatter diagram (plot). Homoscedasticity is a reflection of equal variance of both variables. A *regression line* is the line that best represents the values of the raw scores plotted on a scatter diagram.

Calculation. There are numerous formulas that can be used to compute Pearson's r. With small samples, Pearson's r can be generated fairly easily with a calculator using the following formula:

$$r = \frac{n(\Sigma XY) - (\Sigma X)(\Sigma Y)}{\sqrt{[n(\Sigma X^2) - (\Sigma X)^2][n(\Sigma Y^2) - (\Sigma Y)^2]}}$$

where:

r = Pearson's correlation coefficient
n = number of paired scores
X = score of the first variable
Y = score of the second variable
XY = product of the two paired scores

An example is presented that demonstrates the calculation of Pearson's r. The correlation between the two variables of functioning and coping was calculated. The functional variable (variable X) was operationalized using Karnofsky's scale, and coping was operationalized using a family coping tool. Karnofsky's scale ranges from 1 to 10; 1 is normal function, and 10 is moribund (fatal processes progressing rapidly). The family coping tool (variable Y) was developed using nursing diagnosis terminology and ranges from 1 to 4, with 1 being effective family coping; 2 is ineffective family coping, potential for growth; 3 is ineffective family coping, compromised; 4 is ineffective family coping, disabling. The data for these two variables using 10 subjects are presented in Table 17–26. Usually correlations are conducted on larger samples; this example serves only to demonstrate the process of calculating the Pearson's r.

TABLE 17–26
Data and Computations for Pearson's r

Subjects	X	Y	XY	X^2	Y^2
1	10	4	40	100	16
2	7	3	21	49	9
3	3	2	6	9	4
4	6	3	18	36	9
5	1	1	1	1	1
6	5	2	10	25	4
7	2	2	4	4	4
8	9	4	36	81	16
9	4	1	4	16	1
10	8	4	32	64	16
Sums	55	26	172	385	80

$$r = \frac{(10)\,(172) - (55)\,(26)}{\sqrt{[10(385) - (55)^2]\,[10(80) - (26)^2]}} = \frac{1720 - 1430}{\sqrt{(3850 - 3025)\,(800 - 676)}} =$$

$$\frac{290}{\sqrt{102300}} = \frac{290}{319.844} = 0.907$$

The Pearson product-moment correlation is normally calculated using a computer. Some of the different programs available to generate Pearson's r are identified in Table 17–27.

   Interpretation of the Results. The outcome of the Pearson product-moment correlation analysis is an r value between -1 and $+1$. This r value indicates the degree of relationship between the two variables. A score of zero indicates no relationship.

$$-1 \rule{4cm}{0.4pt} 0 \rule{4cm}{0.4pt} +1$$

A -1 indicates a perfect negative (inverse) correlation. In a negative relation-

TABLE 17–27
Computer Program Information
for Pearson's r

Computer Software	Computer Program Information
SAS	PROC CORR PEARSON page 864
BMDP	P8D page 209
SPSS[x]	PEARSON CORR page 579
ABSTAT	CORR page 73

ship, a high score on one variable is related to a low score on the other variable. A +1 indicates a perfect positive relationship. In a positive relationship, a high score on one variable is related to a high score on the other variable. A positive correlation also exists when a low score on one variable is related to a low score on the other variable. As the negative or positive values of r approach zero, the strength of the relationship decreases. Traditionally, an r of 0.1 to 0.3 is considered a weak relationship, 0.3 to 0.5 a moderate relationship and above 0.5 a strong relationship. However, this interpretation depends to a great extent on the variables being examined and the situation within which they were observed. Therefore, interpretation requires some judgment on the part of the researcher. In the example provided, the r value was 0.907, which indicates a strong positive relationship between the Karnofsky's scale and the family coping tool in this sample.

When Pearson's correlation coefficient is squared, (r^2), the resulting number is the *per cent of variance* explained by the relationship. In the example in Table 17–26, $r = 0.907$, and $r^2 = 0.822$. In this case, the relationship explains 82 per cent of the variability in the two scores. Except for perfect scores, r^2 will always be lower than r.

There has been a tendency to disregard weak correlations in nursing research. However, there is a serious possibility of ignoring a relationship that may have some meaning within nursing knowledge when examined in the context of other variables. This is similar to a Type II error. This situation commonly occurs for three reasons. First, many nursing measurements are not powerful enough to detect fine discriminations. Some instruments may not detect extreme scores. In this case, the relationship may be stronger than indicated by the crude measures available. Second, correlational studies must have a wide range of variance for relationships to be detected. If the study scores are homogeneous or if the sample is small, relationships that exist in the population will not show up as clearly in the sample. Third, in many cases, bivariate analysis does not provide a clear picture of the dynamics in the situation. A number of variables can be linked through weak correlations, but *together* they provide increased insight into situations of interest. Therefore, although one should not overreact to small Pearson's coefficients, the information must be recorded for future reference. If the relationship is intuitively important, one may have to plan better designed studies and reexamine the relationship.

Testing the Significance of a Correlation Coefficient. In order to infer that the sample correlation coefficient applies to the population from which the sample was taken, statistical analysis must be performed to determine whether the coefficient is significantly different from zero (no correlation). In other words, the test will determine whether the coefficient represents a deviation from zero that holds true for the population or, alternatively, that the deviation is likely to be due to sampling error. The test statistic used is the t, distributed according to the t distribution, with $n - 2$ degrees of freedom. The formula for calculating the t statistic follows. This formula was used to calculate the t value for the example where $r = 0.907$.

$$t = \frac{r\sqrt{n-2}}{\sqrt{1-r^2}} \quad t = \frac{0.907\sqrt{10-2}}{\sqrt{1-(0.907)^2}} = \frac{2.565}{\sqrt{0.177}} = \frac{2.565}{0.421} = 6.09$$

where:

r = Pearson's product-moment correlation coefficient
n = sample size of paired scores
$df = n - 2$

The significance of the t obtained from the formula is determined using the t distribution table in Appendix C. With a small sample, a very high correlation coefficient (r) can be nonsignificant. With a very large sample, the correlation coefficient can be statistically significant when the degree of association is too small to be clinically significant. Therefore, in judging the significance of the coefficient, one must consider both the size of the coefficient and the significance of the t test. The t value calculated in the example was 6.09, and the df for the sample was 8. This t value was significant at the 0.001 level.

Cross-Lagged Panel Correlation Analysis

The cross-lagged panel is designed to examine causation of one variable by a second variable. One of the assumptions of causality is that the causal variable must occur prior to the caused variable in time. Cross-lagged panel correlation (CLPC) analysis tests this assumption. In CLPC analysis, only two variables are examined for causality using two or more time periods. Initially, the analysis involves a series of Pearson's product-moment correlations (1) between variables at a single point in time (*synchronous correlations*), (2) between the same variable at two time periods (*autocorrelation*) and (3) between the two variables at two time periods (*cross-lagged correlations*).

Calculation. A step in conducting CLPC analysis is the development of a model of the correlations that will be conducted (Waltz & Bausell, 1981). For example, with two variables and three time periods, 11 correlations are involved. A model of these correlations is presented in Figure 17–12. The CLPC analysis is usually conducted using a computer. The Pearson product-

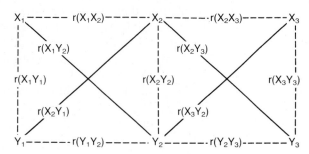

FIGURE 17–12. Model of a cross-lagged panel.

moment correlation programs presented in Table 17–27 are used to conduct this analysis.

Interpretation of Results. The analysis involves comparison of the cross-lagged correlations. Variation in the causal variable is expected to be reflected by variation in the caused variable. These comparisons are expressed as cross-lagged differentials.

$$r\ (X_1Y_2) - r\ (X_2Y_1) = \text{cross-lagged differential 1}$$
$$r\ (X_2Y_3) - r\ (X_3Y_2) = \text{cross-lagged differential 2}$$

If X causes Y, the cross-lagged differential will be positive, and if Y causes X, the cross-lagged differential will be negative. If the cross-lagged differential is not significantly different from zero, causality has not been demonstrated. The possibility of the impact of a third variable on the process must always be considered.

One-Way Analysis of Variance

Analysis of Variance (ANOVA) tests for differences between means. As previously mentioned, the t-test is simply a specialized version of ANOVA in which only two means are examined. Although one-way ANOVA is a bivariate analysis, it is more flexible than other analyses in that it can examine data from two or more groups. This is accomplished by using group membership as one of the two variables under examination and a dependent variable as the second variable. ANOVA has been considered a much more rigorous approach to statistical analysis than regression analysis (which is often mistakenly equated with correlation analysis). However, mathematically, ANOVA is simply a specialized version of regression analysis (Volicer, 1984).

ANOVA compares the variance within each group with the variance between groups. One source of variance is the variance within each group, since individual scores in the group will vary from the group mean. This variance is determined in the same way that variance was calculated earlier in this chapter (see p. 467). The amount of variation about the mean in each group is assumed by ANOVA to be equal. This variance is referred to as the *within* group variance. Another source of variation is variation of the group means around the Grand Mean, which is referred to as the *between* group variance. One could assume that if all the samples were drawn from the same population, there would be little difference in these two sources of variance. The variance from within and between the groups explains all the variance in the data. When these two types of variance are combined, they are referred to as the *total* variance. Assumptions involved in ANOVA include:

1. Homogeneity of variance
2. Independence of observations
3. Normal distribution of the populations from which the samples were drawn
4. Interval level data

Calculation □ Several calculation steps are required for ANOVA because the value of each source of variance must be determined and then compared to other sources of variance. ANOVA is usually calculated using a computer. However, ANOVA is not difficult to calculate by hand with small groups. It is important to understand the process of calculation and the terms used for each step of the analysis. The mathematical logic follows easily from the formulas previously presented. To clarify this connection, the conceptual formulas are used to explain the process.

To begin calculations, scores are separated by group and summed, and a *mean* is calculated for each group. Then scores from all groups are combined and summed, and a mean is obtained for all scores. This mean is referred to as the *Grand Mean*. Next, three different sums of squares are calculated: (1) the total sum of squares, (2) the sum of squares within and (3) the sum of squares between. The sum of squares within and the sum of squares between will equal the total sum of squares. As with any sum of squares, difference scores are used for the calculation. The formula for the *total sum of squares* for three groups is presented as follows:

$$SS_T = \Sigma(X_1 - \overline{\overline{X}})^2 + \Sigma(X_2 - \overline{\overline{X}})^2 + \Sigma(X_3 - \overline{\overline{X}})^2$$

where:

SS_T = total sum of squares
X_1 = single score from group 1
X_2 = single score from group 2
X_3 = single score from group 3
$\overline{\overline{X}}$ = Grand Mean

Mathematically, this formula is expressed more concisely as:

$$SS_T = \Sigma \, \Sigma \, (X - \overline{\overline{X}})^2$$

This formula indicates that the total sum of squares is obtained by summing the sum of squares from each group in the study. The formula for *sum of squares within* (or error) for three groups is:

$$SS_W = \Sigma(X_1 - \overline{X}_1)^2 + \Sigma(X_2 - \overline{X}_2)^2 + \Sigma(X_3 - \overline{X}_3)^2$$

where:

SS_W = sum of squares within
X_1 = single score from group 1
$\overline{X}_1$ = mean from group 1
X_2 = single score from group 2
$\overline{X}_2$ = mean from group 2
X_3 = single score from group 3
$\overline{X}_3$ = mean from group 3

Mathematically, this formula is expressed more concisely as:

$$SS_W = \Sigma \ \Sigma \ (X - \overline{X})^2$$

The formula for *sum of squares between* for these groups is:

$$SS_B = n_1 \ (\overline{X}_1 - \overline{\overline{X}})^2 + n_2 \ (\overline{X}_2 - \overline{\overline{X}})^2 + n_3 \ (\overline{X}_3 - \overline{\overline{X}})^2$$

where:
SS_B = sum of squares between
n_1 = number of scores in group 1
n_2 = number of scores in group 2
n_3 = number of scores in group 3

Mathematically, this formula is expressed more concisely as:

$$SS_B = \Sigma \ n(\overline{X} - \overline{\overline{X}})^2$$

Following these calculations, degrees of freedom are determined for the total, within and between using the following formulas:

$$df_T = n - 1$$
$$df_W = n - N$$
$$df_B = N - 1$$

where:
N = number of groups
n = total number of scores

Using the sum of squares and the degrees of freedom, the mean square between (MS_B) and the mean square within (MS_W) are calculated using the following formulas:

$$MS_B = \frac{SS_{between}}{N - 1}$$

$$MS_W = \frac{SS_{within}}{n - N}$$

From these equations (MS_B and MS_W), the F statistic is calculated as follows:

$$F = \frac{MS_{between}}{MS_{within}}$$

In Table 17–28, the one-way ANOVA formulas previously described are shown in a summary table. Researchers who perform analysis of variance on their data frequently record the results in an ANOVA summary table. Popkess (1981) examined self-image scores between two groups (obese and nonobese). The two variables studied were self-image and group membership. An ANOVA was performed on the data; a summary table of the results is presented in

TABLE 17–28
Summary of One-Way Analysis of Variance Formulas

Source	df	SS	MS	F
Between	$N - 1$	$\Sigma n\,(\overline{X} - \overline{\overline{X}})^2$	$\dfrac{SS_{between}}{N - 1}$	$\dfrac{MS_{between}}{MS_{within}}$
Within	$n - N$	$\Sigma\Sigma\,(X - \overline{X})^2$	$\dfrac{SS_{within}}{n - N}$	
Total	$n-1$	$\Sigma\Sigma\,(\overline{X} - \overline{\overline{X}})^2$		

TABLE 17–29
One-Way Analysis of Variance of Weight Groups and Self-Image

Source	df	SS	MS	F	F Probability
Between Groups	1	776.69	776.69	9.75	0.002
Within Groups	141	11228.74	79.64		
Total	142	12005.43			

From Popkess, S.A.: Assessment scales for determining the cognitive-behavioral repertoire of the obese subject. *Western Journal of Nursing Research*, 3:199, 1981, with permission.

Table 17–29. In this example, the mean square between (MS_B), mean square within (MS_w) and F value were calculated as follows:

$$MS_B = \frac{776.69}{1} = 776.69 \qquad MS_w = \frac{11228.74}{141} = 79.64$$

$$F = \frac{776.69}{79.64} = 9.75$$

ANOVA is frequently performed using the computer. The computer programs used to generate the F statistic in ANOVA are identified in Table 17–30.

TABLE 17–30
Computer Program Information
for ANOVA

Computer Software	Computer Program Information
SAS	PROC ANOVA; page 113
BMDP	P1V page 347
SPSS[x]	ANOVA page 439
ABSTAT	ANOVA page 66

Interpretation of Results □ The test for ANOVA is always two-tailed. The F distribution for determining the level of significance of the F statistic can be found in Appendix D. Use of the table requires knowledge of the degrees of freedom of MS_B and MS_W as well as the desired level of significance. If the F statistic (or ratio) is equal to or greater than the appropriate table value, there is a significant difference between the groups. In the example, the df for MS_B was 1, the df for MS_W was 141 and the F value was 9.75, which is significant at 0.002 level.

If only two groups are being examined, the location of a significant difference is clear. However, if there are more than two groups under study, it is not possible to determine from the ANOVA exactly where the significant differences lie. One cannot assume that *all* the groups examined are significantly different. Therefore, *post hoc analyses* are conducted to determine the location of the differences among groups. There are several options for conducting post hoc analyses. When ANOVA has been conducted using a computer, the computer usually automatically conducts several post hoc analyses and includes their levels of significance on the computer printout. The implications of each analysis must be understood in order to accurately interpret the meaning attached to the outcomes.

Post Hoc Analyses □ One might wonder why a researcher would conduct a test that failed to provide the answer sought—namely, where the significant differences were in a data set. It would seem more logical to perform t-tests or ANOVAs on the groups in the data set in pairs, thus clearly determining whether there is a significant difference between those two groups. However, when this is done with three groups in the data set, the risk of a Type I error increases from 5 per cent to 14 per cent. As the number of groups increases (and with the increase in groups, an increase in the number of necessary comparisons), the risk of a Type I error increases strikingly.

Post hoc tests have been developed specifically to determine the location of differences after ANOVA. These tests were developed to reduce the incidence of a Type I error. The frequently used post hoc tests are: Newman-Keuls test, the Tukey HSD test, the Scheffé test and Dunnett's test. When these tests are calculated, the alpha level is reduced in proportion to the number of additional tests required to locate statistically significant differences. As the alpha level is decreased, reaching the level of significance becomes increasingly more difficult.

The Newman-Keuls test compares all possible pairs of means and is the most liberal of the post hoc tests considered acceptable by publication editors. Liberal means that the alpha level is not as severely decreased.

The Tukey HSD test computes one value to which all means within the data set are compared. It is considered more stringent than the Newman-Keuls test.

The Scheffé test is the most conservative of the post hoc tests and has a good reputation among researchers. However, one must keep in mind that a test that is very conservative increases the risk of a Type II error.

Dunnett's test requires a control group for its use. The mean for each experimental group is then compared to the control group. The test does not require a reduction of alpha and thus is advisable to use when the conditions for the test are met.

Power Analysis □ If the results of the ANOVA are not statistically significant, power analysis should be performed. Power analysis is used to determine the power of the test to detect significance if it is present. Determining effect size (ES) from an ANOVA is relatively easy with the following formula:

$$ES = \sqrt{\frac{SS_B}{SS_W}}$$

To determine the risk of a Type II error, the power table for the F statistic in Appendix M is consulted. The n used is the sample size of a single group, not that of the entire data set. If the groups are of differing sizes, the mean of the sample sizes is used. The degrees of freedom is the number of groups minus one.

Magnitude of Effect □ The magnitude of effect is seldom determined with ANOVA. However, the level of significance alone gives no information about the extent to which the phenomenon is explained by the variables under study. The magnitude is determined by conducting regression analysis. The R^2 resulting from the regression analysis indicates the per cent of variance explained by the difference detected by ANOVA.

Simple Linear Regression

Simple linear regression provides a means to estimate the value of a dependent variable based on the value of an independent variable. The regression equation is a mathematical expression of a causal proposition emerging from a theoretical or conceptual framework. This linkage between the theoretical statement and the equation should be made clear prior to the analysis.

To explain regression analysis we must return to the scatter diagram (see p. 507). Simple linear regression is an effort to explain the dynamics within the scatter plot by drawing a straight line (the line of best fit) through the plotted scores. This line is drawn to provide the best explanation of the relationship between two variables. Knowing that relationship, we can, with some degree of accuracy, predict the value of one variable if we know the value of the other variable. The following assumptions can be made:

1. The presence of homoscedasticity—equal scatter of values of Y above and below the regression line at each value of X (constant variance).
2. The dependent variable is measured at the interval level.
3. The expected value of the residual error is zero.
4. Both variables are normally distributed within the population.

Calculation □ Simple linear regression is a method of determining parameters, a and b. The formula is developed mathematically based on the requirement that the squared deviation values (squared difference scores) be minimized. When squared deviation values are minimized, variance from the line of best fit is minimized. To understand the mathematical process, it is helpful to recall the algebraic equation for a straight line:

$$y = a + bx$$

In regression analysis, the straight line is usually plotted on a graph, with the horizontal axis representing X (the independent, or predictor, variable) and the vertical axis representing Y (the dependent, or predicted, variable). The value represented by the letter a is referred to as the *Y intercept*. This is the point where the regression line crosses (or intercepts) the Y axis. At this point on the regression line, X = 0. The value represented by the letter b is referred to as the *slope* or the coefficient of X. The slope determines the direction and angle of the regression line within the graph. The slope expresses the extent to which Y changes for every change in X. Figure 17–13 is a graph of these points.

In simple, or bivariate, regression, predictions are made using two variables. The score on variable X (independent variable) is predicted based on the same subject's known score on variable Y (dependent variable). The predicted score (or estimate) is referred to as $\hat{Y}$ (expressed Y-hat) or occasionally as Y' (expressed Y-prime).

No single regression line can be used to predict with complete accuracy every Y value from every X value. In fact, one could draw an infinite number of lines through the scattered paired values. However, the purpose of the regression equation is to develop the line to allow the highest degree of prediction possible—the line of best fit. The procedure for developing the line of best fit is the *method of least squares*.

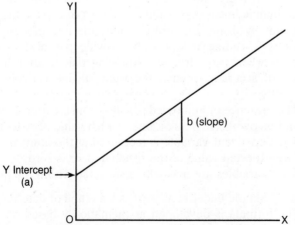

FIGURE 17–13. Graph of a regression line.

To explain the method of least squares, we must return to difference scores. In a real sample in which values on both X and Y are known, the regression line is plotted subject by subject, using both values to determine the placement of each point. The multiple subjects who have a single value on X can have various values on Y. Only the mean of these Y values is located on the regression line. Therefore, at each point on the X axis, one can determine differences scores from the mean on the Y axis. From these difference scores, a sum of squares can be calculated. There can, then, be a sum of squares for each point on the X axis. The sum of squares of all difference scores is an indicator of how good a fit the regression line is to the data. The equations developed to estimate the regression line have been developed in such a way that the value of the sum of squares will be minimized, thus decreasing the variance and maximizing the predictive power of the resulting equation. The three equations for the method of least squares are as follows:

$$b = \frac{n(\Sigma XY) - (\Sigma X)(\Sigma Y)}{n(\Sigma X^2) - (\Sigma X)^2}$$

$$a = \overline{Y} - b\overline{X}$$

$$\hat{Y} = a + bX$$

where:

   b = slope
   n = number of paired values
   X = known value of X
   a = Y intercept
   $\hat{Y}$ = predicted value of Y

The coefficient of X, which is b, can be determined from the analysis of raw data or from the analysis of Z scores. If b is determined from Z scores, it is referred to as *beta*. Beta is preferred when comparisons are made with the results of other analyses. Computer analyses usually provide both values. The computer programs used to conduct regression analysis are presented in Table 17–31.

Interpretation of Results □ A null regression hypothesis suggests that b = 0 (which indicates that Y does not vary based on the score of X). Thus, an alternate hypothesis proposes that b is significantly different from zero. The sampling distribution of b is a t distribution, with 2 degrees of freedom; therefore, the test statistic used to determine the significance of a regression coefficient is t. However, the test uses a different equation than the t-test used to determine significant differences between means. In determining the significance of a regression coefficient, t tends to become larger as b moves further from zero. However, if the sum of squared deviations from regression is large, the t value will decrease. Small sample sizes also decrease the t value.

In reporting the results of a regression analysis, the equation is expressed with the calculated coefficient values. The R^2 value and the t values are also documented. The format for reporting the results of regression is as follows:

$$
\begin{array}{cc}
\text{Y intercept} & \text{b (slope)} \\
\downarrow & \downarrow \\
\end{array}
$$

$$\hat{Y} = 3.45 + 8.72X \qquad\qquad R^2 = 0.63$$
$$\text{(2.79) (4.68)} \longleftarrow \text{t value}$$

The figures in parentheses are not always t values. They may be the standard error of the estimate. Therefore, the report must indicate which values are being reported. If t values are being used, the t value that indicates significance should also be reported. A t value equal to or greater than the table value (Appendix C) indicates significance. From these results, a graph can be developed to illustrate the outcome. Additionally, a table can be developed indicating the changes that are predicted to occur in the value of Y with each increase in the value of X. Names are usually given to identify the variables of X and Y. Using the example where the Y intercept = 3.45 and b = 8.72, a table (Table 17–32) of X and Y values was developed. These values are graphed in Figure 17–14.

After a regression equation has been developed, the equation is tested against a new sample to determine its accuracy in prediction. Some "shrinkage" of R^2 is expected, because the equation was generated to best fit the sample from which it was developed. However, an equation is most useful if it maintains its ability to predict accurately across many and varied samples. The first test of an equation against a new sample should use a sample very similar to the initial sample.

TWO DEPENDENT GROUPS—NOMINAL DATA

Dependent groups implies that the measures taken from the two groups are related in some way. For example, measures may be taken on the same subject at two time periods, such as a pretest and a post-test. If the pretest scores are considered one group and the post-test scores are considered another group, the two sets of scores (and thus the groups) are related. This situation violates the assumptions of many statistical tests and requires the use of tests developed

TABLE 17–31
Computer Program Information for Regression Analysis

Computer Software	Computer Program Information
SAS	PROC REG page 655
BMDP	P1R page 237
SPSS[x]	REGRESSION page 601
ABSTAT	REGR page 83

TABLE 17–32
Predicted Values of Y from
Known Values of X Using
Regression Analysis

Value of X	Predicted Value of Y
0	3.45 (Y Intercept)
1	12.17 (Y Intercept + b)
2	20.89 (+ b)
3	29.61 (+ b)
4	38.33 (+ b)

specifically for these situations. The nonparametric McNemar test is described
in this section.

McNemar Test for Significance of Changes

The McNemar test analyzes changes that occur in dichotomous variables using
a 2 × 2 table. This nonparametric test is particularly appropriate for before
and after or pretest/post-test designs in which the subjects serve as their own
control and the data are nominal. For example, one might be interested in
determining the number of nurses in a sample who changed from hospital

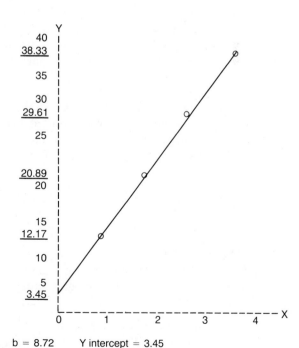

FIGURE 17–14. Regression line
developed from values in Table 17–32.

b = 8.72   Y intercept = 3.45

TABLE 17-33
2 × 2 Contingency Table for
the McNemar Test

		Post-Test	
		−	+
Pretest	+	A	B
	−	C	D

nursing to home health care and vice versa. The two work places in the aforementioned example are nominal, because there is no way to rank one as being better than the other. Pluses and minuses are used to indicate the two conditions, and the assigning of a plus or minus to a variable is at the discretion of the researcher. Data are placed in a 2 × 2 contingency table as exemplified in Table 17-33.

Subjects whose scores changed from positive to negative are tallied in cell A. In the example, those nurses who changed from home health care to hospital nursing were tallied in cell A; there were five nurses. Those who changed from negative to positive are tallied in cell D. If the score remained negative, the subject is tallied in cell C, and if the score remained positive, the subject is tallied in cell B. Only subjects whose scores changed are included in the analysis; therefore, only the tally marks in cells A and D are considered. The null hypothesis is that one half of the subjects changed from negative to positive, and one half changed from positive to negative.

If one were to study the nurses who changed from home health care to hospital nursing, the data might appear as presented in Table 17-34. Cell A contains the number of nurses that changed from home health nursing to hospital nursing; there were five nurses in this category. Fifteen (cell D) nurses changed from hospital nursing to home health care. Five nurses (cell B) stayed in home health nursing, and three nurses (cell C) remained in hospital nursing.

Calculation   □ If $1/2(A + D)$ is 5 or less, the binomial distribution is used to determine the level of probability. Otherwise, the chi-square (χ^2) test with the correction for continuity is used to test the hypothesis. The χ^2 value is calculated for the data presented in Table 17-34.

$$\chi^2 = \frac{(\mid A - D \mid - 1)^2}{A + D}$$

$$\chi^2 = \frac{(\mid 5 - 15 \mid - 1)^2}{5 + 15} = \frac{(10 - 1)^2}{20} = \frac{81}{20} = 4.05$$

The McNemar test for significant changes can also be conducted using the computer. The computer programs for conducting this test are identified in Table 17-35.

Interpretation of Results   □ The significance of the χ^2 value with df = 1 is determined from the χ^2 table in Appendix E. If the value is equal to or greater than the table value, the two groups are considered significantly different. In

TABLE 17–34
Example of 2 × 2 Contingency
Table for McNemar Test

		Post-Test	
		−	+
Pretest	+	A 5	B 5
	−	C 3	D 15

the example, the χ^2 value was 4.05, and the df = 1; the χ^2 value is significant at the 0.05 level.

TWO DEPENDENT GROUPS—ORDINAL DATA

The sign test and the Wilcoxon matched-pairs signed-ranks test are described in this section.

Sign Test

The sign test is a nonparametric test that was developed for data for which it is difficult to assign numerical values. However, the data can be ranked on such dimensions as agree–disagree, easier–harder, earlier–later, more–less, higher–lower. These dimensions must include rankings of three or more possible values. For example, agree–disagree is commonly classified using a Likert scale with five possible values (strongly agree, agree, neutral, disagree and strongly disagree).

The sign test acquired its name from the use of the + sign and the − sign to rank or place value on the variables under study. The variables being examined cannot be dichotomous (*e.g.*, male and female) but must be based on an underlying continuum. The test makes no assumptions about the shape of the underlying distribution or that all subjects are from the same population. The null hypothesis assumes that the same number of subjects will move from positive to negative as will move from negative to positive. Thus, the median is assumed to be zero.

Calculation □ To conduct the sign test, the pretest/post-test or matched-pairs

TABLE 17–35
Computer Program Information
for the McNemar Test

Computer Software	Computer Program Information
BMDP	P4F page 152
SPSS[x]	NPAR MCNEMAR page 679

values are examined to determine whether there was a positive or negative change from the first observation to the second observation. Subjects in whom no change was observed are dropped from the analysis, and the N is reduced accordingly. N is the number of pairs of observations. The number of pluses and minuses for these paired observations are counted. If N is 25 or less, the binomial distribution is consulted for the level of probability. If N is greater than 25, the Z statistic is calculated using the following equation:

$$Z = \frac{(X + 0.5) - 1/2N}{1/2 \sqrt{N}}$$

where:

X = the smaller of either the sum of pluses or the sum of minuses

N = number of paired values retained for analysis

For a two-tailed test, a Z score of 1.96 indicates significance at the 0.05 level. For a one-tailed test, a Z score of 1.643 indicates significance at the 0.05 level. The table for the Z distribution (Cumulative Normal Distribution) can be found in Appendix B. Computer programs are available to calculate the sign test and to determine the significance of the findings. The programs used to conduct this test are presented in Table 17–36.

Wilcoxon Matched-Pairs Signed-Ranks Test

The Wilcoxon matched-pairs signed-ranks test, like the sign test, is a nonparametric test that examines changes that occur in pretest/post-test measures or matched-pairs measures. It is more powerful than the sign test, because it examines both the direction and the magnitude of change that occurs. A pair of scores in which a greater amount of change has occurred is given more weight than a pair in which very little change has occurred. This test requires that the researcher be able to assess the magnitude of a change between the first and second observation. When no change has occurred between the first and second observation, the subject or pair is dropped from the analysis and the sample size is decreased.

Calculation   □ Initially, a difference score (d) is calculated for each pair of

TABLE 17–36
Computer Program Information
for the Sign Test

Computer Software	Computer Program Information
BMDP	P3S page 437
SPSS[x]	NPAR SIGN page 679
ABSTAT	SIGN page 87

scores. If the difference score is zero, the pair is omitted. The plus or minus sign associated with each difference score must be retained. Ignoring the plus and minus signs, the difference scores are ranked, with the lowest difference score ranked 1. If some of the difference scores are tied, the ranks of the tied scores are averaged. For example, if ranks 3, 4 and 5 had the same difference score, the ranks would be summed and divided by the number of ranks [(3 + 4 + 5)/3 = 4], and the resulting rank would be assigned to each of the pairs. The next difference scores would then be assigned the rank of 6.

In the second step of analysis, the *sign* of the difference score is affixed to each rank. This indicates which ranks resulted from a negative change and which ranks resulted from a positive change. If the two groups being examined are not different, the positive and negative ranks should be relatively interspersed, with the greatest difference scores occurring equally among positive and negative ranks. The third step in analysis is to sum the ranks having positive signs and to sum the ranks having negative signs. If there is no difference in the two groups, these two sums should be similar.

Interpretation of Results □ The smallest value of the two sums (T) and the number of pairs (N) are used to determine the significance of the difference in the two sums. If N is 25 or less, the Wilcoxon matched-pairs signed-ranks table in Appendix J is used to determine significance. If T is equal to or less than the table value, the null hypothesis that there is no difference in the values of the two sums is rejected. If N is greater than 25, the Z score is calculated using the following equation:

$$Z = \frac{T - \dfrac{N(N + 1)}{4}}{\sqrt{\dfrac{N(N + 1)(2N + 1)}{24}}}$$

where:

T = the smallest value of the two sums
N = number of matched pairs retained for analysis

In a two-tailed test, a Z score of 1.96 or less indicates a level of significance of 0.05. For a one-tailed test, a Z score of 1.68 or less indicates a level of significance of 0.05. The table for the Z distribution is in Appendix B. Computer programs can be used to calculate the Wilcoxon matched-pairs signed-ranked test and to determine the significance of the findings (Table 17–37).

TWO DEPENDENT GROUPS—INTERVAL DATA

t-Tests for Related Samples

When samples are related, the formula used to calculate the t statistic is different from the formula described on page 503. Samples may be related because matching has been performed as part of the design or because the

TABLE 17–37
Computer Program Information
for the Wilcoxon Matched-Pairs
Signed-Ranks Test

Computer Software	Computer Program Information
BMDP	P3S page 437
SPSS^x	NPAR WILCOXON page 679

scores used in the analysis were obtained from the same subjects under different conditions (*e.g.*, pretest and post-test).

Calculation □ The following formula assumes that scores in the two samples are, in some way, correlated (dependent).

$$t = \frac{\overline{D}}{\sqrt{\dfrac{\Sigma d^2}{n(n-1)}}}$$

where:
$\overline{D}$ = the mean difference between the paired scores
Σd^2 = sum of squared deviation difference scores
n = number of paired scores
df = n − 1

Computer programs are available to calculate the t-test for dependent groups and to determine the significance of the t value. The computer programs used are identified in Table 17–38.

TABLE 17–38
Computer Program Information
for the t-test for
Dependent Groups

Computer Software	Computer Program Information
SAS	PROC MEANS page 799
BMDP	P3D page 94
SPSS^x	T-TEST PAIRS- page 434
ABSTAT	TPAIR page 91

Power Analysis □ When conducting power analysis on related samples, effect size (ES) is first calculated using the formula for independent t-tests. A Pearson's product-moment correlation coefficient must then be calculated on the two samples to determine the degree of relationship; then the following formula is used to calculate ES:

$$\widehat{ES} = \frac{ES}{\sqrt{1 - r}}$$

where:

$\widehat{ES}$ = the effect size for correlated means
ES = the effect size for independent means
r = correlation coefficient

The level of significance, degrees of freedom and ES are then used to determine the power of the test to reject the null, using the power table in Appendix M).

THREE OR MORE INDEPENDENT GROUPS—NOMINAL DATA

The chi-square (χ^2) test of independence can be used with more than two groups. In this case, group membership is used as the independent variable. The χ^2 statistic is calculated using the same formula presented on page 488. If there are more than two categories of the dependent variable, differences in both central tendency and dispersion are tested by the analysis. The computer programs identified in Table 17–12 are used to calculate the chi-square test of independence.

THREE OR MORE INDEPENDENT GROUPS—ORDINAL DATA

The Extension of the Median Test

The extension of the median test determines whether samples have been drawn from populations with equal medians. The assumptions of chi-square must be met in order for the test to be conducted. As with the median test, data for each group are divided into two groups: scores larger than the median, and scores that fall on or below the median. (The description of the median test can be found on pages 493–494.) The data are then placed on a 2 × k contingency table, and the chi-square test for independent groups is performed. The power efficiency is equivalent to that of chi-square. The computer programs for calculating the extension of the median test are presented in Table 17–14. The computer program manuals indicate the specific commands that must be added when the analysis is extended to more than two groups.

The Kruskal-Wallis One-Way Analysis of Variance by Ranks

The Kruskal-Wallis test is the most powerful nonparametric test for examining three independent groups. It has 95 per cent of the power of the F statistic to detect existing differences between groups. The technique tests the null hypothesis that all samples are from the same population. The main assumption with this test is that there is an underlying continuous distribution.

Calculation □ The initial step in analysis is to rank all scores from all samples together, with the smallest score being assigned a rank of 1. N is equal to the largest rank or the total number of observations from all samples. Next, the ranks from each sample are summed. The Kruskal-Wallis test determines whether the sum of ranks from each group is different enough that the samples are not likely to have come from the same population. The statistic used in the Kruskal-Wallis test is H, and the following formula is used to calculate this statistic.

$$H = \frac{12}{N(N + 1)} \sum \frac{R_j^2}{n_j} - 3(N + 1)$$

where:

n_j = number of scores in j sample
N = total number of scores across all samples
R_j = sum of ranks from j sample
$\sum \frac{R_j^2}{n_j}$ indicates that $\frac{R_j^2}{n_j}$ is to be calculated separately for each sample
and the results are to be summed

If there are ties in many of the ranks, a correction factor must be included in the formula (Siegel, 1956, p. 188). The correction factor is incorporated into the H statistic by dividing the H statistic by the following:

$$1 - \frac{\Sigma T}{N^3 - N}$$

where:

$T = t^3 - t$ (t is the number of tied scores in one group of tied scores)
N = number of all scores in all samples

Computer programs are available for calculating the Kruskal-Wallis test and will incorporate the correction factor in the H statistic when appropriate (Table 17–39).

Interpretation of Results □ If there are more than five subjects in each group, the chi-square table in Appendix E can be used to determine levels of significance. Degrees of freedom (df) is calculated as the number of samples minus 1. If the value obtained for H is equal to or greater than the table value, the groups are considered statistically significantly different. If there are three samples and each sample contains fewer than five subjects, exact probabilities for these samples can be found in Appendix K.

TABLE 17–39 Computer Program Information for the Kruskal-Wallis Test	
Computer Software	**Computer Program Information**
BMDP	P3S page 442
SPSS^x	NPAR K-W page 692
ABSTAT	KW page 78

THREE OR MORE DEPENDENT GROUPS—NOMINAL DATA

The Cochran Q Test

The Cochran Q test is an extension of the McNemar test for two related samples (see p. 521). The Cochran Q test can be used in such situations as: (1) when subjects have been matched and several levels of treatment have been administered, (2) when more than one matched control group has been used for comparison or (3) for repeated measures of the dependent variable across time. Measures of the dependent variable must be coded dichotomously. For example, 1 could be coded if an event occurred, 0 if it did not occur; 1 could be coded for yes, 0 for no; + for a positive change, − for a negative change.

Calculation □ Data are arranged in a contingency table where k is equal to the number of columns and N is equal to the number of rows. The null hypothesis is that there is no difference in frequency or proportion of responses by category in each column except that of chance. The computational equation is as follows:

$$Q = \frac{(k - 1) \left[k \, \Sigma \, G_j^2 - (\Sigma G_j)^2 \right]}{K \, \Sigma \, L_i - \Sigma \, L_i^2}$$

where:

$i =$ number assigned to each row
$j =$ number assigned to each column
$k =$ number of columns
$G_j =$ total number of positive responses (yes, 1 or +) in each column
$L_i =$ total number of positive responses (yes, 1 or +) in each row
$N =$ number of rows

The SPSS^x manual includes a program for conducting the Cochran Q test. The programming statement is NPAR COCHRAN and can be found on page 662 of the manual.

Interpretation of Results □ The value of Q is compared to the chi-square table in Appendix E using df = k − 1. If the value of Q is greater than or equal to the table value, the frequency or proportion of subjects coded as positive differs significantly among the samples. The power efficiency of Cochran's Q is not known, because there are no parametric tests with which it can be compared.

THREE OR MORE DEPENDENT GROUPS—ORDINAL DATA

The Friedman Two-Way Analysis of Variance by Ranks

The Friedman two-way ANOVA by ranks may be used with matched samples or in repeated measures. The null hypothesis is that the samples come from the same population. The Friedman test considers magnitude and therefore is more likely than the Cochran Q test to reject the null hypothesis, given the same data.

Calculation □ Data are placed in a contingency table with N rows and k columns. Rows represent groups of subjects, columns represent conditions being studied. Scores within each cell are summed and ranked by row. In Figure 17–15, the scores and the row ranks for these scores are presented in contingency tables. The value of the Friedman test statistic (χ_r^2) can be calculated using the following equation:

$$\chi_r^2 = \frac{12}{Nk\,(k\,+\,1)}\,\Sigma\,(R_j)^2 - 3N\,(k\,+\,1)$$

where:

N = number of rows
k = number of columns
j = column number
R_j = sum of ranks in j column
$\Sigma\,(R_j)^2$ instructs to sum the squares of R_j over all columns

SCORE TOTALS

	Condition			
	I	II	III	IV
Group 1	22	16	8	2
Group 2	41	26	8	12
Group 3	2	8	36	44

ROW RANKS

	Condition			
	I	II	III	IV
Group 1	4	3	2	1
Group 2	4	3	1	2
Group 3	1	2	3	4
R_j	9	8	6	7
R_j^2	81	64	36	49

$(R_j)^2 = 81 + 64 + 36 + 49 = 230$

FIGURE 17–15. Example contingency tables for the Friedman test.

TABLE 17–40
Computer Program Information
for Friedman's Test

Computer Software	Computer Program Information
BMDP	P3S page 411
SPSS^x	NPAR FRIEDMAN page 683

The χ_r^2 value was calculated for the data presented in Figure 17–15.

$$\chi_r^2 = \frac{12}{3(4)\ (4\ +\ 1)}\ [(9)^2\ +\ (8)^2\ +\ (6)^2\ +\ (7)^2]\ -\ (3)\ (3)\ (4\ +\ 1)\ =$$

$$\frac{12}{60}\ (230)\ -\ 45\ =\ (0.2)\ (230)\ -\ 45\ =\ 1.0$$

The computer programs that are available to calculate the Friedman statistic (χ_r^2) are identified in Table 17–40.

Interpretation of Results □ The value of the χ_r^2 statistic is compared to the values in Appendix L. If the value of the test statistic is equal to or greater than the table value for the selected level of significance (*e.g.*, 0.05), the ranks in the various columns differ significantly; therefore, the value of a score depends on the condition. In the example, the $\chi_r^2 = 1.0$, which is not significant, and the null hypothesis would be accepted. If k (number of columns) is greater than 4, the χ_r^2 statistic is compared to the chi-square distribution in Appendix E. The power efficiency to reject the null is equivalent to the F statistic when alpha is 0.05 and 85 per cent of the F statistic when alpha is 0.01.

Multivariate Analysis

Multivariate analysis involves the concurrent statistical examination of more than two variables. This has become increasingly important in nursing research as we have come to recognize the complexity of the phenomena we are studying. As nurse researchers have become more knowledgeable about statistical techniques, more are using these advanced mathematical procedures.

Although use and interpretation of these analyses requires a statistical sophistication not usually acquired before the doctoral level, important studies using the techniques are appearing with increasing frequency in the nursing literature. In this text, our approach is to provide sufficient information to allow the beginning researcher and the nursing research consumer to achieve conceptual understanding of the statistical procedures. From this presentation, the researcher can obtain sufficient information to seek other sources if utilization of the technique is desired. This presentation provides the background that nurses must have in order to conduct critiques of studies with multivariate analyses.

The explanation is directed toward assisting the reader in developing a conceptual understanding of the logic underlying the analyses and the terms used within the procedure. Conceptual formulas will be presented for that purpose. Because the procedures for calculation are very complex and require an understanding of matrix algebra, equations for calculation are not provided.

PARTIAL CORRELATION

Partial correlation is the correlation of two variables while the effect of a third variable, thought to be influencing the relationship between the first two variables, is removed from the analysis (partialed out). This procedure is considered a mechanism of statistical control of variables in situations in which design control is not possible. Whereas the typical correlation procedure is referred to as *zero-order correlation*, the correlation of two variables while controlling a third variable is referred to as *first-order correlation*. The calculations involve conducting correlations between each two of the three variables involved. Then, a single formula, which follows, is used to calculate the partial correlation coefficient.

$$ r_{x2x3.x1} = \frac{r_{x2x3} - r_{x2x1}r_{x3x1}}{\sqrt{(1 - r^2_{x2x1})(1 - r^2_{x3x1})}} $$

where:

$r_{x2x3.x1}$ = partial correlation coefficient
r_{x2x1} = correlation coefficient between variable X and variable Y
r_{x3x1} = correlation coefficient between variable X and variable Z
r_{x2x3} = correlation coefficient between variable Y and variable Z

The t statistic is used to test the significance of the partial correlation coefficient using the following formula:

$$ t = \frac{r_{x2x3.x1}\sqrt{n - 3}}{\sqrt{1 - r^2_{x2x3.x1}}} $$

where:

$r_{x2x3.x1}$ = partial correlation coefficient
$df = n - 3$

The computer programs used to calculate the partial correlation coefficient and to determine the significance of this coefficient are identified in Table 17–41. Second-order correlations can be conducted in which two variables are partialed out. In fact, more than two variables can be partialed out. However, for each variable added, a degree of freedom is lost, which increases the size of the critical t value necessary to reach significance. Because of these factors, larger sample sizes are necessary in order for these complex relationships to be examined.

If the results of the zero-order correlations are significant but the partial correlation is not significantly different from zero, the relationship between the

TABLE 17–41
Computer Program Information
for the Partial Correlation
Coefficient

Computer Software	Computer Program Information
BMDP	P6R page 509
SPSS[x]	PARTIAL CORR page 589

two variables of interest is due only to their correlation with the variable being partialed out. If the first-order correlation is significantly different from zero, the relationship between the two variables of interest is a true reflection of reality or is due to the effect of another variable not tested. In some cases, both the zero-order correlation and the first-order correlation will be significant; however, the first-order correlation will be lower than the zero-order correlation. This indicates that a portion of the relationship is due to the partialed out variable but that the relationship between the two variables of interest has not been completely explained by the third variable.

MULTIPLE REGRESSION

Multiple regression is an extension of the simple linear regression described on page 517. However, in multiple regression, more than two variables are entered into the analysis. The dependent variable (or predicted variable) is represented by Y in the regression equation. The independent variables (or indicators) are represented by X_i in the regression equation. Regression, unlike correlation, is one way. The independent variables can predict the dependent variable, but the dependent variable cannot be used to predict the independent variables. The coefficient of the independent variable can be reported as a *b weight* (based on raw scores) or a *beta weight* (based on Z scores). These two weights are discussed on page 519.

There are many versions of regression analyses that are used in a variety of research situations. Some versions have been developed particularly for analyses in which some of the following assumptions are violated:

1. Variables are measured at the interval level.
2. The independent variables are not correlated.
3. Dependent variable scores come from a normal distribution.
4. Scores are homoscedastic (equally dispersed about the line of best fit); thus, there is a normal distribution of Y scores at each value of X.
5. Y scores have equal variances at each value of X; thus, difference scores (residuals or error scores) are random and equal at each value of X.

Selection of Independent Variables

Independent variables should be selected based on theoretical grounds. Thus, the researcher should be able to justify theoretically why the variables selected were included in the analysis. The analysis, then, tests a hypothesis emerging from the theoretical stance. The word theory is used broadly here and can include conceptual frameworks, in some cases derived from previous research. Thus, the variables selected may, to some extent, come from previous studies that suggest that variable X_i is an effective predictor of Y.

The number of variables included will dictate a minimal sample size for a particular analysis, because at least 30 subjects should be included for each independent variable in the analysis. In general, the larger the sample size, the more accurate the prediction will be (Cohen & Cohen, 1983).

Independent variables selected for the analysis should have strong correlations with the dependent variable but only weak correlations with other independent variables to be used; thus, multiple correlations are usually performed prior to regression analyses. When the independent variables are strongly correlated, this is referred to as *multicollinearity*. In nursing studies, some multicollinearity is inevitable; however, as multicollinearity decreases, the predictive power of the analysis increases. This is because uncorrelated predictor variables explain a greater amount of the variance in the dependent variable than occurs with correlated predictor variables. This is illustrated by the Venn diagram in Figure 17–16. The overlapped area of X_1 with Y indicates

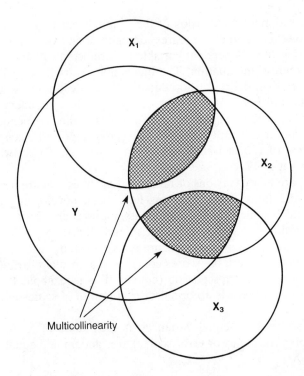

Multicollinearity

FIGURE 17–16. Variance of Y explained by three independent variables showing the effect of multicollinearity.

the amount of variance of Y explained by X_1. As can be seen, some of this same variance is also explained by X_2 which is demonstrated by a black area in the figure. The same situation occurs with X_3 and X_2 and is demonstrated by a black area. These black areas represent multicollinearity among these three variables. The greater the correlation between X_1, X_2 and X_3, the less *new* variance explained by the second variable.

The primary approach to analysis in the field of economics is regression analysis, which is considered by economists to be superior to advanced ANOVA techniques. Multiple regression estimates the parameters of a population and is considered to be equivalent to experimental designs in its power to examine causality. When multiple regression is used in this way, large samples are used rather than randomization to obtain an accurate estimate of the population.

The outcome of regression analysis is referred to as a *prediction equation*. This equation is similar to that described for simple linear regression except that making a prediction is more complex. Consider the following example equation:

$$\text{DURATION} = 10.6 + 0.3\text{AGE} + 2.4\text{INCOME} + 3.5\text{COPING}$$
$$(4.56) \quad (2.78) \quad\quad (4.43) \quad\quad\quad (7.52)$$
$$R^2 = 0.51 \quad n = 350 \quad F = 1.832 \quad p < 0.001$$

If duration were measured in the number of days that the patient received care, the Y intercept would be 10.6 days. For each increase in 1 year of age, the patient would receive 0.3 days more of care. For each increase in income level, the patient would receive an additional 2.4 days of care. For each increase in coping ability measured on a scale, the patient would receive an additional 3.5 days of care. In this example, $R^2 = 0.51$, which means that these variables explain 51 per cent of the variance in the duration of care that the patient receives. The regression analysis of variance indicates that the equation is significant at the $p < 0.001$ level.

Relating these findings to real situations requires additional work. First, it is necessary to know how the variables were coded for the analysis; for example, one would need to know the range of scores on the coping scale, the income classifications and the range of ages in the sample. Then, possible patient situations would be proposed and duration of care would be predicted for a patient with those particular dimensions of each independent variable. For example, suppose a patient is 64 years of age, in income level 3 and in coping level 5. In this case, the patient's predicted duration would be $10.6 + (64 \times 0.3) + (3 \times 2.4) + (5 \times 3.5)$, or 54.5 days of care.

Cross-Validation

To determine the accuracy of the prediction, the predicted values must be compared to actual values obtained from a new sample of subjects. This analysis is conducted on the difference scores between predicted values and the means of actual values. Thus, in the new sample, the number of days of care for all patients 64 years of age, in income level 3 and in coping level 5 would be averaged, and the mean would be compared with 54.5 days of care. Each possible case within the new sample would be compared in this manner. An R^2 is obtained on the new sample and compared to the original sample. In most cases, the R^2 will be lower in the new sample, because the original equation was developed to most precisely predict scores in the original sample. This is referred to as the *shrinkage of R^2*. Shrinkage of R^2 is greater in small samples and when multicollinearity is great.

Dummy Variables

Regression analysis can be conducted using categorical variables. Categorical variables of interest in nursing that might be used in regression analysis include gender, income, race, social status, level of education and diagnosis. To use categorical variables in regression analysis, a coding system must be developed to represent group membership. If the variable is dichotomous, such as gender, members of one category are assigned the number 1, and all others are assigned the number 0. In this case, for gender, the coding could be as follows:

$1 =$ female
$0 =$ male

The variable, gender, can then be used as an independent variable in the regression equation.

If the categorical variable has three values, two dummy variables must be used; for example, social class could be classified as lower class, middle class or upper class. The first dummy variable (X_1) would be classified as:

$1 =$ lower class
$0 =$ not lower class

The second dummy variable (X_2) would be classified as:

$1 =$ middle class
$0 =$ not middle class

The three social classes would then be specified in the equation in the following manner:

Lower Class $X_1 = 1,$ $X_2 = 0$
Middle Class $X_1 = 0,$ $X_2 = 1$
Upper Class $X_1 = 0,$ $X_2 = 0$

When more than three categories must be used to define the values of the variable, increased numbers of dummy variables are used. The number of dummy variables is always one less than the number of categories.

Regression analysis can be used for time-series analysis by coding time in a categorical form and using it as an independent variable. For example, if 5 years of data were available, the following coding system could be used:

$-2 =$ subjects cared for in the first year
$-1 =$ subjects cared for in the second year
$0 =$ subjects cared for in the third year
$+1 =$ subjects cared for in the fourth year
$+2 =$ subjects cared for in the fifth year

If minutes of care given to each subject were available, this could be used as the dependent variable. The regression equation could then test whether minutes of care had changed over time.

Multiplicative Terms

Multiple regression assumes that all independent variables have an additive effect on the dependent variable. This means that each independent variable has the same relationship with the dependent variable at each value of the other independent variables. Thus, if variable X_1 increased as X_2 increased in lower values of X_2, X_1 would be expected to continue to increase at higher values of X_2. However, in some analyses, this does not prove to be the case. For example, in a study conducted by one of the authors, minutes of care (MC) was used as the dependent variable. Duration (DUR), or number of days, of care and age (AGE) were included as independent variables. When duration was short, minutes of care increased as age increased. However, when duration was long, minutes of care decreased as age increased.

In this situation, better prediction can occur if multiplicative terms are included in the equation. In this case, the regression model takes the following form:

$$\hat{Y} = a + b_1X_1 + b_2X_2 + b_3X_1X_2$$

The last term $(b_3X_1X_2)$ takes the form of a multiplicative term and is the product of the first two variables (X_1 multiplied by X_2). This term expresses the joint effect of the two variables. For example, duration (DUR) might be expected to interact with the subject's age (AGE). The third term would show the combined effect of the two variables (DURAGE). The example equation would then be expressed as:

$$MC = a + b_1DUR + b_2AGE + b_3DURAGE$$

This procedure is similar to multivariate ANOVA, in which main effects and interaction effects are considered.

Ordinary Least Squares Multiple Regression

The most elementary form of multiple regression is referred to as *ordinary least squares (OLS)*. The equation for OLS builds upon that of simple linear regression with a term (b_iX_i) added to the equation for each independent variable. An example equation with three independent variables follows:

$$\hat{Y} = a + b_1X_1 + b_2X_2 + b_3X_3$$

In OLS, all independent variables (based on a proposed model and derived from theory) are entered into the analysis simultaneously. Thus, the outcome gives the amount of variance explained by the sum of the independent variables.

Computer programs used to conduct ordinary least squares multiple regression are presented in Table 17–42.

Stepwise Regression

The most common approach to regression analysis in nursing research is stepwise regression. Stepwise regression is not based on theory and therefore is useful only in exploratory or descriptive studies designed to develop theory. There are several approaches to stepwise regression. In *forward stepwise regression*, independent variables are entered into the analysis one at a time, and an analysis is made of the effect of including that variable on R. Thus, the computer printout indicates the increase in R with the addition of the new variable and the statistical significance (F value) of the change. In *backward stepwise regression*, all the independent variables are initially included in the analysis. Then, one variable at a time is removed from the equation and the effect of that removal on R is evaluated. In either approach, the researcher is able to determine the order of entering or removing variables. Otherwise, the independent variables are entered into the regression equation or removed from the regression equation by the computer program based on the amount of additional variance of the dependent variable explained by that particular independent variable. Computer programs used to calculate stepwise regression analysis are identified in Table 17–43.

During the process of stepwise regression analysis, partial correlations are performed, so that the amount of variance of Y explained by X_1 is "partialed out" before the variance explained by X_2 is analyzed. This partialing out continues throughout the analysis. Each additional variable included in the analysis will tend to explain a smaller additional amount of the variance in Y. As more variables are included, the increase in R is less and the degrees of freedom decrease, making it more difficult to obtain a significant F statistic for the increase in R.

Although using stepwise regression is intuitively appealing and may be useful in initial explorations of phenomena not previously well examined, there are several problems that must be considered in using this analysis approach.

TABLE 17–42
Computer Program Information
for Ordinary Least Squares
Multiple Regression

Computer Software	Computer Program Information
SAS	PROC REG page 655
BMDP	P1R page 237
ABSTAT	REGR page 83

TABLE 17–43
Computer Program Information for Stepwise Regression Analysis

Computer Software	Computer Program Information
SAS	PROC STEPWISE page 763
BMDP	P2R page 251
SPSS[x]	REGRESSION page 601

First, the strategy is somewhat akin to "fishing" in the data to find whatever significance is there. This is similar to conducting t-tests between each two variables in a data set that includes many variables. Both strategies run a great risk of detecting significant differences present in the data that are the result of random error. This greatly increases the risk of a Type I error. The shrinkage of R when cross-validation is conducted is likely to be great; thus, the value of R in stepwise regression is likely to be inflated.

Second, in forward stepwise regression, the first variable to be included in the equation is the one that explains the greatest amount of variance in the dependent variable. This first step limits the possibility of inclusion of other variables that initially explain a lesser portion of the variance but joined with a different combination of variables would together explain a greater portion.

Third, the variables selected in the procedure may be effective in *predicting* values of the dependent variable, but not very effective in *explaining* the variance in the dependent variable. From a theoretical point of view, this is not satisfactory. Knowing why part of the variance of the dependent variable is explained by a particular independent variable is important. Being able to explain changes in values of the dependent variable is an important prerequisite to being able to control those values.

Nonlinear Relationships

The typical regression model assumes a linear regression in which the relationship between X and Y can be illustrated on a graph as a straight line. However, in some cases, the relationship is not linear. In these cases, deviations from the regression line will be great and predictive power will be low. The fact that the scores are curvilinear can sometimes be demonstrated by graphing the values. Otherwise, a Type II error might be made, because the F ratio will not be significant and R^2 will be low. In this situation, the independent variable can be squared, which provides a quadratic term. This strategy will improve the predictive capacity of the analysis. An example of a mathematical model that includes a squared independent variable follows:

$$\hat{Y} = a + b_1 X + b_2 X^2$$

This equation states that $\hat{Y}$ is related to both X and X^2 in such a way that changes in $\hat{Y}$'s values are a function of both X and X^2. The nonlinearity analysis can be extended beyond the squared term to add more terms; thus, the values of X^3, X^4 and so on can be included in the equation. Each term adds another curve in the regression line. Using this strategy, very complicated relationships can be modeled.

If this approach is used with OLS, the terms are introduced simultaneously for analysis. The t values are used to determine the significance of the coefficient of the term. If the equation provides better prediction, the R^2 will be increased and the F ratio will be significant.

If the approach is used with stepwise regression analysis, the simple term would first be entered into the analysis. At the second step, X^2 would be included. Terms would continue to be added one step at a time. Each step would be examined to see whether prediction had been significantly improved, as evidenced by an increase in R^2 and a larger F ratio.

Power Analysis

Power analysis for partial correlation and multiple regression involves two steps prior to entering the table. First the effect size (ES) is calculated using the following equation:

$$ES = \frac{R^2}{1 - R^2}$$

next, H is calculated using the following equation:

$$H = ES\,(N - g - 1)$$

where:
$$(N - g - 1) = \text{df for error}$$
$$g = \text{number of predictor variables}$$

The ES and H values are compared with the values in the F power table in Appendix M. The power analysis is useful in determining the probability of a Type II error.

PATH ANALYSIS

Path analysis is designed to test the causal relationships proposed in a theoretical model. Inference is from the data to the model, rather than to a population. Consistency of the findings with the proposed relationships does not prove the accuracy of the model but supports it. This modeling process was initially described in Chapter 10; the same model is used to describe the analysis process. The path diagram clearly displays the proposed relationships among the variables (Fig. 17–17).

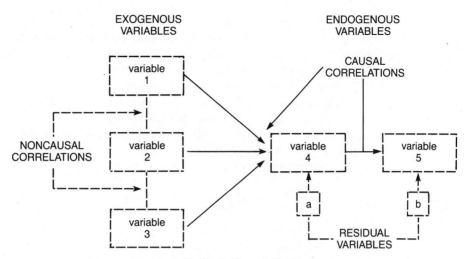

FIGURE 17–17. Path analysis diagram.

In the aforementioned model, variables 1, 2 and 3 are expected to be causally related to variable 4. Variable 4 is expected to be a cause of variable 5. However, variable 5 would *not* be considered a cause of variable 4. The model demonstrates unidirectional causal flow. Because the causal relationships will not explain all the variance in the model, residual variables (shown here as a and b) are introduced to indicate the effect of variables not included in the analysis. Noncausal relationships such as those between variables 1 and 2, 1 and 3, and 2 and 3 are not included in the causal model. The following assumptions can be made:

1. The relationships examined in the model are causal, linear and additive.
2. The residual variables are not correlated with other residual variables or with variables being examined in the model.
3. Causal pathways are unidirectional.
4. Variables are measured at the interval level.

As with regression analysis, a large sample is desirable, with at least 30 subjects for each variable being considered. Larger samples are more likely to yield statistically significant path coefficients needed to validate the model. Because of the importance of model building to theory development, the risk of a Type II error must be reduced. Using a large sample is a means of reducing the risk of a Type II error.

Path analysis requires a series of regression analyses between the variables in the model. In the analysis, a *path coefficient* indicates the effect of an independent variable on the dependent variable. The symbol for a path coefficient is P with two subscripts. The first subscript indicates the dependent variable; the second subscript indicates the independent variable. For example, the direct effect of variable 4 on variable 5 would be symbolized as P_{54}. Path coefficients are usually expressed in the form of beta weights. Beta weights were discussed in the section on simple linear regression.

The model in Figure 17–17 would require two regression analyses to identify the path coefficients. In the first analysis, path coefficients would be obtained by regressing variable 4 on variables 1, 2 and 3. Then, variable 5 would be regressed on variable 4. Computer programs used to conduct path analysis are the same as those for the ordinary least squares multiple regression, which were identified in Table 17–42. Currently, specific computer programs are being developed to conduct path analysis.

In interpreting the results of a path analysis, the weight of the coefficient and its level of statistical significance are considered. A large coefficient that is highly significant validates the causal pathway.

FACTORIAL ANALYSIS OF VARIANCE

Factorial analysis of variance is simply a specialized version of multiple regression. ANOVA was developed from the perspective of decision theory, whereas multiple regression is based on estimation. There are a number of types of factorial ANOVAs that have been developed to analyze data from specific experimental designs. These include two-way ANOVA developed for studies with two independent variables, multifactorial ANOVA for studies with more than two independent variables, randomized block ANOVA, repeated measures ANOVA and multivariate ANOVA for studies with more than one dependent variable (MANCOVA). The following assumptions can be made:

1. The dependent variable is measured at the interval level.
2. At least one independent variable must have values that are categorical rather than continuous.
3. The variance of the dependent variable must be equal in the various groups included in the analysis.
4. Subjects should be randomly selected.
5. The sample size in each group must be equal.

ANOVA has generally been robust to violation of its assumptions. However, it is relatively sensitive to variations in sample sizes between groups. This becomes an increasing problem as the complexity of the design increases and, with it, the number of groups. Although computerized forms of ANOVA have included modifications of the analysis to control for different group sizes, there remains a problem of interpreting interaction effects when group sizes vary.

In each type of ANOVA, the mathematical equations differ slightly. However, one element is characteristic of them all: a partitioning of the sum of squares. The result of this partitioning is a lessening of the error term, or the amount of unexplained (within-group) variance. With the decrease in the unexplained (within-group) variance comes an increased probability of detecting existing differences in the variables under study. Additionally, the partitioning provides the opportunity to examine interactions between variables, which may illustrate effects not initially considered.

Two types of effects are considered in interpreting the results of a factorial ANOVA. *Main effects* are the effects of a single factor. *Interaction effects* are the multiplicative effects of two or more factors. In complex designs, the interaction effects can be difficult to interpret, particularly when they are the combined effect of three or more variables. The results of multivariate ANOVA are generally exhibited in contingency tables as well as in an ANOVA summary table.

The summary table is used to report both main effects and interaction effects, the F value of each and the level of significance of the F value. The sum of squares for each portion of the analysis is provided, as well as the degrees of freedom and the mean square.

Although the contingency table is used to organize results, the terminology is somewhat different. In ANOVA, an independent variable is referred to as a *factor*; thus, in a 2 × 2 ANOVA, there is a row factor and a column factor. The rows and columns in the contingency table are referred to as *levels*; thus, in a 2 × 2 contingency table, there would be a first level row factor and a second level row factor, a first level column factor and a second level column factor.

Interaction effects are evaluated prior to consideration of main effects, because interaction effects may render main effects meaningless. On the contingency table, the interaction effects are found by comparing cell means. Main effects are determined by examining column and row means. When the analysis becomes more complex than a 2 × 2 ANOVA, post hoc analyses are necessary to determine the location of significant differences. Computer programs for calculating factorial ANOVA can be found in Table 17–30.

ANALYSIS OF COVARIANCE

Analysis of Covariance (ANCOVA) is designed to reduce the error term (or the variance within groups) using a somewhat different strategy than that of factorial ANOVA. ANCOVA partials out the variance resulting from a confounding variable by performing regression analysis prior to performing ANOVA. This strategy removes the effect of differences between groups that is due to a confounding variable. This technique is sometimes used as a method of statistical control, which is an alternative to design control. ANCOVA allows the researcher to examine the effect of the treatment apart from the effect of the confounding variable; for example, such variables as age, education, social class or anxiety level may appear to explain initial differences between groups in a study. These variables, which can affect subjects' responses to a treatment, can be partialed out using ANCOVA.

ANCOVA is a useful approach to analysis in pretest-post-test designs in which differences occur in groups on the pretest. For example, individuals who achieve low scores on a pretest will tend to have lower scores on the post-test than those whose pretest scores were higher, even if the treatment had a significant effect on post-test scores. Conversely, if an individual achieves a high pretest score, it is doubtful that the post-test will indicate a strong change as a result of the treatment. ANCOVA maximizes the capacity to detect differences in such cases.

By using multiple regression, it is also possible to partial out the effects of several covariates. For each covariate, a degree of freedom is lost, somewhat decreasing the possibilities of achieving significance, especially with small samples. Therefore, researchers should be cautious in their use of multiple covariates. ANCOVA can be used with the more advanced types of ANOVA, such as factorial designs and repeated measures designs.

FACTOR ANALYSIS

Factor analysis is mathematically related to regression analysis. In both analyses, equations are developed that are linear combinations of the variables. Regression analysis tests hypotheses involving dependent and independent variables. Factor analysis examines interrelationships among large numbers of variables and disentangles those relationships to identify clusters of variables that are most closely linked together. These closely related variables are grouped together into a "factor." Several factors may be identified within a data set.

Once the factors have been identified mathematically, the researcher must explain why the variables are grouped as they are. Thus, factor analysis aids in the identification of theoretical constructs. Factor analysis is also used to confirm the accuracy of a theoretically developed construct. For example, a theorist might state that the concept (or construct) "hope" consisted of the elements (1) anticipation of the future, (2) belief that things will work out for the best and (3) optimism. Ways could be developed to measure these three elements, and a factor analysis could be conducted on the data to determine whether subject responses clustered into these three groupings.

Factor analysis is frequently used in the process of developing measurement instruments, particularly those related to psychological variables such as attitudes, beliefs, values or opinions. The instrument operationalizes a theoretical construct. Factor analysis can also be used to attempt to sort out meaning from large numbers of questions on survey instruments.

There are two types of factor analysis: exploratory and confirmatory. *Exploratory factor analysis* is similar to stepwise regression in which the variance of the first factor is partialed out before analysis is begun on the second factor. It is performed when the researcher has few prior expectations about the factor structure. *Confirmatory factor analysis* is more closely related to ordinary least squares regression analysis. It is based on theory and tests a hypothesis about the existing factor structure. In confirmatory factor analysis, statistical significance of the analysis outcomes is determined and the parameters of the population are estimated. Confirmatory factor analysis is usually conducted after examination of the correlation matrix or after initial development of the factor structure through exploratory factor analysis.

Exploratory Factor Analysis

The first step in exploratory factor analysis is the development of a correlation matrix of the scores on all variables to be included in the factor analysis. This matrix is usually developed automatically by the computer program conducting the analysis. Although there are multiple procedures for the actual factor analysis, the procedure described here is the one most commonly reported in the literature.

The second step is a *principal components analysis*, which provides preliminary information needed by the researcher in order for decisions to be made prior to the final factoring. The computer printout of the principal components analysis will give (1) the eigenvalues, (2) the amount of variance explained by each factor and (3) the weight for each variable on each factor. The weights (loadings) express the extent to which the variable is correlated with the factor. The weightings on the variables from a principal components factor analysis are essentially uninterpretable and are generally disregarded (Nunnally, 1978).

Eigenvalues are the sum of the squared weights for each factor. The researcher examines the eigenvalues to decide how many factors will be included in the factor analysis. To decide the number of factors to include, the researcher must determine the minimal amount of variance that must be explained by the factor to add significant meaning. This decision is not straightforward and has resulted in some criticism of the analysis as being subjective. Several strategies have been proposed for determining the number of factors to be included in a construct. One approach is to select factors that have an eigenvalue of 1.00 or above. Another strategy used is the scree-test. *Scree* is a geological term that refers to the debris that collects at the bottom of a rocky slope. This test, which is considered by some to be the most reliable, requires that the eigenvalues be graphed (Fig. 17–18).

From this graph, one can see a change in the angle of the slope. A steep drop in value from one factor to the next indicates a large difference score between the two factors and an increase in the amount of variance explained. When the slope begins to become flat, indicating small difference scores between factors, little additional information will be obtained by including more factors.

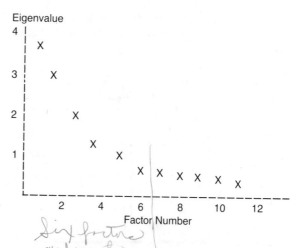

FIGURE 17–18. Graphed eigenvalues from a factor analysis.

In Figure 17–18, the slope begins to flatten at factor six; therefore, six factors would be extracted to explain the construct.

The third step in exploratory factor analysis is *factor rotation*. The purpose of factor rotation is to obtain the best fit between variables to form the clusters or factors. The procedure most commonly used is referred to as the *varimax rotation*. In the varimax rotation, the factors are rotated for the best fit (best factor solution), and the factors are uncorrelated. The process of factor analysis is actually a series of multiple regression analyses. A *factor* is a linear combination of variables in a data matrix (Kim & Mueller, 1978a; 1978b). The equation for a factor could be expressed as:

$$F = b_1X_1 + b_2X_2 + b_3X_3 + \cdots \cdots b_kX_k$$

where:

    F = factor score
    X_k = original variables from the matrix
    b_k = weights of the individual variables in the factor. If the scores used are standardized, b is a beta weight.

In exploratory factor analysis, regression analysis is performed for the first factor. Then, the variance of each variable explained by the first factor is partialed out. Next, a second regression analysis is performed on the residual variance. The variance from that analysis is then partialed out, and a regression is performed on the third factor. This process is continued until all the factors have been developed. The computer printout will include a rotated factor matrix that will contain information similar to that in Table 17–44.

Factor Loadings □ A factor loading is actually the regression coefficient of the variable on the factor. The factor loading indicates the extent to which a single variable is related to the cluster of variables. On variable 1, the factor loading is 0.76 on Factor I and 0.27 on Factor II. Squaring the factor loadings ($[0.76]^2 = 0.578$, and $[0.27]^2 = 0.073$) will give the amount of variance in variable 1, which explains Factors I and II.

Communality □ Communality (h^2) is the squared multiple regression coefficient for each variable and is closely related to the R^2 in regression. Thus, the

---

TABLE 17–44
Factor Loadings and Variance for Two Factors

Variable	Factors I	Factors II	h^2
1	0.76*	0.27	0.65
2	0.91*	0.03	0.83
3	0.64*	0.29	0.49
4	0.14	0.67*	0.47
5	0.22	0.59*	0.40
6	0.07	0.77*	0.60
Sum of squared loadings	1.89	1.55	
Variance	0.22	0.13	Total = 0.35

*Indicates the variables to be included in each factor.

communality coefficient describes the amount of variance in a single variable that is explained across all the factors in the analysis. The communality for a variable can be obtained by summing the squared factor loadings on the variable for each factor. In Table 17–44, the communality coefficient for variable 1 is $(0.76)^2 + (0.27)^2 = 0.65$. Factor analysis is conducted using the computer, and the programs are identified in Table 17–45.

Identifying the Relevant Variables in a Factor □ Only variables with factor loadings that indicate that a meaningful portion of the variable's variance is explained within the factor are included as elements of the factor. A cutoff point is selected for the purpose of identifying these variables. The minimum cutoff point that is acceptable is 0.30; however, it is acceptable to have a higher cutoff point, such as 0.50. In Table 17–44, the factor loadings with asterisks indicate the variables that will be included in each factor. In this example, which uses a 0.50 cutoff, variables 1, 2 and 3 would be included in Factor I, and variables 4, 5 and 6 would be included in Factor II. Ideally, a variable will "load" on only one factor. If the variable does have high loadings on two factors, the lowest loading is referred to as a *secondary loading*. When many secondary loadings occur, it is not considered a "clean" factoring, and the researcher must reexamine the variables included in the analysis. Sometimes, researchers will attempt to set the cutoff point high enough to avoid secondary loadings of a variable.

"Naming" the Factor □ At this point, the mathematics of the procedure take a back seat, and the theoretical reasoning of the researcher takes over. The researcher examines the variables that have clustered together in a factor and explains that clustering. Variables with high loadings on the factor must be included, even if they do not fit the preconceived theoretical notions of the researcher. The purpose is to identify the broad construct of meaning that has caused these particular variables to be so strongly intercorrelated. Naming this construct is a very important part of the procedure, because the naming of the factor provides theoretical meaning.

Factor Scores □ After the initial factor analysis, additional studies are conducted to examine changes in the phenomenon in various situations and to

TABLE 17–45
Computer Program Information
for Factor Analysis

Computer Software	Computer Program Information
SAS	FACTOR page 335
BMDP	P4M page 480
SPSS[x]	FACTOR page 647

determine the relationships of the factors with other concepts. Factor scores are used during data analysis in these additional studies. To obtain factor scores, the variables included in the factor are identified, and the scores on these variables are summed for each subject. Thus, each subject will have a score for each factor in the instrument. Because some variables explain a larger portion of the variance of the factor than others, additional meaning can be added by multiplying the variable score by the weight (factor loading) of that variable in the factor. Using the example in Table 17–44, variable 1 had a factor loading of 0.76 on Factor I. If the subject score on variable 1 were 7, the score would be "weighted" by multiplying the variable score by the factor loading as follows:

$$7 \times 0.76 = 5.32$$

These weighted scores can be generated using the computer. If comparisons between studies are to be made, standardized (Z) scores (for variable scores) and beta weights (for factor loadings) should be used. Once analysis is complete, factor scores can be used as independent variables in multiple regression equations.

Confirmatory Factor Analysis

Confirmatory factor analysis is a fairly recent development and is extremely complex mathematically. Interpretation of results requires a high level of sophistication in statistical analyses. In confirmatory factor analysis, the researcher develops hypotheses about the factor structure. Because the elements of each factor are set in the analysis, factor rotation and partialing out of variance are not performed. Cutoff points for representation within the factor may also be preset and included in the analysis. As an outcome of the analyses, estimation of the population parameters for the factor structure are made. The statistical significance of the results of the analyses are tested. Nunnally (1978) has provided an extensive section on this analysis technique in *Psychometric Theory*.

DISCRIMINANT ANALYSIS

Discriminant analysis is closely related to both factor analysis and regression analysis. However, in discriminant analysis, the dependent variable values are categorical in form. Each value of the dependent variable is considered a group. When the dependent variable is dichotomous, multiple regression is performed. However, when there are more than two groups, analysis becomes much more complex. The dependent variable in discriminant analysis is referred to as the *discriminant function*. It is equivalent in many ways to a factor.

Two similar data sets are required for a complete analysis. The first data set must contain measures on all the variables to be included in the analysis and the group membership of each subject. The purpose of the analysis of the first data set is to identify variables that most effectively discriminate between groups. Variables are selected for the analysis based on the researcher's expectation that they will be effective in this regard. An effort is made in the analysis to maximize between-group variance while minimizing within-group variance. Variables that are expected to achieve this maximization and minimization of variance are selected for the discriminant function. The variables can be entered in a stepwise manner if desired. Those variables most effective in discriminating are retained. Weightings on each variable are included in the computer printout. The variables selected for the discriminant function are then tested on a second set of data to determine their effectiveness in predicting group membership. Two sources for referral for discriminant analysis are Nunnally (1978) and Volicer (1984). The computer programs used to conduct discriminant analysis are presented in Table 17–46.

CANONICAL CORRELATION

Canonical correlation is an extension of multiple regression in which there is more than one dependent variable. Researchers using the technique should be very familiar with both regression analysis and factor analysis. The purpose of the test is to analyze the relationships between two or more dependent variables and two or more independent variables. The least squares principle is used to partition and analyze variance. Two linear composites are developed: one associated with the dependent variables, and the other associated with the independent variables. The relationship between the two linear composites is then examined and expressed by the value R_c. The square of this canonical correlation coefficient indicates the proportion of variance explained by the analysis. When there is more than one source of covariation, more than one cannonical correlation can be identified. The minimal sample size with which canonical correlation can be used is 200. With smaller samples, results are not likely to be replicable (Levine, 1977; Waltz & Bausell, 1981). The computer programs used to conduct the canonical correlation are identified in Table 17–47.

TABLE 17–46
Computer Program Information for Discriminant Analysis

Computer Software	Computer Program Information
SAS	PROC DISCRIM page 317
BMDP	P7M page 519
SPSS[x]	DISCRIMINANT page 623

TABLE 17–47
Computer Program Information
for Canonical Correlation

Computer Software	Computer Program Information
SAS	PROC CANCORR page 139
BMDP	P6M page 500

Other Approaches to Analysis
TIME-SERIES ANALYSIS

In the past, the analysis of time-series data has been problematic because computer programs designed for this purpose were not easily accessible. The most common approach to analysis was ordinary least squares multiple regression. However, this approach has been, for the most part, unsatisfactory.

A new approach to the analysis of time-series data was developed and described by McCain and McCleary (1979), McCleary and Hay (1980) and McDowall, McCleary, Meidinger and Hay (1980). This section relies heavily on their descriptions of the analysis process. The most commonly used time-series analysis model is the *Autoregressive Integrated Moving Average (ARIMA) Model*, which is based on work by Box and Jenkins (1976). A model is an equation or series of equations that explains a naturally occurring process (McCain & McCleary, 1979). The computer programs available to conduct this analysis technique are identified in Table 17–48.

The terminology and the problems that must be dealt with in time-series analysis are different from those that we are more familiar with in analyzing conventional data. There are two components to a time series: the deterministic component, and the stochastic component. The *deterministic component* represents all the parameters of time series that are not dependent on error (or random variation in the data). However, this parameter cannot perfectly predict the values in a time series, because even though the underlying process may

TABLE 17–48
Computer Program Information
for the ARIMA Model

Computer Software	Computer Program Information
SAS/ETS	PROC ARIMA page 127
BMDP	P2T page 639
SPSS[x]	BOX-JENKINS page 697

be systematic, a single observation will deviate from the expected value. The *stochastic component* describes what is referred to as "noise" (or random variance) in the data. There are two parts to the stochastic component, the systematic part and the unsystematic part. The systematic part is related to the autocorrelation inherent in time-series data. *Autocorrelations*, as the term implies, are repeated occurrences in the data that are systematic and to some extent patterned. Each one of these events is correlated with both past and future occurrences of the same event. The unsystematic part is the typical error variance that leads to differences from measures of central tendency found in all data. The unsystematic part is the element in time series from which such measures as standard deviations are calculated.

The ARIMA (p,d,q) models describe time series as stochastic or "noise" processes. The null hypothesis is that only the noise component is present and that no change has occurred. There are three parameters to an ARIMA model: p, d and q. The integer values of these parameters must be identified through a simple statistical analysis called *identification*. However, first it is important to understand the parameters.

Stationarity

To use an ARIMA (p,d,q) model, the data must be either stationary or nonstationary in a homogeneous sense. The noise in a time series "drifts" up and down across time. If the data are stationary, it means that there is no decrease or increase in the level of the series as it drifts. However, most data in the social sciences are nonstationary. Nonstationary "in the homogeneous sense" means that "differencing" can be used to make the data stationary. To accomplish this, difference scores are calculated between the sequences in the time series. The value of the first observation is subtracted from the second, the value of the second is subtracted from the third, and so on. For example, consider the following series of numbers as a time series:

$$2, 4, 6, 8, 10, 12. \ldots$$

This series is nonstationary. But note the effect of differencing the series:

$$4 - 2 = 2$$
$$6 - 4 = 2$$
$$8 - 6 = 2$$
$$10 - 8 = 2$$

Now the series is stationary:

$$2, 2, 2, 2, 2, 2, \ldots \ldots 2.$$

Fortunately, most social science data can be differenced to achieve stationarity. Differencing has no effect on the deterministic parameters of the model, which will be used in the analysis to detect changes. The model parameter d indicates the number of times a series must be differenced before it becomes stationary. A zero in the model (ARIMA [p,0,q]) indicates that the time series is stationary and does not require differencing.

Autoregressive Models

The parameter p indicates the autoregressive order of the model. There are two elements in the parameter p: 0_1 and a_t. The 0_1 is a correlation coefficient that describes the degree of dependency between observations. If there is a direct relationship between adjacent observations, the value of p exceeds zero. This direct relationship between observations means that the observations are dependent. If they are dependent, the current value can be predicted based on the previous value in the series, and the present value can be used to predict future values. The p parameter of the model indicates the number of autoregressive terms included in the model. The a_t is the error term and describes what is referred to as "white noise" or "random shock." This is the unsystematic element in the stochastic component of the model. In equations calculating this parameter, the 0_1 and a_t must be summed.

Moving Average Models

The q parameter in the ARIMA (p,d,q) model is an indication of the moving average order. In some time series, there is persistence of a random shock beyond a single observation. This persistence is similar to the effect of dropping a pebble in water. If this occurs, q exceeds zero. The statistic ϕ (phi) is a correlation coefficient which expresses the extent to which the current time series observation can be predicted from preceding random shocks. Phi (ϕ) is used as the weight in a weighted term in a prediction equation. In some models, more than one weighted term may be used.

Noise Model Identification

The systematic part of the stochastic component in an ARIMA (p,d,q) model is identified by using two functions: the autocorrelation function (ACF), and the partial autocorrelation function (PACF). When a likely model has been identified, the parameters are estimated using special nonlinear computer software. Then the ACF and the PACF are used to diagnose the adequacy of the model. If the model is inadequate, a new ARIMA (p,d,q) model must be identified, the parameters must be estimated and the residuals must be diagnosed. This procedure continues until an adequate model is generated.

Hypothesis Testing

When the first three steps of the modeling strategy—identification, estimation and diagnosis—have been satisfactorily completed, then hypothesis testing can be performed. For this purpose, the *transfer function* is specified. This transfer function is added to the previously identified ARIMA noise model. Together they form a tentative joint transfer function–ARIMA model. The parameters for this joint model are then estimated, and the data are tested for signs of change. Three types of change can be detected: abrupt, constant change;

gradual, constant change; and abrupt, temporary change. In some cases, the researcher will have some idea as to which type of change has occurred. If so, a transfer function appropriate to test this particular type of change is selected. In an adequate model, the residuals act like white noise, allowing the model to detect differences between the white noise and the effects of change. If the change effect size detected by the model is large, the fit of the joint model should be tested to ensure that the effect size given is accurate. This is a concern because previous approaches to time-series analyses have tended to overestimate effect sizes. The effect sizes are tested for significance, and a decision is made to reject or accept the null hypothesis.

Because of its newness, time-series analysis (ARIMA model) has not been used in nursing research, but it has potential for providing us with important information about processes in nursing practice. Most phenomena of interest in nursing occur over time. It is often difficult to differentiate the effect of a particular intervention from all the other changes happening in the nursing situation.

Although the analysis process itself does not require extreme degrees of statistical sophistication, it will require some changes in the way that studies are designed. For this type of analysis, a minimum of 50 observations are necessary for each subject. As the number of variables included in the analysis increases, the number of observations must increase. At first, this seems unrealistic; however, we may have to consider different approaches to making observations. If a care process is being examined, each element of that care is an observation. Each behavioral response of the patient is an observation. Thus, the process of observation may require that the situation be broken down into very discrete elements (McCain & McCleary, 1979; McCleary & Hay, 1980; McDowall, McCleary, Meidinger & Hay, 1980; Metzger & Schultz, 1982).

META-ANALYSIS

Meta-analysis is the examination of research findings across studies in order to make more accurate estimates of population parameters than is possible from a single study. Meta-analysis is also useful in resolving conflicting findings of studies that examine the same phenomenon. Meta-analysis is statistically based, objective and replicable and provides a much more accurate way to summarize existing research than has been done in the past with written summaries. This analysis technique should lead to an increase in theory development that is empirically based.

Meta-analysis has been developed in the past 10 years and has just begun to influence nursing research. Two primary approaches to the analysis are currently available: (1) that of Glass, McGaw and Smith (1981) and (2) that of Hunter, Schmidt and Jackson (1982). The strategy of Hunter, Schmidt and Jackson is described here.

Meta-analysis is most effective when large numbers of studies have been reported in which the same phenomenon has been examined. However, Hunter, Schmidt and Jackson state that the technique can be used with as few as two studies. Conducting a thorough search for studies is an important part of the process. Studies examined should include dissertations and papers presented at meetings to the extent that this is possible. Contrary to Glass and colleagues' (1981) position, Hunter and colleagues (1982) do not believe that it is necessary to delete poorly designed studies from the analysis, because labeling a study as poorly designed is merely someone's value judgment and tends to be biased.

Hunter and colleagues discount the value of correlating study characteristics such as sex, age and so on with study outcomes. The coding required to do this is massive, and, because of the small sample sizes (fewer than 500 subjects), there is a high risk of one's jumping to false conclusions. After sampling error and other artifacts have been removed, they have found that little important variation is left to be explained by study characteristics.

Calculation or "cumulation" of results across studies is performed using the following steps described by Hunter and colleagues (1982):

1. Calculate the desired descriptive statistic for each study available, and average that statistic across studies.
2. Calculate the variance of the statistic across studies.
3. Correct the variance by subtracting the amount due to sampling error.
4. Correct the mean and variance for study artifacts other than sampling error.
5. Compare the corrected standard deviation to the mean to assess the size of the potential variation in results across studies in qualitative terms. If the mean is more than two standard deviations larger than 0, then it is reasonable to conclude that the relationship considered is always positive. (p. 28)

Hunter and colleagues have developed cumulation formulas for correlation coefficients and effect sizes. They are continuing their work and plan an expanded second edition to include additional cumulation formulas. An explanation of use of the analysis procedure is available in Hunter, Schmidt and Jackson (1982).

Qualitative Analysis Techniques

Qualitative analysis techniques use words rather than numbers as the basis of analysis. Until very recently, qualitative analysis has been poorly defined, communicated primarily by word of mouth to the initiated and, to some extent, researcher specific. The analysis process relies heavily upon intuitive processes. The approach is emotionally appealing and appears much easier than quantitative analysis.

Qualitative research, however, requires essentially the same careful skills in analytic reasoning as those required of the researcher by quantitative analysis. It is more difficult in a sense because much of the analytic process performed mathematically in quantitative data goes on in the head of the qualitative researcher, although perhaps not always in a conscious sense. The analytic reasoning process guides the organization, reduction and clustering of the findings and leads to the development of theoretical explanations.

The most complete description of qualitative analysis strategies currently available was written by Miles and Huberman (1984). This excellent presentation of qualitative data analysis approaches is used as the basis for this section. Although space does not allow a complete listing of the strategies proposed by Miles and Huberman, the following should provide a sufficient understanding of the process of data analysis to allow the reader to comprehend the process and to facilitate the critique of qualitative research. The strategies described by Miles and Huberman were developed for analysis of data from grounded theory research. However, many of these strategies are used in the analysis of data from other qualitative approaches. Researchers wishing to conduct qualitative research are referred to Miles and Huberman's (1984) text. The content presented includes references to relevant pages in Miles and Huberman.

Miles and Huberman identify three concurrent "flows of activity" involved in the analysis of qualitative data: (1) data reduction, (2) data display and (3) conclusion drawing/verification. *Data reduction* is "the process of selecting, focusing, simplifying, abstracting, and transforming the 'raw' data that appear in written-up field notes" (Miles & Huberman, 1984, p. 21). *Data display* is the organized assembly of information using such forms as tables, graphs and matrices. This is considered part of the process of analysis, not the outcome of analysis. *Conclusion drawing/verification* involves attaching meaning to the findings. The process begins with the initiation of data collection and ends with the writing of the final report. All three processes occur simultaneously. There are multiple data analysis strategies associated with each of the three processes.

DATA REDUCTION

Massive amounts of data are collected during a qualitative study. In a large study, one might have 5000 pages of notes. These notes are generally narrative descriptions of field observations. Strategies to reduce the data are essential to extracting the meaning inherent within these extensive notes.

Contact Summary Sheet

The contact summary is a one-page form with focused questions that assist the data collector in considering the implications of recently written field notes. Questions suggested by Miles and Huberman (1984) include:
- What people, events, or situations were involved?
- What were the main themes or issues in the contact?
- Which research questions did the contact bear most centrally on?
- What new hypotheses, speculations, or guesses about the field situations were suggested by the contact?
- Where should the fieldworker place most energy during the next contact, and what sorts of information should be sought? p. 50

The form should be completed soon after the field notes have been reviewed and corrected. This allows reflection over the contact, which is the beginning of analysis.

Document Summary Form

In field research, researchers often collect documents from the site. These documents may include such things as meeting agendas, minutes of meetings, memos, evaluation reports, rosters, brochures, lunch menus and so on. The documents often require explaining and summarizing. The document summary form can be used to indicate the significance of the document and to place it in context (Miles & Huberman, 1984, p. 51).

Codes and Coding

Field notes from the data collection process accumulate with amazing rapidity. It soon becomes difficult to find specific notations that have been recorded or to connect one note with another note. A code is a symbol or abbreviation used to classify the words. Coding is a means of categorizing. Miles and Huberman suggest creating a "start list" of codes at the beginning of data collection and then adding to it as needed.

There are three types of codes: descriptive, interpretative and explanatory. *Descriptive codes* simply classify the words; for example, the researcher might wish to categorize some notes as TCH (teaching). This could be separated into PT-TCH (patient teaching) and ST-TCH (staff teaching).

Interpretative codes are usually developed later in the data collecting process as the researcher gains some insight into the processes occurring. For example, some patient teaching might be done because of institutional requirements. When this type of teaching is being done, the nurse might shift into an automatic semimemorized speech addressed to the patient with little concern about the patient's response to the information. This might be coded AUTO-TCH. In other cases, the nurse might be observed in dialogue with the patient as new information is shared and its impact is being explored. This might be coded DIAL-TCH.

Explanatory codes are developed late in the data collection process after theoretical ideas from the study have begun to emerge. The explanatory codes are part of the researcher's attempt to unravel the meanings inherent in the situation. These codes connect the data to the emerging theory, and the codes used may be specific to the theory or more general, such as PATT (pattern), TH (theme) or CL (causal link). A list of codes and their definitions should be available to all data collectors in the study. Typically, codes will not stay the same throughout the study. Some codes will have to be broken down into subclassifications. Other codes may be discontinued because they do not work.

Codes are generally placed in the left-hand margin of the field notes; therefore, a wide left-hand margin should be maintained in the field notes. The codes may be placed there as the notes are taken or entered later when the notes are reviewed shortly after the data collection process (Miles & Huberman, 1984, pp. 54–64).

Reflective Remarks

While the field notes are being written, the researcher often has thoughts or insights that emerge into consciousness. These thoughts are generally included within the field notes and are separated from the rest of the notes by ((double parentheses)). Later, they may need to be extracted and used for memoing (Miles & Huberman, 1984, p. 64).

Marginal Remarks

As the field notes are being reviewed, observations about the notes should be written immediately. These remarks are usually placed in the right-hand margin of the notes. The remarks often connect the notes with other parts of the data or suggest new interpretations. Reviewing field notes can become boring, which is a signal that thinking has ceased. Making marginal notes assists the researcher in "retaining a thoughtful stance" (Miles & Huberman, 1984, p. 65).

Memoing

A memo is a write-up of ideas about field notes, codes or remarks made on the notes that move the researcher toward theorizing. Memos are conceptual rather than factual. They may link pieces of data together or use a specific piece of data as an example of a conceptual idea. The memo may be written to someone else in the study or just a note to oneself. The important thing is to value one's ideas and to get them written down quickly.

Any time an idea emerges, even if it is vague and not well thought out, it should be written down immediately. One's initial feeling is that the idea is so clear in one's mind that it can be written later. However, the thought is soon forgotten and often cannot be retrieved again.

As one becomes immersed in the data, these ideas will occur at odd times, such as 2 A.M., when one is driving or when one is preparing a meal. Therefore, it is advisable to keep paper and pencil handy. If one is awakened with an idea, it should be written down immediately; it will be gone by morning.

Memos should be dated, titled with the key concept discussed and connected by codes with the field notes or forms that generated the thoughts. The memo should be filed under the concept but separately from the field notes (Miles & Huberman, 1984, pp. 69–71).

Developing Propositions

As the study progresses, the need for organization of ideas into a cohesive framework becomes more prominent. One way to do this is by generating propositions and making connections between propositions. Everyone involved in the study can participate in the development of propositions. Statements or propositions can be written on index cards and sorted into categories. A working list can then be typed and shared among the researchers, generating further discussion (Miles & Huberman, 1984, pp. 71–72).

Data Accounting Sheet

In field research, one can easily lose track of where one is in the study. An accounting sheet lists each research question and the data sources needed to obtain information related to that question. A checklist can be developed from this information to indicate what information has been obtained and the areas of missing or incomplete data (Miles & Huberman, 1984, pp. 77–78).

DISPLAYS

Displays contain highly condensed versions of the outcomes of qualitative research. They are equivalent to the summary tables of statistical outcomes developed in quantitative research and allow the researcher to "get across" the main ideas of the research to individuals not willing to take the time to read narrative accounts of the study. The strategies for achieving displays are limited only by the imagination of the researcher. Some suggested ideas follow.

Context Chart

One of the main tenets of qualitative research is that data must not be interpreted "out of context." Finding ways to succinctly clarify the context of the study is important. One strategy is to develop an organizational chart that indicates each subject's role and level of involvement in areas of interest. The chart could also show the character of relationships between subjects in the study (Miles & Huberman, 1984, pp. 91–95).

Variable-Specific Context Chart

Sometimes, the researcher is interested in understanding variations in a particular variable within the context of the study. For example, if the dynamics of social support had emerged as an important variable, one might wish to know to whom and in what situations social support was provided. This information could be summarized in a context chart. How the support was received could also be illustrated (Miles & Huberman, 1984, p. 95).

Matrices

An important characteristic of qualitative researchers is an open-minded reception to manifestations of reality. There is an avoidance of placing positive and negative values or numbers on data. However, qualitative researchers do more of this than they are generally willing to admit. If researchers are willing to let go of enough of their aimlessness to collect predetermined data and enter the data into a prespecified analysis form, matrices can be used to summarize the findings.

For a matrix to be useful, the variable of interest must be unbundled into indicators or codable components; for example, if teaching on the nursing unit were the variable of interest, elements necessary for teaching to occur might be commitment, knowledge, materials, teaching skills, time allocation, administrative support and peer support. These elements could constitute the rows in a matrix. The columns could consist of classifications of nursing staff. The researcher then uses the matrix to summarize the findings. This technique alerts the researcher to data in a particular cell that have not been collected. The matrix provides a broad point of view from which to perform analysis of the data.

Matrices can be time-ordered, with columns arranged by time period. For example, teaching techniques could be examined from the initiation of a new teaching program, from the point of employment of a nurse or from the point of graduation. This type of matrix allows one to see when a phenomenon occurred. A matrix can also be role-ordered to allow analysis of differing patterns of behavior or differing values of individuals with specific roles in an organization. Role-and-time or role-and-group can be combined in the same matrix.

On another plane, matrices can be developed to clarify the concepts in the study or the outcomes of a change that is of interest in the study. An explanatory effects matrix can assist in answering questions such as why an outcome was achieved or what caused the outcome. A process-outcome matrix can allow the researcher to trace the processes that led to differing outcomes. An event-time matrix can facilitate comparisons of the events occurring in different sites during particular time periods (Miles & Huberman, 1984, pp. 95–128).

Critical Incident Chart

In some studies, the researcher wishes to identify key events occurring in the course of a process. A matrix listing critical incidents in relation to time could provide increased insight into the dynamics of the process. This is sometimes referred to as *mapping*.

Causal Network

As the data are collected and analyzed, the researcher gains increasing understanding of the dynamics involved in the process under study. Miles and Huberman refer to this understanding as a "mental map." The first mental maps are vague and poorly pieced together. In some cases, they are altogether wrong. The best way to verify a mental map is to share it with others, particularly informants in the study situation. Informants have their own mental maps, which have never been clearly expressed. Developing a good causal map is difficult and requires some hard work. The outcome is a model, similar to those described in Chapter 7. Miles and Huberman (1984, pp. 130–142) provide some excellent suggestions for causal network analysis.

Making and Testing Predictions

The validity of predictions developed in a causal model must be tested. However, finding effective ways to achieve this is difficult. Predictions are usually developed near the end of the study. Since the findings are often context specific, the predictions must be tested on the same sample or on a sample that is very similar. One strategy suggested is to predict outcomes expected to occur 6 months after the completion of the study. Six months later, these predictions can be sent to informants who participated in the study. The informants can be asked to respond to the accuracy of (1) the predictions and (2) the explanation of why the prediction was expected to occur (Miles & Huberman, 1984, pp. 142–150).

DRAWING AND VERIFYING CONCLUSIONS

Strategies for generating meaning from the data have been general to this point. The specific processes involved in these generalizations have not been clear in the literature. Miles and Huberman have identified 12 tactics that can be used in qualitative data analysis.

Counting

Qualitative researchers have tended to avoid any use of numbers. However, when judgments of qualities are made, counting is occurring. The researcher states that a pattern occurs "frequently" or "more often." Something is considered "important" or "significant." These judgments are made in part by counting. If the researcher is counting, it should be recognized and planned. Counting can help researchers "see" what they have; it can help verify a hypothesis; and it can help keep one intellectually honest. Qualitative researchers work by insight and intuition; however, their conclusions can be wrong. It is easier to see confirming evidence than to see disconfirming evidence. Comparing insights with numbers can be a good method of verification (Miles & Huberman, 1984, pp. 215–216).

Noting Patterns, Themes

People easily identify patterns, themes and gestalts from their observations—almost too easily. The difficulty is in seeking *real* additional evidence of that pattern while remaining open to disconfirming evidence. Any pattern that is identified should be subjected to skepticism—that of the researcher and that of others (Miles & Huberman, 1984, p. 216).

Seeing Plausibility

Very often during analysis, a conclusion is seen as plausible. It seems to "fit"; "it makes good sense." When asked how one arrived at that point, the researcher may state that it "just feels right." These intuitive feelings are important in both qualitative and quantitative research. However, plausibility cannot stand alone. After plausibility comes systematic analysis, which means that first intuition occurs, then examination (Miles & Huberman, 1984, pp. 216–218).

Clustering

Clustering is the process of sorting elements into categories or groups. It is the first step in inductive theorizing. In order to cluster objects, people or behavior into a group, one must first conceptualize them as having similar patterns or characteristics. Clustering is very familiar to those researchers who perform content analysis. Clusters, however, like patterns, must be viewed with caution, and they must be verified. There may be alternative ways to cluster that are much more meaningful (Miles & Huberman, 1984, pp. 218–221).

Making Metaphors

Miles and Huberman suggest that qualitative researchers should think and write metaphorically. They believe that metaphors add meaning to the findings and use the example of the "mother's separation anxiety," which is "less appealing, less suggestive, and less theoretically powerful" (p. 221) than "the empty nest syndrome." Metaphors are also *data-reducing devices* that involve generalizing from the particulars. They are *pattern-making devices* that place the pattern into a larger context. Metaphors are very effective *decentering devices*. They force the viewer to step back from the mass of particular observations to see the larger picture. Metaphors are also ways of *connecting findings to theory*. They are what initiates the researcher to thinking in more general terms. A few suggestions about developing metaphors follow: (1) It is unwise to look for metaphors early in the study. (2) In order to develop metaphors, one must be cognitively playful, moving from the denotative to the connotative. Interacting with others in a "cognitively playful environment" can be very useful. (3) Metaphors can be taken too far in terms of meaning; therefore, one must know when to stop.

Splitting Variables

Qualitative research is strongly oriented toward integrating concepts. However, is some cases, researchers must recognize the need for differentiation. They must have the courage to question; Miles and Huberman refer to this early integration as "premature parsimony." Splitting variables is particularly important during the initial stages of the analysis to allow more detailed examination of the processes that are occurring. It also often occurs with the development of matrices. During theorizing, if the variable does not seem to relate well with the rest of the framework, it may have to be split to allow a more coherent, integrated model to be developed (Miles & Huberman, 1984, p. 222).

Subsuming Particulars into the General

This process is similar to clustering, in that it involves the clumping of things together. Clustering tends to be intuitive and is similar to coding. Subsuming particulars into the general is a move from the concrete to the abstract and theoretical.

Factoring

The idea of factoring is taken from the quantitative procedure of factor analysis. If one has a list of characteristics, are there general themes within the list that allow one to explain more clearly what is going on? As with factor analysis, when clusters have been identified, they must be named. Factoring can occur at several levels of abstraction in the data. The important consideration is that they make a meaningful difference in clarity (Miles & Huberman, 1984, pp. 223–224).

Noting Relations Between Variables

The development of relationships between variables was discussed previously. However, at this point, it is important to go beyond verifying that, in fact, a relationship exists to explain the relationship. Relationships that might occur include:

(1) A+, B+ (both are high, or both low at the same time)

(2) A+, B− (A is high, B is low, or vice versa)

(3) A↑, B↑ (A has increased, and B has increased)

(4) A↑, B↓ (A has increased, and B has decreased)

(5) A↑ then ⟶B↑ (A increased first, then B increased)

(6) A↑ then ⟶B↑ then A↑ (A increased, then B increased, then A increased some more) (Miles & Huberman, p. 225)

Finding Intervening Variables

In some cases, the researcher believes that two variables should go together; however, findings do not verify this thinking. In other cases, two variables are found during data analysis to go together, but their connection cannot be explained. In both of these situations, a third variable may be responsible for the confusion. Therefore, the third variable must be identified. The matrices described earlier can be very useful in the search for this variable, and the search often requires some careful detective work. Finding an intervening variable is easiest when there are multiple cases of the two-variable relationship to examine (Miles & Huberman, 1984, pp. 226–227).

Building a Logical Chain of Evidence

At first glance, this would seem to be the same activity described earlier that resulted in the development of a theoretical model; however, this activity assumes the prior development of a theoretical model. Building a logical chain of evidence involves testing that model. The researcher must go back and carefully trace evidence from the data through the entire theoretical model; then, the elements, relationships and propositions of the model are tested against new data. The researcher looks for cases that closely fit the model and for those that clearly do not fit the model. The model may then be modified. This process is referred to as *analytic induction* and uses two interlocking cycles. The first cycle is *enumerative induction*, in which a number and variety of instances are collected that verify the model. *Progressive focusing*, sometimes referred to by qualitative researchers, is another term for this activity. The second cycle, *eliminative induction*, requires that the hypothesis be tested against alternatives. The researcher is required to carefully check for limits to the generalizability of the model. The process of "constant comparisons" and "structural corroborations" are activities related to eliminative induction. The diagnostic process in nursing switches back and forth between the two activities of enumerative and eliminative induction (Miles & Huberman, 1984, pp. 227–228).

Making Conceptual/Theoretical Coherence

The previous steps have described a gradual move from empirical data to a conceptual overview of the findings. Inferences have been made as the analysis moved from the concrete to the more abstract. The steps then moved from metaphors to interrelationships, then to constructs and from there to theories. The theory must now be connected with other existing theories in the body of knowledge. In order to accomplish this step, one must develop a familiarity with a wide variety of theories that could be used to explain the current phenomenon. If connections can be made with other theories, it further strengthens the present theoretical explanation (Miles & Huberman, 1984, pp. 228–230).

Summary

Most nursing research involves statistical analyses using mathematical formulas. A solid background in mathematical logic and statistical techniques is essential for conducting quality research. Statistics can be used for a variety of purposes, including (1) to summarize, (2) to compare or contrast descriptively, (3) to test the proposed relationships in a theoretical model, (4) to infer that the findings from the sample are indicative of the entire population, (5) to establish causality, (6) to predict or (7) to infer from the sample to a theoretical model.

Data analysis begins with summary statistics in any study in which the data is numeric. For some exploratory and descriptive studies, summary statistics will be the only approach to analysis of the data. Summary statistics also provide a means for describing the characteristics of the sample from which the data were collected. Summary statistics discussed in this chapter include frequency distributions, measures of central tendency (mode, median and mean) and measures of dispersion (modal percentages, range, difference scores, sum of squares, variance and standard deviation).

The shape of a distribution provides very important information about the sample under study. Several terms are used to describe the shape of the curve. A symmetrical curve is one in which the left side of the curve is a mirror image of the right side. Any curve that is not symmetrical is referred to as skewed, or asymmetrical. Most curves are unimodal, which means that there is one mode and that frequencies progressively decline as they move away from the mode. Kurtosis explains the degree of peakedness of the curve shape, which is related to the spread of variance of scores. Because of differences in the characteristics of various distributions, comparing a score in one distribution with a score in another distribution is difficult. To facilitate this comparison, a mechanism has been developed to transform raw scores into standard (or Z) scores. The normal curve, a product of mathematical theory, is symmetrical, unimodal and has continuous values. The mean, median and mode are equal.

A statistic is a numerical figure obtained from the sample. The parameter is the same value within the population. The most commonly used statistical analyses are parametric statistics. The three assumptions of parametric statistics are (1) the sample was drawn from a normal distribution, (2) random sampling techniques were used to obtain the sample and (3) the data were measured at the interval level. Nonparametric statistical analyses do not meet one or more of these assumptions.

There are two mathematical theory approaches to statistical analysis: estimation and decision theory. An estimator estimates the parameter of a population. Using this approach, the researcher develops confidence intervals to estimate the population parameters. In hypothesis testing, which uses decision theory, sample statistics from each sample are compared through statistical analysis to determine whether the statistics from the different samples are similar enough to suggest that the samples probably come from the same population. The researcher must make a decision about whether the hypothesis is to be accepted or rejected. The level of significance, developed from decision theory, is the cutoff point used to determine whether the samples being tested are members of the same population or are from different populations. Two types of error can occur in making decisions about the meaning of a value obtained from a statistical test. A Type I error occurs when the researcher concludes that the samples tested are from different populations when, in fact, the samples are from the same population. A Type II error occurs when the researcher concludes that there is no significant difference between the samples examined when, in fact, a difference exists.

Bivariate analysis involves the comparison of summary values from two groups on the same variable or of two variables within a group. Selection of the statistical analysis will depend on the level of measurement (nominal, ordinal, interval or ratio) of the data and the subproblems posed in the study. Bivariate analysis for both independent groups and dependent groups was discussed.

Multivariate analysis involves the concurrent statistical examination of more than two variables. Use and interpretation of these analyses requires a statistical sophistication not usually acquired before the doctoral level. Sufficient information on the various statistical techniques has been provided to allow the beginning researcher and the nursing research consumer to achieve conceptual understanding of the procedures.

Other approaches to analysis discussed in the chapter include time-series analysis, meta-analysis and qualitative analysis techniques. Qualitative analysis requires essentially the same careful skills in analytic reasoning as those required by quantitative analysis. Qualitative analysis is more difficult in a sense because much of the analytic process performed mathematically in quantitative analysis goes on in the head of the qualitative researcher. Analytic reasoning processes guide the organization, reduction and clustering of the findings and lead to the development of theoretical explanations. Strategies described by Miles and Huberman (1984) were used as the basis for discussion of qualitative analysis.

References

Abraham, I. & Schultz, S. II (1983). Univariate statistical models for meta-analysis. *Nursing Research*, <u>32</u>(5), 312–315.

Allison, P. D. (1984). *Event history analysis: regression for longitudinal event data*. Beverly Hills: Sage Publications.

Asher, H. B. (1983). *Causal modeling* (2nd ed.). Beverly Hills: Sage Publications.

Barnett, V. (1982). *Comparative statistical inference*. New York: John Wiley & Sons.

Box, G. E. P. & Jenkins, G. M. (1976). *Time-series analysis: forecasting and control* (rev. ed.). San Francisco: Holden-Day.

Brogan, D. R. (1981). Choosing an appropriate statistical test for a nursing research hypothesis or question. *Western Journal of Nursing Research*, 3(4), 337–368.

Burt, R. S. & Minor, M. J. (1983). *Applied network analysis: a methodological introduction*. Beverly Hills: Sage Publications.

Cohen, J. (1977). *Statistical power analysis for the behavioral sciences*. New York: Academic Press.

Cohen, J. & Cohen, P. (1983). *Applied multiple regression/correlation analysis for the behavioral sciences*. Hillsdale, New Jersey: Lawrence Erlbaum Associates, Publishers.

Cohen, M. Z. & Loomis, M. E. (1985). Linguistic analysis of questionnaire responses: methods of coping with work stress. *Western Journal of Nursing Research*, 7(3), 357–366.

Conover, W. J. (1971). *Practical nonparametric statistics*. New York: John Wiley & Sons.

Curlette, W. L. & Cannella, K. S. (1985). Going beyond the narrative summarization of research findings: the meta-analysis approach. *Research in Nursing & Health*, 8(3), 293–301.

Egger, M. J. & Miller, J. R. (1984). Testing for experimental effects in the pretest-posttest design. *Nursing Research*, 33(5), 306–312.

Feldman, M. J. & Ventura, M. R. (1984). Evaluating change using noninterval data. *Nursing Research*, 33(3), 182–184.

Ferketich, S. L. & Verran, J. A. (1984). Residual analysis for causal model assumptions. *Western Journal of Nursing Research*, 6(1), 41–76.

Glass, G. V., McGaw, B. & Smith, M. L. (1981). *Meta-analysis in social research*. Beverly Hills: Sage Publications.

Glass, G. V. & Stanley, J. C. (1970). *Statistical methods in education and psychology*. Englewood Cliffs, New Jersey: Prentice-Hall, Inc.

Good, I. J. (1983). *Good thinking: the foundations of probability and its applications*. Minneapolis: University of Minnesota Press.

Goodman, L. A. & Kruskal, W. H. (1954). Measures of association for cross classifications. *Journal of the American Statistical Association*, 49, 723–764.

Goodman, L. A. & Kruskal, W. H. (1959). Measures of association for cross classifications, II: further discussion and references. *Journal of the American Statistical Association*, 54, 123–163.

Goodman, L. A. & Kruskal, W. H. (1963). Measures of association for cross classifications, III: approximate sampling theory. *Journal of the American Statistical Association*, 58, 310–364.

Goodman, L. A. & Kruskal, W. H. (1972). Measures of association for cross classifications, IV: simplification of asymptotic variances. *Journal of the American Statistical Association*, 67(338), 415–21.

Goodwin, L. D. (1984). The use of power estimation in nursing research. *Nursing Research*, 33(2), 118–120.

Harris, R. J. (1975). *A primer of multivariate statistics*. New York: Academic Press.

Hinshaw, A. S. (1984). Theoretical model testing: full utilization of data. *Western Journal of Nursing Research*, 6(1), 5–10.

Hinshaw, A. S., Gerber, R. M., Atwood, J. R. & Allen, J. R. (1983). The use of predictive modeling to test nursing practice outcomes. *Nursing Research*, 32(1), 35–42.

Hinshaw, A. S. & Schepp, K. (1984). Problems in doing nursing research: how to recognize garbage when you see it! *Western Journal of Nursing Research*, 6(1), 126–130.

Holm, K. & Christman, N. J. (1985). Post hoc tests following analysis of variance. *Research in Nursing and Health*, 8(2), 207–210.

Hunter, J. E., Schmidt, F. L. & Jackson, G. B. (1982). *Meta-analysis: cumulating research findings across studies*. Beverly Hills: Sage Publications.

Jackson, D. J. & Borgatta, E. F. (1981). *Factor analysis and measurement in sociological research: a multi-dimensional perspective*. Beverly Hills: Sage Publications.

James, L. R., Mulaik, S. A. & Brett, J. M. (1982). *Causal analysis: assumptions, models, and data*. Beverly Hills: Sage Publications.

Kenny, D. A. (1979). *Correlation and causality*. New York: John Wiley & Sons.

Kerlinger, F. N. (1972). *Foundations of behavioral research* (2nd ed.). New York: Holt, Rinehart and Winston.

Kerlinger, F. N. & Pedhazur. (1973). *Multiple regression in behavioral research*. New York: Holt, Rinehart and Winston.

Kim, J. & Mueller, C. W. (1978a). *Introduction to factor analysis: what it is and how to do it*. Beverly Hills: Sage Publications.

Kim, J. & Mueller, C. W. (1978b). *Factor analysis: statistical methods and practical issues*. Beverly Hills: Sage Publications.

Knafl, K. A. (1985). How families manage a pediatric hospitalization. *Western Journal of Nursing Research*, 7(2), 151–176.

Knapp, R. G. (1985). *Basic statistics for nurses* (2nd ed.). New York: John Wiley & Sons.

Kviz, F. J. & Knafl, K. A. (1980). *Statistics for nurses: an introductory text*. Boston: Little, Brown and Company.

Leininger, M. M. (1985). *Qualitative research methods in nursing*. New York: Grune & Stratton, Inc.

Levine, M. S. (1977). *Canonical analysis and factor comparison*. Beverly Hills: Sage Publications.

Liebetrau, A. M. (1983). *Measures of association*. Beverly Hills: Sage Publications.

McArt, E. W. & McDougal, L. W. (1985). Secondary data analysis—a new approach to nursing research. *Image: The Journal of Nursing Scholarship*, 17(2), 54–57.

McCain, L. J. & McCleary, R. (1979). The statistical analysis of the simple interrupted time-series quasi-experiment. In T. D. Cook & D. T. Campbell (Eds.), *Quasi-experimentation: design & analysis issues for field settings*, pp. 233–293. Chicago: Rand McNally College Publishing Company.

McCleary, R. & Hay, R. A. Jr. (1980). *Applied time-series analysis for the social sciences*. Beverly Hills: Sage Publications.

McDowall, D., McCleary, R., Meidinger, E. E. & Hay, R. A. Jr. (1980). *Interrupted time-series analysis*. Beverly Hills: Sage Publications.

Marascuilo, L. A. (1971). *Statistical methods for behavioral science research*. New York: McGraw-Hill Book Company.

Marascuilo, L. A. & McSweeney, M. (1977). *Nonparametric and distribution-free methods for the social sciences*. Monterey, California: Brooks/Cole Publishing Company.

Metzger, B. L. & Schultz, S. II (1982). Time-series analysis: an alternative for nursing. *Nursing Research*, 31(6), 375–378.

Miles, M. B. & Huberman, A. M. (1984). *Qualitative data analysis: a sourcebook of new methods*. Beverly Hills: Sage Publications.

Munro, B. H., Visintainer, M. A. & Page, E. B. (1986). *Statistical methods for health care research*. Philadelphia: J. B. Lippincott Company.

Nunnally, J. C. (1978). *Psychometric theory* (2nd ed.). New York: McGraw-Hill Book Company.

O'Flynn, A. I. (1982). Meta-analysis. *Nursing Research*, 31(5), 314–316.

Ostrom, C. W. Jr. (1978). *Time-series analysis: regression techniques*. Beverly Hills: Sage Publications.

Popkess, S. A. (1981). Assessment scales for determining the cognitive—behavioral repertoire of the obese subject. *Western Journal of Nursing Research*, 3(2), 199–215.

Powers, M. J., Murphy, S. P. & Wooldridge, P. J. (1983). Validation of two experimental nursing approaches using content analysis. *Research in Nursing and Health*, 6(1), 3–9.

Reynolds, H. T. (1984). *Analysis of nominal data*. Beverly Hills: Sage Publications.

Roscoe, J. T. (1969). *Fundamental research statistics for the behavioral sciences*. New York: Holt, Rinehart and Winston.

Shelley, S. I. (1984). *Research methods in nursing and health*. Boston: Little, Brown and Company.

Siegel, S. (1956). *Nonparametric statistics for the behavioral sciences*. New York: McGraw-Hill Book Company.

Smith, M. C. & Naftel, D. C. (1984). Meta-analysis: a perspective for research synthesis. *Image: The Journal of Nursing Scholarship*, 16(1), 9–13.

Van Maanen, J. (1983). *Qualitative methodology*. Beverly Hills: Sage Publications.

Verran, J. A. & Ferketich, S. L. (1984). Residual analysis for statistical assumptions of regression equations. *Western Journal of Nursing Research*, 6(1), 27–40.

Volicer, B. J. (1984). *Multivariate statistics for nursing research*. New York: Grune & Stratton, Inc.

Waltz, C. & Bausell, R. B. (1981). *Nursing research: design, statistics and computer analysis*. Philadelphia: F. A. Davis Company.

Waltz, C. F., Strickland, O. L. & Lenz, E. R. (1984). *Measurement in nursing research*. Philadelphia: F. A. Davis Company.

18

Interpreting Research Outcomes

When data analysis is complete, there is a feeling that "the answers" are in and the study is finished. However, the results of statistical analysis, alone, are inadequate to complete the study. The researcher may "know" the results, but without careful intellectual examination, these results are of little use to others or to nursing's body of knowledge. To be useful, the evidence from data analysis must be carefully examined, organized and given meaning. This process is referred to as *interpretation*.

Data collection and data analysis are action-oriented activities. However, when the results of the study have been obtained, activity moves back to abstract thought processes. The creative use of introspection, reasoning and intuition again becomes the key focus of the process. In some ways, these last steps in the research process are the most difficult. They require a synthesis of the logic used to develop the research plan, strategies used in the data collection phase and the mathematical logic or insight and gestalt formation used in data analysis. Evaluation of the entire research process, the organization of meaning of the results and forecasting of the usefulness of the findings, all of which are involved in interpretation, require very high-level intellectual processes.

In general usage, the concept of interpretation is used in reference to language, although it can be thought of more broadly in terms of communication. Another concept, *translation*, is frequently thought of as being synonymous with interpretation. Abstract theoretical statements are sometimes referred to as being translated into more concrete meaning, as, for example, in the operationalization of a variable. Although the two words translate and interpret are similar, there are subtle differences in their meanings. *Translation* means to transform from one language to another or to use terms that can be more easily understood. *Interpreting* involves explaining the meaning of information. Interpretation seems to include translation and to go beyond it to explore and impart the meaning within the communication. Thus, in this segment of research, the researcher translates the results of analysis into findings and then interprets by attaching meaning to the findings.

Within the process of interpretation are several intellectual activities that can be isolated and explored. These activities include examining evidence, forming conclusions, considering implications, exploring the significance of the findings, generalizing the findings and suggesting further studies. Each of these activities is discussed in this chapter. The material presented in this chapter is usually included in the final chapter of theses and dissertations and in the final sections of research articles and presentations.

Examining Evidence

The first step in interpretation is a consideration of all the evidence available that supports or contradicts the validity of results related to the research subproblems. In order to consider the evidence, one must first determine what the evidence is and then gather it together. The impact of each bit of evidence on the validity of results must be carefully considered; then, the evidence as a whole must be synthesized for a final judgment.

EVIDENCE FROM THE RESEARCH PLAN

The initial evidence of the validity of the study results is derived from a reexamination of the research plan. The reexamination requires a reexploration of the logic of the methodology. This exploration will involve analyzing the logical links between the problem statement, framework, subproblems, variables, design, methods of observation, methods of measurement and types of analyses. These elements of the study logically link together and are consistent with the research problem. Remember the old adage, a chain is only as strong as its weakest link? This is also true of studies. Therefore, the study must be examined to identify its weakest links.

These weak links must then be examined in terms of the results of analysis. Could the results, or some of the results, be a consequence of a weak link in the methodology rather than a true test of the hypotheses? Can the research objectives or questions be answered from the methodology used? For example, could the results be a consequence of an inappropriate operationalization of the conceptual definition of the variable? Do the research subproblems clearly emerge from the framework? Can the results be related back to the framework? Are the analyses logically planned to test the subproblems?

If the types of analysis are inappropriate to examine the research subproblems, what do the results of analysis mean? If the design failed to control extraneous variables, could some of these extraneous variables explain the results rather than their being explained by the variable measures examined through statistical analysis? Was the population to be tested a logical group on which to test the hypotheses? Each link in the design must be carefully evaluated in this way to determine potential weaknesses. Every link is clearly related to the meaning given to the study results.

EVIDENCE FROM MEASUREMENT VALIDITY AND RELIABILITY

One of the assumptions often made in interpreting study results is that the study variables were adequately measured. Although reliability and validity of measurement strategies should be determined prior to their use in the study, the measures must be reexamined to determine the strength of evidence available from results. For example, did the scale that was used to measure anxiety truly reflect the anxiety experienced in the study population? The validity and reliability of measurement is critical to the validity of results. If the instruments used do not measure the variables as defined conceptually and operationally in the study, the results of analyzed measurement scores mean little. Unfortunately, many nursing studies use instruments with little or no reported validity. This means that we do not know whether the instrument measures what it is reported to measure. It is difficult to know what meaning to give to the reported findings of these studies; thus, they add little to the body of knowledge.

The reliability of the instrument is also critical. An instrument that does not give the same score or measure each time a specific level of the variable is tested is of no use. For example, a thermometer that measures temperature as 97.8 and 3 minutes later indicates a measure of 101 when no changes have occurred is not reliable. Likewise, an anxiety scale that shows a high level of anxiety and 15 minutes later, on retest, with no changes, measures anxiety as low is not reliable.

Reliability and validity of research instruments are often available in published reports of previous studies. In some cases, the author must be contacted to obtain validity and reliability data. If validity and reliability information is not available on study instruments, studies to determine reliability and validity should be conducted before the study is conducted. Validity and reliability of research instruments are discussed in Chapter 11.

Scores from measurement instruments without validity and reliability can be used for statistical analyses just as easily as those with validity and reliability. The mathematical formula or the computer cannot detect the difference. Results of the analyses give the same information regardless of the validity and reliability. The difference is in the meaning given to the results. This difference is detectable only by scientists, not by computers.

Studies specifically designed to improve the validity and reliability of instruments designed to measure nursing variables are needed in nursing research. These studies are referred to as methodology studies. Studies to improve the reliability and validity of existing instruments are appropriate for master's students conducting thesis research.

EVIDENCE FROM THE DATA COLLECTION PROCESS

Many activities that occur during the data collection process affect the meaning of results. Was the sample size sufficient? Did unforeseen events occur during the study that might have changed or had an impact on the data? Did strategies for acquiring a sample eliminate important groups whose data would have influenced results? Were measurement techniques consistent? If measurement techniques were not consistent, each measure may have a different meaning. If questionnaires are completed by one subject and another subject's spouse completes the questionnaires for him or her, it is difficult to justify analyzing the scores to obtain a single meaning. If an anxiety scale is given to one subject immediately before a painful procedure and to another subject upon awakening in the morning, the scores cannot be considered comparable. These types of differences are seldom reported and sometimes are not even recorded. To some extent, only the researcher knows how consistently the measurements were taken. The preciseness of the data collection process is dependent on the integrity of the researcher. Consistency in data collection techniques strengthens the meaning of data analysis results.

EVIDENCE FROM THE DATA ANALYSIS PROCESS

The process of data analysis is an important factor in evaluating the meaning of results. A number of pertinent questions can be asked that are related to the meaning of results. How many errors were made in entering the data into the computer? How many subjects have missing data that could affect statistical analyses? Were the analyses accurately calculated? Were statistical assumptions violated? Were the statistics used appropriate to the data?

Except in very simple studies, data analysis in quantitative studies is usually performed using a computer. Using prepared statistical analysis programs, multiple analyses can be performed on the data that are not well understood by the researcher. To the unknowing researcher, the computer spits out reams of paper with incomprehensible printed information and, in the end, gives a level of significance. The appropriateness of the data and the logic behind the program may remain unknown, but the level of significance may be considered by this researcher as absolute "proof" of an important finding.

The analysis process in qualitative studies is usually conducted manually and is, to some degree, subjective. The process itself, however, requires great skill and can seldom be learned by reading a journal article. Sorting, organizing and developing theoretical formulations from the data require great care and experience, yet the meaning derived from the analysis is dependent on the skill of conducting the analysis. The analysis and interpretation of qualitative data are discussed in Chapter 17.

In gathering evidence for the implications of the study results, it is critical to reexamine the data analysis process. The researcher must examine the sufficiency of personal knowledge of the statistics and proficiency in the analyses used. Data should be reexamined for accuracy and completeness. Mathematical operations performed manually should be rechecked for accuracy. Computer printouts should be reexamined for meaningful information that may have been overlooked. Tables of data should be rechecked for accuracy and clarity. The researcher should be as confident as possible in the results as they are reported.

EVIDENCE FROM DATA ANALYSIS RESULTS

The outcomes of data analysis are the most direct evidence available on the results related to the research subproblems. The validity of these results is dependent on the evidence previously discussed. In exploratory, descriptive and correlational studies, the validity of the results is dependent on how accurately the research process has explained the variables that are being examined in the samples. The value of evidence in any study is dependent on the amount of variance in the phenomenon explained within the study, a factor that is often not considered in interpreting the results. In quasi-experimental and experimental studies, in which hypothesized differences in groups are being examined, the differences or lack of differences do not indicate the amount of variance explained. Magnitude testing (discussed in Chapter 17) is required for this purpose. Interpretation of results from quasi-experimental and experimental studies is traditionally based on decision theory, with five possible results: (1) significant results that are in keeping with those predicted by the researcher, (2) nonsignificant results, (3) significant results that are opposite to those predicted by the researcher, (4) mixed results and (5) unexpected results.

Significant and Predicted Results

Results that are in keeping with those predicted by the researcher are the easiest to explain and, unless there are weak links that belie them, validate the proposed logical links between the elements of the study. These results support the logical links developed by the researcher between the framework, subproblems, variables and measurement tools. This is very satisfying to the researcher. However, in this situation, the researcher must consider alternate explanations for the positive findings. What other elements could possibly have led to the significant results?

Nonsignificant Results

Nonsignificant or inconclusive results are the most difficult to explain. These results are often referred to as negative results. The negative results could be a true reflection of reality. In this case, the reasoning of the researcher or the theory used by the researcher to develop the hypothesis is in error. If so, the negative findings are an important addition to the body of knowledge.

The results could also be due to inappropriate methodology, a deviant sample, a small sample, problems with internal validity, inadequate measurement, use of weak statistical measures or faulty analysis. This result may be a Type II error, which may mean that in reality the findings are significant but, because of weaknesses in the methodology, the significance was not detected. Unless these weak links are detected, the reported results could lead to faulty information in the body of knowledge. It is easier for the researcher to blame faulty methodology for nonsignificant findings than to admit to failures in theoretical or logical reasoning. Therefore, the tendency is to be very critical of methodology if findings are negative. If faulty methodology is blamed, the researcher should explain exactly how the breakdown in methodology led to the negative results. Negative results, in any case, do *not* mean that there are no relationships among the variables; they indicate that the study failed to find any. Nonsignificant results lead to a lack of evidence of either the truth *or* falsity of the hypothesis.

Significant and Not Predicted Results

Significant results opposite to those predicted can be embarrassing to report because of the reflection on the logic of the researcher and the logic of the theory being tested. However, if the results are valid, they are an important addition to the body of knowledge. An example would be a study in which social support and ego strength were proposed to be positively related. If the study showed that high social support was related to low ego strength, the result would be opposite to that predicted. Results such as this, when verified by other studies, indicate that we are headed in the wrong direction theoretically. Since these types of studies direct nursing practice, it is important to know the truth. In some of these cases, the researcher believes so strongly in the theory that the results are not believed. The researcher remains convinced that there was a problem in the methodology. Sometimes this belief remains entrenched in the minds of scientists for a number of years.

Mixed Results

Mixed results are probably the most common outcome of studies. In this case, one variable may uphold predicted characteristics while another does not; or, two dependent measures of the same variable may show opposite results. These differences may be due to methodology problems, such as differing reliability or sensitivity of two methods of measuring variables. The mixed results may also indicate the need to modify existing theory.

Unexpected Results

Unexpected results are usually relationships found between variables that were not hypothesized and not predicted from the framework being used. Most researchers examine as many elements of data as possible in addition to those directed by the subproblems. These findings can be very useful in theory development or modification of existing theory and in the development of later studies. In addition, serendipitous results are important as evidence in developing the implications of the study. However, serendipitous results must be dealt with carefully in considering meaning because the study was not designed to examine these results (see Chapter 16).

EVIDENCE FROM PREVIOUS STUDIES

The results of the present study should always be examined in light of previous findings. It is important to know whether results are consistent with past research. Consistency in findings across studies is extremely important in theory development and scientific progress. Therefore, any inconsistencies should be explored to determine reasons for the differences.

Findings

Results in a study are translated and interpreted; then they become findings. Findings are a consequence of evaluating evidence. Although much of the process of developing findings from results occurs in the mind of the researcher, evidence of the thinking can be found in published research reports. Walsh's (1985) study "Health beliefs and practices of runners versus nonrunners" presents the following hypotheses, results and findings.

Hypothesis 1 □ There is a difference between runners and nonrunners in the relative value placed on personal health. (p. 354)

Results □ The first hypothesis...was tested using the Mann-Whitney U, with alpha set at .05, and was accepted, $p < .019$. The value of U was found to be 1876.5; of U', 4990.5. (p. 354)

Findings □ Greater value was placed on personal health by the runners than by the nonrunners. (p. 354)

Hypothesis 2 □ There are differences in the number of specific health-related behaviors undertaken by runners and nonrunners. (p. 354)

Results □ It (second hypothesis) was tested with the two-sample t test for independent groups, with alpha set as .05, and was accepted, $t < .001$. (p. 354)

Findings □ ...the major differences between groups (were) nutrition, exercise, and medical awareness and self-care. (pp. 354–355)

Forming Conclusions

Conclusions are derived from the findings and are a synthesis of findings. Forming these conclusions requires a combination of logical reasoning, creative formation of a meaningful whole from pieces of information obtained through data analysis and findings from previous studies, receptivity to subtle clues in the data and utilization of an open context in considering alternative explanations of the data.

In forming conclusions, it is important to remember that research never proves anything; rather, research offers support for a position. Proof is a logical part of deductive reasoning but not of the research process. Because of this, formulation of causal statements is risky. For example, the causal statement that A *causes* B (absolutely, in all situations) cannot be scientifically proved. It is more credible to state conclusions in the form of conditional probabilities that are qualified. For example, one could say that, in the study described, if A occurred, then B occurred under conditions x, y and z (Kerlinger, 1973). If the following study had been conducted (which it has not), one could say that if preoperative teaching were given, postoperative anxiety was lowered as long as pain was controlled, complications did not occur and family contacts were high.

Walsh (1985) concluded that "Runners placed a higher value on health and performed more health-related behaviors than did nonrunners" (p. 355). The findings are related to findings from previous research and theoretical literature. "The findings from this investigation, however, are congruent with those of Blair et al. (1981), in that runners exert tighter control over the types of nutrients they consume than do nonrunners" (p. 355). Congruence of findings with theoretical literature was also examined. "The findings regarding running while ill or in pain, incidence of injuries, and negative feelings when unable to run are in keeping with descriptions of compulsion and addiction to running (Hartung & Farge, 1981; Morgan, 1979)" (p. 355). The methodology of the study was examined in drawing conclusions from the findings.

> It might have been expected that these runners would represent the extreme ends of the scales in terms of mileage and frequency of runs, by virtue of their membership in a running club and presumed greater commitment to the sport. This was not found to be the case...There was no stipulation that the runners be limited to running as their sole form of exercise. Sampling frame alterations and more stringent controls might have produced different results. (p. 355)

In spite of the researcher's higher motives to be objective, subjective judgments and biases will creep into the conclusions. The researcher must remain on the alert for these and keep them under control. Students sometimes want to have positive findings so much that they will misinterpret statistical results on computer printouts to be significant when they are clearly nonsignificant.

One of the risks in developing conclusions in research is "going beyond the data." This means forming conclusions that are not warranted by the data. The most common example is a study that examines relationships between A and B by correlational analysis and then concludes that A causes B. Going beyond the data is due to faulty logic and occurs more frequently in published studies than one would like to believe. Once a study is published, it is there forever for anyone and everyone to see. Therefore, the researcher should check the validity of logical arguments related to conclusions before the findings are revealed publicly.

Considering Implications

Implications are the meanings of conclusions for the body of knowledge, for theory and for practice. Implications are based on the conclusions and are more specific than conclusions. They provide specific suggestions for implementing the findings. The researcher must consider the areas of nursing for which the study findings would be useful. For example, suggestions could be made about how nursing practice should be modified. If a study indicated that a specific solution was effective in decreasing stomatitis, the implications would state that the findings had implications for caring for patients with stomatitis. It would *not* be sufficient to state that the study had implications for nurses practicing in oncology.

Walsh's (1985) study suggested the following implications:

A runner may require assistance in formulating and adhering to a reasonable training program, in light of the runners' tendency to run despite pain and the addictive nature of running for some individuals. The health practitioner, therefore, should be aware of the signs of compulsion and obsession within this population. Further, nurses should be familiar with abnormal signs and symptoms relating to early stages of injury.

The runner also needs to know that running while ill creates more hazards than benefits. Similarly, the nurse should teach the importance of the cool-down period following running, particularly to an individual with coronary risk factors. Finally, in dealing with negative feelings, the nurse should assess runners and determine who might need counseling by a mental health professional experienced in sports medicine and make the referral. (p. 355)

Exploring the Significance of Findings

There are two ways in which the word significance is used in research. Statistical significance is related to the results of the study. To be important, the results of quantitative studies that use statistical analysis must be statistically significant. *Statistical significance* means that the results were not due to chance. However, statistically significant results are not necessarily important in clinical practice. The results can indicate a real difference that is not necessarily an important difference clinically. For example, Yonkman (1982, p. 356), in reporting results from her study of the effect of cool or heated aerosol on oral temperature, reported that "The statistical tests yielded small values which implied that differences were statistically significant. It is not clear that these differences in temperature are clinically significant."

The *significance of a study* is associated with its importance to the body of knowledge. Significance is not a dichotomous characteristic, because studies contribute in varying degrees to the body of knowledge. Significance may be associated with the amount of variance explained, control in the study design to eliminate unexplained variance or detection of statistically significant differences. To the extent possible at the time that the study is reported, the researcher is expected to clarify the significance. The areas of significance may be more obvious to the researcher who has been immersed in the study than to the reader or listener. Therefore, the researcher cannot assume obvious significance; he or she must point it out.

A few studies, referred to as landmark studies, become important referent points in the discipline (Johnson, 1972; Lindeman & Van Aernam, 1971; Passos & Brand, 1966; Williams, 1972). The true importance of a particular study may not become apparent for years after publication. However, there are some characteristics associated with the significance of studies. Significant studies make an important difference in peoples' lives. It is possible to generalize the findings far beyond the study sample so that the findings have the potential of affecting large numbers of people. The implications of significant studies go beyond concrete facts to abstractions and lead to the generation of theory or revisions in existing theory. A very significant study has implications for one or more disciplines in addition to nursing. The study is accepted by others in the discipline and is frequently referenced in the literature. Over a period of time, the significance of a study is measured by the number of studies it generates.

Generalizing the Findings

One of the key differences between research and evaluation is the ability to generalize. Findings of studies that have no capacity to be generalized are of little use to the body of scientific knowledge. Generalization extends the implications of the findings from the sample studied to a larger population. The findings may be extended from the situation studied to a larger situation. For example, if the study was conducted on diabetic patients, it may be possible to generalize the findings to persons with other illnesses or to well individuals. Walsh's (1985, p. 355) study of runners had the following statement of generalization: "This group of runners was typical of runners across America in terms of variables for which verifiable normative data were available."

How far can generalizations be made? This is a debatable question. From a very narrow perspective, one cannot really generalize from the sample on which the study was done. Any other sample is likely to be different in some way. The conservative position, represented by Kerlinger (1973), recommends caution in considering the extent of generalization. Generalization is considered particularly risky by conservatives if the sample was not randomly selected. According to Kerlinger (1973, p. 325), "Unless special precautions are taken and special efforts made, the results of research are frequently not representative, and hence not generalizable" (p. 325).

Generalizations based on accumulated evidence from many studies are called *empirical generalizations*. These generalizations are important for the verification of theoretical statements or the development of new theory. Empirical generalizations are the base of a science and contribute to scientific conceptualization. Nursing has few empirical generalizations at this time.

Suggesting Further Studies

The completing of a study and the examination of implications should culminate in the consideration of future studies that logically emerge from the present study and from previous studies in the same area of interest. Suggested studies or recommendations for further study may include replications or repeating the design with a different or larger sample. In every study, the researcher gains knowledge and experience that can be used to design a "better study next time." This section of the study allows that thinking to become more specific and stimulates the researcher to more clearly define how to make the study "better." From a logic or theoretical point of view, the findings should lead directly to more hypotheses to further test the framework in use. The suggestions made in this section should not be just for other researchers but should also move the researcher in the direction of planning the next research endeavor.

Kurzuk-Howard, Simpson, and Palmieri (1985), in a comparative study of decubitus ulcer care, built their study on Gerber and Van Ort's (1979) study and made recommendations for further study.

> Because of the encouraging results with a relatively small number of subjects, studies on the safety and effectiveness of moist wound healing should be continued. The results of this study indicate that it should be repeated using a larger sample. Questions to be addressed are: (1) Is the rate of healing when using Op-Site superior to other treatments that provide a moist environment? (2) How effective is Op-Site when used in treating patients in other settings, that is, nursing homes and the community? A more precise means of measuring the rate of healing of ulcers is also needed. (p. 74)

Summary

To be useful, the evidence from data analysis must be carefully examined, organized and given meaning. This process is referred to as *interpretation*. Data collection and data analysis are action-oriented activities. However, when the results of the study have been obtained, activity moves back to abstract thought processes. Within the process of interpretation are several intellectual activities that can be isolated and explored. These activities include examining evidence, forming conclusions, considering implications, exploring the significance of the findings, generalizing the findings and suggesting further studies.

The first step in interpretation is a consideration of all the evidence available that supports or contradicts the validity of results related to the research subproblems. The evidence is obtained from a variety of sources, including the research plan, measurement validity and reliability, data collection process, data analysis process, data analysis results and previous studies. Evidence of the validity of the results is derived from a reexamination of the research plan. The reliability and validity of measurement strategies should be determined prior to their use in a study, and these measures must be reexamined to determine the strength of evidence available from results. Many activities can occur during the data collection process that affect the meaning of results, such as insufficient sample size, inappropriate sampling strategies or unforeseen events that occur during data collection. The evidence from data analysis is dependent on the researcher's knowledge of statistics and the proficiency of the analysis methods used.

The outcomes of data analysis are the most direct evidence available on the results related to the research subproblems. The validity of these results is dependent on the evidence previously discussed. There are five possible results: (1) significant results that are in keeping with those predicted by the researcher, (2) nonsignificant results, (3) significant results that are opposite to those predicted by the researcher, (4) mixed results and (5) unexpected results. The results of a study should always be examined in light of previous findings.

The results of a study are translated and interpreted and then become findings. *Findings* are a consequence of evaluating evidence. *Conclusions* are derived from the findings and are a synthesis of findings. Forming conclusions requires a combination of logical reasoning, creative formation of a meaningful whole from pieces of information obtained through data analysis and findings from previous studies, receptivity to subtle clues in the data and utilization of an open context in considering alternative explanations of the data.

Implications are the meanings of conclusions for the body of knowledge, for theory and for practice. The *significance of a study* is associated with its importance to the body of knowledge. Significance is not a dichotomous characteristic, because studies contribute in varying degrees to the body of knowledge. *Generalization* extends the implications of the findings from the sample studied to a larger population. The completing of a study and the examination of implications should culminate in the consideration of future studies that logically emerge from the present study and from previous studies in the same area of interest. Suggested studies or recommendations for further study may include replications or repeating the design with a different or larger sample.

References

Gerber, R. M. & Van Ort, S. R. (1979). Topical application of insulin in decubitus ulcers. *Nursing Research*, 28(1), 16–19.

Johnson, J. E. (1972). Effects of structuring patients' expectations on their reactions to threatening events. *Nursing Research*, 21(6), 499–503.

Kerlinger, F. N. (1973). *Foundations of behavioral research* (2nd ed.). New York: Holt, Rinehart and Winston.

Kurzuk-Howard, G., Simpson, L. & Palmieri, A. (1985). Decubitus ulcer care: a comparative study. *Western Journal of Nursing Research*, 7(1), 58–79.

Lindeman, C. A. & Van Aernam, B. (1971). Nursing intervention with the presurgical patient— the effects of structured and unstructured preoperative teaching. *Nursing Research*, 20(4), 319–332.

Neale, J. M. & Liebert, R. M. (1980). *Science and behavior: an introduction to methods of research* (2nd ed.). Englewood Cliffs, New Jersey: Prentice-Hall, Inc.

Passos, J. Y. & Brand, L. M. (1966). Effects of agents used for oral hygiene. *Nursing Research*, 15(3), 196–202.

Walsh, V. R. (1985). Health beliefs and practices of runners versus nonrunners. *Nursing Research*, 34(6), 353–356.

Williams, A. (1972). A study of factors contributing to skin breakdown. *Nursing Research*, 21(3), 238–243.

Yonkman, C. A. (1982). Cool and heated aerosol and the measurement of oral temperature. *Nursing Research*, 31(6), 354–357.

19

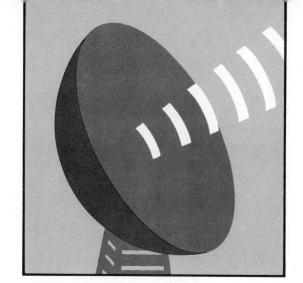

Communicating Research Findings

Imagine a nurse researcher conducting a study in which a unique phenomenon has been described or a link has been detected that was previously unrecognized. Knowing this information might make a difference in nursing practice. However, the nurse feels unskilled in presenting information and overwhelmed by the idea of publishing. She places the study in a bottom drawer with an intent to communicate the findings "some day." What are the consequences of the decision to not communicate findings for nursing and for the individual nurse? This decision has been made by too many nurses, and many studies lay unpublished at the bottom of someone's drawer.

Communication of findings is the final step of the research process and is essential for the utilization of findings in practice. When research findings are communicated, nurses have the opportunity to critique the studies. The shared research findings stimulate others to replicate studies and develop additional research problems. Many research activities are conducted alone, and communicating findings is a time for researchers to interact with others and share their knowledge. Through communication of findings, researchers are rewarded for their work by receiving personal recognition, professional advancement and other psychological and financial compensations. These rewards are essential to the continuation of research.

Many researchers fail to plan for this step during the development of their research project. A plan for communicating findings should be developed during the proposal and should include the designation of time and money necessary to share the findings. Some researchers communicate their findings, but only to very limited audiences of other nurse researchers and scholars. Practicing nurses, other health professionals and health care consumers are often not aware of research findings because they do not attend nursing research conferences or read nursing research journals (Butts, 1982). Nurses must broaden their options for communicating findings to reach larger audiences of greater variety. This is a difficult task for which some options are discussed in this chapter.

Communicating research findings involves the development of a research report that is disseminated effectively and efficiently to a selected audience (King, Barnard & Hoehn, 1981). The research report includes an introduction and a description of the research methods and results and concludes with a discussion of the findings. A variety of oral and visual presentations and written reports can be developed to disseminate research findings. Research findings should be shared with audiences of nurse researchers, educators and practitioners; other health professionals; and health care consumers. In this chapter, the content of a research report is described, the audiences for communication of nursing research findings are identified and the processes for presenting and publishing research findings are given in detail.

Content of the Research Report

Both quantitative and qualitative research reports include four basic sections: (1) introduction, (2) methods, (3) results and (4) discussion. However, the depth of the content and the emphasis placed on certain sections of the report vary with the audience and the mechanism for disseminating the report. For example, theses and dissertations are research reports that are usually developed in depth to demonstrate the student's understanding of the research process to faculty members. Research articles for publication are concisely written to efficiently and effectively communicate the findings of a study to nurses and health professionals.

The content of a research report should be well organized and clearly and concisely written. A clear, concise report is legible. It has no punctuation, spelling or sentence structure errors; confusing words; cliches; jargon; or wordiness (Kolin & Kolin, 1980). A well-organized report includes the logical development of ideas and leads to a scholarly conclusion. Therefore, the introduction section should provide a basis for the development of the methods section, and both these sections should serve as a basis for the presentation of the results. The introduction, methods and results sections should provide a background for the discussion of the findings, identification of the implications for nursing and development of recommendations for further research.

INTRODUCTION

The introduction of a research report briefly identifies which problem was studied and the rationale for studying that problem. The introduction includes a problem statement, significance of the problem, study purpose, a review of relevant literature, frame of reference, assumptions and research subproblems. Depending on the type of research report, the review of literature and theoretical framework might be separate sections or even separate chapters.

The review of literature should document the current knowledge of the problem investigated. The sources included in the literature review are those that were used to develop the study and those that served as a basis for comparison of the study findings. A review of literature can be two or three paragraphs or several pages in length. In journal articles, the review of literature is very concise and usually includes between three and eight sources. Theses and dissertations frequently include an extensive literature review to document the student's knowledge of the research problem.

The research report should clearly indicate the frame of reference for the study. A model can be developed to clarify the logic within the framework. The major concepts in the framework are conceptually defined. If a particular proposition is being tested, that proposition should be clearly stated. The connection between the frame of reference and the research subproblems should be evident in the research report. The subproblems (objectives, research questions or hypotheses) must be clearly stated. Operational definitions must be provided for the variables identified in the research problem and subproblems. The assumptions relevant to the study should also be identified.

METHODS

The methods section of a research report describes in detail how the study was conducted. This section should provide sufficient information for nurses to critique and/or replicate the study procedures. Included in the methods section is the design, setting, sample, methodological limitations and the data collection process used in the study. If the research project included a pilot study, the planning, implementation and results obtained from the pilot study should be presented briefly. In addition, the changes made in the research project based on the pilot study should be described.

Design

The specific type of quantitative or qualitative study conducted should be identified in the research report. In reporting qualitative research, the researcher should describe the flexible, dynamic implementation of the research project (see Chapter 4). In describing a quantitative study, the report should specify the structural framework within which the study was implemented (see Chapter 10). A complex study design might be presented using a table or figure. Osguthorpe, Roper and Saunders (1983, p. 208) presented their research design in a table (Table 19–1). The purpose of this quasi-experimental study was to determine the most effective method for teaching psychiatric patients about their medication. There were three treatment groups (A, B and C) and one control group (D). The structural framework for this study was a pretest-post-test control group design.

Sample and Setting

The research report should include the criteria for selecting the sample and the sample size. If the subjects were divided into groups (experimental and control groups), the method for assigning subjects to groups and the number of subjects in each group should be identified. Many journal editors now require a statement about how the subjects' anonymity and confidentiality were protected. The setting of the study should be described in one or two sentences, and agencies should not be identified by name unless agency permission has been obtained. For example, the setting might be described as a large, urban hospital in the Southwest. The study was conducted on four general medical-surgical units in this hospital.

Data Collection Process

The description of the data collection process in the research report should detail who collected the data, what data collection tools were used, and how these tools were used. In describing who collected the data, the report should indicate the experience of the data collector and any training provided for the data collection process. If more than one person collected data, the precautions taken to ensure consistency in the data collection process should be described.

The details about data collection tools and the use of these tools in the data collection process are critical for nurses to critique and replicate a study. The report should describe what information is collected by each tool, the frequency with which the tool has been used in previous research and any reliability and validity information previously published on the tool. In addition, the report should include the reliability of the tool for the study conducted and should describe any further development of the validity that was done.

In reports on qualitative research, a variety of data collection "tools" might be described, such as observation guides, open-ended interviews, direct participation, documents, open frames, guides, life histories, audiovisual media (photographs, videotapes), biographies and diaries (Leininger, 1985). The

Table 19–1
Quasi-Experimental Design

Study Group	Observation	Intervention	Observation
A	Pretest	Drug Information Sheet	Post-test
B	Pretest	Drug Information Sheet Videotaped Nurse Explanation	Post-test
C	Pretest	Videotaped Nurse Explanation	Post-test
D	Pretest	None	Post-test

(From Osguthorpe, N., Roper, J. & Saunders, J.: The effect of teaching on medication knowledge. *Western Journal of Nursing Research, 5*, 205, 1983; with permission.)

flexible, dynamic way in which a qualitative researcher collects data frequently requires an extensive, complex description. For example, if the data collection involved participant-observation, the number and length of the observation and participation periods should be described as well as the structure and focus of each of these periods. In addition, the tools for recording the information gained from these periods of observation and participation should be presented.

Certain types of quantitative studies involve the implementation of a treatment. In reporting these types of studies, the researcher should describe the research treatment, procedures for administering these treatments and the measurement devices used to determine the effects of these treatments.

Methodological Limitations

The methodological limitations that were identified in the proposal and during the conduct of the study should be included in the research report. For example, a study might have limitations related to sample size or sample characteristics (such as age, race or socioeconomic status). There might be limitations related to design or instrumentation of a study.

RESULTS

The results section describes the data analyses that were performed and presents the results generated from these analyses. In qualitative research, the data analysis methods (content, symbolic, structural, interactional, philosophical, ethnographic, phenomenological, semantic, historical, inferential, grounded theory, perceptual and reflexive) are performed during and after the data collection process (Leininger, 1985). Data analysis methods are discussed in Chapter 17. The results section should identify which analysis procedures were performed and when.

In quantitative research, data analyses are performed when all the data have been collected and involve various statistical methods. In the research report, the data analyses performed and the computer programs used to perform these analyses are identified. The level of significance selected should be clearly stated. If there are subproblems in the study, the data analyses that were conducted to generate results for each subproblem should be identified.

Presentation of Results

The results section of the research report should include a description of the characteristics (*e.g.*, age, race, gender) of the sample and a presentation of the results generated to accomplish the research purpose. If the study includes subproblems, they provide an excellent organization for presenting the results. A good approach is to list a subproblem and describe the data analyses and results related to it, then list another subproblem and describe its analyses and results. This approach clarifies the purpose for each analysis technique and ensures that each subproblem has been addressed.

The results from quantitative and qualitative research can be presented in narrative format and/or organized into illustrations and tables. The method used to present the results depends on the end product of data analysis and the researcher's preference. In reporting the results of some studies, a narrative description provides the clearest method of communication. For example, in qualitative research, the results include gestalts, patterns and theories that are developed to describe life experiences, which are frequently expressed in narrative format.

Tables and illustrations are used to concisely and clearly present a large amount of detailed information. They are also useful in demonstrating relationships and reducing the amount of discussion needed in the text of the report (Mirin, 1981). In many research reports, some findings are presented in narrative format, and others are presented in tables or illustrations, whichever is thought to best express the information to the reader. Tables and illustrations can be revealing and convincing if they are appropriate for the data collected and the purpose of the study and are well constructed. When illustrations and tables are developed for a report, certain precautions should be taken:

1. Use tables and illustrations to explain or support only the major points of the report. Using too many tables and illustrations can overwhelm the rest of the report, but a few tables and illustrations receive attention and are convincing in conveying the main findings. In addition, statistically nonsignificant findings are usually not presented in tables.

2. Keep the tables and illustrations simple; do not try to convey too much information in a single table. If a table or illustration is cluttered, it will not clearly convey the main findings. Two simple tables are better than one complex one.

3. Design the table or illustration to focus on the meaning you are trying to convey. The title of the table and the labels on the table should clearly indicate what findings are being presented. In fact, the reader should be able to completely understand the table or illustration without returning to the body of the text.

4. Tie the table or illustration into the written text by referring to it and by placing it as close as possible to the section of the text where you discuss it (Shurter, Williamson & Broehl, 1965).

The discussion of a table or illustration in the written portion of the report should reinforce the major point for which the table or illustration was developed. In some reports, the researcher describes the variable that is presented in the table or illustration and/or indicates the variation that occurs within each variable. If the table or illustration includes more than one variable, the researcher should discuss the relationships (significant and nonsignificant) noted among the variables. In addition, the discussion should indicate any unusual patterns that appear in the data (Abdellah & Levine, 1979).

Illustrations □ Illustrations provide the reader with a picture of the results. Some common illustrations used in research reports include diagrams and graphs. Illustrations are identified as figures, are numbered sequentially and are discussed in the text of the research report. Many researchers use computers to generate a variety of black and white and colored illustrations.

The pie diagram is used to show the component parts that make up a whole. The wedge-shaped pieces can be labeled and can include the percentage of the whole represented. If the wedges in the diagram are very small, colors, shading or patterns can be used to represent variables or sample groups. A key is then included with the illustration to indicate what the colors, shading or patterns represent. Clinton (1982, p. 288) used a pie diagram (Fig. 19–1) to present the findings generated to address the research questions: "How strongly do you feel a part of an ethnic group? Would you say you identify very strongly, somewhat strongly, or not strongly?" The wedges of this pie diagram are labeled with the subjects' responses and the percentage of the sample and specific number of subjects (N) making that response.

There are a variety of graphs that can be developed to present results, but those commonly used in published nursing reports include bar graphs and line graphs. The bar graphs can have horizontal or vertical bars; these bars represent the size or amount of the group or variable studied. The bar graph is also a means of comparing one item with another. In Clinton's (1982, p. 284) study of ethnicity, the subjects were asked "What is your ethnic origin?" The findings to this question are presented in Figure 19–2. The discussion of this bar graph in the text would identify the countries included in each region and focus on any unusual patterns in the data, such as regions with unexpectedly large or small numbers of subjects.

In bar graphs, the bars can be grouped together to compare different

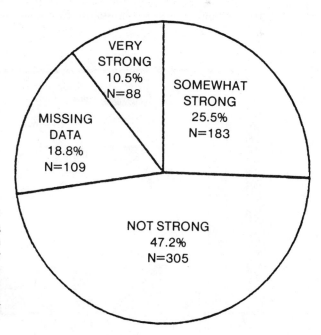

FIGURE 19–1. Strength of ethnic ties (N=845). (From Clinton, J.: Ethnicity: The development of an empirical construct for cross-cultural health research. *Western Journal of Nursing Research*, 4(3), 281, 1982. Copyright 1982 by Western Journal of Nursing Research. Reprinted by permission of Sage Publications, Inc.)

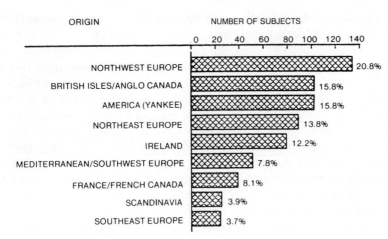

FIGURE 19–2. Claimed region of ethnic origin (N=645). (From Clinton, J.: Ethnicity: The development of an empirical construct for cross-cultural health research. *Western Journal of Nursing Research*, 4(3), 281, 1982. Copyright 1982 by Western Journal of Nursing Research. Reprinted by permission of Sage Publications, Inc.)

but related sets of data. Kalisch and Kalisch (1981, p. 137) examined the statements made in the newspapers about nurses in 1978. They developed a bar graph (Fig. 19–3) that includes the positive, negative, mixed and neutral statements of three groups (nurses, patients and others). A discussion of this graph might focus on the relationships demonstrated. For example, nurse made the most positive statements about nurses when compared with statements made by patients and others.

Another form of graph that is frequently used in research reports is the line graph. The line graph is developed by joining a series of points with a line and shows how a quantity of something varied from one time to the next. In

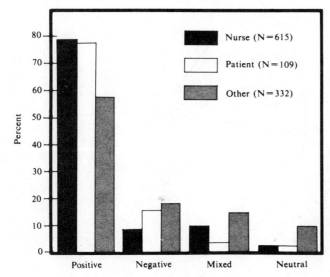

FIGURE 19–3. Statements about nurses made by nurses, patients, and others in 1978 newspaper articles. (Reprinted with permission from Kalisch, B.J., and Kalisch, P.A.: Communicating clinical nursing issues through the newspaper. *Nursing Research*, 30(3), 137, May/June 1981. Copyright 1981 by American Journal of Nursing Company.)

this type of graph, the horizontal scale is used to measure time and the vertical scale is used to measure number and quantity (Shurter, Williamson & Broehl, 1965).

Figure 19–4 is a line graph developed by Swain and Steckel (1981, p. 219) to demonstrate the effect of three treatments (routine clinical care, health education and contingency contracting) upon patients' blood pressure. The horizontal scale is labeled with four visits or the four different times at which the blood pressure was taken. The vertical scale represents the quantity of the diastolic blood pressure. This graph presents the fluctuation of patients' blood pressures over four visits for three treatment groups. The discussion of this graph would include a comparison of the variance in blood pressure readings for the three treatment groups and identify the treatment group that had a controlled blood pressure.

Development of Tables ☐ Tables are used more frequently in research reports than are illustrations, and they can be developed to present results from numerous statistical analyses. In tables, the results are presented in columns and rows for easy review by the reader. The example tables included in this chapter present characteristics of a sample, measures of central tendency, standard deviations (SDs), t values, F values, correlations and chi-square values.

Lowery and Jacobsen (1985, p. 83) used a table to present the characteristics of their sample of chronically ill subjects, who had arthritis, diabetes or hypertension (Table 19–2). The discussion of this table might focus on specific sample characteristics that the researcher believed were unusually high

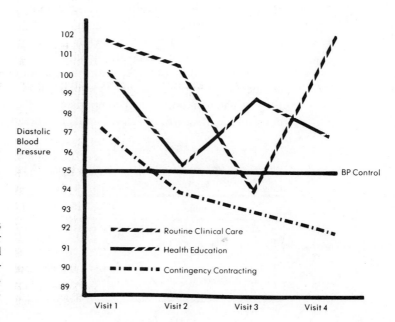

FIGURE 19–4. Blood pressures by treatment group across four visits. (From Swain, M.A., and Steckel, S.B.: Influencing adherence among hypertensives. *Research in Nursing & Health,* 4:213, 1981; with permission.)

TABLE 19–2
Characteristics of Sample by Chronic Disease (N = 296)

	Chronic Disease		
Variables	**Arthritis** **(n = 77)**	**Diabetes** **(n = 113)**	**Hypertension** **(n = 106)**
Age (mean)	58.5 yr	57.0 yr	55.3 yr
Length of illness (mean)	14.6 yr	12.7 yr	12.6 yr
Number in household (mean)	2.5	2.8	3.0
*Sex			
Female	87%	78%	58%
Marital status			
Married	36%	46%	51%
Divorced/separated/widowed	55%	46%	37%
Never married	9%	8%	12%
Ethnic group			
Black (not Hispanic)	81%	81%	78%
White	18%	17%	20%
Other	1%	2%	2%
Education			
Less than high school	57%	58%	43%
Retired	36%	35%	30%
*Employed	23%	29%	49%
*Clinic patients	95%	78%	32%
*Other major illness	55%	57%	33%

*p < 0.05
(From Lowery, B. J. & Jacobsen, B. S.: Attributional analysis of chronic illness outcomes. *Nursing Research, 34*:82, 1985; with permission.)

or low. In addition, the researcher would probably discuss the characteristics of the sample that differed significantly among the three groups of subjects.

Tables can be used to present results from a frequency analysis, which includes measures of central tendency, standard deviations and ranges. Andrews and Andrews (1983) tabled the findings that were generated from a frequency analysis of the data obtained from the measurement of six descriptive characteristics of a sample of pregnant women (Table 19–3). The discussion of Table 19–3 might include a brief comparison of the unusual differences that were noted in the measures of central tendency (mean, median and mode) for certain

TABLE 19–3
Measures of Central Tendency, Standard Deviations, and Range of Descriptive Data (N = 100)

Variable	**Mean**	**SD**	**Median**	**Mode**	**Range**
Age (Yr)	26.33	4.12	25.93	22	19–38
Estimated fetal weight (lb.)	6.95	.83	7.00	7.5	4.5–9
Subject's weight (lb.)	156.57	20.07	154.70	134	114–216
Height (in.)	62.69	9.84	64.02	63	59–71.5
Fundal height (cm)	37.03	1.83	37.26	38	32–40
Torso (cm)	44.40	7.87	45.50	48	33–56

(From Andrews, C. M. & Andrews, E. C.: Nursing, maternal postures, and fetal position. *Nursing Research, 32*:336, 1983; with permission.)

characteristics. The research report might also include a discussion of any unexpected ranges or standard deviations.

Tables provide a concise presentation of results obtained from t tests and analysis of variance (ANOVA). Tables of t-test results frequently provide the means ($\overline{X}$), standard deviations and t values. These tables should clearly indicate the degrees of freedom (df) and the level of significance for each t-test. Jalowiec and Powers (1981, p. 12) measured the stress of hypertensive and emergency room patients, conducted a t-test on the data and tabled the findings (Table 19–4). The discussion of Table 19–4 might include that the most stressful life events were reported by the emergency room patients in the personal and social category and that the least number of stressful life events were reported by both groups in the financial category. The research report might also focus on the level of significance of the t values.

Tables of the results obtained from analysis of variance frequently identify the degrees of freedom, sum of squares (SS), mean squares (MS) and F value(s). The table should also indicate the level of significance for the F values. Swain and Steckel (1981, p. 219) tabled the findings from an analysis of variance performed on the diastolic blood pressure readings of three treatment groups over a period of four clinic visits (Table 19–5). A line graph of the treatment groups' diastolic blood pressure readings was presented in Figure 19–4 of this chapter. A discussion of Table 19–5 might identify the data analysis performed, the computer program used to perform the analysis and any unexpected results that were obtained.

Tables are used to identify correlations among variables, and often the table presents the correlation matrix generated from the data analysis. Brown, Muhlenkamp, Fox and Osborn (1983, p. 160) tabled the correlations they found among the total health promotion activity, health value and subscales of the Multidimensional Health Locus of Control Scale (MHLC) of a selected sample. Table 19–6 indicates the degree of the correlations among the variables and

TABLE 19–4
Means, Standard Deviations, and t Values for Types of Stressful Life Events Reported for 25 Emergency Room and 25 Hypertensive Patients

Stressful Life Event Category[1]	Emergency Room Patients		Hypertensive Patients		t Values[2]
	$\overline{X}$	SD	$\overline{X}$	SD	
Health (6)	1.48	1.32	2.36	0.99	2.65†
Work (16)	1.68	1.52	1.04	1.24	1.63
Home and family (30)	2.64	1.91	1.52	1.36	2.39*
Personal and social (18)	3.52	2.95	1.80	1.68	2.53†
Financial (6)	1.00	0.76	0.52	0.59	2.49†

[1]Numbers in parentheses indicate number of items per category
[2]df = 48
*p < 0.05
†p < 0.02
(From Jalowiec, A. & Powers, M. J.: Stress and coping in hypertensive and emergency room patients. *Nursing Research, 30,* 10, 1981; with permission.)

TABLE 19–5
ANOVA Diastolic Blood Pressures for Treatment Groups
Across Four Clinic Visits

Source	df	SS	MS	F
Mean	1	1919192.0	1919192.00	4466.68
Groups	2	2912.12	1456.06	3.39*
Error	49	21053.74	429.67	4.90†
Visits	3	1598.80	532.93	1.52
Visits X Groups	6	992.35	165.39	
Error	147	15984.48	108.74	

*$p < 0.05$
†$p < 0.005$
(From Swain, M. A. & Steckel, S. B.: Influencing adherence among hypertensives. *Research in Nursing and Health,* 4:213, 1981; with permission.)

the level of significance of these correlations. The discussion of this table might focus on the positive and negative correlations and on significant and insignificant correlations.

Tables are an effective method for presenting the results from nonparametric data analyses as well as from parametric analyses. Rudy and Estok (1983, p. 331) investigated the research question "What reported physical symptoms of female joggers are related to the intensity of jogging?" Table 19–7 identifies the significant values that were obtained when different symptoms of jogging were related to the intensity of jogging. The discussion of this table might identify the data analysis performed and focus on the significance level of the chi-square values that were obtained.

DISCUSSION

The discussion section ties the other sections of the research report together and gives them meaning. This section includes the major findings, conclusions drawn from the findings, implications of the findings for nursing and recommendations for further research. The major findings, which are generated

TABLE 19–6
Correlations Between Total Health Promotion Activity,
Health Value, and MHLC Subscales

	IHLC	PHLC	CHLC	HV
Total Health Promotion Activity	0.023	0.145	−0.325*	0.056
IHLC		−0.395*	−0.246	0.204
PHLC			0.402*	0.030
CHLC				0.113

*$p < 0.01$
Note: IHLC = Internal Health Locus of Control
      PHLC = Powerful Other Health Locus of Control
      CHLC = Chance Health Locus of Control
(From Brown, N., Muhlenkamp, A., Fox, L. & Osborn, M.: The relationship among health beliefs, health values, and health promotion activity. *Western Journal of Nursing Research,* 5:155, 1983; with permission.)

TABLE 19–7
Physical Symptoms Significantly Related to the Intensity of
Jogging in Women

Symptom	Chi-square (X^2)	Significance Level
Appetite change	19.240	0.001
Stress fractures	12.43	0.010
Scant menstrual flow	11.910	0.010
Hematuria	9.480	0.010
Missed or skipped menstrual flow	8.02	0.020
Hip problems	6.440	0.050

(From Rudy, E. B. & Estok, P. J.: Intensity of jogging: its relationship to selected physical and psychosocial variables in women. *Western Journal of Nursing Research,* 5:325, 1983; with permission.)

through an interpretation of the results (see Chapter 18), should be discussed in relationship to the research problem, purpose and subproblems (if applicable). Frequently, a study's findings are compared with the findings from previous research and are discussed in light of the study's frame of reference and the existing theoretical knowledge base. The discussion of the findings should also identify the limitations of the study and the generalizability of the findings.

The research report includes the conclusions or the knowledge that was generated from the findings. Conclusions are frequently stated in tentative or speculative terms, because one study does not produce conclusive findings (Tornquist, 1983). The researcher might provide a brief rationale for accepting certain conclusions and rejecting others. The study conclusions should be discussed in light of the conceptual limitations of the study.

The conclusions should be discussed in terms of their implications or usefulness for nursing knowledge, theory and practice. The researcher should describe how the findings and conclusions might be implemented in specific areas of nursing. The research report concludes with recommendations for further research. Specific problems that require investigation are identified, and/or the procedures for replicating the study are described. The discussion section of the research report should demonstrate the value of conducting the study and stimulate the reader to use the findings in practice and/or to conduct additional research.

THESES AND DISSERTATIONS

Theses and dissertations are research reports that are developed in depth by students as part of the requirements for a degree. The content included in a thesis or dissertation depends on the members of the student's research committee, but the organization of the content usually follows the outline included in Table 19–8. The Introduction, Review of Relevant Literature and the Methods and Procedures sections of this outline are described in Chapter 13. The content of sections IV, Results, and V, Discussion, is very similar to the content just described.

TABLE 19–8
Outline for Developing Theses and Dissertations

I. Introduction
  A. Statement of the problem
  B. Background and significance of the problem
  C. Statement of the purpose
II. Review of Relevant Literature
  A. Review of relevant theoretical literature
  B. Review of relevant research
  C. Summary
III. Frame of Reference
  A. Development of the conceptual or theoretical framework
  B. Formulation of research subproblems
  C. Definition of major variables
  D. Identification of assumptions
III. Methods and Procedures
  A. Description of the research design
  B. Description of the population and sample
  C. Description of the setting
  D. Presentation of ethical considerations
  E. Description of the pilot study
  F. Description of data collection methods and procedures
  G. Identification of methodological limitations
IV. Results
  A. Description of data analysis procedures
  B. Presentation of results
V. Discussion
  A. Major findings
  B. Conclusions
  C. Implications for nursing
  D. Recommendations for further research

Audiences for Communication of Research Findings

Before writing a research report, the researcher must determine "who" needs to know about the findings. The greatest impact on nursing practice can be achieved by communicating nursing research findings to nurses, other health professionals and health care consumers. Nurses need to be aware of research findings for use in practice and for conducting additional studies. Other health professionals need to be aware of the knowledge generated by nurse researchers and to facilitate the use of that knowledge in health care. Consumers need to be aware of the knowledge generated by nurse researchers and to know that their care is based on research findings.

MECHANISMS FOR COMMUNICATING FINDINGS TO DIFFERENT AUDIENCES

Research findings can be communicated through written reports and oral and visual presentations. The different mechanisms for communicating findings to nurses, health care professionals and consumers are outlined in Table 19–9.

Audience of Nurses

The most common mechanism used by nurses to communicate research findings with their peers is presentations at conferences and meetings. An increasing number of nursing organizations and institutions are sponsoring research conferences. The American Nurses' Association and many state associations sponsor annual nursing research conferences. The Western Council of Higher

TABLE 19–9
Audiences and Mechanisms for Communicating Findings

Audience	Mechanisms for Communicating Findings

Nurses–Researchers, educators, and practitioners	Oral and Visual Presentations
	  Nursing research conferences
	  Professional nursing meetings and conferences
	  Collaborative nursing groups—researchers, educators, practitioners
	  Thesis and dissertation defenses
	  Videotaped presentations
	Written Reports
	  Nursing journals
	  Nursing books
	  Monographs
	  Nursing theses and dissertations
	  Research newsletters
	  Foundation reports

Other health care professionals	Oral and Visual Presentations
	  Professional conferences and meetings
	  Interdisciplinary collaboration
	  Videotaped presentations
	Written Reports
	  Professional journals and books
	  Newsletters
	  Foundation reports

Health care consumers	Oral and Visual Presentations
	  Television and radio
	  Community meetings
	  Patient and family teaching
	  Presentations to legislators
	Written Reports
	  Newspapers
	  News magazines
	  Popular magazines
	  Reports to funding agencies
	  Reports to legislators

Education for Nursing has been sponsoring annual research conferences since 1968, and the proceedings from these conferences are published in a volume entitled *Communicating Nursing Research Findings*. The national honor society, Sigma Theta Tau, and many of the organization's local chapters sponsor research conferences. Sigma Theta Tau also sponsors an international research conference to facilitate the sharing of research findings with other countries. Many universities and some health care agencies are sponsoring or co-sponsoring research conferences.

For a variety of reasons, many nurses are unable to attend research conferences. To increase the communication of research findings, many conference sponsors are now providing tapes or videotapes of the research presentations. Some conference sponsors are publishing abstracts of studies with the conference proceedings. For example, since 1981, the *Western Journal of Nursing Research* has published the proceedings of the Communicating Nursing Research Conference, which is sponsored by the Western Society for Research in Nursing, a division of the Western Council on Higher Education for Nursing (Brink & Kearns, 1984).

There are currently more opportunities for nurses to publish their studies because the number of nursing research journals has increased in the last 10 years. Many of the specialty journals now publish research findings. Some researchers are publishing books or chapters in books in order to communicate their findings; however, many studies are still not being published, such as the studies conducted by masters and doctorate students.

Newsletters and monographs are being developed to communicate research findings. Many universities and hospitals publish regular newsletters, which include abstracts of the research conducted by their members. The American Nurses' Association Council of Nurse Researchers publishes a newsletter. This newsletter reports studies that have been presented at conferences and identifies the ongoing studies of the council members. Some universities and professional organizations are developing monographs to communicate findings from research projects. The monographs are usually paperback publications that include approximately 10 research reports. Sometimes these monographs focus on a specific research topic or research problem.

Foundations and federal government agencies publish reports of studies that have been conducted or are in progress. The American Nurses' Foundation publishes a newsletter, *Nursing Research Report*, which identifies the studies that were funded and includes abstracts of research and complete research reports. The Division on Nursing, Public Health Service, U.S. Department of Health and Human Services publishes reports on their grants, which include project titles, names and addresses of researchers, period of support, a brief description of each project and publication citations (Carnegie, 1977).

Audience of Health Care Professionals

Most nursing research findings are never made available to other health professionals. However, some nurse researchers are making an effort to bridge that gap by presenting their research findings at meetings and conferences sponsored by other health professionals, such as the conferences sponsored by the American Heart Association, American Public Health Association, American Cancer Society and National Hospice Organization. The proceedings from the Seventh Annual Symposium on Computer Applications in Medical Care included papers presented by nurse researchers. We must believe in the value of our findings and make an attempt to present these findings at conferences that attract a variety of health care professionals.

A variety of professional journals are potential sources for publication of nursing research, and we must seek publication in these journals. Nurse researchers and other health professionals conducting research on the same or similar problems might publish a journal article, book chapter or even a book together. This type of interdisciplinary collaboration might increase the communication of research findings and the impact of the findings on health care.

Audience of Health Care Consumers

An audience that is highly neglected by nurse researchers is the health care consumer. The findings from nursing studies can be communicated to the public through news releases that could be picked up by one or one hundred syndicated newspapers across the United States. For example, Elizabeth H. Winslow, R.N., Ph.D.; Lynda D. Lane, R.N., B.S.N.; and Andrew Gaffney, M.D. developed a news release to communicate the findings from their study, which focused on the problem: "Which is more difficult for the patient—using the bedpan or using the bedside commode?" The *Dallas Morning News* published the researchers' findings in an article entitled "Research suggests bedpans should be banned" on August 19, 1985 in the Discovery Section (Rubin, 1985). This article was then published in other papers across the country, and the study findings reached many potential health care consumers.

Nursing research findings could be communicated to consumers by being published in news magazines (*Time* and *Newsweek*) or popular women's and health magazines. Television and radio are other valuable sources for communicating nursing research findings. The findings from many medical studies are covered through these media; thus nursing research findings should also be communicated by these means.

Nurse researchers need to communicate their findings with legislators through written reports and personal presentations, so that their findings have an impact on the health policies that are developed. Nancy Burns, R.N., Ph.D. and Kim Carney, Ph.D. (Professor of Economics) have been studying hospice care since 1981. These researchers have written representatives and senators in Washington, D.C. informing them of their research findings. Dr. Burns and Dr. Carney are trying to communicate their findings to legislators who are involved with the development of hospice health care policies.

Another important but often overlooked method of communicating research findings to consumers is through patient and family teaching. Consumers need to know if the information and nursing care that they are receiving are based on research. Nursing interventions that are based on research are probably more credible to consumers than are unresearched nursing actions.

Presenting Research Findings

Research findings are presented at conferences and meetings through verbal presentations and poster presentations. Presentations allow the audience the opportunity to interact with the researcher and to ask questions about the study. With presentations, there is frequently little delay between the completion of the research project and the communication of findings. By the time research findings are published, there usually has been a 1- to 3-year delay.

VERBAL PRESENTATIONS

Many researchers are communicating their findings through verbal presentations at nursing conferences. To present findings at a conference, the researcher must be accepted as a presenter, develop a research report and deliver the report. Most research conferences require the submission of an abstract, and the selection of the presenters is based on the abstracts. Many research journals as well as research newsletters include "calls for abstracts." In addition, conference sponsors send "calls for abstracts" to universities and major health care agencies.

The "call for abstracts" will indicate the format for the development of the abstract. Frequently, abstracts are limited to a one-page, single-spaced format and include a statement of the research problem and subproblems, frame of reference, sample size, major findings, conclusions, implications for nursing and recommendations for further research. Writing an abstract requires practice; frequently, a researcher will rewrite an abstract many times until it meets all the criteria outlined by the conference sponsors. An abstract must clearly and concisely describe the study that was conducted and "sell" that study to the committee selecting the studies that will be presented. An example of an abstract is presented in Figure 19–5.

Developing a Research Report

The report developed depends on the time designated for each presentation. The major sections of a research report (introduction, methods, results and discussion) must be addressed. Some conferences focus on certain sections of the research report, such as tool development, data analyses, results or the implications of the results for nursing practice.

The focus of the conference directs the researcher in the development of the research report. Many researchers develop a typed script of their study for presentation and include visuals, such as transparencies or slides. The script for the research presentation should indicate when a slide or transparency is to be shown. The information presented on transparencies and slides should be limited and should include only major points. A single visual should contain information that can be easily read and examined in 30 seconds or a minute. The use of color on a visual can increase the clarity of the information presented and can be appealing to the audience. Preparing the written report and the visuals for a presentation is difficult, and the assistance of an experienced

Title: Perceived Competency Behaviors for the Clinical
         Nurse Specialist Role

Investigators: Mary Ellen Wyers, R.N., Ed.D.
                 Susan K. Grove, R.N., Ph.D.

During the past 10 years, the perceived competency behaviors for the role of the clinical nurse specialist (CNS) have differed among nurse administrators, graduate nurse educators, and CNSs. The purpose of this descriptive study was to describe the competency behaviors for the CNS role as perceived by the nurse administrators, graduate nurse educators, and CNSs and to identify the subroles that constitute the CNS role. The conceptual framework focused on the concepts perception and role from Hardy and Conway's (1978) role theory.

The design involved the development of a questionnaire of the competency behaviors for the CNS role. A pilot was conducted to refine this list of behaviors. Then a 40-item questionnaire was sent to a national sample of 161 nursing administrators, 233 graduate nurse educators, and 133 CNSs. The subjects were asked to rank the behaviors on the questionnaire on a six-point scale from most essential to least essential.

A frequency analysis was conducted, and the means for the behaviors ranged from 4.50 to 5.78 on a six-point scale. An ANOVA indicated no significant difference among the administrators, educators, and CNSs regarding their responses on the 40-item questionnaire. Exploratory factor analysis was conducted and four factors were identified. Factor 1 accounted for 64 per cent of the variance and was named practitioner; factor 2 (teacher) accounted for 15.7 per cent of the variance; factor 3 (researcher), 10.7 per cent of the variance; and factor 4 (consultant), 9.5 per cent of the variance. The reliability alpha for the questionnaire was 0.910.

The results of this study have implications for all three groups. These behaviors can guide nurse administrators in effectively utilizing and evaluating CNSs. Graduate nurse educators can use these behaviors in curriculum development. CNSs can clarify their role and develop a job description based on these behaviors.

FIGURE 19–5. Example abstract.

researcher can be valuable. Access to experts in audiovisual materials is also helpful; blurred or poorly constructed audiovisuals detract from the presentation. Print should be large enough and dark enough to be easily read. Typed pages from a thesis, dissertation or report should not be used on an overhead projector because the print is very difficult to read.

Delivering a Research Report and Responding to Questions

A novice researcher should attend several conferences and examine the presentation style of other researchers. Researchers should develop their own presentation style, but observing others can promote the development of an effective style. The script (developed for the presentation) guides the presenter's delivery. If the time frame for the presentation is limited, a researcher often reads the script; however, a presenter should never just read a script without making eye contact with the audience. Sometimes the research report is given from an outline or delivered using the slides or transparencies.

An effective presentation requires practice. If you are planning a research presentation, practice your presentation several times using the script until you are comfortable with the timing, content and your presentation style. In practicing a presentation, use the slides or transparencies so that you are comfortable with the audiovisual equipment. The presentation of the study should be within the designated time frame, which is identified by the sponsors of the conference. At many conferences, the researcher has 15 to 30 minutes to present his or her study and 5 to 10 minutes for questions. Some conferences include a presentation by the researcher, a critique of the study by another researcher and a question period. When preparing for a presentation, you should speculate about the questions that might be asked related to your study. You might want to present your study to colleagues and ask them to raise questions. If you practice making clear, concise responses to specific questions, you may not be as anxious during the actual presentation.

POSTER PRESENTATIONS

Researchers can elect to present their findings at a poster session. A poster presentation frequently includes the research problem, subproblems, frame of reference, data collection instruments, major findings, conclusions, implications for nursing and recommendations for further research. The poster usually includes tables and illustrations to communicate the results of a study. The poster should be easy to transport and assemble at the conference setting.

Poster presentations last from 1 to 2 hours; the researcher should remain with the poster during this time. Anyone passing the poster should be able to read the content in 3 to 5 minutes and have the opportunity to ask the researcher questions about the study. An advantage of a poster presentation is the opportunity for one-to-one interaction between the researcher and those viewing the poster. Many researchers write abstracts and give them to interested individuals.

Publishing Research Findings

Presentations are valuable means of communicating findings, but their impact is limited. Published research findings are permanently recorded in a journal or book and usually reach a larger audience than do presentations (Diers, 1981). However, the research report developed for presentation can serve as a basis for the development of an article for publication. Many researchers present their findings at a meeting and then never submit the paper for publication. Studies in which the findings show no significant difference or the absence of a relationship that was hypothesized are most likely not presented at meetings or submitted for publication. However, these negative findings are as important to the development of knowledge as are findings that support hypotheses.

Publishing research findings is a very rewarding experience, but the process of publishing demands a great deal of time and mental energy. The manuscript rejections that all authors receive can be discouraging. However, one can take certain steps to increase the probability of developing a successful manuscript or one that is accepted for publication. Plans for publishing a study should be outlined during the development of the proposal. At this time, the investigators should discuss and, if possible, determine authorship (McLaughlin, 1981). Some researchers develop the entire manuscript and are then faced with the decision of who will be first author, second author and so on. There are many ways for determining authorship credit, but the decision should be one that is acceptable to all investigators involved. Werley, Murphy, Gosch, Gottesmann and Newcomb (1981) studied the issue of authorship credit assignment; their article provides some suggestions for the assignment of credit in research publications.

PUBLISHING JOURNAL ARTICLES

The steps involved in developing a manuscript for publication include (1) selection of a journal, (2) development of a query letter, (3) preparation of the manuscript, (4) submission of the manuscript and (5) review and revision of the manuscript.

Selecting a Journal

Selecting a journal for publication of a study requires knowledge of the basic requirements of the journal, the journal's refereed status and the recent articles published in the journal. McCloskey and Swanson (1982) studied the publishing opportunities for nurses by conducting a comparison of 100 journals. In their article, they included a table of the basic requirements of 100 nursing and health care journals. The table includes the circulation, frequency of publication, article length, query letter, number of copies submitted, author reprints and payments, authorship preference, subject preference, waiting period for acceptance and publication, and solicited and unsolicited manuscripts for the 100 journals.

The refereed status of a journal should be determined in selecting a site for publication. A *refereed journal* uses referees or expert reviewers to determine the acceptance or rejection of a manuscript. In nonrefereed journals, the editor makes the decisions for acceptance or rejection, but these decisions are usually made after consultation with a nursing expert (Carnegie, 1975). Most refereed journals require that the manuscripts submitted to them be reviewed anonymously by three reviewers. The reviewers are asked to determine the strengths and weaknesses of a manuscript, and these comments or a summary of these comments is sent to the author (Johnson, 1982). Most academic institutions support the refereed system and will only recognize those publications that are in refereed journals. The refereed status and some basic publishing information for three nursing research journals are outlined in Table 19–10.

The researcher should review the articles recently published in the journal to which he or she is submitting a manuscript. This review will indicate whether the research topic has recently been covered and if the research findings would be of interest to the audience of the journal. This selection process enables researchers to identify a few journals that would be appropriate for publishing their findings. The researcher should then send query letters to the editors of these journals.

Developing a Query Letter

A query letter is developed to determine an editor's interest in reviewing a particular manuscript. The query letter should include the research problem

TABLE 19–10
Nursing Research Journals—Publishing Information

Journal	Issue Fre-quency	Article Length	Format for Report	Copies Sub-mitted	Referred
Nursing Research	6	14–16 pages	American Psychological Association	3	Yes
Research in Nursing and Health	4	10–15 pages	American Psychological Association	4	Yes
Western Journal of Nursing Research	4	25 pages	American Psychological Association	4	Yes

studied, a brief discussion of the major findings, the significance of the findings and the researcher's qualifications for writing the article (Mirin, 1981). The query letter should be addressed to the current editor of the journal. Frequently, three or four letters are sent to different journals at the same time. The query letter enables the researcher to make the final selection of a journal for submission of a manuscript. An example of a query letter is presented in Figure 19–6.

January 26, 1987

Florence S. Downs, Ed.D., F.A.A.N.
Editor Nursing Research
Associate Dean, School of Nursing
University of Pennsylvania
420 Service Drive, S2
Philadelphia, Pennsylvania 19104

Dear Dr. Downs:

An increasing number of nursing studies are focusing on clinical problems and specifically on the effectiveness of certain nursing interventions. Currently, many nursing interventions are implemented in the hospital setting without adequate research; one such intervention is pain management. Pain management involves many possible nursing actions, and knowledge of the impact of one or a combination of these actions is important in providing nursing care. The purpose of this study was to examine the effects of heat therapy and relaxation therapy on hospitalized patients who are experiencing low back pain.

The framework for this study was Margo McCaffery's theory of pain management. The independent variables of heat therapy and relaxation therapy were defined using McCaffery's theory. The patients' responses to the therapy were recorded using a magnitude scale. The study had a sample of 100 subjects; and the subjects were randomly assigned to four groups: control group and three experimental groups. An ANOVA was used to analyze the data. One experimental group was exposed to heat therapy, another to relaxation therapy and a third to heat and relaxation therapy. The experimental group that received both heat and relaxation therapy had a significantly different response as measured by the magnitude scale than the control group. The responses from the other two experimental groups were not significantly different from the control group response. This information is important for the development of nursing knowledge regarding pain management. If you are interested in reviewing this manuscript, I would be happy to send it to you upon your request.

Sincerely,

Susan K. Grove, R.N., Ph.D.
Associate Professor, School of Nursing
University of Texas at Arlington

FIGURE 19–6. Example query letter.

Preparation of the Manuscript

The manuscript is written according to the format outlined by the journal. When a manuscript is developed, the guidelines should be read and followed carefully. Guidelines for the development of a manuscript for *Nursing Research* are presented in Figure 19–7. Writing research reports for publication requires skills in technical writing that are not used in other types of publications. Technical writing condenses information and is stylistic. *The Chicago Manual of Style* (1982) is considered to be the primary source for quality technical writing. Cook (1985) and Strunk and White (1979) are two other sources that might be helpful in developing expertise in technical writing.

Knowledge of the guidelines provided by the journal and a background in technical writing facilitate the development of an outline for the proposed manuscript. The outline will include the content identified for a research report that was presented earlier in this chapter. The initial brief outline must be developed into a detailed outline that will guide the writing of the manuscript. A rough draft of the article is developed from the outline and is revised

INFORMATION FOR AUTHORS

The Editor of NURSING RESEARCH welcomes manuscripts of relevance and interest to those concerned with the conduct or results of research in nursing. Manuscripts should be sent to Florence S. Downs, Ed.D., F.A.A.N., Editor, NURSING RESEARCH, Associate Dean, School of Nursing, University of Pennsylvania, 420 Service Drive/S2, Philadelphia, Pa. 19104. It is understood that manuscripts submitted for consideration were prepared specifically and solely for NURSING RESEARCH, and that NURSING RESEARCH will have exclusive rights to the article and to its reproduction and sale in all countries.

• **Procedure.** It is advisable to precede submission with a letter of inquiry to the Editor, describing the article.

Manuscripts contributed to NURSING RESEARCH that are appropriate to the purpose of the journal are forwarded to members of a review panel who are experts in the subject matter of the particular study reported. The decision with regard to acceptance for publication is based on the evaluation of the referees. NURSING RESEARCH is concerned that the rights and dignity of all subjects involved in research be protected. No manuscript will be considered for publications unless it contains an explicit statement in this regard.

• **Preparing the Manuscript.** The author should submit three double-spaced copies of the manuscript on 8½- x 11-inch paper using generous margins; 14-16 typewritten pages is a desirable length. Authors should use a good bond paper for the copy; do not use "erasable" paper. Because manuscripts are refereed anonymously, authors should list their names only on the title page. Accepted manuscripts become the property of NURSING RESEARCH and may be reproduced in other publications, in whole or in part, only with the permission of the Editor of NURSING RESEARCH. Rejected manuscripts will not be returned; therefore, authors should be sure to keep at least one copy for their files.

NURSING RESEARCH reserves the right to edit all manuscripts to its style and space requirements and to clarify the presentation. Edited copy is submitted to the author(s) for approval. Authors are responsible for checking the accuracy of the material as it appears in the edited copy. Authors will be billed for alterations in the galley proof that follows.

• **Style and Format.** Authors should follow the American Psychological Association *Publication Manual*. Format should correspond to that used in NURSING RESEARCH. Titles should be short, and descriptive headings should be used to indicate the divisions of an article. Abbreviations should be spelled out the first time they are used, with the abbreviation placed in parentheses following the word. Greek letters or other special symbols should be identified in the margin the first time they are used. (This does not apply to the standard symbols used in statistical tests.) Addenda and appendixes are not used. The article should be accompanied by a 100- to 200-word factual abstract of the work presented.

• **Footnotes and References.** Incidental comments, qualifications, and the like, other than references to published sources, ordinarily are worked into the text. Personal communications and unpublished material should not be included in the references; if necessary to the article, they may be included in footnotes. Acknowledgements should be limited to persons making a substantial contribution to the author's work.

For information regarding treatment of references, see the APA *Publication Manual*.

• **Tables and Figures.** Tables and figures are printed only when they express more, and do so more clearly and briefly, than can be done by words in the same amount of space. All tables and figures should be referred to in the text, but should be largely self-explanatory and should not duplicate the text. They should be typed double-spaced on separate sheets of 8½- x 11-inch paper and should be numbered consecutively, have descriptive titles, and indicate the source of the data. Any inconsistencies in marginal totals or other figures should be explained in a footnote. Charts and tables should be complete.

• **Reprints.** The authors will receive a few "tear sheets" of the article. Reprints may be ordered by the authors at a reasonable price. Order forms for reprints are sent routinely at the time of publication.

FIGURE 19–7. *Nursing Research*: Information for authors. (From Nurs Res, 1986; with permission.)

numerous times. The content in the article should be logically and concisely developed and organized under clear subheadings. The title selected for the manuscript should reflect the content.

The development of a concise, clear manuscript is difficult to accomplish. Often, universities and other agencies offer writing seminars to assist students and other researchers in the development of a research report for publication. Some faculty members who chair theses and dissertation committees will assist their students in the development of an article for publication. In this situation, the faculty member is frequently the second author for the article.

When the researcher is satisfied with the manuscript, he or she should ask one or two colleagues to review it for organization, completeness of content and writing style. Colleagues' comments can be used to make the final revisions in the manuscript (Hagemaster & Kerrins, 1984). The manuscript should be expertly typed according to the format identified by the journal to which the manuscript will be submitted. Most journals will accept papers written on a word processor and printed on a dot matrix printer. Currently, there is a trend to send the disk to the publisher. In some cases, information can be transmitted from the computer to the journal editors' offices using a modem.

Submission of the Manuscript

Guidelines in each journal will indicate the name of the editor and the address for submission of a manuscript. A manuscript must be submitted to only one journal. The researcher should submit the number of copies of the manuscript requested and the original manuscript, if required. The editor of the journal frequently sends a postcard to the author to indicate that the manuscript was received and how long the review process might take.

Review and Revision of the Manuscript

The review of a manuscript results in one of three possible decisions: (1) acceptance of the manuscript as submitted, (2) tentative acceptance of the manuscript pending revisions or (3) rejection of the manuscript. The editor will send the author a letter that indicates the acceptance of the manuscript as submitted and a possible issue of publication.

About 90 per cent of submitted manuscripts are returned for revision. Many of these returned manuscripts are never rewritten. The author interprets it as a rejection and assumes that the revised manuscript will also be rejected; this is not necessarily true. Also, the act of revising based on reviewers' comments can improve the author's skills in writing. When editors return a manuscript for revisions, they include the actual comments of the reviewers or a summary of the comments to direct the revision. The researcher must carefully review the comments and make those revisions that improve the quality of the research report without making inaccurate statements about the study. Sometimes a paper must be revised more than once before it is published.

The author who receives a rejection is very disappointed, but he or she is not alone. Every author, even very famous authors, has had his or her manuscripts rejected. There are a variety of reasons why manuscripts are rejected. McCloskey and Swanson (1982) listed the following eight reasons for manuscript rejection that were identified by journal editors: (1) the subject was covered recently, (2) the content is scheduled for future publication, (3) the content is too technical, (3) the content is inaccurate, (4) the content is undocumented, (5) the research design is poor, (6) the content is not important and (6) the manuscript is poorly written. If you receive a rejection notice, you should view it as a learning experience and determine why the manuscript was rejected. Then, revise and resubmit the manuscript to another journal.

PUBLISHING RESEARCH FINDINGS IN BOOKS

Some researchers publish their findings in books or selected chapters of books. Qualitative studies and large, complex quantitative studies are sometimes published in book form. Publishing a book requires extensive commitment on the part of the researcher and that the researcher select a publisher and convince that publisher to support the book project. A prospectus must be developed that identifies the proposed content of the book, describes the market for the book and includes a rationale for publishing the book. The publisher and researcher must negotiate a contract that is acceptable to both regarding: (1) the content and length of the book, (2) the time required to complete the book, (3) the percentage of royalties to be received and (4) the advances to be offered (Evans, 1981). The researcher must fulfill the obligations of the contract by producing the proposed book in the time frame agreed upon. Publishing a book is a significant accomplishment and an effective means of communicating research findings.

Summary

Communication of findings is the final step of the research process and is essential for the utilization of findings in practice. Communicating research findings involves the development of a research report that is disseminated effectively and efficiently to a selected audience. Both quantitative and qualitative research reports include four basic sections: (1) introduction, (2) methods, (3) results and (4) discussion. The introduction includes a problem statement, significance of the problem, study purpose, a review of relevant literature, frame of reference, assumptions and research subproblems. The methods section includes the design, setting, sample, methodological limitations and the data collection process used in the study. The results section describes the data analyses that were performed and presents the results generated from these analyses. The discussion section ties the other sections of the research report together and gives them meaning. This section includes the major findings, conclusions drawn from the findings, implications of the findings for nursing and recommendations for further research.

Before writing a research report, the researcher must determine "who" needs to know about the findings. The greatest impact on nursing practice can be achieved by communicating nursing research findings to nurses, other health professionals and health care consumers. A variety of mechanisms for communicating to these audiences have been discussed in this chapter. Research findings can be communicated through written reports and oral and visual presentations. Research findings are presented at conferences and meetings through verbal presentations and poster presentations. Presentations allow the audience the opportunity to interact with the researcher and to ask questions about the study. Presentations are valuable means of communicating findings, but the impact of a presentation is limited.

Published research findings are permanently recorded in a journal or book and usually reach a larger audience than presentations. The steps involved in developing a manuscript for publication include (1) selection of a journal, (2) development of a query letter, (3) preparation of the manuscript, (4) submission of the manuscript and (5) review and revision of the manuscript. Publishing research findings is a very rewarding experience, but the process of publishing demands a great amount of time and mental energy. Some specific information for publishing in the nursing research journals has been provided. It is hoped that the information in this chapter will stimulate researchers to present and publish their findings.

References

Abdellah, F. G. & Levine, E. (1979). *Better patient care through nursing research*. New York: Macmillan Publishing Company, Inc.

Andrews, C. M. & Andrews, E. C. (1983). Nursing, maternal postures, and fetal position. *Nursing Research*, 32(6), 336–341.

Brink, P. J. & Kearns, J. M. (1984). Editorial: reporting research findings. *Western Journal of Nursing Research*, 6(3), 319–320.

Brown, N., Muhlenkamp, A., Fox, L. & Osborn, M. (1983). The relationship among health beliefs, health values, and health promotion activity. *Western Journal of Nursing Research*, 5(2), 155–163.

Butts, P. A. (1982). Dissemination of nursing research findings. *Image*, 14(2), 62–64.

Carnegie, M. E. (1975). The referee system *Nursing Research*, 24(4), 243.

Carnegie, M. E. (1977). Avenues for reporting research. *Nursing Research*, 26(2), 83.

Clinton, J. (1982). Ethnicity: the development of an empirical construct for cross-cultural health research. *Western Journal of Nursing Research*, 4(3), 281–300.

Cook, C. K. (1985). *Line by line: how to edit your own writing*. Boston: Houghton Mifflin Company.

Diers, D. (1981). Why write? Why publish? *Image*, 13(1), 3–8.

Evans, N. (1981). Authors and publishers—the mutual selection process. *American Journal of Nursing*, 81(2), 350–352.

Hagemaster, J. N. & Kerrins, K. M. (1984). Six easy steps to publishing. *Nurse Educator*, 9(4), 32–34.

Jalowiec, A. & Powers, M. J. (1981). Stress and coping in hypertensive and emergency room patients. *Nursing Research*, 30(1), 10–15.

Johnson, S. H. (1982). Selecting a journal. *Nursing and Health Care*, 3(5), 258–263.

Kalisch, B. J. & Kalisch, P. A. (1981). Communicating clinical nursing issues through the newspaper. *Nursing Research*, 30(3), 132–138.

King, D., Barnard, K. E. & Hoehn, R. (1981). Disseminating the results of nursing research. *Nursing Outlook*, 29(3), 164–169.

Kolin, P. C. & Kolin, J. L. (1980). *Professional writing for nurses in education, practice, and research*. St. Louis: The C.V. Mosby Company.

Leininger, M. M. (1985). *Qualitative research methods in nursing*. New York: Grune & Stratton, Inc.

Lowery, B. J. & Jacobsen, B. S. (1985). Attributional analysis of chronic illness outcomes. *Nursing Research*, 34(2), 82–87.

McCloskey, J. C. (1977). Publishing opportunities for nurses: a comparison of 65 journals. *Nurse Educator*, 11(4), 4–13.

McCloskey, J. C. & Swanson, E. (1982). Publishing opportunities for nurses: a comparison of 100 journals. *Image*, 14(2), 50–56.

McLaughlin, F. E. (1981). The publication of nursing research. *Journal of Nursing Administration*, 11(5), 37–40.

Mirin, S. K. (1981). *The nurse's guide to writing for publication*. Wakefield, Massachusetts: Nursing Resources.

Osguthorpe, N., Roper, J. & Saunders, J. (1983). The effect of teaching on medication knowledge. *Western Journal of Nursing Research*, 5(3), 205–216.

Rubin, R. (August 19, 1985). Research suggests bedpans should be banned. *Dallas Morning News*, Discovery Section.

Rudy, E. B. & Estok, P. J. (1983). Intensity of jogging: its relationship to selected physical and psychosocial variables in women. *Western Journal of Nursing Research*, 5(4), 325–336.

Shurter, R. L., Williamson, J. P. & Broehl, W. G. (1965). *Business research and report writing*. New York: McGraw-Hill Book Company.

Strunk, W. & White, E. B. (1979). *The elements of style* (3rd ed.). New York: Macmillan Publishing Company, Inc.

Swain, M. A. & Steckel, S. B. (1981). Influencing adherence among hypertensives. *Research in Nursing and Health*, 4(1), 213–222.

The University of Chicago Press (1982). *The Chicago Manual of Style* (13th ed.). Chicago: The University of Chicago Press.

Tornquist, E. M. (1983). Strategies for publishing research. *Nursing Outlook*, 31(3), 180–183.

Werley, H. H., Murphy, P. A., Gosch, S. M., Gottesmann, H. & Newcomb, B. J. (1981). Research publication credit assignment: nurses' views. *Research in Nursing and Health*, 4(2), 261–279.

IV

THE IMPLICATIONS OF RESEARCH FOR NURSING

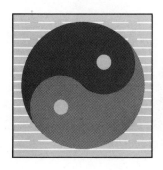  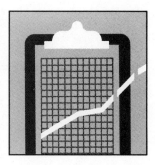

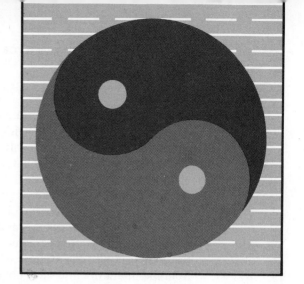

20

Critical Analysis of Nursing Studies

The critique of studies is an essential process in the development of a body of knowledge; yet, this is probably one of the least understood of the processes related to research. The word *critique* is often linked with the word *criticize*, which has negative connotations. In nursing, criticism is generally considered to be untherapeutic and to lead to feelings of inadequacy and rejection. To criticize another is thought to be unkind, mean and self-centered and is often interpreted as a personal attack.

In the arts and sciences, however, criticism takes on another meaning. It is associated with critical thinking and appraisal and requires carefully developed intellectual skills. This type of critique is sometimes referred to as *intellectual critique*. An intellectual critique is directed not at the person who created but at the element of creation. For example, one might critique an art object, an architectural design, a ballet performance, a philosophical essay, a theory or a study. It is even possible to critique a critique. An intellectual critique is the carefully thought out examination of all aspects of the object of the analysis. This critiquing process involves judging both the merits and the faults and the meaning and significance of the object being examined. This judgment is made in light of experience with previous objects. Conducting a critique requires both a thorough background in critical analysis and skills in logical reasoning processes.

Research Critique Within Nursing

Nurses, as individuals, and the nursing profession, as a whole, have had and continue to have difficulty with the critique process. A useful process for critiquing research has not evolved in nursing because of the incomplete way in which the critique process has been implemented and the inadequate numbers of nurses prepared to conduct critiques. During the early period of nursing research, verbal presentations of research were followed by critiques of the study. The early critiques involved examining only the faults of studies and tended to be severely critical, harsh and emotionally traumatic for the researcher (Meleis, 1985). As a consequence of these early unpleasant experiences, nurse researchers moved to a strategy of protecting and sheltering their nurse scientists from the threat of criticism. Public critiques, written or verbal, rarely occurred. Those responding to research presentations limited their remarks to praise of the investigator. Faults in these studies either were not mentioned or were minimized. The impact that the faults had on the meaning and significance of the study was often lost. Both of these situations resulted in incomplete critiques.

During the last 20 years, most studies have been presented or published without a formal critique. Nurses have lacked the expertise and/or the willingness to perform thorough critiques. Nursing education, both undergraduate and graduate, has provided a weak base for conducting research critiques. At local research conferences, finding sufficient numbers of researchers to present their studies has been and continues to be difficult. Finding equally qualified persons to critique the studies being presented is often an impossible task.

Incomplete critiques or the absence of critiques may have served a purpose as nurses gained rudimentary skills in the conduct of research. However, the discipline of nursing is moving past this point, and intellectual critiques will facilitate scientific investigation and the utilization of findings in nursing practice. More nurses now have the preparation and expertise for conducting intellectual critiques. Nursing research textbooks have moved past the point of being mere cookbooks of the mechanics of conducting research and provide information on the critiquing process. Nursing research skills, including critique, are now being introduced at the baccalaureate level of nursing education. Faculty are teaching the critiquing process and are requiring students to perform critiques.

In the development and refinement of nursing knowledge, an intellectual critique of studies is essential. Nurses must look closely at the meaning of the study findings and raise searching questions. Are the findings a good reflection of reality? Do they lead to increased understanding of the nature of phenomena that are important in nursing? Can nursing practice be based on the information provided by the findings? How do findings from the present study relate to those from previous studies? The answers to these questions for a particular study depend on a careful examination of the research problem and the way in which the study was designed and conducted. Not only must the mechanics of the conduct of the study be examined, but the abstract and logical reasoning used by the researcher in planning the study must also be critiqued. If there are flaws in the reasoning processes used to develop the study, there are probably flaws in the interpretation of the findings.

All studies have flaws. If all flawed studies were discarded, there would be no scientific base for practice; in fact, science itself is flawed. Science does not completely or perfectly describe, explain, predict and control reality. However, better understanding, increased ability to predict and control and further theory development depend on the recognition of the flaws in studies and in science. New studies must be planned so that the flaws of earlier studies are diminished. This means that the researcher must be familiar with previous studies conducted in the particular field and must perform critiques on these studies to determine existing flaws. Study findings must be interpreted in light of identified flaws. These flaws can lead to inaccurate data, inaccurate outcomes of analyses or limits in the ability to generalize the findings; however, study findings are utilized recognizing that knowledge is not absolute and certain. Confidence in nursing's knowledge base increases as more and better-designed studies are conducted.

All studies have strengths as well as flaws. Recognition of these strengths is critical to the generation of scientific knowledge and the utilization of findings in practice. If only flaws are identified, nurses will discount the value of the study and refuse to invest time in examining research. The continued work of the researcher also depends on the recognition of the study's strengths. Points of strength in a study, added to points of strength from multiple other studies, slowly build a knowledge base.

In nursing, a critique is often seen as a first step in learning the research process. In order to learn the research process, one must be able to read and comprehend published reports of studies. However, comprehension of the research report is dependent on a prior understanding of the research process and familiarity with the current body of knowledge. The neophyte in research usually has an inadequate background in theory and previous research in the area of the study to place the findings within the context of existing knowledge. Inadequacies in these areas impair the capacity to conduct a good critique. Conducting a critique is not a basic skill, and the content presented in previous chapters in this book is essential for implementation of the critiquing process.

Use of Critique in Nursing

There are several points in time during which the critique of studies is an important activity. These events include learning experiences for the student; examination of studies by the practicing nurse, the educator and the researcher; verbal critique after a verbal research presentation; written critique to follow a written research report; critiques for the purpose of selecting abstracts for presentations; editorial critiques for the purpose of selecting papers for publication; and critique for the purpose of evaluating proposals to conduct research.

STUDENT CRITIQUES

Basic knowledge of the research process and of the critique process should be provided early in the education of professional nurses. More advanced critique skills must be taught at the master's and doctoral level. Written critiques should be a required activity within undergraduate and graduate courses. These critiques should be designed to progressively increase students' skills in the five stages of critique (discussed in this chapter) as their knowledge of the research process increases. Conducting critiques should facilitate the utilization of research findings, which form a scientific base for nursing practice.

CRITIQUES BY THE PRACTICING NURSE

Critiques of studies by practicing nurses are essential to the utilization of research. The professional role requires the continual updating of nursing practice with the current body of knowledge. This body of knowledge is derived and evolves from current research and theory development. However, at present, clinical nurses tend to depend on the inservice coordinator or other authority figures within the institution to keep them informed of the existence and value of research. These nurses seem to believe that if something is important to know, someone will tell them. This attitude is not consistent with the view of the nurse as a responsible professional.

Individual nurses must accept responsibility for and design methods to remain current in a selected practice area. A bulletin board for posting current studies can be helpful but is not sufficient for critique to occur. Discussion groups, in which studies are presented and critiqued by a member of the group, can be effective. These groups can be conducted at the hospital nursing unit level and also among middle management nurses within a hospital. This activity is just as critical in community nursing; for example, in home health care, hospice, school nursing or occupational nursing, meetings should be held for the explicit purpose of critiquing current nursing research related to a specific area of practice.

CRITIQUES BY NURSING EDUCATORS

Educators use critiques for expansion of their knowledge base and development and refinement of the educational process. The careful critique of current nursing studies leads to the continual updating of curricular content taught in clinical and classroom settings. The educator models for the student by placing a positive value on examining new studies. In addition, the educator critiques and uses research findings in clinical practice and role models these activities for students. The educator's responsibility to generate and conduct research also requires the critique of previous studies.

CRITIQUES BY RESEARCHERS

Researchers conduct critiques in the preparation for a study and while it is being carried out. Most researchers continue to conduct research within the same field of study and seek out new studies reported in their area of expertise. These studies are then critiqued by the researcher, and the outcome of the critique influences the selection of research problems, development of methodology and interpretation of findings. Critiques of previous studies are presented in the review of literature for a particular study.

CRITIQUE AFTER VERBAL PRESENTATION OF STUDIES

Verbal critiques should be considered part of a research presentation. Through verbal critique, researchers can gain increased understanding of the strengths and flaws of their studies and generate ideas for further research. Participants who hear critiques can gain insight into the conduct of research. Experiencing the critique process can increase the participant's ability to critique studies and to judge the usefulness of the findings for nursing practice.

CRITIQUE AFTER A PUBLISHED RESEARCH REPORT

Currently, only one nursing research journal, *The Western Journal of Nursing Research*, includes commentaries (a partial critique) after a published research report. In this journal, authors receive feedback on their work and have an opportunity to respond to the critiques. Published critiques increase the reader's understanding of the study and abilities to critique research. If more journals incorporated published critiques, the quality of research conducted and the utilization of findings in clinical practice might increase.

CRITIQUE FOR ABSTRACT SELECTION

One of the most difficult types of critique to perform is that of examining abstracts. The amount of information available is usually very limited; yet, the reviewer must select the best-designed studies with the most significant outcomes for presentation at nursing meetings. This process requires an experienced researcher who requires fewer cues to determine the quality of a study.

CRITIQUE FOR EDITORIAL SELECTION

Nurse researchers serve as reviewers for professional journals to evaluate the quality of research papers submitted for publication. The role of these scientists is to examine the quality of the study to ensure that studies accepted for publication are well designed and contribute to the body of knowledge. Most of these reviews are conducted "blind" (anonymously) so that friendship relationships, contacts with the editor or reputation do not interfere with the selection process. In most refereed journals, the research report is examined by three reviewers and the researcher is provided with feedback.

EVALUATING RESEARCH PROPOSALS

There are three purposes for the critique of research proposals: (1) to approve student research projects, (2) to permit data collection in an institution and (3) to select the best studies for funding. The peer review process in federal funding agencies involves an extremely complex critique. At present, few nurses are qualified for this level of research review. Therefore, few nursing representatives review nursing studies submitted to federal agencies.

The Critique Process for Quantitative Studies

Many nursing research textbooks have approached the process of critique with a list of questions to be addressed in conducting the critique. Although a list of questions can serve as a useful guide in conducting a critique, the list often requires a sophistication in research knowledge not yet acquired by the neophyte. Conducting a critique is a complex mental process that is stimulated only by raising questions; therefore, the level of critique conducted is influenced by the level of sophistication of the individual doing the critique. A critique conducted by an undergraduate nursing student is different from one conducted by a graduate nursing student. The initial critique of an undergraduate student often involves only the comprehension step of the critique process. The critique of a doctoral nursing student is more thorough than that of less educated nurses but does not provide the strength of a critique by an experienced researcher. Written critiques, when comprehensive, may be more extensive than the research report being examined.

There are five steps in the process of critique, and, within each step, there are varying degrees of depth. The steps are comprehension, comparison, analysis, evaluation and conceptual clustering. The steps occur in sequence and presume accomplishment of the preceding steps. However, the person who is experienced in critiquing frequently performs several steps of this process simultaneously. In this section, the five steps are described and questions on which to focus the critique process are provided. The questions listed for each step are not comprehensive. They have been selected as a means for stimulating the abstract reasoning necessary for the conduct of a critique. Persons experienced in critiquing formulate additional unique questions as part of their reasoning processes. As knowledge of research increases, more searching questions are raised.

STEP I—COMPREHENSION

Initial attempts to comprehend research reports are often frustrating; thus, many practicing nurses refuse to read them. The experience of reading research reports can be like reading a nursing textbook in a foreign language, because the terminology and stylized manner of the report are unfamiliar. Skills in reading and comprehending research reports must be taught, just as reading in a foreign language is taught. The stylized manner of the report and the concepts inherent in the research process (which have been described in earlier chapters of this book) must be understood in order to identify elements of a study and to comprehend the study meaning.

Comprehension is the first step in performing a critique of the written or verbal research report. Comprehension involves identifying study elements and grasping the nature, significance and meaning of these elements. The reviewer must be able to identify and understand the meaning of the explicit and implicit elements of the study. In addition, comprehension requires that the person critiquing the study interpret the meanings of the terms and concepts used in the report similar to the way in which the researcher used them.

Guidelines and Questions

A. Read the study from beginning to end.
B. Mark unfamiliar words and determine their meaning.
C. State the research problem (paraphrase if necessary).
D. State the purpose of the study (paraphrase if necessary).
E. Examine the literature review.
   1. Are previous studies related to the research problem identified and described?
   2. Are the references current?
   3. Are the studies critiqued by the researcher?
   4. Is the current knowledge of the research problem described?
F. Examine the framework.
   1. Is the framework explicitly expressed, or must the reviewer extract the framework from implicit statements in the literature review?
   2. Does the study have a conceptual or theoretical framework?
   3. Does the framework describe and define the concepts of interest, relate them to the variables of the study and show relationships between the concepts discussed?
   4. Is a model of the framework provided for clarity?
   5. Is the framework related to the nursing body of knowledge?
   6. State the framework, clearly but briefly.
   7. If a model is not presented, develop a model that shows the variables under study and the proposed relationships from which the study has emerged.
G. List the subproblems.
H. Identify and define the variables.
   1. Independent variable(s)
   2. Dependent variable(s)
   3. Research variables
   4. Attribute variables
   5. Extraneous variables
I. Describe the sample.
   1. Size
   2. Description of subjects
   3. Sampling technique
   4. Response rate
J. Identify the design.

1. Draw a model similar to those in Chapter 10 illustrating the design.
2. Were pilot study findings used to design the major study?

K. Describe measurement strategies.
   1. Identify and describe methods of measurement.
   2. Identify the origin of the measurement tools.
   3. Describe reliability and validity of measurement tools.

L. Describe procedures used for data collection.

M. Describe the statistics used.
   1. Are the statistics primarily descriptive, correlational or inferential?
   2. Are differences or relationships being examined?
   3. Name the statistical techniques used.
   4. Identify the outcome of each statistical analysis.

N. Discuss the researcher's interpretation of findings.
   1. Explain the meaning of each outcome.
   2. Which findings were in keeping with those expected?
   3. Which findings were not expected?
   4. Are serendipitous findings described?

O. Describe the researcher's generalization of the findings.

P. Identify the researcher's suggestions for implications of the findings.

Q. List the researcher's suggestions for further studies.

R. Identify missing elements of the study.

S. Is the description of the study sufficiently clear to allow replication of the study?

STEP II—COMPARISON

The second step, comparison, requires knowledge of what each step of the research process should be like. The ideal is compared to the real. During the comparison step, one examines the extent to which the researcher followed the "rules" for an ideal study. The reviewer must also gain a sense of how clearly the researcher grasped the study situation and expressed it. The clarity of the researcher's explanation of the elements of research is a beginning demonstration of the researcher's skill in using and expressing ideas that require abstract reasoning.

Guidelines and Questions

A. Review the chapters of this textbook related to elements of the research process.

B. Compare the elements in the study to criteria established for each element in this textbook.
   1. Statement of the research problem and purpose
      a. Does the purpose narrow and clarify the focus of the problem to be studied and identify the research variables, subjects and setting?

     b. Is the identified problem researchable?

2. Research subproblems

     a. Are the hypotheses, questions or objectives appropriately expressed?

3. Sample and population

     a. Is the sampling design adequate to produce a representative sample?

     b. What are the potential biases in the study?

     c. Is the sample size sufficient to avoid a Type II error?

     d. If more than one group is used, do the groups appear to be equivalent?

     e. Were the rights of human subjects protected?

     f. Is the target population to which the findings will be generalized defined?

4. Measurements

     a. Scales and questionnaires

        (1) Are the data collection instruments clearly described?

        (2) Are the techniques used to complete and score the instruments given?

        (3) How are validity and reliability of the instruments described?

        (4) Did the researcher examine the validity and reliability of instruments in the present sample?

        (5) If the instrument was developed for the study, is the instrument development process described?

     b. Observation

        (1) Are the elements being observed clearly defined?

        (2) Is interrator reliability described?

        (3) Are the techniques for recording the observations described?

     c. Interviews

        (1) Do interview questions address concerns expressed in the problem statement?

        (2) Does the design of the questions tend to bias the subject's responses in a specific direction?

        (3) Does the sequence of questions tend to bias the subject's responses?

5. Design

     a. Is the design used in the study the most appropriate way to obtain the needed data?

     b. Does the design provide a means to examine all the subproblems?

6. Data collection

     a. Is the data collecting procedure clearly described?

     b. Is the training of data collectors clearly described and adequate?

    c. Did the data collection procedure appear to be conducted in a consistent manner?

    d. Was the data collection method ethical?

7. Data analysis

    a. Were data analysis procedures appropriate to the type of data collected?

    b. Were data analysis methods clearly described?

    c. Were the results presented in an understandable way?

8. Interpretation of findings

    a. Are findings discussed in relation to each subproblem?

    b. Are various explanations for the findings examined?

    c. Does the interpretation of findings appear biased?

STEP III—ANALYSIS

The analysis step involves a critique of the logic links connecting one study element with another. For example, the logical link of the problem and purpose must be analyzed. In addition, the overall flow of logic in the study must be examined. The variables identified in the research subproblems should be conceptually defined in light of the study framework. The conceptual definitions should provide the basis for the development of the operational definitions, and the study design must be appropriate for the investigation of the identified subproblems.

    Most of the faults in a study result from breakdowns in logical reasoning. For example, the biases due to sampling and design impair the logical flow from design to interpretation of findings. Examination of logic requires the identification of expressed and unexpressed assumptions of the researcher. The previous levels of critique have addressed concrete aspects of the study. During analysis, the process moves into the examination of abstract dimensions of the study, thus requiring a greater familiarity with the logic behind the research process and increased skills in abstract reasoning.

Guidelines and Questions

A. Reread the research report, with increased alertness for the logical links among the elements of a study.

    1. Is the literature review organized to demonstrate the progressive development of ideas through previous research?

    2. Does the literature review provide a rationale for the study?

    3. Are the subproblems logically linked to the research purpose?

    4. Are there uncontrolled extraneous variables that may have influenced the findings?

    5. Is the framework logically linked with the research purpose, variables and subproblems?

    6. Would another framework fit more logically with the study?

    7. Are the subproblems derived from the framework?

    8. Are the variables reflective of the framework?

9. Are the variables defined based on previous research and/or theories?
10. Is the conceptual definition of a variable consistent with the operational definition?
11. Are the instruments sufficiently sensitive to detect small differences between subjects?
12. Do the data collected address the subproblems?
13. Was the setting used in the study typical of clinical settings?
14. Are the sampling techniques, design and statistical analyses logically linked?
15. Are biases that are present in the study identified?
16. Do the conclusions fit with the findings from the analyses?
17. Identify the types of validity and reliability used in the development of the measurement tools.
18. Is instrument validity and reliability adequate for its use in the study?
19. Examine the validity of the design using the discussion in Chapter 10. Identify probable threats to the validity of the design.
20. Is the sample size sufficient to detect significant differences if they are present? Was power analysis used to determine sample size?
21. Did data analyses address the subproblems?
22. Were the analyses of data appropriate for the type of study and data obtained?
23. Were the analyses interpreted correctly?
24. Are the conclusions reached based on statistically significant results?
25. Are there limitations not identified by the researcher?
26. Are there inconsistencies in the report?

STEP IV—EVALUATION

Evaluation examines the meaning and significance of the study according to set criteria. During this step of the critique, the internal and external validity of the study are examined. The links between the study process, study findings and previous studies are also examined. Evaluation must build upon conclusions reached during the first three stages of the critique and provides the basis for the conceptual clustering step of the process.

The evaluation step involves comparing the present study with previous studies conducted in the field of interest. Evaluation must be made between the elements of this study and previous studies, such as an evaluation between previous hypotheses and present hypotheses, previous designs and the present design and previous methods of operationalizing variables and present approaches to operationalization. The findings of the present study must be considered in the light of findings of previous studies.

Guidelines and Questions

A. Reexamine the findings, conclusions and implications sections of the study and the researcher's suggestions for further study.
1. What rival hypotheses can be suggested for the findings?
2. How much confidence can be placed in the study findings?
3. To what populations can the findings be generalized?
4. What research questions emerge from the findings? Were these questions identified by the researcher?
5. What future research can be envisioned?
6. Do data collection instruments used in the study need further research?
7. Are the findings related back to the framework?
8. What implications do the findings have in relation to current theory of the phenomenon of interest?
9. In what ways do the findings add to the current body of knowledge?
10. When the findings are examined in the light of previous studies, what is now known about the phenomenon under study?
11. Summing up the critique findings, what were the strengths and faults of the study? Could the faults have been corrected?

B. Read previous studies conducted in the area of the research being examined.
1. Are the findings of previous studies used to generate the research problem and purpose?
2. Do subproblems emerge from the findings of previous studies?
3. Does the current research build upon previous measurement strategies so that measurement is more precise or more reflective of the variables?
4. Do sampling strategies show an improvement over previous studies?
5. Does the sample selection have the potential for adding diversity to samples previously studied?
6. Is the design an advancement over previous designs?
7. How do statistical analyses compare with those used in previous studies?
8. Do the findings build upon findings of previous studies?
9. Does the author address previous findings in discussing present findings?

STEP V—CONCEPTUAL CLUSTERING

The last step of the critique process is the clustering of present knowledge within a given area of study. Through the merging of existing findings, nurses are able to add to the existing knowledge base for nursing. This clustering can lead to new information being included in nursing textbooks and classroom lectures and changes in clinical practice. Conceptual clustering is a means of generating new research questions and developing and refining theory. Skills in this process should begin during basic nursing education.

Until recently, conceptual clustering was seldom addressed in the nursing literature. *Annual Review of Nursing Research* presents conceptual clustering of specific phenomena of interest to nursing (Werley & Fitzpatrick, 1983, 1984, 1985). These publications and others like them hold great promise for stimulating further research and for the utilization of research findings in nursing practice. Research findings should be utilized in practice only after a clustering of the findings has been accomplished.

During conceptual clustering, current knowledge in a specific area of study is carefully analyzed, relationships are examined and the knowledge is organized theoretically. Conceptual clustering maximizes the meaning attached to research findings, highlights gaps in knowledge and generates new research questions.

Guidelines and Questions

   A. Drawing a model that shows the concepts and the relationships found by the studies will increase the ease in detecting gaps in understanding relationships.

   B. The model can also be compared with current theory in the area of study.
   1. Is it consistent?
   2. Are differences that are found upheld by well-designed research? If so, modification of existing theory should be considered.
   3. Are there concepts and relationships in existing theory that have not been examined in the studies under consideration? If so, studies should be developed to examine these gaps.
   4. Are there conflicting theories within the field of study? Do existing study findings tend to support one of the theories?
   5. Are there existing theories to explain the phenomenon under consideration?
   6. Can current research findings be used to begin the development of nursing theory to more completely explain the phenomenon?

   C. Utilization of findings in practice.
   1. Is there sufficient information to utilize the findings in nursing practice?
   2. If the information is not sufficient, what further knowledge is needed before the findings can be utilized?
   3. How will patient outcomes be affected by utilization of the findings?
   4. Would the changes in outcomes make a significant difference in the health of clients?

Critique of Qualitative Research

Many of the elements involved in the critique of qualitative research are the same as those required for the critique of quantitative research. The quality of the critique is dependent on the reviewer's knowledge of the specific research process being examined. However, there are some differences in the critique because of differing designs, data collection techniques and data analysis techniques.

The reputation of the researcher conducting the study should be examined. Qualitative studies require specialized skills and carefully developed analytical capacities. The outcome of the study relies heavily on the capabilities of the researcher. The expertise of the researcher can be ascertained by examining the impact of previous theory developed by that researcher.

Details related to the data collection process must be spelled out more carefully than in quantitative studies. The process by which information was acquired for analysis is very significant to the meaning attached to the emerging theory. The emerging theory is equivalent to the findings in a quantitative study. See the data collection description in Germain's ethnographic study in Chapter 4.

The process of data analysis is often conducted manually and to some extent intellectually. Data are sorted and organized, resorted and then reorganized, repeatedly. Although the process is well understood by those conducting qualitative research, it is often not clearly described in qualitative study reports. To some extent, this is justifiable. The outcome of the analysis is much more important than the process. The process itself may vary from one researcher to another.

Examination of the emerging theory is the critical point in a critique of qualitative research. The emerging theory should clearly be derived from the data and should easily "make sense" to the reviewer. If the theory has been carefully developed, it will be succinct and will increase understanding of the phenomenon being examined. Often, the theory will be explained so simply that those reading or hearing it will have the feeling that they have always known that. However, the explanation is frequently not known, and knowing it may make a difference in clinical practice situations.

Summary

An intellectual critique is the carefully thought out examination of all aspects of the object of the analysis. This critiquing process involves judging both the merits and the faults and the meaning and significance of the object being examined. Judgment during the critique is made in light of experience with previous objects. In the development and refinement of nursing knowledge, an intellectual critique of studies is essential. Conducting a critique is not a basic skill, and understanding the content presented in previous chapters of this book is necessary for implementing the critiquing process.

There are several points in time during which the critique of studies is an important activity. These events include learning experiences for the student; examination of studies by the practicing nurse, the educator and the researcher; verbal critique after a verbal research presentation; written critique following a written research report; critiques for the purpose of selecting abstracts for presentations; editorial critiques for the purpose of selecting papers for publication; and critique for the purpose of evaluating proposals to conduct research.

There are five steps in the critique process, and, within each step, there are varying degrees of depth. The steps are comprehension, comparison, analysis, evaluation and conceptual clustering. The steps occur in sequence and presume accomplishment of the preceding steps. However, the person experienced in critiquing frequently performs several steps of this process simultaneously. Each step of the process was described in this chapter, and questions were provided to aid in achieving each step of the critique.

References

Ackerman, W. B. & Lohnes, P. R. (1981). *Research methods for nurses*. New York: McGraw-Hill Book Company.

Barritt, E. R. (1981). Critique: historical study. In S. D. Krampitz & N. Pavlovich (Eds.), *Readings for nursing research* (pp. 161–163). St. Louis: The C. V. Mosby Company.

Binder, D. M. (1981). Critique: experimental study. In S. D. Krampitz & N. Pavlovich (Eds.), *Readings for nursing research* (pp. 152–160). St. Louis: The C. V. Mosby Company.

Castles, M. R. (1975). Continuing education: a practitioner's guide to utilization of research findings. *JOGN Nursing*, 4(1), 50–53.

Downs, F. S. (1984). *A source book of nursing research* (3rd ed.). Philadelphia: F. A. Davis Company.

Duffy, M. E. (1985). A research appraisal checklist for evaluating nursing research reports. *Nursing and Health Care*, 6(10), 538–540.

Fleming, J. W. & Hayter, J. (1974). Reading research reports critically. *Nursing Outlook*, 22(3), 172–175.

Fox, D. J. (1982). *Fundamentals of research in nursing*. Norwalk, Connecticut: Appleton-Century-Crofts.

Halloran, E. J. (1984). Editorial: the need for writing reactions to research. *CNR*, 11(4), 2.

Horsley, J. A., Crane, J., Crabtree, M. K. & Wood, D. J. (1983). *Using research to improve nursing practice: a guide—CURN project*. New York: Grune & Stratton, Inc.

Komnenich, P. & Noack, J. A. (1981). The process of critiquing. In S. D. Krampitz & N. Pavlovich (Eds.), *Readings for nursing research* (pp. 145–151). St. Louis: The C. V. Mosby Company.

Meleis, A. I. (1985). *Theoretical nursing*. Philadelphia: J. B. Lippincott Company.

Norbeck, J. S. (1979). The research critique: a theoretical approach to skill development and consolidation. *Western Journal of Nursing Research*, 1(3), 296–306.

Notter, L. E. (1978). *Essentials of nursing research*. New York: Springer Publishing Company.

Phillips, L. R. F. (1986). *A clinician's guide to the critique and utilization of nursing research*. Norwalk, Connecticut: Appleton-Century-Crofts.

Sherman, K. M. & Kirsch, A. K. (1978). Research Q & A. Can nursing educators deal effectively with nursing students' difficulty in critiquing nursing research articles? How can critical thinking be fostered? *Nursing Research*, 27(1), 69–70.

Sherwen, L. N. & Toussie-Weingarten, C. (1983). *Analysis and application of nursing research: parent-neonate studies*. Monterey, California: Wadsworth Health Sciences Division.

Stetler, C. B. & Marram, G. (1976). Evaluating research findings for applicability in practice. *Nursing Outlook*, 24(9), 559–563.

Sweeney, M. A. & Olivieri, P. (1981). *An introduction to nursing research: research, measurement, and computers in nursing*. Philadelphia: J. B. Lippincott Company.

Treece, E. W. & Treece, J. W. Jr. (1982). *Elements of research in nursing* (3rd ed.). St. Louis: The C. V. Mosby Company.

Ward, M. J. & Fetler, M. E. (1979). Research Q & A: What guidelines should be followed in critically evaluating research reports? *Nursing Research*, 28(2), 120–125.

Werley, H. H. & Fitzpatrick, J. J. (1983). *Annual review of nursing research* (Vol. 1). New York: Springer Publishing Company.

Werley, H. H. & Fitzpatrick, J. J. (1984). *Annual review of nursing research* (Vol. 2). New York: Springer Publishing Company.

Werley, H. H. & Fitzpatrick, J. J. (1985). *Annual review of nursing research* (Vol. 3). New York: Springer Publishing Company.

21

Utilization of Research in Nursing Practice

The preceding chapters of this book describe what nursing research is, the thinking processes associated with research, the techniques of developing and conducting studies and the skills needed to critique studies. Implicit in all these chapters is the belief that the expected outcome of nursing research activities is to improve nursing practice. In order for research to have an impact on practice, the findings of studies must be utilized by practitioners.

Very little of our current nursing practice is based on research findings. Until the last decade, little research had been conducted on nursing practice; most nursing studies focused on nursing education and characteristics of nurses. Many of the initial clinical studies were not well designed; tools to measure needed variables were inadequate or unavailable; and existing well-designed studies were not replicated. However, in the past 10 years, the number of clinical studies has gradually increased, study designs are improving and an increasing number of replications are being reported in the literature. We now have research findings that could improve nursing practice.

Most people believe that a good idea will sell itself—the word will spread rapidly and the idea will quickly be used. Unfortunately, this is seldom true. Even today, research findings that clearly warrant utilization are not being used. Ketefian (1975) studied the extent to which widely reported findings of a series of studies on the procedure for correctly determining oral temperature were being utilized in nursing practice. Of 87 registered nurses located in two states, only one nurse knew the time needed to accurately record an oral temperature.

These findings about taking oral temperatures would be comparatively simple to implement. The decision could be made by the nurse alone; no physician's order would be needed. Administrative personnel would not have to give approval. No added cost would be involved, and additional nursing time would be minimal. At the time of Ketefian's study, the study findings had been available in the literature for 5 to 10 years. Why were they not utilized? Had the nurses not read the information? Was it not taught in the nursing schools? Or was the suggested change in nursing practice not considered important by those who did read the information? Although these findings are not of great importance in our present era of electronic thermometers, they are an indication of a research utilization problem that is clearly evident throughout nursing.

With alterations in reimbursement for health care, nursing is currently in the process of making major changes in practice. Society is demanding more of us than ever before. We have the attention of the policymakers of health care for the future. Meeting their expectations will require increased acceptance of responsibilities throughout nursing, including high-quality research and the utilization of those findings to develop a scientific base for our practice. Understanding the process of research utilization and developing strategies to achieve it are critical to nursing. To address these concerns, in this chapter, we examine what is known about knowledge utilization in general, techniques that have been used in nursing, problems we face in utilization of nursing studies and potential ways to address these problems.

Knowledge Utilization

TIME LAGS

Nursing is not the only discipline concerned about inadequate utilization of new knowledge. Knowledge is expanding rapidly in many disciplines, but its use does not seem to be keeping pace. The utilization of knowledge was also a concern in the past, when wide acceptance of a new idea or finding could take as long as 50 years. The time lag between the discovery of citrus juice as a preventive measure for scurvy and its use on British ships was 264 years.

Glaser, Abelson & Garrison (1983) presented a table of the span of time between the first conception of 10 ideas and initial utilization of them (Table 21–1). The table suggests that the average length of time between discovery and utilization is almost 20 years. Enos (cited in Glaser, Abelson & Garrison, 1983) reports an average time interval of between 11 and 14 years. Lynn (cited in Glaser, Abelson & Garrison, 1983) reports a decrease in time for utilization of discoveries made in the period between 1885 and 1950 from 30 years (1885 to 1919) to 9 years (1945 to 1964). Why some findings require much longer to

TABLE 21–1
Span of Time Between Idea and Utilization

Innovation	Year of First Conception	Year of First Realization	Duration in Years
Heart pacemaker	1928	1960	32
Input-output economic analysis	1936	1964	28
Hybrid corn	1908	1933	25
Electrophotography	1937	1959	22
Magnetic ferrites	1933	1955	22
Hybrid small grains	1937	1956	19
Green revolution: wheat	1950	1966	16
Organophosphorus insecticides	1934	1947	13
Oral contraceptive	1951	1960	9
Videotape record	1950	1956	6
Average duration			19.2

(From Glaser, E. M., Abelson, H. H. & Garrison, K. N.: *Putting knowledge to use.* San Francisco: Josey-Bass, 1983; with permission.)

implement than others is not clearly understood. Historical events, attitudes toward the researcher and research in general, and the necessity with some innovations to change attitudes and values before the findings can be accepted and utilized seem to influence the time required.

THE STUDY OF UTILIZATION

The concern about the span of time between discovery and utilization became more intense in the early 1970s when it was discovered that many of the findings from research funded by the federal government were not being used. A think tank of experts in the area of research utilization was convened by the government to examine reasons for the lack of utilization and to propose strategies to improve utilization.

From the work done by this group, there evolved a field of study that examines the process of utilization. Researchers and theorists across disciplines began addressing the problem. The processes of utilization in agriculture, education, industry and medicine have been closely scrutinized. As a consequence, measures have been taken to decrease the time lag and improve the utilization of research findings in these fields. In agriculture, the Agricultural Extension Department was expanded. In education, the National Diffusion Network was established through the U. S. Department of Education. Computer networks have been developed to speed the communication of scientific and technical information. Scientists are gaining increased insight into the process that occurs in the diffusion and utilization of new knowledge, and a new professional journal, *Knowledge: Creation, Diffusion, Utilization,* has been established to publish their works.

In the following sections of this chapter, three current theories about diffusion and adoption of innovations are described: Rogers' theory of diffusion of innovations; Lewin's field theory, which describes the process of change; and Havelock's theory of linker systems. These three theories have been the framework for most research in the area of utilization. The theories also provide a means for planning strategies to increase utilization of research in nursing. Only recently has nursing entered the search to understand utilization of research. Currently, three projects have been undertaken within nursing to improve the adoption of innovations within nursing practice: the WCHEN Regional Program for Nursing Research Development, The Conduct and Utilization of Research in Nursing (CURN) project and the Nursing Child Assessment Satellite Training (NCAST) project. These three theories were used as the theoretical frameworks for the projects. These projects, their outcomes and implications for nursing are discussed in the following sections.

ADOPTION OF INNOVATIONS

An expert and noted theorist in the field of knowledge diffusion and utilization is E. M. Rogers (1983), who developed a theory of the process of adoption of innovations. Rogers has conducted research related to diffusion for 25 years. His theory is a synthesis of the findings from his research and those of many other scientists in this field of study. Rogers' theory can provide a framework within which we can gain an understanding of the dynamics of utilization within nursing. Familiarity with Rogers' definitions of concepts is important in order to understand his process of utilization.

DIFFUSION

According to Rogers (1983), "*Diffusion* is the process by which an innovation is communicated through certain channels over time among the members of a social system" (p. 5). The word *dissemination* is considered synonymous with diffusion. The main elements of diffusion are (1) the innovation, (2) communication channels, (3) time and (4) the social system.

Innovations

Rogers defines an innovation as "an idea, practice, or object that is perceived as new by an individual or other unit of adoption" (p. 11). The idea might not necessarily *be* new, but must be *perceived* as new by those considering adoption. Characteristics of an innovation that determine the probability and speed of its adoption include (1) relative advantage, (2) compatibility, (3) complexity and (4) trialability. *Relative advantage* is the extent to which the innovation is perceived to be better than current practice. *Compatibility* is the degree to which the innovation is perceived to be consistent with current values, past experience and priority of needs. *Complexity* is the degree to which the innovation is perceived to be difficult to understand or use. If the innovation requires the development of new skills, complexity increases. *Trialability* is the extent to which an individual or agency can try out the idea on a limited basis with the option of returning to previous practices. Innovations that have great relative advantage, are compatible, have flexible trialability and are not complex will be adopted more quickly than innovations that do not meet these criteria.

Uncertainty is another important factor in decision making in regard to an innovation. *Uncertainty* is the degree to which one can predict that an expected or desired outcome will result from utilization of an innovation. Information reduces uncertainty, and evaluative information from near-peers further reduces uncertainty.

Communication Channels

Communication channels may include one-to-one communication, one individual communicating to several others or mass media such as books, journals, newspapers and television. Mass media are effective for achieving diffusion; however, interpersonal channels involving face-to-face exchange have been found to be more effective in achieving adoption of the innovation. The communication is more effective when the two interacting individuals are similar in such characteristics as beliefs, values, education, social status and profession. Rogers refers to these individuals as *near-peers*. If this is true, a doctorally prepared researcher would not be the most effective person to persuade a staff nurse to adopt an innovation.

Time

Time is an important element in understanding diffusion and adoption. There are three time periods of interest in understanding diffusion-adoption: (1) the time span from the point at which an individual first hears about an innovation to the point at which a decision is made to accept or reject the innovation, (2) the innovativeness of the individual or agency that determines the time needed to achieve adoption and (3) the number of individuals within a social system who adopt an innovation within a given time period.

Decision-Making Steps

The decision-making time period has been conceptualized by Rogers as consisting of five steps: (1) knowledge, (2) persuasion, (3) decision, (4) implementation and (5) confirmation. *Knowledge* is the first awareness of the existence of the innovation. *Persuasion* occurs when the individual forms an attitude toward the innovation. *Decision* occurs when the individual chooses to adopt or reject the innovation. *Implementation* occurs when the individual uses the innovation. *Confirmation* occurs when the individual seeks reinforcement of the decision. The individual may reverse the previous decision if exposed, at this point, to conflicting information.

During the knowledge stage, effective communication can occur through mass media, because the individual seeks information in order to reduce uncertainty. However, at the persuasion stage and throughout the rest of the innovation-decision process, mass media are less effective. Rather than information, the individual seeks evaluative statements related to the innovation. Have you used it? How do you feel about it? What are the consequences of using it? What are the advantages-disadvantages of using it in my situation? Would you advise me to use it? Will I still be approved of and accepted if I use it? Interpersonal networks with near-peers are much more likely to influence the individual during these latter phases. This same process occurs when the decision maker is an agency or organization rather than an individual.

Innovativeness

Innovativeness is the "degree to which an individual or other unit of adoption is relatively earlier in adopting new ideas than are the other members of a system" (Rogers, 1983, p. 22). Rogers uses five categories to describe adopters, based on their degree of innovativeness: (1) innovators, (2) early adopters, (3) early majority, (4) late majority and (5) laggards.

Innovators are active information seekers about new ideas. They have a high level of mass media exposure and interpersonal networks that are widely extended, reaching beyond their local social system. From these sources, they receive early information about innovations. Innovators usually function outside the existing social structures and tend to have cosmopolitan relationships. Their social support system is diverse and not tightly linked. Innovators can cope with higher levels of uncertainty related to an innovation than can other adopters and are the first to adopt a new idea. They do not rely on subjective evaluations of the innovation by other system members. Because innovators are less closely linked with the local social system, they have less influence on adoption of the innovation within the system than do early adopters.

Early adopters tend to be leaders in existing social structures. They tend to learn of new ideas rapidly, utilize them and then serve as role models in their use. The *early majority* rarely are leaders but are active followers. They will follow willingly in the use of a new idea. The *late majority* are skeptical about new ideas and will adopt them only if group pressure is great. The *laggards* tend to be isolates without a strong support system. They are security oriented and cling to the past. By the time they adopt a new idea, it is considered by most to be an old idea.

The rate of adoption is measured by the length of time involved in adoption of the innovation by a certain percentage of the individuals within a social system. Initially, a few innovators adopt the innovation. Diffusion at this point is slow. However, over time, diffusion becomes more rapid and the rate of adoption increases. Then, the rate of adoption slows as fewer and fewer individuals remain who have not adopted. Rates of adoption for the same innovation vary in different social systems.

The Social System

Rogers (1983) defines a social system as "a set of interrelated units that are engaged in joint problem solving to accomplish a common goal" (p. 24). Diffusion occurs within a social system, and the social structure of the system affects the diffusion of the innovation. A social system has both formal and informal structure. Formal structure is related to authority and power. Informal structure is related to who interacts with whom under what circumstances. The norms or expected behavior patterns within the social system also affect diffusion. Norms can serve as a barrier to change. Within the social system are opinion leaders who have informal leadership roles. When the social system is oriented toward change, the opinion leaders tend to be innovative. When the norms are opposed to change, so also are the opinion leaders. When innovations are diffused and adopted or rejected within a social system, social change occurs.

There are centralized and decentralized diffusion systems. Centralized diffusion systems involve group decision making within organizations and usually involve activities by a change agent. A decentralized diffusion system involves one-to-one communication and individual decisions regarding utilization of the innovation.

In any system, there are leaders who are in favor of innovations and leaders who oppose change. These leaders are at the center of the system's interpersonal communication networks and tend to reflect the norms of the system. In seeking adoption of an innovation within a social system, one must identify the opinion leaders and seek their acceptance of the innovation.

Change agents are professionals outside the social system who enter it for the purpose of achieving adoption of an innovation by the social system. Change agents tend to use opinion leaders in their diffusion campaigns. However, if the opinion leader deviates too far from the norms of the group, he or she will lose status as an opinion leader.

There is a general assumption that diffusion and utilization of innovations are desirable. This may not always be the case. In some instances, an innovation may be desirable for one individual or agency but not for another. Innovations may have one set of consequences for one element of the social system and another set of consequences for another element. The consequences of innovations are often not considered for the poor, the aged and minorities—those without power within the system.

TYPES OF UTILIZATION

Direct Application

Another interest in the field of utilization research has been the way in which innovations are utilized. Our general expectation is that the innovation will be used exactly as it has been developed. In fact, some scientists would not consider the innovation to have been adopted unless its original form has been kept intact. For example, if a study demonstrated that a particular care activity, conducted in exactly defined steps, was effective in achieving a specific outcome, adoption would require that the nurse perform those steps in exactly the same way in which they were described in the study. This expectation reflects the narrow, precise definition of an innovation that is necessary to the scientific endeavor. However, this preciseness is not in keeping with typical practice behavior, and research has indicated that maintenance of the original innovation does not always occur.

Reinvention

Adopters often modify the innovation to best meet their own needs. Rogers refers to this process as *reinvention*. Using this strategy, the steps of a procedure might be changed, or some of the steps might be combined with care activities emerging from previous experience. To a researcher, adding to or deleting steps in a procedure means that it is no longer the same innovation. Thus, adoption has not occurred. From the practitioner's viewpoint, the innovation has been adopted.

Indirect Effects

The way in which new knowledge is used is not well understood. The expectation is that the new knowledge will directly modify the actions of the individual, either in the original suggested way or as reinvention. However, it would seem that, in a larger number of cases, the knowledge is incorporated into the knowledge base of the individual and used in more diffuse ways. The findings are discussed among practitioners and researchers, cited in clinical papers and textbooks and used to provide strength to arguments. Thus, the knowledge would be incorporated into the individual's thinking and combined with past experience, previous education and current values and, in this form, would influence actions. In this instance, determining that the innovation was being utilized would be more difficult. Thus, we may be underestimating the extent of utilization.

Weiss (1980), another theorist in the field of knowledge utilization, suggests considering utilization as a continuum, with one extreme being findings that have a direct effect on decisions and activities, and the other extreme being findings that have a more diffuse or indirect effect. This indirect effect involves awareness, insight or cumulative understanding that may lead to gradual changes in behavior that are less specific and not easy to pinpoint in time. The middle of the continuum indicates a modified impact of the findings in which the findings are combined with many other factors and other types of information for the purpose of problem solving and decision making.

Rogers' theory has the potential to direct the utilization of nursing research findings. Rogers' descriptions of adoption strategies by various individuals allows you the opportunity to examine your role, alter your role and assess the roles of others within your system. Using Rogers' theory as a framework, findings can be utilized precisely or merged with other knowledge to more indirectly affect nursing practice.

LINKER SYSTEMS

Havelock (1970, 1973, 1974) added a new dimension to the current knowledge of utilization theory by proposing the development of a linker system. This linker system is used to transfer new knowledge, skills or products (innovations) from resource systems (the researchers and their publications) to user systems (the practitioners) for dissemination. Havelock's model (Fig. 21–1) illustrates his ideas.

The transfer would involve *packaging* the innovation in a form that would increase its acceptability to the user system and, thus, increase utilization. The idea of packaging comes from the research and development programs (R

The Linkage Process

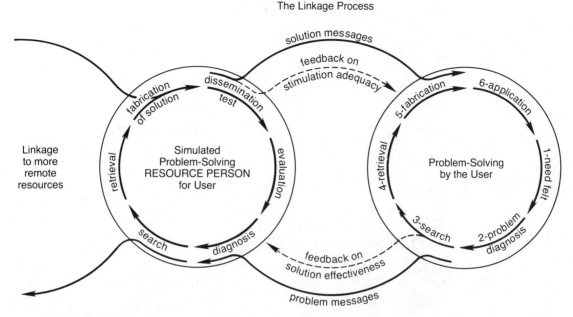

FIGURE 21–1. Havelock's linker system. From Havelock, R. G.: Ideal systems for research utilization: four alternatives. U.S. Department of Health, Education and Welfare. Washington, D.C. (1974); with permission.

& D) of technology in which researchers make a discovery. Then another group (the linker system) takes the new idea and develops practical ways to use it. The linker system is involved in the transmission of user needs to the resource systems, thus increasing the probability of new studies addressing practitioner concerns. This idea was borrowed from industry's use of research and is associated with its continual drive to "build a better mousetrap." Figure 21–2 illustrates how the entire linker system is expected to function to increase the production and utilization of useful research.

Havelock also suggests the establishment of a linker, an individual who could serve as a connection between the user system and the resource system. The linker would have a broader range of knowledge of research findings and strategies for implementing them and could serve in an advisory or helper capacity to the user system in implementing new ideas. The linker could also communicate user needs to the resource system. Translating or packaging of new ideas for use in practice could be accomplished by the linker. This theory introduces the idea of packaging, which could be useful in the preparation of nursing research findings for utilization.

CHANGE THEORY

Change theory was developed from Kurt Lewin's field theory and describes the strategies necessary to successfully achieve change. Change theory adds the element of change agent, which is not addressed by Rogers or Havelock. A *change agent* is an individual or group, external to the system, that is used to

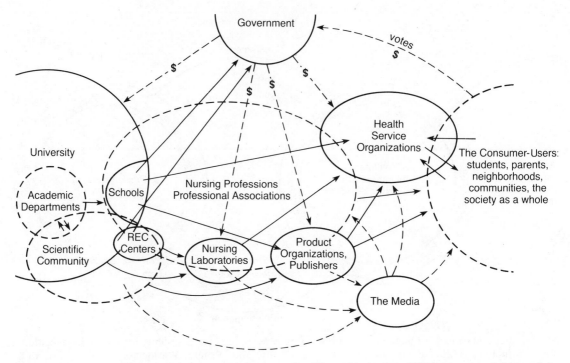

FIGURE 21–2. Transmission of ideas between systems. See Figure 21–1, page 633, for source of this model.

initiate and facilitate the change process. When the change has been adopted by the majority of the members, the agent leaves the system. Using a change agent, the change is carefully planned. The change agent (sometimes a committee) identifies clearly and in detail the desired outcome. Steps to achieve the outcome are developed. Persons, groups or factors that will facilitate the change and persons, groups or factors that will resist the change are identified. Careful plans are made to facilitate, strengthen and promote those factors facilitating the change. Strategies are designed to counter factors resisting the change. The change agent seeks to diffuse the innovation throughout the system, and working through opinion leaders, the agent modifies attitudes toward the change and implements the findings into the practice pattern of the system. Unfortunately, in some cases, when the change agent is withdrawn, continuation of the innovation gradually declines.

Motivation for Utilization

What are the reasons that a practitioner utilizes new knowledge? This varies with the individual. Innovators and early adopters have an interest in new knowledge for the sake of knowledge itself. These individuals read research journals, attend research conferences and seek continuing education programs to increase their general knowledge base. Other practitioners have a specific practice problem for which they have no satisfactory solution. They may search the research literature for effective practice strategies to resolve their problem. These individuals may also seek advice from near-peers, who may inform them of an innovation. Groups or committees often use this strategy for problem solving. If the knowledge is not available, the search may lead to the generation of studies to increase the specific knowledge sought. This action involves interaction between practitioner and researcher to meet a clinical practice need.

In other situations, a change agent, external to the social system, may directly or indirectly generate an awareness or need for the innovation. The change agent may be a speaker in an inservice or continuing education program, a consultant employed by the institution or a sales representative demonstrating a new product.

Research findings may also indirectly affect clinical practice. Sundquist (1978) describes the role of research "brokers" who "repackage" research knowledge for use by policymaking bodies. Health policymakers may use the information in modifying policies governing reimbursement or levels of care required. These health policies then influence practice by facilitating specific approaches to care and imposing the constraints within which nursing is practiced.

Barriers to Utilization

SOCIAL SYSTEM BARRIERS

Within any social system, there are forces that promote stability and oppose change as well as forces that promote change. The strength of these forces varies with the social system. Generally, social systems that have existed over a long period of time, value tradition and have an authoritative management style with a strongly centralized power structure will be strongly resistant to change. In this type of social system, innovators are not well tolerated and opinion leaders support the institutional stance.

Some social systems take pride in being innovative and actively encourage the utilization of new ideas. In these organizations, management patterns and communication patterns will facilitate rapid dissemination of new ideas and support efforts to implement them. Resources needed for diffusion and implementation will be readily available. Innovators and early adapters are nurtured in these settings.

Social systems that are in disarray tend to be more receptive to change and the utilization of innovations because the forces resisting change have little power. Currently, the entire health care system is in disarray because of the major changes in reimbursement patterns. Although currently there are greater economic constraints, the potential for change has increased.

Nursing is difficult to place, as a social system, within these categories. Many changes have occurred in nursing. However, the changes were probably imposed on the system by external powers. Nursing has tended to be traditional and to rely on authorities, which are characteristics related to resistance to innovativeness. Perhaps this can explain the unwillingness to use new nursing knowledge. If this is so, the values and norms of nursing as a social system will need to change before innovations will be utilized. Researchers, who tend to be innovators in the nursing social system, may be in opposition to the opinion leaders, who tend to prefer stability.

LACK OF COMMUNICATION

A frequent concern expressed in the literature is the communication gap between the university-based researcher and the institutionally based practitioner. This concern is not limited to nursing; it was a major topic of discussion at the think tanks originated by the federal government. Criticisms included the following: (1) Researcher-originated studies do not solve pressing clinical problems, (2) findings from researcher-originated studies often cannot be utilized in practice, (3) findings are communicated primarily to other researchers, (4) findings are not expressed in terms understood by practitioners, (5) practitioners do not value research, (6) practitioners are unwilling to read research reports and (7) practitioners have inadequate education related to the research process. There are clearly differences between doctorally prepared university-based researchers and less educated practitioners. Reference groups, values and norms of the two groups are clearly different. Duffy (1985c) has described the situation well:

> Most researchers live easily with the tentative and the hypothetical. Even in research reports, they use probability statements to answer hypothetical questions about relationships among variables. During research planning and implementing, they tend to communicate only with immediate colleagues—usually other researchers. When they've completed their studies, they disseminate findings in formal presentations and through publication, usually in a research journal. These presentations and articles are full of academic and research jargon that is familiar only to other researchers. Because of their academic orientation, many researchers believe they have "done their job" when they've reported findings to other colleagues through these presentations or publications. Although these communication lines are appropriate among researchers, practitioners looking for practice implications are hard-pressed to find that information.
>
> Practitioners, on the other hand, are more pragmatic. They tend to seek prescriptions—what to do in given situations. Clinicians view each case as unique. They're not interested in discovering common patterns within a population, or in tentative conclusions. Their immediate goals are to find answers that will improve patient care. Basically, practitioners want the answer to "how?" while researchers what to know "why?" Practitioners also tend to rely on precedent, on common sense, and on previous experience more than on research findings. They do not think of the scientific method and research as holding a key position in their work, so they assign it and its use a low priority.
>
> The most regrettable outcome of the disparity between groups is the tendency of both to stereotype the other. Researchers become "ivory-

tower idealists"—out of touch with the real world; practitioners "won't" use research "to improve patient care." (p. 238)

Research Utilization Strategies in Nursing

Although nursing's interest in utilization strategies is fairly recent, three programs have been developed to attempt to increase utilization of nursing research findings. The nurse researchers involved in these activities, with federal funding for their work, have designed and implemented strategies for utilization based on existing literature from other fields of practice. These programs are The WCHEN Regional Program for Nursing Research Development, The Conduct and Utilization of Research in Nursing (CURN) project and The Nursing Child Assessment Satellite Training (NCAST) project.

WCHEN

The WCHEN project, initiated in the mid-1970s, was the first major nursing project to address research utilization in nursing. The project was directed by Krueger and colleagues (Krueger, 1978; Krueger, Nelson & Wolanin, 1978). The 6-year project was funded by the Division of Nursing, within the U.S. Department of Health, Education and Welfare. The initial goal of the project was to increase nursing research activities within the Western region of the United States. Havelock's linkage model, Lewin's strategies of planned change and Rogers' diffusion of innovations were used as theoretical bases for the project.

The project had three major activities, only one of which directly addressed research utilization. The utilization focus involved the presentation of a series of workshops in three sites. At the workshop, participants were organized into dyads composed of a nurse educator and a clinician. Teaching focused on developing skills in critiquing research, by using change theory and diffusion of innovations. Each dyad selected research findings addressing a particular clinical problem that they were willing to attempt to implement within an institution. The dyad was to function as a change agent.

The project staff and participants had difficulty identifying clinical studies with findings appropriate to implement into practice. Findings that were identified tended to be merged with other activities by the dyad and then implemented as a package. Since the project staff expected the findings to be implemented in purer form, this strategy was viewed with some disfavor. Reports of the three projects from this activity were published: Axford and Cutchen (1977) developed a preoperative teaching program; Dracup and Breu (1978) devised a care plan for grieving spouses and tested its effectiveness; Wichita (1977) developed a program to treat and prevent constipation in nursing home residents by increasing the fiber in their diet.

CURN

The CURN project, directed by Horsley (Horsley, Crane & Bingle, 1978; Horsley, Crane, Crabtree & Wood, 1983), was awarded to the Michigan Nurses Association by the Division of Nursing in the U.S. Department of Health, Education and Welfare. The 5-year (1975 to 1980) project was developed to increase the utilization of research findings in the following ways: (1) disseminating findings, (2) facilitating organizational modifications necessary to implementation and (3) encouraging collaborative research that was directly transferable to clinical practice. The theoretical base included Lewin's planned change and Rogers' diffusion of innovations. Research utilization was seen as an organizational process rather than as a process to be implemented by an individual practitioner. The activities involved in the process of utilization were described as:

> (1) the identification and synthesis of multiple research studies in a common conceptual area (research base); (2) the transformation of the knowledge derived from a research base into a solution or clinical protocol; (3) the transformation of the clinical protocol into specific nursing actions (innovations) that are administered to patients; and (4) a clinical evaluation of the new practice to ascertain whether it produced the predicted result. (Horsley, Crane, Crabtree & Wood, 1983, p. 2)

Existing clinical studies were critiqued, and the following 10 areas, considered to have sufficient *quality* research to warrant implementation, were selected.

1. Structured preoperative teaching
2. Reducing diarrhea in tube-fed patients
3. Preoperative sensory preparation to promote recovery
4. Preventing decubitus ulcers
5. Intravenous cannula change
6. Closed urinary drainage systems
7. Distress reduction through sensory preparation
8. Mutual goal setting in patient care
9. Clean intermittent catheterization
10. Pain: deliberative nursing interventions

Protocols were developed from the findings, and implementation was initiated on a test unit within a hospital. The outcome of the implementation was evaluated using baseline data and comparison groups. Follow-up questionnaires were sent to the 17 participating hospitals for a 4-year period to determine the long-term impact of the implementation on the organization. Pelz and Horsley (1981) reported that prior to the project, research utilization was low in both comparison and experimental groups. One year after the intervention, significant differences were found, with experimental organizations having higher levels of utilization. The second year after the intervention, there were still differences between the groups, but differences were not significant on all 10 utilization activities. The third year, experimental units continued to perform the protocols. The rate of diffusion of the innovations to other units was not reported. The clinical protocols developed during the project have been published (CURN Project).

NCAST

The NCAST project, developed by King, Barnard and Hoehn (1981), was originally a 2-year (1976 to 1978) project funded jointly by the Division of Nursing and the National Foundation/March of Dimes. Funding was continued through the Harris Foundation of Chicago. The theoretical framework for the project was Rogers' Diffusion of Innovations. The program's focus was educational and was directed at the individual nurse practitioner. A four-component process was used involving (1) recruitment, (2) translation, (3) dissemination and (4) evaluation. Recruitment involved selection of appropriate learners. The research findings were translated from research terminology to terms more familiar to practicing nurses. The content that was disseminated addressed findings derived from a longitudinal study of nurse-child assessment, indicating the importance of assessment of caregiver-child interactions and the infant's environment.

Practicing nurses were taught specific assessment procedures that identified and evaluated the animate and inanimate environment of the infant. A satellite communication system was used to send the information to various settings across the United States. Four alternative communication modes were used: (1) "the duplex mode, involving two-way communication; (2) the simplex mode, involving one-way communication; (3) the videotape mode; and (4) the conventional or control mode" (King, Barnard, and Hoehn, 1981, p. 165). The duplex mode involved two-way interactions between the nurse researcher and the clinical nurses. Both the researcher and the clinical practitioners were able to see each other by television. The simplex mode involved one-way satellite transmission from the university to the two clinical sites. The learners were able to see and hear the researcher. The researcher could communicate with the learners by telephone hookup. In the videotape mode, there was no interaction between the researcher and the learner. The learners viewed videotape recordings of the content. The nurses exposed to the conventional or control mode were given only reference lists and documents with information used to develop NCAST.

The teaching was provided through one of the communication modes using a satellite communication system. The communication was directly from the researcher to the practitioner. Although the model is still being developed and final outcomes have not been reported, Barnard (1982) reports that 85 per cent of nurses exposed to the protocols adopted the assessment procedure. Four years after the program was initiated, the high adoption rate has continued. From this experience, Barnard suggests that every innovation needs a missionary (Barnard, 1982).

Stetler/Marram Model

Stetler's model of research utilization (Fig. 21–3) was developed inductively and initially published in 1976. Since then it has been further developed by Stetler (1983, 1985).

Stetler (1985) proposes that utilization involves a series of judgmental activities by the individual nurse in the role of caregiver, educator or manager or as a leader making decisions that will mandate the actions of other nurses. These judgments involve (1) validation, (2) comparative evaluation and (3) decision making. In the *validation* phase, the nurse conducts a critique of the study. In *comparative evaluation*, the nurse "explores scientific criteria that, as a whole, help to determine whether or not any use can be made of the findings or other study components" (p. 42). During *decision making*, alternative types of application are considered. Alternatives for utilization include direct action and cognitive application. *Direct action* includes using the study to "support the need for change, as impetus for evaluation of services, and/or a model for practice" (p. 42). *Cognitive application* would involve uses that affect the "nurse's way of thinking, approaching and/or observing situations" (p. 42). Cognitive application may improve the nurse's understanding of a situation or allow analysis of practice dynamics.

According to Stetler's model, the organization may or may not be involved in the utilization process, depending on the specific innovation being considered. However, the model considers utilization as an essential component of professional nursing practice. Thus, professional nursing practice requires that the nurse continually seek the outcomes of current research, evaluate their potential for use in practice and modify practice continually as new knowledge becomes available. Change, in this case, is not the focus. Utilization is continuous and is the norm. Stetler (1985) refers to the paper by Clark & Lenburg (1980) in which it is suggested that the professional nurse is knowledge oriented rather than rule oriented and functions as a critical thinker, using

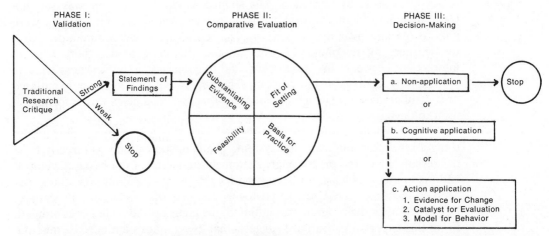

FIGURE 21–3. Stetler's model of research utilization. From Stetler, C. B.: Research utilization: defining the concept. *Image: The Journal of Nursing Scholarship, 17*, 40, 1985; with permission.

research to "more scientifically provide care, teach, and/or manage" (Stetler, 1985, p. 42).

Where Do We Go From Here?

From an examination of utilization theory and previous attempts to increase the utilization of nursing research, we have gained some understanding of the problems we face and become familiar with some proposed alternatives. Examination of the information also generates questions. What is the most effective strategy for implementing findings? How should research be utilized? How is research being utilized? Do we have research that is ready to be utilized? Whose responsibility is it to promote the implementation of findings?

We suggest that effective strategies for implementing findings will require a multifaceted approach, taking into consideration the researcher, the educator, the individual practitioner and the organizations within which nursing functions. In the following section, we examine problems in and possible approaches toward increasing the utilization of findings in nursing practice using Roger's five decision-making steps: (1) knowledge, (2) persuasion, (3) decision, (4) implementation and (5) confirmation.

KNOWLEDGE

Problems

There is a serious problem in nursing with diffusion of research information, and this problem has a number of facets. Nursing research that is conducted as theses or dissertations is usually not published. Most theses are not microfilmed or abstracted and, thus, are not listed in computerized data bases. These findings are, for all practical purposes, lost to nursing's body of knowledge; they cannot be implemented into practice.

Professional nursing education is not providing adequate information to basic nursing students about research to allow them to make intelligent judgments about using research in practice. This capacity requires a more than surface knowledge of the research process and competency in critiquing research. Part of this problem is due to the inadequate educational preparation of many nursing faculty in relation to research.

Nursing textbooks do not make clear whether the information being provided is based on research, tradition or experience or is derived from other professions. Research reports on which the text information is based are seldom cited in nursing textbooks. Classroom teaching seldom includes content from nursing research. If the content is included, the student is not usually informed that the information was obtained through nursing research. Thus, in basic nursing education, students are not enculturated to utilizing nursing research in their practice.

Published research reports are seldom read by the practicing nurse. The reasons for this are multiple and include lack of understanding, valuing and time. Understanding and values begin in basic nursing education. However, expectations of the professional nurse by both the profession of nursing and the health care system influence education and the attitudes of the nurse.

Institutions within which nurses work are not familiar with current nursing research findings. This is reflected in multiple dimensions of institutional functioning. For example, the procedure manual that guides many of the tasks performed by nurses is often not congruent with findings reported in the literature. Standards of care and nursing care plans also may not reflect current nursing research–based knowledge.

Solutions

Immediately obvious solutions to the aforementioned problems include increasing the research-related educational content of the basic nursing student, increasing the research knowledge competence of the nursing educator and including nursing research findings in nursing textbooks. This strategy may in turn increase the congruence between current nursing research and procedure manuals, standards of care and care plans.

Diffusion Strategies

Professional organizations, linkers, researchers or change agents might work through the inservice coordinator, usually an opinion leader within the organization, to diffuse research information through the nursing staff. Current research reports could be reviewed by the inservice coordinator, copied and distributed to the appropriate nursing personnel.

Comprehension

Because some researchers view the utilization problem as being due to inability of the practitioner to read and comprehend research reports, one proposed strategy to increase utilization is to translate research findings into a more popularized form for publication in clinical practice journals. Although this idea has some appeal, it also has some drawbacks. The clinician would have to accept the validity of the findings with little or no opportunity to evaluate the quality of the research or the degree of similarity between the study setting, the study sample and the current clinical situation. It would seem much more advisable to provide the nurse with the skills necessary to comprehend existing research reports.

Currently, some clinical practice journals have a special section for reporting recent research findings. These "news items" generally cite the research journal in which the original research report can be found; thus, the clinician can identify findings that seem relevant and seek out the study for additional information.

Another potentially helpful strategy is the publication of papers by clinicians reporting effective clinical use of research findings. Wichita's (1977) paper is a good example of this strategy. This type of communication tends to move the reader from the information stage to the persuasion stage.

Clustering

The question of what is the most appropriate form in which to diffuse research findings must be addressed. We believe that the practitioner must be aware of individual findings. As was mentioned previously, findings are often used cognitively or indirectly. They have the potential for increasing the practitioner's insight into the situation, and thus influencing nursing actions indirectly. However, we believe that all the findings on a specific topic should be examined

TABLE 21–2
Nausea and Vomiting: Summary of Descriptive Studies

Author(s) and Purpose	Subjects and Procedures	Major Findings
Scogna and Smalley Study selected factors that might influence degree of nausea and vomiting experienced by patients receiving chemotherapy	41 patients: 33 female; 8 male; 16–77 yr; mean age = 50 yr Variety of cytotoxic agents No control for antiemetic therapy Self-administered questionnaire: attitude about therapy effectiveness; hours of sleep before therapy; activity levels (24 hr); food intake (24 hr)	None of the four factors (attitude, sleep, activity, food intake) was shown to influence degree of nausea and vomiting 11 patients experienced nausea and vomiting in the 24-hr period prior to administration of chemotherapy

Welch
Describes radiation-related emesis and determine variables that may influence occurrence of vomiting
	24 patients receiving external beam radiation to abdomen, pelvis or posterior spine
	No control for antiemetic therapy
	Interviewed during first and last courses of radiation therapy
	Five variables studied:
	  Characteristics of nausea and vomiting
	  Type and extent of disease
	  Extent of radiation therapy
	  Nutritional status
	  Psychological factors
		Patients being radiated for recurrent disease had more nausea and vomiting
		46% vomited within 24 hr of therapy
		79% experienced some degree of nausea and vomiting
		Greater reduction in appetite in those receiving short and long duration radiation therapy
		Weight loss occurred from time of initiation of therapy to final course of treatment
		All 9 subjects receiving radiation in AM experienced emesis: decline in emesis incidence for those receiving radiation in the afternoon

Zook and Yasko
Investigate relationship between anxiety, hopelessness, pain, specific demographic characteristics and degree of nausea and vomiting experienced by patients receiving chemotherapy
	26 patients: 17 males; 9 females; 19–78 yr; mean age = 57 yr
	Variety of cytotoxic agents
	Receiving chemotherapy for first time
	Variety of antiemetics
	Self-administered instruments given pre-therapy and within 24 hr post-therapy:
	  Spielberger State-Trait Inventory
	  Beck Hopelessness Scale
	  McGill-Melzack Pain Questionnaire
	  Nausea and Vomiting Scale
	  Demographic Data Sheet
		Anxiety, hopelessness, pain, and age were not significantly correlated with nausea and vomiting
		Negative perceptions of past experience with others treated with chemotherapy were significantly correlated with degree of nausea experienced
		Women experienced more vomiting than men
		Vomiting and nausea occur as separate phenomena

(From Lindsey, A. M.: Building the knowledge base for practice, part 1: nausea and vomiting. *Oncology Nursing Forum,* 12, 49, 1985; with permission.)

TABLE 21-3
Nausea and Vomiting: Quasi-Experimental and Experimental Antiemetic Studies

Author(s) and Purpose	Subjects and Procedures	Major Findings
Gathercole, Connolly & Birdsall Confirm that dexamethasone administered IV possesses antiemetic, antinausea properties	20 patients: 11 males, mean age = 57 yr; 9 females, mean age = 52 yr Receiving first cycle of chemotherapy Variety of cytotoxic agents All received prochlorperazine at time of chemo administration and took home for prn use Half received 10 mg IV dexamethasone Half received 2.5 ml NS (placebo) Completed self-administered questionnaire at 4-hr intervals for 36 hr posttherapy	6 had no nausea or vomiting; 8 had decreased incidence of nausea and vomiting Study discontinued due to side effects of tingling
Daniels & Belt Evaluate efficacy of metoclopramide given IV at high doses in patients receiving cis-platinum	31 patients: 29–76 yr Majority had prior chemotherapy or radiation 15 received only cis-platinum 16 received cis-platinum and other agents Metoclopramide given at 2 mg/kg as IV bolus 30 min before initiation of cytotoxic agent and at 2-hr intervals during 6-hr infusion Nausea and vomiting evaluated over 24 hr by observation and interview	No nausea or vomiting observed in 54.5% of 55 courses of therapy in 21 patients 6 vomited in association with eating; 12 patients in 14 courses had spontaneous vomiting without nausea
Lamb & Cox Determine effectiveness of droperidol as antiemetic agent	20 males: 26–81 yr 9 had prior chemotherapy Variety of chemotherapy agents 2.5 droperidol given 30 min prior to chemo; repeated at 3-hr intervals × 2 Nausea and vomiting evaluated by nurse observation and patient self-report of number and duration of episodes	12 had no vomiting; 4 had only 1 vomiting episode Vomiting associated with food intake after chemotherapy
Berry-Opersteny & Heusinkveld Investigate effects of prophylactic administration of the antiemetic droperidol on chemotherapy	15 patients: 10 males; 5 females; 17–83 yr; 8 experimental group; 7 control group Some had prior chemotherapy Variety of chemotherapeutic agents Experimental group received 0.5 mg droperidol 30 min prior to chemo and 2 additional doses at 4-hr intervals Control group received the same antiemetic prn Self-report of nausea and vomiting 12–24 hr following chemotherapy	Found trend of decreased perception of nausea in experimental group Decrease in vomiting in experimental group (statistically significant) Found correlation between severity and duration of nausea and frequency of vomiting

(From Lindsey, A. M.: Building the knowledge base for practice, part 1: nausea and vomiting. *Oncology Nursing Forum,* 12, 49, 1985; with permission.)

TABLE 21–4
Nausea and Vomiting: Quasi-Experimental and Experimental Studies

Author(s) and Purpose	Subjects and Procedures	Major Findings

Moore
Investigates influence of time of day of administration of cis-platinum on nausea and vomiting and identify other variables influencing extent of nausea and vomiting
	13 patients: 10 females; 3 males; 49–68 yr
	Receiving cis-platinum and other agents
	Some had prior chemotherapy
	Time chemo administered:
	  2 AM
	  4 PM
	  6 PM
	  1 AM
	Structured interviews
	Anxiety measure prior to chemo
	Self-report nausea and vomiting for 17 hr after chemo administered
		No significant correlation between time of day cis-platinum was administered and nausea and vomiting
		Significant negative correlation between hours of sleep night before chemo and severity of vomiting
		Significant negative correlation between hours of sleep night before chemo and anxiety
		Degree of nausea had significant positive correlation with number of previous chemotherapy treatments
		6 of 13 had nausea or vomiting at home before chemotherapy; 5 vomited in hospital before treatment

Cotanch
Tests use of progressive muscle relaxation (PMR) in reducing nausea and vomiting and psychological averseness associated with chemotherapy
	12 patients: 5 females; 7 males; 17–49 yr: mean age = 34 yr
	All experiencing refractory drug-induced nausea and vomiting
	Variety of experimental cytotoxic agents
	All receiving antiemetic agents
	Behavior intervention of PMR
	Baseline data for one drug cycle
	Measured for 2 days postchemotherapy:
	  Physiological arousal
	  State-trait anxiety
	  Food and fluid intake
	  Degree and frequency of nausea and vomiting
	  Antiemetic therapy used
		9 of 12 subjects showed some decrease in nausea and vomiting after PMR training (only 1 had a 100% response; 5 had greater than 25% response; 3 had no response)
		Caloric intake was greater in all patients 48 hr after chemotherapy

Scott, Donahue, Mastrovito and Hakes
Evaluate effectiveness of relaxation protocol on nausea and vomiting
	10 women receiving chemo for ovarian carcinoma
	Relaxation Protocol:
	  Slow stroke back massage
	  Guided imagery
	  Progressive relaxation
	  Coaching by investigator during 4–6 hr of chemo administration
		Relaxation did not entirely block vomiting
		Reduction in duration, frequency and intensity of vomiting
		Decrease in amount of emesis

(From Lindsey, A. M.: Building the knowledge base for practice, part 1: nausea and vomiting. *Oncology Nursing Forum,* 12, 49, 1985; with permission.)

to determine what is currently known, considering all findings. Barnard (1984) refers to this as *cognitive clustering*. Lindsey (1985) illustrates this strategy well in her paper examining the current knowledge base related to treatment-induced nausea and vomiting in cancer patients. She examined representative studies published in the previous 5 years, critiqued the studies and summarized the findings. Her summaries can be found in Tables 21–2, 21–3 and 21–4. From this review, Lindsey (1985) came to the following conclusions:

> Building upon observations from the previous work, it may be important to develop and test clinical therapies aimed at desensitizing those patients who hold negative perceptions received from other previously treated cancer patients and aimed at those who may have a conditioned averseness to therapy.
>
> Managing or relieving the human responses of therapy-related nausea and vomiting is a complex clinical problem that involves consideration of various factors. There are competing notions about the effectiveness of sedation and quiet, restful environmental conditions, versus the use of distractive techniques in decreasing the nausea and vomiting experienced. Perhaps the effectiveness of these clinical therapies will depend on the personal preferences of the patients for quiet or for distraction. The influence of the position of the patient during administration of chemotherapy on the nausea and vomiting experienced remains unknown. The influence of activity and food and fluid intake on the occurrence and severity of nausea and vomiting also remain as questions. There is some accumulating evidence across studies, as serendipitous observations, that vomiting occurs in direct association with food and fluid intake. There is need for more accurate descriptions of these side effects in greater numbers of subjects, with similar tumor types, undergoing similar therapies, and under more controlled conditions. (p. 55)

Pillemer and Light (1980) suggest that we must go beyond even this approach to conducting statistical analyses of the outcomes of relevant studies. This type of analysis is referred to as *meta-analysis*. This approach allows consideration to be given to such factors as sample size, level of significance and variables examined. This approach would allow one to make objective rather than subjective evaluations of the existing findings, leading to more valid conclusions.

Packaging

Others believe that we must go beyond even this approach to developing a "package" such as is done in industry. Using this strategy, we would synthesize the findings and develop a step-by-step description of how the findings are to be used in the practice setting. This package would then be published in the clinical journals or developed in a more sophisticated way to be sold to health care institutions. The CURN project packaged its programs and published them in book form.

If findings are to be translated or "packaged," whose responsibility is it? There is some justification for arguing that it is the responsibility of the profession. The CURN project was conducted by the Michigan Nurses Association. Perhaps our professional organizations should address this problem. Sigma Theta Tau, for example, with its emphasis on research, could consider this an addition to its goals.

If the research is funded, should the funding source provide sufficient funds for the researcher to perform this activity? If so, researchers who write grant proposals must include this activity as a budget item and explain what activities will be conducted to achieve diffusion, packaging and adoption. This makes the researcher accountable for these activities. However, would funding sources provide additional money for this activity or simply decrease the amount provided for the actual research process? Another possible consequence would be that funding sources would increase grant funding to achieve diffusion but would then fund fewer proposals. Since cognitive clustering and packaging require different and additional skills and time, the researcher may be unable to accomplish these new tasks without external funding.

Groups of professional colleagues within an institution or within a nursing organization could be effective in gathering the findings from a specific topic of nursing research and synthesizing the findings. The group could then package the findings for use within the institution or by the members of the nursing organization. Within an institution, the group could then include the clustered findings in such institutional guidelines as procedure manuals, standards of care and outcome measures. The inservice coordinator could assist by offering a program to allow presentation of the clustered findings to the nursing staff. This same type of procedure could occur on a nursing unit that provided a specialized type of care.

Research conferences are being held with increasing frequency. The purpose of the conferences is to communicate research findings to nurse clinicians. If cognitive clustering or packaging is necessary to the clinical use of research findings, part of each conference should be devoted to presentations in which clustering or packaging is discussed. Written materials should be prepared for distribution to the clinicians. Group discussions after such a presentation might facilitate problem solving related to utilization of the findings. These discussions would help move participants from the knowledge stage to the persuasion stage.

Using a Linker

The "linker" described by Havelock (1970) would be in an ideal position for translation and packaging of research findings. But who, in nursing, would be the linker? What educational level would be necessary for effective functioning in this capacity? The clinically based, doctorally prepared nurse researcher could be effective in these activities; however, there are few nurses with these credentials who are working with clinical facilities. The clinical nurse specialist may be a more available linker. The inservice coordinator might also serve in this capacity, particularly if the individual were educationally prepared at the masters level.

Frequently, staff nurses within an institution look to the inservice coordinator to keep them informed of innovations in nursing practice. Yet, inservice coordinators usually do not view the communication of research findings as one of their responsibilities, and thus, have not usually "kept up" with current nursing research, much less attempted to synthesize or package it. Perhaps an organized group of inservice coordinators could consider accepting that responsibility as a group.

A new role might be developed within the health care institution that would have one major responsibility: the packaging of current research for utilization by practicing nurses within the institution. This idea might be particularly useful to the new complex hospital systems that own and operate a number of hospitals and other health care programs.

PERSUASION

Persuasion assumes prior knowledge of the innovation and is associated with values, attitudes and norms. The extent of persuasion necessary is related to the degree of uncertainty associated with the particular innovation. According to Rogers, persuasion is most effective in one-to-one interactions with near-peers. In order to persuade, one must first be convinced of the value of something and then must have used the innovation. To be a near-peer, one must be working closely with a person and be similar in education, values and social status.

Hospital-Based Nurses

Who is a near-peer of the front line clinical nurse? Obviously, the closest near-peer is another clinical nurse. However, unless the clinical nurse has used the innovation, persuasion is out of the question. Other reasonably close peers in the hospital setting are the supervisors, clinical specialists and inservice coordinators, although these individuals are likely to have a higher educational level. Of this group, the clinical specialist is most likely to be knowledgeable about research, to value its use and to have used a specific clinical innovation. However, this has not been an expectation of the clinical specialist role in the past. If the clinical specialist is to function in this manner, relevant content on utilization must be included in the educational program designed to prepare clinical specialists. The behavior must be accepted and the skills must be developed in order to achieve it.

Community-Based Nurses

Outside the institution, professional colleagues would be the most probable near-peers. Where do near-peers interact outside institutional settings? How do we facilitate persuasive interactions about research findings during these interactions? In areas of practice such as home health care, school nursing, industrial nursing and other dimensions of community health care, nurses tend to interact during the period when activities of patient care are being recorded and when the staff gathers for regularly scheduled group conferences. This is appropriate timing for the introduction of discussions about innovations in care. Nurses tend to be at desks in close proximity to one another. Bulletin boards are available, and there are usually tables at which discussions can occur. Interactions about innovations could occur in these situations. Knowledge of innovations can be introduced by the posting, sharing and discussing of research reports. Moving from this point to persuasion would require that an innovator or early adopter choose to utilize the findings and bring that experience back to the group for further discussion.

The nurse practitioner in a clinic setting and other nurses who tend to be rather isolated in their work often have established opportunities, both social and professional, to meet with nursing colleagues. These meetings can provide opportunities for sharing experiences about clinical practice and can lead to discussions about innovations in practice.

Persuasion Situations

In what situations can planned persuasion activities occur? At professional nursing meetings, presentations could be made by nurses who have utilized a specific set of research findings. The presentation could be followed by group discussion. An even more effective approach would be to encourage nurses at the meeting to implement the innovation and share their experiences at the next meeting.

Committees or groups within an institution, after synthesizing a set of findings, could implement them within their own practice or on a selected nursing unit. The results could then be presented to a larger group of nursing staff. Since the nurses work within the same institution, there are opportunities for later contacts by interested nurses or those attempting to implement the findings.

DECISION

When an individual practitioner is making a decision to use an innovation, the decision itself usually occurs within the person's thinking process. It is not public and may not be verbally expressed except, perhaps, to close colleagues. However, taking a public stand and committing oneself to an action increases the probability that the action will actually be taken. Therefore, at meetings at which persuasion has been part of the activity, seeking commitment to attempt the innovation may increase the incidence of attempts. However, too much pressure could have the opposite effect.

When institutional committees or groups of nurses are considering implementing an innovation, the decision point may be more clearly evident. In some cases, a vote may be taken. A shift in action may occur, with activities beginning for planning the methods of implementation. When the innovation is institutional, decision making may be distributed through several levels of the hierarchy. Thus, a decision at one level may lead to contact with another official who must approve the action.

In keeping with the guidelines of planned change, institutional changes are more likely to be effective if all those affected by the change have a voice in the decision and/or in planning the change. Thus, decision making may also be extended downward in the hierarchy. Nurses involved in the initial work may have to shift back to the knowledge and persuasion stages with the staff nurses prior to the request for a decision if the staff nurses have not been aware of the activities of the committee.

IMPLEMENTATION

Implementing an innovation can be very simple or extremely complex, depending on the innovation. In some cases, a long period of time will be spent in planning the implementation after the decision is made. In other cases, implementation can begin immediately. Usually, a great deal of support is needed during initial implementation of an innovation. As with any new activity, the unexpected will often occur. The new innovator often does not know how to interpret events that occur. Contact with a person more experienced in the innovation can make the difference between continuation and rejection of the innovation.

CONFIRMATION

After the innovation has been implemented, the clinician will continue to seek feedback from near-peers related to the innovation. Even if near-peers have not used the innovation, they will often have observed the activity or discussed it with their colleagues. Their reactions to the change in nursing practice will greatly influence the nurse attempting an innovation. If near-peers disapprove or provide negative feedback, the nurse will often abandon the innovation. This is most likely to occur when using the innovation requires a change in attitude or norms. Only the innovator, who has sources of support outside the social system or the very determined nurse with a strong ego will be able to continue an innovation when there is group disapproval.

Do We Have Nursing Research That Is Ready For Clinical Implementation?

There is disagreement among the scholars in nursing about the appropriateness of clinical utilization of nursing research at its present stage in development. Many studies in the literature are exploratory or descriptive, not prescriptive. However, we believe that the profession of nursing must begin a careful examination of exactly what clinical studies are available and to determine what steps should be taken before the information can be useful in clinical practice. In addition, students and practicing nurses must learn how to search the literature for available research on a selected topic, critique it and cluster the findings.

Conclusions

Nursing's work in the area of utilization of research is just beginning. Our decisions in relation to utilization will have a major impact on the direction of nursing in the future. Nursing is changing rapidly at the present time. The nurse is becoming more autonomous, more accountable and more highly educated. A shift in the site of nursing practice is occurring, with nursing practice moving from hospital settings into the community. There is a greater emphasis on health, health practices and health promotion. As these changes occur, the institution will play less of a role in controlling the practice of the nurse. Responsibilities for diffusion and adoption activities will fall increasingly upon the profession and the individual nurse. These responsibilities must be carefully considered by both the individual nurse and by the profession as a whole. An appendix is provided with this chapter that includes major research topics and studies conducted in these areas. These studies were identified to facilitate the clustering of findings for utilization in practice.

Summary

Most people believe that a good idea will sell itself. Unfortunately, this is seldom true. There are nursing research findings that clearly warrant utilization that are not being used. Understanding the process of research utilization and developing strategies to achieve it are critical to nursing. There are three theories that have been the framework for most research in the area of utilization. These theories are Rogers' theory of diffusion of innovations, Havelock's theory of linker systems and Lewin's field theory, which describes the process of change. Rogers is an expert and noted theorist in the field of knowledge diffusion and utilization. He has conducted research related to diffusion for 25 years. The key elements of *diffusion* are innovation, communication channels, time, decision making, innovativeness and social system. The types of *utilization* identified by Rogers include direct application, reinvention and indirect effects. Havelock added a new dimension to current knowledge of utilization theory by proposing the development of a *linker system*. This linker system is used to transfer new knowledge, skills or products (innovations) from resource systems (researchers and their publications) to user systems (practitioners) for dissemination. Lewin's theory includes the facet of *change agent*. Change agent is an individual or group, external to the system, that is used to initiate and facilitate the change process.

Practitioners have a variety of reasons for utilizing research findings. Some practitioners read research and attend research conferences just to increase their general knowledge base. Other practitioners seek research findings to answer a practice problem. Consultants sometimes provide practitioners with research findings. There are barriers, however, to the utilization of research findings. One barrier is a social system that promotes stability and opposes change. Another barrier is the lack of communication between the university-based researcher and the institutionally based practitioner.

Although nursing's interest in utilization strategies is fairly recent, three programs have been developed to attempt to increase utilization of nursing research findings. These projects are the WCHEN Regional Program for Nursing Research Development, the Conduct and Utilization of Research in Nursing (CURN) project and the Nursing Child Assessment Satellite Training (NCAST) project. Rogers, Havelock and Lewin's theories were used as the theoretical frameworks for these projects. The WCHEN project was the first major nursing project to address research utilization in nursing. A part of this project focused on developing skills in critiquing research, using change theory and diffusion of innovations. Research findings were examined and merged with other activities for implementation in practice. The CURN project was developed to increase the utilization of research findings in the following ways: dissemination of findings, facilitating organizational modifications necessary to implementation and encouraging collaborative research that was directly transferable to clinical practice. Clinical studies were critiqued, protocols were developed from the findings and implementation was initiated on a test unit within a hospital. The protocols developed during this project have been published. The focus of the NCAST project was educational and directed at the individual nurse practitioner. The intent of the project was to examine methods of translating and disseminating research findings in practice.

Stetler, a nursing theorist, developed a model for research utilization. Stetler proposed that utilization involves a series of judgmental activities by the individual nurse in the role of caregiver, educator or manager or as a leader making decisions that will mandate the actions of other nurses. These judgments involve validation, comparative evaluation and decision making. The model considers utilization as an essential component of professional nursing practice. The professional nurse must continually seek the outcomes of current research, evaluate their potential for use in practice and modify practice continually as new knowledge becomes available. The problems of and possible approaches toward increasing the utilization of findings in nursing were examined using Rogers' five decision-making steps: knowledge, persuasion, decision, implementation and confirmation. Nursing's work in the area of utilization of research is just beginning. Decisions related to utilization will have a major impact on the direction of nursing in the future.

References

Axford, R. & Cutchen, L. (1977). Using nursing research to improve preoperative care. *Journal of Nursing Administration*, 7(10), 16–20.

Barbichon, G. (1968). The diffusion of scientific and technical knowledge. *Journal of Social Issues*, 24(2), 157–159.

Barnard, K. E. (1980). Knowledge for practice: directions for the future. *Nursing Research*, 29(4), 208–212.

Barnard, K. E. (1982). Proceedings of the 1982 Conference of the Western Society for Research in Nursing. The research cycle: nursing, the profession, the discipline. *Western Journal of Nursing Research*, 4(3), 1–12.

Barnard, K. E. (1984). MCN keys to research: knowledge development. *MCN*, 9(3), 175.

Barnes, B. (1982). On the implications of a body of knowledge. *Knowledge: Creation, Diffusion, Utilization*, 4(1), 95–110.

Batey, M. V. (1975). Research: its dissemination and utilization in nursing practice. *Washington State Journal of Nursing*, 47, 6–9.

Breu, C. (1983). President's message: the research process in the intensive care unit: where does it break down? *Heart and Lung*, 12(6), 30A, 32A.

Breu, C. & Dracup, K. (1976). Implementing nursing research in a critical care setting. *Journal of Nursing Administration*, 6(10), 14–17.

Brooten, D. A. (1982). Guest editorial: Is soft sell enough? *Nursing Research*, 31(4), 195.

Burr, W. R., Mead, D. E. & Rollins, B. C. (1973). A model for the application of research findings by the educator and counselor: research to theory to practice. *The Family Coordinator*, 22(3), 285–290.

Butts, P. A. (1982). Dissemination of nursing research findings. *Image*, 14(2), 62–64.

Castles, M. R. (1975). Continuing education: a practitioner's guide to utilization of research findings. *JOGN Nursing*, 4(1), 50–53.

Clark, N. M. & Lenburg, C. B. (1980). Knowledge-informed behavior and the nursing culture: a preliminary study. *Nursing Research*, 29(4), 244–249.

Coe, R. M. & Barnhill, E. A. (1967). Social dimensions of failure in innovation. *Human Organization*, 26(3), 149–156.

Cohen, J. (1959). Factors of resistance to the resources of the behavioral sciences. *Journal of Legal Education*, 12, 67–70.

Crane, D. (1970). The nature of scientific communication and influence. *International Social Science Journal*, 22(1), 28–41.

CURN Project. *Using research to improve nursing practice*. New York: Grune & Stratton, Inc. Series of Clinical Protocols: *Clean intermittent catheterization* (1982), *Closed urinary drainage systems* (1981), *Distress reduction through sensory preparation* (1981), *Intravenous cannula change* (1981), *Mutual goal setting in patient care* (1982), *Pain: deliberative nursing interventions* (1982), *Preventing decubitus ulcers* (1981), *Reducing diarrhea in tube-fed patients* (1981), *Structured preoperative teaching* (1981).

Dexter, L. A. (1965). On the use and abuse of social science by practitioners. *The American Behavioral Scientist*, 9(3), 25–29.

Diers, D. (1972). Application of research to nursing practice. *Image*, 5(1), 2–11.

Dracup, K. A. & Breu, C. S. (1978). Using nursing research findings to meet the needs of grieving spouses. *Nursing Research*, 27(4), 212–216.

Duffy, M. E. (1985a). Research in practice: the time has come. *Nursing and Health Care*, 6(3), 127.

Duffy, M. E. (1985b). Research utilization: what's it all about? *Nursing and Health Care*, 6(9), 474–475.

Duffy, M. E. (1985c). Strengthening communication signals to build a research-based practice. *Nursing and Health Care*, 6(5), 238–239.

Dunn, W. N. (1983). Measuring knowledge use. *Knowledge: Creating, Diffusion, Utilization*, 5(1), 120–133.

Engstrom, J. L. (1984). University, agency, and collaborative models for nursing research: an overview. *Image: The Journal of Nursing Scholarship*, 16(3), 76–80.

Fawcett, J. (1980). A declaration of nursing independence: the relation of theory and research to nursing practice. *Journal of Nursing Administration*, 10(6), 36–39.

Fawcett, J. (1982). Utilization of nursing research findings. *Image*, 14(2), 57–59.

Fawcett, J. (1983). Contemporary nursing research: its relevance for nursing practice. In N. L. Chaska (Ed.), *The nursing profession: a time to speak* (pp. 169–182). New York: McGraw-Hill Book Company.

Glaser, E. M. (1973). Knowledge transfer and institutional change. *Professional Psychology*, 4, 434–444.

Glaser, E. M., Abelson, H. H. & Garrison, K. N. (1983). *Putting knowledge to use*. San Francisco: Josey-Bass.

Gortner, S. R. (1975). Research for a practice profession. *Nursing Research*, 24(3), 193–197.

Gortner, S. R., Bloch, D. & Phillips, T. P. (1976). Contributions of nursing research to patient care. *Journal of Nursing Administration*, 6(3), 22–28.

Hakel, M. D., Sorcher, M., Beer, M. & Moses, J. L. (1982). *Making it happen: designing research with implementation in mind*. Beverly Hills: Sage Publications.

Haller, K. B., Reynolds, M. A. & Horsley, J. A. (1979). Developing research-based innovation protocols: process, criteria, and issues. *Research in Nursing and Health*, 2(1), 45–51.

Harrell, J. S. (1986). Needed: nurse engineers to link theory and practice. *Nursing Outlook*, 34(4), 196–198.

Havelock, R. G. (1970). *A guide to innovation in education*. Center for Research on Utilization of Scientific Knowledge, Institute for Social Research, The University of Michigan, Ann Arbor, Michigan.

Havelock, R. G. (1973). *The change agent's guide to innovation in education*. Englewood Cliffs, New Jersey: Educational Technology Publications.

Havelock, R. G. (1974). *Ideal systems for research utilization: four alternatives*. Contract 22-P-55893/5-01, Social and Rehabilitation Service, U. S. Department of Health, Education & Welfare, Washington, D. C.

Havelock, R. G. & Lingwood, D. A. (1973). *R&D utilization strategies and functions: an analytical comparison of four systems*. Center for Research on Utilization of Scientific Knowledge, Institute for Social Research, University of Michigan, Ann Arbor, Michigan.

Horsley, J. A., Crane, J. & Bingle, J. D. (1978). Research utilization as an organizational process. *Journal of Nursing Administration*, 8(7), 4–6.

Horsley, J. A., Crane, J., Crabtree, M. K. & D. J. Wood. (1983). *Using research to improve nursing practice: a guide, CURN Project*. New York: Grune & Stratton, Inc.

Jacox, A. & Prescott, P. (1978). Determining a study's relevance for clinical practice. *American Journal of Nursing*, 78(11), 1882–1889.

Johnson, J. E. (1978). Translating research to practice. In American Nurses' Association (Ed.), *Power, nursing's challenge for change* (pp. 125–133). Kansas City, Missouri: American Nurses' Association.

Jung, C. & Lippitt, R. (1966). The study of change as a concept in research utilization. *Theory Into Practice*, 5(1), 25–29.

Ketefian, S. (1975). Application of selected nursing research findings into nursing practice: a pilot study. *Nursing Research*, 24(2), 89–92.

Ketefian, S. (1980). Using research in practice: selected issues in the translation of research to nursing practice. *Western Journal of Nursing Research*, 2(1), 429–431.

King, D., Barnard, K. E. & Hoehn, R. (1981). Disseminating the results of nursing research. *Nursing Outlook*, 29(3), 164–169.

Krone, K. P. & Loomis, M. E. (1982). Developing practice-relevant research: a model that worked. *Journal of Nursing Administration*, 12(4), 38–41.

Krueger, J. C. (1978). Utilization of nursing research: the planning process. *Journal of Nursing Administration*, 8(1), 6–9.

Krueger, J. C., Nelson, A. H. & Wolanin, M. O. (1978). *Nursing research: development, collaboration, and utilization*. Germantown, Maryland: Aspen Systems Corporation.

Lindeman, C. A. & Krueger, J. C. (1977). Increasing the quality, quantity, and use of nursing research. *Nursing Outlook*, 25(7), 450–454.

Lindsey, A. M. (1985). Building the knowledge base for practice, part 1: nausea and vomiting. *Oncology Nursing Forum*, 12(1), 49–56.

Loomis, M. E. (1985). Knowledge utilization and research utilization in nursing. *Image: The Journal of Nursing Scholarship*, 17(2), 35–39.

Mayo, C. & LaFrance, M. (1977). *Evaluating research in social psychology: a guide for the consumer*. Monterey, California: Brooks/Cole Publishing Company.

Mercer, R. T. (1984). Nursing research: the bridge to excellence in practice. *Image: The Journal of Nursing Scholarship*, 16(2), 47–51.

Miller, J. R. & Messenger, S. R. (1978). Obstacles to applying nursing research findings. *American Journal of Nursing*, 78(4), 632–634.

Mulkay, M. J. (1972). Conformity and innovation in science. *The Sociological Review Monograph*, 18, 5–23.

Murdaugh, C. (1982). Using research in practice: can (cardiac) patients be taught effectively in the critical care setting? *Focus on AACN*, 9, 11–14.

Nuckolls, K. B. (1972). Nursing research—good for what? *Nursing Forum*, 11(4), 374–384.

O'Connell, K. A. & Duffey, M. (1976). Research in nursing practice: its nature and direction. *Image*, 8(1), 6–12.

Pelz, D. & Horsley, J. (1981). Measuring utilization of nursing research. In J. Ciarlo, (Ed.), *Utilizing evaluation*. Beverly Hills: Sage Publications.

Phillips, L. R. F. (1986). *A clinician's guide to the critique and utilization of nursing research*. Norwalk, Connecticut: Appleton-Century-Crofts.

Pillemer, D. B. & Light, R. J. (1980). Synthesizing outcomes: how to use research evidence from many studies. *Harvard Educational Review*, 50(2), 176–195.

Rogers, E. M. (1983). *Diffusion of innovations* (3rd ed.). New York: The Free Press.

Rogers, E. M. & Shoemaker, F. F. (1971). *Communication of innovations: a cross-cultural approach*. New York: The Free Press.

Roper, N. (1977). Justification and use of research in nursing. *Journal of Advanced Nursing*, 2(4), 365–371.

Ropka, M. E. (1983). Utilization of research in nursing practice. *Oncology Nursing Forum*, 10(1), 92–94.

Rothman, J. (1979). Conversion and design in the research utilization process. *Journal of Social Service Research*, 2(1), 117–131.

Sherwen, L. N. & Toussie-Weingarten, C. (1983). *Analysis and application of nursing research: parent-neonate studies*. Monterey, California: Wadsworth Health Sciences Division.

Smoyak, S. A. (1976). Is practice responding to research? *American Journal of Nursing*, 76(7), 1146–1150.

Stetler, C. B. (1983). Nurses and research: responsibility and involvement. *Journal of the National Intravenous Therapy Association*, 6(3), 207–212.

Stetler, C. B. (1985). Research utilization: defining the concept. *Image: The Journal of Nursing Scholarship*, 17(2), 40–44.

Stetler, C. B. & Marram, G. (1976). Evaluating research findings for applicability in practice. *Nursing Outlook*, 24(9), 559–563.

Stevenson, J. S. (1977). Editorial: Nursing research and the industrial community. *Image*, 9(1), 3.

Stokes, J. E. (1981). Utilization of research findings by staff nurses. In S. D. Krampitz & N. Pavlovich (Eds.), *Readings for nursing research* (pp. 227–234). St. Louis: The C. V. Mosby Company.

Sundquist, J. L. (1978). Research brokerage: the weak link. In L. E. Lynn Jr. (Ed.), *Knowledge and policy: the uncertain connection* (pp. 126–144). Washington, D. C.: National Academy of Sciences.

Towell, D. (1979). A 'social systems' approach to research and change in nursing care. *International Journal of Nursing Studies*, 16(1), 111–121.

Van De Vall, M. (1975). Utilization and methodology of applied social research: four complementary models. *The Journal of Applied Behavioral Science*, 11(1), 14–38.

Walker, L. O. (1983). Theory and research in the development of nursing as a discipline: retrospect and prospect. In N. L. Chaska (Ed.), *The nursing profession: a time to speak* (pp. 406–415). New York: McGraw-Hill Book Company.

Weiss, C. J. (1980). Knowledge creep and decision accretion. *Knowledge: Creation, Diffusion, Utilization*, 1(3), 381–404.

Wichita, C. (1977). Treating and preventing constipation in nursing home residents. *Journal of Gerontological Nursing*, 3(6), 35–39.

Zaltman, G. & Wallendorf, M. (1983). *Consumer behavior: basic findings and managerial implications* (2nd ed.). New York: John Wiley & Sons.

Appendix

Blood Pressure

Dawson, C. (1985). Hypertension, perceived clinician empathy, and patient self-disclosure. *Research in Nursing and Health*, 8(2), 191–198.

Hellmann, R. & Grimm, S. A. (1984). The influence of talking on diastolic blood pressure readings. *Research in Nursing and Health*, 7(4), 253–256.

Swain, M. A. & Steckel, S. B. (1981). Influencing adherence among hypertensives. *Research in Nursing and Health*, 4(1), 213–222.

Tachovsky, B. J. (1985). Indirect auscultatory blood pressure measurement at two sites in the arm. *Research in Nursing and Health*, 8(2), 125–129

Thomas, S. A., Friedmann, E., Lottes, L. S., Gresty, S., Miller, C. & Lynch, J. J. (1984). Changes in nurses' blood pressure and heart rate while communicating. *Research in Nursing and Health*, 7(2), 119–126.

Breast Engorgement

Bristol, W. M. (1966). Comparative effectiveness of compressional and supporting breast binders in suppressing lactation. *Nursing Research*, 15(3), 203–206.

Brooten, D. A., Brown, L. P., Hollingsworth, A. O., Tanis, J. L. & Donlen, J. (1983). A comparison of four treatments to prevent and control breast pain and engorgement in nonnursing mothers. *Nursing Research*, 32(4), 225–229.

Dickson, E. K. & Post, C. W. (1981). Breast engorgement in non-nursing mothers following administration of estrogen-containing lactation suppressant medication. *Issues in Health Care of Women*, 3(2), 71–80.

Meserve, Y. (1982). Management of postpartum breast engorgement in nonbreastfeeding women by mechanical extraction of milk. *Journal of Nurse-Midwifery*, 27(3), 3–8.

Breastfeeding

Albers, R. M. (1981). Emotional support for the breast-feeding mother. *Issues in Comprehensive Pediatric Nursing*, 5(2), 109–124.

Arafat, I., Allen, D. E. & Fox, J. E. (1981). Maternal practice and attitudes toward breastfeeding. *JOGN Nursing*, 10(2), 91–95.

Atkinson, L. D. (1979). Prenatal nipple conditioning for breastfeeding. *Nursing Research*, 28(5), 267–271.

Beske, E. J. & Garvis, M. S. (1982). Important factors in breast-feeding success. *MCN*, 7(3), 174–179.

Brown, M. S. & Hurlock, J. T. (1975). Preparation of the breast for breast-feeding. *Nursing Research*, 24(6), 448–451.

Chapman, J. J., Macey, M. J., Keegan, M., Borum, P. & Bennett, S. (1985). Concerns of breast-feeding mothers from birth to 4 months. *Nursing Research*, 34(6), 374–377.

Cohen, S. A. (1980). Postpartum teaching and the subsequent use of milk supplements. *Birth and the Family Journal*, 7(3), 163–167.

Crowder, D. S. (1981). Maternity nurses' knowledge of factors promoting successful breast-feeding: a survey of two hospitals. *JOGN Nursing*, 10(1), 28–30.

Gulick, E. E. (1982). Informal correlates of successful breast-feeding. *MCN*, 7(6), 370–375.

Hall, J. M. (1978). Influencing breastfeeding success. *JOGN Nursing*, 7(6), 28–30.

Hayes, B. (1981). Inconsistencies among nurses in breast-feeding knowledge and counseling. *JOGN Nursing*, 10(6), 430–433.

Hughes, R. B. (1984). Satisfaction with one's body and success in breastfeeding. *Issues in Comprehensive Pediatric Nursing*, 7(2/3), 141–153.

Whitley, N. (1978). Preparation for breastfeeding: a one-year follow-up of 34 nursing mothers. *JOGN Nursing*, 7(3), 44–48.

Wiles, L. S. (1984). The effect of prenatal breastfeeding education on breastfeeding success and maternal perception of the infant. *JOGN Nursing*, 13(4), 253–257.

Childbirth Education

Beck, N. C., Siegel, L. J., Davidson, N. P., Kormeier, S., Breitenstein, A. & Hall, D. G. (1980). The prediction of pregnancy outcome: maternal preparation, anxiety and attitudinal sets. *Journal of Psychosomatic Research*, 24(3/4), 343–351.

Bernardini, J. Y., Maloni, J. A. & Stegman, C. E. (1983). Neuromuscular control of childbirth-prepared women during the first stage of labor. *JOGN Nursing*, 12(2), 105–111.

Bowen, S. M. & Miller, B. C. (1980). Paternal attachment behavior as related to presence at delivery and preparenthood classes: a pilot study. *Nursing Research*, 29(5), 307–311.

Dalzell, I. (1965). Evaluation of a prenatal teaching program. *Nursing Research*, 14(2), 160–163.

Furr, P. A. & Kirgis, C. A. (1982). A nurse-midwifery approach to early mother-infant acquaintance. *Journal of Nurse-Midwifery*, 27(5), 10–14.

Gaziano, E. P., Garvis, M. & Levine, E. (1979). An evaluation of childbirth education for the clinic patient. *Birth and the Family Journal*, 6(2), 89–94.

Glazer, G. (1980). Anxiety levels and concerns among pregnant women. *Research in Nursing and Health*, 3(3), 107–113.

Halstead, J. & Fredrickson, T. (1978). Evaluation of a prepared childbirth program. *JOGN Nursing*, 7(3), 39–42.

Humenick, S. S. & Marchbanks, P. (1981). Validation of a scale to measure relaxation in childbirth education classes. *Birth and the Family Journal*, 8(3), 145–150.

Nunnally, D. M. & Aguiar, M. B. (1974). Patients' evaluation of their prenatal and delivery care. *Nursing Research*, 23(6), 469–474.

Perry, S. E. (1983). Parents' perceptions of their newborn following structured interactions. *Nursing Research*, 32(4), 208–212.

Thordarson, L. & Costanzo, G. A. (1976). An evaluation of the effectiveness of an educational program for expectant parents. *Canadian Journal of Public Health*, 67(8), 117–121.

Timm, M. M. (1979). Prenatal education evaluation. *Nursing Research*, 28(6), 338–342.

Whitley, N. (1979). A comparison of prepared childbirth couples and conventional prenatal class couples. *JOGN Nursing*, 8(2), 109–111.

Willmuth, R., Weaver, L. & Borenstein, J. (1978). Satisfaction with prepared childbirth and locus of control. *JOGN Nursing*, 7(3), 33–37.

Communication

Stetler, C. B. (1977). Relationship of perceived empathy to nurses' communication. *Nursing Research*, 26(6), 432–438.

Wallston, K. A. & Wallston, B. S. (1975). A role-playing simulation approach toward studying: nurses' decisions to listen to patients. *Nursing Research*, 24(1), 16–22.

Decubitus Ulcers

Becker, L. & Goodmote, C. (1984). Treating pressure sores with or without antacid. *American Journal of Nursing*, 84(3), 351–352.

Childs, L. & Rimmington, P. M. (1983). Decubitus ulcers: a survey picture at two hospitals. *Australian Nurses Journal*, 13(1), 35, 52.

Diekmann, J. M. (1984). Use of dental irrigating device in the treatment of decubitus ulcers. *Nursing Research*, 33(5), 303–305.

Gerber, R. M. & Van Ort, S. R. (1979). Topical application of insulin in decubitus ulcers. *Nursing Research*, 28(1), 16–19.

Goldstone, L. A. & Roberts, B. V. (1980). A preliminary discriminant function analysis of elderly orthopedic patients who will or will not contract a pressure sore. *International Journal of Nursing Studies*, 17(1), 17–23.

Gosnell, D. J. (1973). An assessment tool to identify pressure sores. *Nursing Research*, 22(1), 55–59.

Hayter, J. & McPhetridge, L. M. (1976). Study of decubitus care. *Journal of Gerontological Nursing*, 2(3), 24–25.

Lee, L. K. & Ambrus, J. L. (1975). Collagenase therapy for decubitus ulcers. *Geriatrics*, 30(5), 91–93, 97–98.

Porreca, R. C. & Chagares, R. M. (1983). Op-Site: a treatment for pressure sores in the orthopedic patient population. *Orthopedic Nursing*, 2(5), 30–36.

Roberts, B. V. & Goldstone, L. A. (1979). A survey of pressure sores in the over sixties on two orthopedic wards. *International Journal of Nursing Studies*, 16(4), 355–364.

Steffel, P. E. S., Schenk, E. A. P. & Walker, S. L. (1980). Reducing devices for pressure sores with respect to nursing care procedures. *Nursing Research*, 29(4), 228–230.

Taylor, V. (1979). Intact heel decubitus: an innovative treatment with a special cleansing sponge. *ARN Journal*, 4, 9–10.

Van Ort, S. R. & Gerber, R. M. (1976). Topical application of insulin in the treatment of decubitus ulcers: a pilot study. *Nursing Research*, 25(1), 9–12.

Verhonick, P. J. (1961). Decubitus ulcer observations measured objectively. *Nursing Research*, 10(4), 211–214.

Verhonick, P. J., Lewis, D. W. & Goller, H. O. (1972). Thermography in the study of decubitus ulcers. *Nursing Research*, 21(3), 233–237.

Williams, A. (1972). A study of factors contributing to skin breakdown. *Nursing Research*, 21(3), 238–243.

Discharge Planning

Cagan, J. (1983). Evaluation of a discharge planning tool for use with families of high-risk infants. *JOGN Nursing*, 12(4), 275–281.

Chamorro, I. L., Davis, M. L., Green, D. & Kramer, M. (1973). Development of an instrument to measure premature infant behavior and care-taker activities. *Nursing Research*, 22(4), 300–309.

Given, B., Given, C. W. & Simoni, L. E. (1979). Relationships of processes of care to patient outcomes. *Nursing Research*, 28(2), 85–93.

Watkins, J. D., Williams, T. F., Martin, D. A., Hogan, M. D. & Anderson, E. (1967). A study of diabetic patients at home. *American Journal of Public Health*, 57(3), 452–459.

Electronic Fetal Monitoring

Applegate, J., Haverkamp, A. D., Orleans, M. & Tayler, C. (1979). Electronic fetal monitoring: implications for obstetrical nursing. *Nursing Research*, 28(6), 369–371.

Empathy

Hardin, S. B. & Halaris, A. L. (1983). Nonverbal communication of patients and high and low empathy nurses. *Journal of Psychosocial Nursing and Mental Health Services*, 21(1), 14–20.

Hills, M. D. & Knowles, D. (1983). Nurses' levels of empathy and respect in simulated interactions with patients. *International Journal of Nursing Studies*, 20(2), 83–87.

Margaret, M. H. (1981). Empathic ability in a psychiatric setting. *Nursing Journal of India*, 72(11), 311–314.

Staller, C. B. (1977). Relationship of perceived empathy to nurses' communication. *Nursing Research*, 26(6), 432–435.

Hypoxia During Endotracheal Suctioning

Baun, M. M. (1984). Physiological determinants of a clinically successful method of endotracheal suctioning. *Western Journal of Nursing Research*, 6(2), 213–225.

Belling, D., Kelley, R. R. & Simon, R. (1978). Use of the swivel adaptor aperture during suctioning to prevent hypoxemia in the mechanically ventilated patient. *Heart and Lung*, 7(2), 320–322.

Jung, R. C. & Newman, J. (1982). Minimizing hypoxia during endotracheal airway care. *Heart and Lung*, 11(3), 208–212.

Indwelling Urinary Catheters

Castle, M. & Osterhout, S. (1974). Urinary tract catheterization and associated infection. *Nursing Research*, 23(2), 170–174.

Cleland, V., Cox, F., Berggren, H. & MacInnis, M. R. (1971). Prevention of bacteriuria in female patients with indwelling catheters. *Nursing Research*, 20(4), 309–318.

Kennedy, A. P. & Brocklehurst, J. C. (1982). The nursing management of patients with long-term indwelling catheters. *Journal of Advanced Nursing*, 7(5), 411–417.

Kennedy, A. P., Brocklehurst, J. C. & Lye, M. D. W. (1983). Factors related to the problems of long-term catheterization. *Journal of Advanced Nursing*, 8(3), 207–212.

Infection Control in IV Therapy

Amonsen, S. & Gren, J. E. (1978). Relationship between length of time and contamination in open intravenous solutions. *Nursing Research*, 27(5), 372–374.

Arras, B. & McKnight, T. (1978). Catheter materials and associated complications from a nursing standpoint. *American Journal of Intravenous Therapy*, 5(5), 32, 37, 42.

Bair, J. N. & Petersen, R. V. (1979). The status of the IV therapy team in the genesis of intravenous therapy complications. *American Journal of Intravenous Therapy and Clinical Nutrition*, 6(5), 39, 43–44, 53–56, 58.

Begala, J. E., Maher, K. & Cherry, J. D. (1982). Risk of infection associated with the use of Broviac and Hickman catheters. *American Journal of Infection Control*, 10(1), 17–23.

Beideman, M. E., Herman, A., Peeples, O. S. & Terry, T. (1979). A clinical overview study of infusion phlebitis. *American Journal of Intravenous Therapy*, 6(2), 23–26, 31–32, 34.

Brown, B. J., Mackowiak, P. A. & Smith, J. W. (1980). Care of veins during intravenous therapy: incidence of phlebitis as related to knowledge and performance. *American Journal of Infection Control*, 8(4), 107–111.

Geiger, E. M. & Jansen, G. A. (1976). Complications associated with the use of plastic catheters. *American Journal of Intravenous Therapy*, 3(6), 42–44, 46.

Hanson, R. L. (1977). Nursing research priorities: choice or chance. A comparison of the rate of complications with heparin-lock and keep-open IVs. WICHE Publication. *Communicating Nursing Research*, 8, 188–200.

Johnstone, J. D. (1982). Infrequent infections associated with Hickman catheters. *Cancer Nursing*, 5(2), 125–129.

Nichols, E. G., Barstow, R. E. & Cooper, D. (1983). Relationship between incidence of phlebitis and frequency of changing IV tubing and percutaneous site. *Nursing Research*, 32(4), 247–252.

Ross, S. A. (1972). Infusion phlebitis: selected factors. *Nursing Research*, 21(4), 313–318.

Samson, O. D. & Watson, C. L. (1977). A question of safety. The catheter vs the needle. *American Journal of Intravenous Therapy*, 4(3), 7–8, 11–12.

Trent, B. A. (1984). The effects of utilization of an IV therapy team upon the incidence of IV peripheral-associated phlebitis. *NITA*, 7(4), 295–306.

Management of Hypotensive Crisis in Hemodialysis

Chrystal, C. & Weinzerl, C. (1978). The creation and correction of blood pressure crises in hemodialysis patients. *Journal of the American Association of Nephrology Nurses and Technicians*, 5(2), 89–96.

Coons, M. H. (1984). Evaluation of hypotensive episodes during maintenance hemodialysis in patients with impaired cardiovascular function. *ANNA Journal*, 11(5), 45–51.

Williams, J. A. (1981). Hypotensive crises: identifying the high-risk patient on hemodialysis. *Heart and Lung*, 10(2), 309–316.

Maternal Role Development

Avant, K. C. (1981). Anxiety as a potential factor affecting maternal attachment. *JOGN Nursing*, 10(6), 416-419.

Cannon, R. B. (1977). The development of maternal touch during early mother-infant interaction. *JOGN*, 6(2), 28–33.

Censullo, M., Lester, B. & Hoffman, J. (1985). Rhythmic patterning in mother-newborn interaction. *Nursing Research*, 34(6), 342–346.

Crawford, G. (1985). A theoretical model of support network conflict experienced by new mothers. *Nursing Research*, 34(2), 100–102.

Curry, M. A. (1979). Contact during the first hour with the wrapped or naked newborn: effect on maternal attachment behaviors at 36 hours and three months. *Birth and the Family Journal*, 6(4), 227–235.

Curry, M. A. (1982). Maternal attachment behavior and the mother's self-concept: the effect of early skin-to-skin contact. *Nursing Research*, 31(2), 73–78.

Gottleib, L. (1978). Maternal attachment in primiparas. *JOGN* Nursing, 7(1), 39–44.

Kontos, D. (1978). A study of the effects of extended mother-infant contact on maternal behavior at one and three months. *Birth and the Family Journal*, 5(3), 133–140.

Lenz, E., Soeken, K. L., Rankin, E. A. & Fischman, S. H. (1985). Sex-role attributes, gender, and postpartal perceptions of the marital relationship. *Advances in Nursing Science*, 7(3), 49–62.

Majewski, J. L. (1986). Conflicts, satisfactions, and attitudes during transition to the maternal role. *Nursing Research*, 35(1), 10–14.

Mercer, R. T. (1985). The process of maternal role attainment over the first year. *Nursing Research*, 34(4), 198–204.

Mercer, R. T. (1986). Predictors of maternal role attainment at one year post birth. *Western Journal of Nursing Research*, 8(1), 9–32.

Mercer, R. T. (1986). The relationship of developmental variables to maternal behavior. *Research in Nursing and Health*, 9(1), 25–33.

Schroeder, M. A. (1977). Is the immediate postpartum period crucial to the mother-child relationship? *JOGN* Nursing, 6(3), 37–40.

Walker, L. O., Crain, H. & Thompson, E. (1986). Maternal role attainment and identity in the postpartum period: stability and change. *Nursing Research*, 35(2), 68–71.

Medication Compliance

Batey S. R. & Ledbetter, J. E. (1982). Medication education for patients in a partial hospitalization program. *Journal of Psychosocial Nursing and Mental Health Services*, 20(7), 7–10.

Battle, E. H., Halliburton, A. & Wallston, K. A. (1982). Self medication among psychiatric patients and adherence after discharge. *Journal of Psychosocial Nursing and Mental Health Services*, 20(5), 21–28.

Chang, B. L., Uman, G. C., Linn, L. S., Ware, J. E. & Kane, R. L. (1985). Adherence to health care regimens among elderly woman. *Nursing Research*, 34(1), 27–31.

Craig, H. M. (1985). Accuracy of indirect measures of medication compliance in hypertension. *Research in Nursing and Health*, 8(1), 61–66.

Davidhizar, R. E. (1982). Compliance by persons with schizophrenia: a research issue for the nurse. *Issues in Mental Health Nursing*, 4(3), 233–255.

De Von, H. A. & Powers, M. J. (1984). Health beliefs, adjustment to illness, and control of hypertension. *Research in Nursing and Health*, 7(1), 10–16.

Durel, S. M. & Munjas, B. A. (1982). Client perception of role in psychotropic drug management. *Issues in Mental Health Nursing*, 4(1), 65–76.

Kucera-Bozarth, K., Beck, N. C. & Lyss, L. (1982). Compliance with lithium regimens. *Journal of Psychosocial Nursing and Mental Health Services*, 20(7), 11–15.

McKay, E. A. (1984). Schizophrenia and the effect of patient education. *Nursing Papers*, 16(1), 55–68.

Osguthorpe, N., Roper, J. & Saunders, J. (1983). The effect of teaching on medication knowledge. *Western Journal of Nursing Research*, 5(3), 205–216.

Whiteside, S. E. (1983). Patient education: effectiveness of medication programs for psychiatric patients. *Journal of Psychosocial Nursing and Mental Health Services*, 21(10), 16–21.

Witt, R. (1981). Medication compliance among discharged psychiatric patients. *Issues in Mental Health Nursing*, 3(4), 305–317.

Neonatal Thermoregulation

Britton, G. B. (1980). Early mother-infant contact and infant temperature stabilization. *JOGN Nursing*, 9(2), 84–86.

Fardig, J. A. (1980). A comparison of skin-to-skin contact and radiant heaters in promoting neonatal thermoregulation. *Journal of Nurse-Midwifery*, 25(1), 19–28.

Gardner, S. (1979). The mother as incubator—after delivery. *JOGN Nursing*, 8(3), 174–176.

Hill, S. T. & Shronk, L. K. (1979). The effect of early parent-infant contact on newborn body temperature. *JOGN Nursing*, 8(5), 287–290.

Nurse-Patient Relationship

Drew, N. (1986). Exclusion and confirmation: a phenomenology of patients' experiences with caregivers. *Image: Journal of Nursing Scholarship*, 18(2), 39–43.

Flaskerud, J. H. (1986). On toward a theory of nursing action: skills and competency in nurse-patient interactions. *Nursing Research*, 35(4), 250–252.

Johnson, M. N. (1979). Self-disclosure and anxiety in nurses and patients. *Issues in Mental Health Nursing*, 2(1), 41–56.

Johnson, M. N. (1980). Self-disclosure: a variable in the nurse-client relationship. *Journal of Psychiatric Nursing and Mental Health Services*, 8(1), 17-20.

Karshmer, J. F., Kornfeld-Jacobs, G. & Carr, A. (1980). Causal attributions: bias in the nurse-patient relationship. *Journal of Psychiatric Nursing and Mental Health Services*, 18(5), 25–30.

Kasch, C. R. (1986). Establishing a collaborative nurse-patient relationship: a distinct focus of nursing action in primary care. *Image: Journal of Nursing Scholarship*, 18(2), 44–47.

Kasch, C. R. (1986). Toward a theory of nursing action: skills and competency in nurse-patient interaction. *Nursing Research*, 35(4), 226–230.

Krikorian, D. A. & Paulanka, B. J. (1982). Self-awareness—the key to a successful nurse-patient relationship? *Journal of Psychosocial Nursing and Mental Health Services*, 20(6), 19–21.

Lindell, A. R. (1979). Congruence—a necessary behavior in the nurse-patient relationship. *Issues in Mental Health Nursing*, 2(1), 27–40.

Webster-Stratton, C., Glascock, J. & McCarthy, A. M. (1986). Nurse practitioner-patient interactional analyses during well-child visits. *Nursing Research*, 35(4), 247–249.

Williams, C. L. (1979). Empathic communication and its effect on client outcome. *Issues in Mental Health Nursing*, 2(1), 15–26.

Oral Care

Beck, S. (1979). Impact of a systematic oral care protocol on stomatitis after chemotherapy. *Cancer Nursing*, 2(3), 185–199.

Daeffler, R. (1980). Oral hygiene measures for patients with cancer: Part I. *Cancer Nursing*, 3(5), 347–356.

Daeffler, R. (1980). Oral hygiene measures for patients with cancer: Part II. *Cancer Nursing*, 3(6), 427–432.

Daeffler, R. (1981). Oral hygiene measures for patients with cancer: Part III. *Cancer Nursing*, 4(1), 29–35.

DeWalt, E. M. (1975). Effect of timed hygienic measures on oral mucosa in a group of elderly subjects. *Nursing Research*, 24(2), 104–108.

DeWalt, E. M. & Haines, A. Sr. (1969). The effects of specified stressors on healthy oral mucosa. *Nursing Research*, 18(1), 22–27.

Drimmelen, J. V. & Rollins, H. F. (1969). Evaluation of a commonly used oral hygiene agent. *Nursing Research*, 18(4), 327–332.

Klocke, J. M. & Sudduth, A. G. (1969). Oral hygiene instruction and plaque formation during hospitalization. *Nursing Research*, 18(2), 124–130.

Passos, J. Y. & Brand, L. M. (1966). Effects of agents used for oral hygiene. *Nursing Research*, 15(3), 196–202.

Oral Temperature Monitoring

Baker, N., Cerone, S. B., Gaze, N. & Knapp, T. R. (1984). The effect of type of thermometer and length of time inserted on oral temperature measurements of afebrile subjects. *Nursing Research*, 33(2), 109–111.

Cooper, K. H. & Abrams, R. M. (1984). Attributes of the oral cavity as a site for basal body temperature measurements. *JOGN Nursing*, 13(2), 125–129.

Durham, M. L., Swanson, B. & Paulford, N. (1986). Effect of tachypnea on oral temperature estimation: a replication. *Nursing Research*, 35(4), 211–214.

Erickson, R. (1976). Thermometer placement for oral temperature measurement in febrile adults. *International Journal of Nursing Studies*, 13(4), 199–208.

Erickson, R. (1980). Oral temperature differences in relation to thermometer and technique. *Nursing Research*, 29(3), 157–164.

Graves, R. D. & Markarian, M. F. (1980). Three-minute time interval when using an oral mercury-in-glass thermometer with or without J-temp sheaths. *Nursing Research*, 29(5), 323–324.

Kirkpatrick, M. & Stanley, S. M. (1976). Evaluation of a new single-use thermometer. *Occupational Health Nursing*, 24(12), 9–18.

Nichols, G. A., Fielding, J. J. & McKevitt, R. K. (1969). Taking oral temperatures of febrile patients. *Nursing Research*, 18(5), 448–450.

Nichols, G. A. & Kucha, D. H. (1972). Oral measurements. *American Journal of Nursing*, 72(6), 1091–1093.

Nichols, G. A., Ruskin, M. M., Glor, B. A. & Kelly, W. H. (1966). Oral, axillary, and rectal temperature determinations and relationships. *Nursing Research*, 15(4), 307–310.

Nichols, G. A. & Verhonick, P. J. (1968). Placement times for oral thermometers: a nursing study replication. *Nursing Research*, 17(2), 159–161.

Takacs, K. M. & Valenti, W. M. (1982). Temperature measurement in a clinical setting. *Nursing Research*, 31(6), 368–370.

Oxygen Inhalation Effect on Oral Temperature

Dressler, D. K., Smejkal, C. & Ruffolo, M. L. (1983). A comparison of oral and rectal temperature measurement on patients receiving oxygen by mask. *Nursing Research*, 32(6), 373–375.

Graas, S. (1974). Thermometer sites and oxygen. *American Journal of Nursing*, 74(10), 1862–1863.

Hasler, M. E. & Cohen, J. A. (1982). The effect of oxygen administration on oral temperature assessment. *Nursing Research*, 31(5), 265–268.

Lim-Levy, F. (1982). The effect of oxygen inhalation on oral temperature. *Nursing Research*, 31(3), 150–152.

Yonkman, C. A. (1982). Cool and heated aerosol and the measurement of oral temperature. *Nursing Research*, 31(6), 354–357.

Pain Management

Austin, C., Cody, C. P., Eyres, P. J., Hefferin, E. A. & Krasnow, R. W. (1986). Hospice home care pain management: four critical variables. *Cancer Nursing*, 9(2), 58–65.

Bafford, D. C. (1977). Nursing research priorities: choice or chance. Progressive relaxation as a nursing intervention: a method of controlling pain for open-heart surgery patients. WICHE Publication. *Communicating Nursing Research*, 8, 284–290.

Bagley, C. S., Falinski, E., Garnizo, N. & Hooker, L. (1982). Pain management: a pilot project. *Cancer Nursing*, 5(3), 191–199.

Bruegel, M. A. (1971). Relationship of preoperative anxiety to perception of postoperative pain. *Nursing Research*, 20(1), 26–31.

Ceccio, C. M. (1984). Postoperative pain relief through relaxation in elderly patients with fractured hips. *Orthopedic Nursing*, 3(3), 11–19.

Chambers, W. G. & Price, G. G. (1967). Influence of nurse upon effects of analgesics administered. *Nursing Research*, 16(3), 228–233.

Diers, D., Schmidt, R. L., McBride, M. A. B. & Davis, B. L. (1972). The effect of nursing interaction on patients in pain. *Nursing Research*, 21(5), 419–428.

Fagerhaugh, S. Y. & Strauss, A. (1977). *Politics of pain management: staff-patient interaction.* Menlo Park, California: Addison-Wesley Publishing Co.

Flaherty, G. G. & Fitzpatrick, J. J. (1978). Relaxation technique to increase comfort level of postoperative patients: a preliminary study. *Nursing Research*, 27(6), 352–355.

Geden, E., Beck, N. C., Brouder, G., Glaister, J. & Pohlman, S. (1985). Self-report and psychophysiological effects of Lamaze preparation: an analogue of labor pain. *Research in Nursing and Health*, 8(2), 155–165.

Geden, E., Beck, N., Hauge, G. & Pohlman, S. (1984). Self-report and psychophysiological effects of five pain-coping strategies. *Nursing Research*, 33(5), 260–265.

Hartfield, M. T., Cason, C. L. & Cason, G. J. (1982). Effects of information about a threatening procedure on patients' expectations and emotional distress. *Nursing Research*, 31(4), 202–206.

Hauck, S. L. (1986). Pain: problem for the person with cancer. *Cancer Nursing*, 9)2), 66–76.

Jacox, A. K. (1979). Assessing pain. *American Journal of Nursing*, 79(5), 895–900.

Johnson, J. E. (1972). Effects of structuring patients' expectations on their reactions to threatening events. *Nursing Research*, 21(6), 499–504.

Johnson, J. E., Kirchhoff, K. T. & Endress, M. P. (1975). Altering children's distress behavior during orthopedic cast removal. *Nursing Research*, 24(6):404–410.

Johnson, J. E. & Rice, V. H. (1974). Effects of accurate expectations and behavioral instructions on reactions during a noxious medical examination. *Journal of Personality and Social Psychology*, 29(5), 710–718.

Johnson, J. E. & Rice, V. H. (1974). Sensory and distress components of pain: implications for the study of clinical pain. *Nursing Research*, 23(3), 203–209.

Johnson, J. E., Rice, V. H., Fuller, S. S. & Endress, M. P. (1978). Sensory information, instruction in a coping strategy, and recovery from surgery. *Research in Nursing and Health*, 1(1), 4–17.

McBride, M. A. B. (1967). Nursing approach, pain, and relief: an exploratory experiment. *Nursing Research*, 16(4), 337–341.

Mason, D. J. (1981). An investigation of the influences of selected factors on nurses' inferences of patient suffering. *International Journal of Nursing Studies*, 18(4), 251–259.

Minckley, B. B. (1968). A study of noise and its relationship to patient discomfort in the recovery room. *Nursing Research*, 17(3), 247–250.

Mogan, J. (1984). Using relaxation to manage postoperative pain. *Canadian Nurse*, 80(10), 15.

Moss, F. T. & Meyer, B. (1966). The effects of nursing interaction upon pain relief in patients. *Nursing Research*, 15(4), 303–306.

Padilla, G. V., Grant, M. M., Rains, B. L., Hansen, B. C., Bergstrom, N., Nong, H. L., Hanson, R. & Kubo, W. (1981). Distress reduction and the effects of preparatory teaching films and patient control. *Research in Nursing and Health*, 4(4), 375–387.

Rankin, M. A. & Snider, B. (1984). Nurses' perceptions of cancer patients' pain. *Cancer Nursing*, 7(2), 149–155.

Taylor, A. G., Skelton, J. A. & Butcher, J. (1984). Duration of pain condition and physical pathology as determinants of nurses' assessments of patients in pain. *Nursing Research*, 33(1), 4–8.

Valentine, A. S., Steckel, S. & Weintraub, M. (1978). Pain relief for cancer patients. *American Journal of Nursing*, 78(12), 2054–2056.

Wells, N. (1982). The effect of relaxation on postoperative muscle tension and pain. *Nursing Research*, 31(4), 236–238.

Young, D. M. S. (1982). Guided imagination as an intervention in hopelessness. *Journal of Psychosocial Nursing and Mental Health Services*, 20(6), 29–32.

Paternal Role Development

Bills, B. J. (1980). Enhancement of paternal-newborn affectional bonds. *Journal of Nurse-Midwifery*, 25(5), 21–26.

Bowen, S. M. & Miller, B. C. (1980). Paternal attachment behavior as related to presence at delivery and preparenthood classes: a pilot study. *Nursing Research*, 29(5), 307–311.

Cronenwett, L. R. & Newmark, L. L. (1974). Fathers' responses to childbirth. *Nursing Research*, 23(3), 210–217.

Gabel, H. (1982). Childbirth experiences of unprepared fathers. *Journal of Nurse-Midwifery*, 27(2), 5–8.

Jones, C. (1981). Father to infant attachment: effects of early contact and characteristics of the infant. *Research in Nursing and Health*, 4, 183–192.

Jones, L. C. & Lenz, E. R. (1986). Father-newborn interaction: effects of social competence and infant state. *Nursing Research*, 35(3), 149–153.

Klein, R. P., Gist, N. F., Nicholson, J. & Standley, K. (1981). A study of father and nurse support during labor. *Birth and the Family Journal*, 8(3), 161–164.

MacLaughlin, S. (1980). First-time fathers' childbirth experience. *Journal of Nurse-Midwifery*, 25(3), 17–21.

Nicholson, J., Gist, N. F., Klein, R. P. & Standley, K. (1983). Outcomes of father involvement in pregnancy and birth. *Birth*, 10(1), 5–9.

Taubenheim, A. M. (1981). Paternal-infant bonding in the first-time father. *JOGN Nursing*, 10(4), 261–264.

Toney, L. (1983). The effects of holding the newborn at delivery on paternal bonding. *Nursing Research*, 32(1), 16–19.

Wandersman, L. P. (1980). The adjustment of fathers to their first baby: the roles of parenting groups and marital relationship. *Birth and the Family Journal*, 7(3), 155–161.

Weaver, R. H. & Cranley, M. S. (1982). An exploration of paternal-fetal attachment behavior. *Nursing Research*, 32(2), 68–72.

Positioning for Intramuscular Injections

Keen, M. F. (1986). Comparison of intramuscular injection techniques to reduce site discomfort and lesions. *Nursing Research*, 35(4), 207–210.

Kruszewski, A. Z., Lang, S. H. & Johnson, J. E. (1979). Effect of positioning on discomfort from intramuscular injections in the dorsogluteal site. *Nursing Research*, 28(2), 103–105.

Levin, R. F. (1982). Choice of injection site, locus of control, and the perception of momentary pain. *Image*, 14(1), 26–32.

Rettig, F. M. & Southby, J. R. (1982). Using different body positions to reduce discomfort from dorsogluteal injection. *Nursing Research*, 31(4), 219–221.

Positioning the Patient With Intracranial Hypertension

Lipe, H. P. & Mitchell, P. H. (1980). Positioning the patient with intracranial hypertension: how turning and head rotation affect the internal jugular vein. *Heart and Lung* 9(6), 1031–1037.

Mitchell, P. H. & Mauss, N. K. (1978). Relationship of patient-nurse activity to intracranial pressure variations: a pilot study. *Nursing Research*, 27(1), 4–10.

Mitchell, P. H., Ozuna, J. & Lipe, H. P. (1981). Moving the patient in bed: effects on intracranial pressure. *Nursing Research*, 30(4), 212–218.

Postcardiotomy Delirium

Budd, S. & Brown, W. (1974). Effect of a reorientation technique on postcardiotomy delirium. *Nursing Research,* 23(4), 341–348.

Sadler, P. D. (1979). Nursing assessment of postcardiotomy delirium. *Heart and Lung*, 8(4), 745–750.
Sadler, P. D. (1981). Incidence, degree, and duration of postcardiotomy delirium. *Heart and Lung*, 10(6), 1084–1091.

Pregnancy

Brouse, S. H. (1985). Effect of gender role identity on patterns of feminine and self-concept scores from late pregnancy to early postpartum. *Advances in Nursing Science*, 7(3), 32–48.
Brown, M. A. (1986). Social support during pregnancy: a unidimensional or multidimensional construct? *Nursing Research*, 35(1), 4–9.
Brown, M. A. (1986). Social support, stress, and health: a comparison of expectant mothers and fathers. *Nursing Research*, 35(2), 72–76.
Fawcett, J., Bliss-Holtz, V. J., Haas, M. B., Leventhal, M. & Rubin, M. (1986). Spouses' body image changes during and after pregnancy: a replication and extension. *Nursing Research*, 35(4), 220–223.
Fawcett, J. & York, R. (1986). Spouses' physical and psychological symptoms during pregnancy and the postpartum. *Nursing Research*, 35(3), 144–148.
Lee, P. A. (1986). Health beliefs of pregnant and postpartum Hmong Women. *Western Journal of Nursing Research*, 8(1), 83–93.

Premature Infant Stimulation

Brown, J. V., LaRossa, M. M., Aylward, G. P., Davis, D. J., Rutherford, P. K. & Bakeman, R. (1980). Nursery-based intervention with prematurely born babies and their mothers: are there effects? *Journal of Pediatric Psychology*, 97(9), 487–491.
Hays, J. S. (1980). Premature infant development: the relationship of neonatal stimulation, birth condition and home environment. *Pediatric Nursing*, 6(6), 33–36.
Jay, S. S. (1982). The effects of gentle human touch on the clinical improvement of mechanically ventilated very-short-gestation infants. *Maternal-Child Nursing Journal*, 11(4), 199–256.
Johnson, S. H. (1981). Comparison of interactional deprivation of the mother with a transported versus nontransported premature infant. *Journal of Nurse-Midwifery*, 26(2), 30–32.

Preoperative Teaching

Abrams, L. (1982). Resistance behaviors and teaching media for children in day surgery. *AORN Journal*, 35(2), 244–255.
Bruegel, M. A. (1971). Relationship of preoperative anxiety to perception of postoperative pain. *Nursing Research*, 20(1), 26–31.
Christopherson, B. & Pfeiffer, C. (1980). Varying the timing of information to alter preoperative anxiety and postoperative recovery in cardiac surgery patients. *Heart and Lung*, 9(5), 854–861.
Devine, E. C. & Cook, T. D. (1983). A meta-analytic analysis of effects of psychoeducational interventions on length of postsurgical hospital stay. *Nursing Research*, 32(5), 267–274.
Devine, E. C. & Cook, T. D. (1986). Clinical and cost-saving effects of psychoeducational interventions with surgical patients: a meta-analysis. *Research in Nursing and Health*, 9(2), 89–105.
Dumas, R. G. & Leonard, R. C. (1963). The effect of nursing on the incidence of postoperative vomiting. *Nursing Research,* 12(1), 12–15.
Dziurbejko, M. M. & Larkin, J. C. (1978). Including the family in pre-operative teaching. *American Journal of Nursing*, 78(11), 1892–1894.
Felton, G., Huss, K., Payne, E. A. & Srsic, K. (1976). Preoperative nursing intervention with the patient for surgery: outcomes of three alternative approaches. *International Journal of Nursing Studies*, 13(2), 83–96.
Ferguson, B. F. (1979). Preparing young children for hospitalization: a comparison of two methods. *Pediatrics*, 64(5), 656–664.
Fortin, F. & Kirouac, S. (1976). A randomized controlled trial of preoperative patient education. *International Journal of Nursing Studies*, 13(1), 11–24.
Girouard, S. (1978). The role of the clinical specialist as change agent: an experiment in preoperative teaching. *International Journal of Nursing Studies*, 15(2), 57–65.
Graham, L. E. & Conley, E. M. (1971). Evaluation of anxiety and fear in adult surgical patients. *Nursing Research*, 20(2), 113–122.

Hinshaw, A. S., Gerber, R. M., Atwood, J. R. & Allen, J. R. (1983). The use of predictive modeling to test nursing practice outcomes. *Nursing Research*, 32(1), 35–42.

Johnson, J. E., Christman, N. J. & Stitt, C. (1985). Personal control interventions: short- and long-term effects on surgical patients. *Research in Nursing and Health*, 8(2), 131–145.

Johnson, J. E., Dabbs, J. M. & Leventhal, H. (1970). Psychosocial factors in the welfare of surgical patients. *Nursing Research*, 19(1), 18–29.

King, I. & Tarsitano, B. (1982). The effect of structured and unstructured pre-operative teaching: a replication. *Nursing Research*, 31(6), 324–329.

Kinney, M. R. (1977). Effects of preoperative teaching upon patients with differing modes of response to threatening stimuli. *International Journal of Nursing Studies*, 14(1), 49–59.

Kishi, K. I. (1983). Communication patterns of health teaching and information recall. *Nursing Research*, 32(4), 230–235.

Lamontagne, L. L. (1984). Children's locus of control beliefs as predictors of preoperative coping behaviors. *Nursing Research*, 33(2), 76–79, 85.

Lindeman, C. A. (1972). Nursing intervention with the presurgical patient; effectiveness and efficiency of group and individual preoperative teaching—phase two. *Nursing Research* 21(3), 196–209.

Lindeman, C. A. (1973). Symposium: education of patients. Influencing recovery through preoperative teaching. *Heart and Lung*, 2(4), 515–521.

Lindeman, C. A. & Aernam, B. V. (1971). Nursing intervention with the presurgical patient—the effects of structured and unstructured preoperative teaching. *Nursing Research*, 20(4), 319–332.

Lindeman, C. A. & Stetzer, S. L. (1973). Effect of preoperative visits by operating room nurses. *Nursing Research*, 22(1), 4–16.

Melamed, B. G. & Siegel, L. J. (1975). Reduction of anxiety in children facing hospitalization and surgery by use of filmed modeling. *Journal of Consulting Psychology*, 43(4), 511–521.

Miller, P. Sr. & Shada, E. A. (1978). Preoperative information and recovery of open-heart surgery patients. *Heart and Lung*, 7(3), 486–493.

Rice, V. H. & Johnson, J. E. (1984). Preadmission self-instruction booklets, postadmission exercise performance, and teaching time. *Nursing Research*, 33(3), 147–151.

Schmitt, F. E. & Wooldridge, P. J. (1973). Psychological preparation of surgical patients. *Nursing Research*, 22(2), 108–116.

Shimko, C. (1981). The effect of preoperative instruction on state anxiety. *Journal of Neurosurgical Nursing*, 13(6), 318–322.

Sime, A. M. & Libera, M. B. (1985). Sensation information, self-instruction and responses to dental surgery. *Research in Nursing and Health*, 8(1), 41–47.

Visintainer, M. A. & Wolfer, J. A. (1975). Psychological preparation for surgical pediatric patients: the effect on children's and parents' stress responses and adjustment. *Pediatrics*, 56(2), 187–202.

Volicer, B. J. (1974). Patients' perceptions of stressful events associated with hospitalization. *Nursing Research*, 23(3), 235–238.

Voshall, B. (1980). The effects of preoperative teaching on postoperative pain. *Topics in Clinical Nursing*, 2(1), 39–43.

Weiler, M. C. (1968). Postoperative patients evaluate preoperative instruction. *American Journal of Nursing*, 68(7), 1465–1467.

Wolfer, J. A. & Davis, C. E. (1970). Assessment of surgical patients' preoperative emotional condition and postoperative welfare. *Nursing Research*, 19(5), 402–414.

Ziemer, M. M. (1983). Effects of information on postsurgical coping. *Nursing Research*, 32(5), 282–287.

Rape-Trauma Care

Burgess, A. W. & Holmstrom, L. L. (1974). Crisis and counseling requests of rape victims. *Nursing Research*, 23(3), 196–202.

Damrosch, S. P. (1981). How nursing students' reactions to rape victims are affected by a perceived act of carelessness. *Nursing Research*, 30(3), 168–170.

Ipema, D. K. (1979). Rape: the process of recovery. *Nursing Research*, 28(5), 272–275.

Relaxation

Bohachick, P. (1984). Progressive relaxation training in cardiac rehabilitation: effect on psychological variables. *Nursing Research*, 33(5), 283–287.

Ceccio, C. M. (1984). Postoperative pain relief through relaxation in elderly patients with fractured hips. *Orthopedic Nursing*, 3(3), 11–19.

Fehring, R. J. (1983). Effects of biofeedback-aided relaxation on the psychological stress symptoms of college students. *Nursing Research*, 32(6), 362–366.

Flaherty, G. G. & Fitzpatrick, J. J. (1978). Relaxation technique to increase comfort level of postoperative patients: a preliminary study. *Nursing Research*, 27(6), 352–355.

Lamontagne, L. L., Mason, K. R. & Hepworth, J. T. (1985). Effects of relaxation on anxiety in children: implications for coping with stress. *Nursing Research*, 34(5), 289–292.

Pender, N. J. (1984). Physiologic responses of clients with essential hypertension to progressive muscle relaxation training. *Research in Nursing and Health*, 7(3), 197–203.

Pender, N. J. (1985). Effects of progressive muscle relaxation training on anxiety and health locus of control among hypertensive adults. *Research in Nursing and Health*, 8(1) 67–72.

Rice, V. H., Caldwell, M., Butler, S. & Robinson, J. (1986). Relaxation training and response to cardiac catheterization: a pilot study. *Nursing Research*, 35(1), 39–43.

Wells, N. (1982). The effect of relaxation on postoperative muscle tension and pain. *Nursing Research*, 31(4), 236–238.

Reminiscing

Bramwell, L. (1984). Use of the life history in pattern identification and health promotion. *Advances in Nursing Science*, 7(1), 37–44.

Stress of Transfer

Minckley, B. B., Burrows, D., Ehrat, K., Harper, L., Jenkin, S. A., Minckley, W. F., Page, B., Schramm, D. E. & Wood, C. (1979). Myocardial infarct stress-of-transfer inventory: development of a research tool. *Nursing Research*, 28(1), 4–10.

Schwartz, L. P. & Brenner, Z. R. (1979). Critical care unit transfer: reducing patient stress through nursing interventions. *Heart and Lung*, 8(3), 540–546.

Smith, M. C. (1976). Patient responses to being transferred during hospitalization. *Nursing Research*, 25(3), 192–196.

Suicide Prevention

Harris, R. A. (1966). Factors related to continued suicidal behavior in dyadic relationships. *Nursing Research*, 15(1), 72–75.

Inman, D. J., Bascue, L. O., Kahn, W. J. & Shaw, P. A. (1984). The relationship between suicide knowledge and suicide interviewing skill. *Death Education*, 8(2/3), 179–184.

Kumler, F. R. (1964). Communication between suicide attemptors and significant others: an exploratory study. *Nursing Research*, 13(3), 268–270.

Teaching Breast Self-Examination

Edwards, V. (1980). Changing breast self-examination behavior. *Nursing Research*, 29(5), 301–306.

Fink, R., Shapiro, S. & Roester, R. (1972). Impact of efforts to increase participation in repetitive screening for early breast cancer detection. *American Journal of Public Health*, 62(3), 328–336.

Hallal, J. C. (1982). The relationship of health beliefs, health locus of control, and self concept to the practice of breast self-examination in adult women. *Nursing Research*, 31(3), 137–142.

McLendon, M. S., Fulk, C. H. & Starnes, D. C. (1982). Effectiveness of breast self-examination teaching to women of low socioeconomic class. *JOGN Nursing*, 11(1), 7–10.

Michalek, A. M., Walsh, D., Burns, P. & Mettlin, C. (1981). Report on a BSE educational program for lay audiences conducted by nurse health educators. *Cancer Nursing*, 4(5), 385–388.

Schlueter, L. A. (1982). Knowledge and beliefs about breast cancer and breast self-examination among athletic and nonathletic women. *Nursing Research*, 31(6), 348–353.

Stillman, M. J. (1977). Women's health beliefs about breast cancer and breast self-examination. *Nursing Research*, 26(2), 121–127.

Turnbull, E. M. (1978). Effect of basic preventive health practices and mass media on the practice of breast self-examination. *Nursing Research*, 27(2), 98–102.

Temperature Monitoring in Neonates

Eoff, M. J. F., Meier, R. S. & Miller, C. (1974). Temperature measurement in infants. *Nursing Research*, 23(6), 457–460.

Fleming, M., Hakansson, H. & Svenningsen, N. W. (1983). A disposable new electronic temperature probe for skin temperature measurements in the newborn infant nursery. *International Journal of Nursing Studies*, 20(2), 89–96.

Schiffman, R. F. (1982). Temperature monitoring in the neonate: a comparison of axillary and rectal temperatures. *Nursing Research*, 31(5), 274–277.

Therapeutic Use of Pets

Baun, M. M., Bergstrom, N., Langston, N. F. & Thoma, L. (1984). Physiological effects of human/companion animal bonding. *Nursing Research*, 33(3), 126–129.

Friedmann, E., Katcher, A. H., Lynch, J. J. & Thomas, S. A. (1980). Animal companions and one-year survival of patients after discharge from a coronary care unit. *Public Health Reports*, 95(4), 307–312.

Lapp, C. A. & Scruby, L. (1982). Responsible pet relationships: a mental health perspective. *Health Values: Achieving High Level Wellness*, 6(4), 20–25.

Tracheostomy Care

Harris, R. B. (1984). National survey of aseptic tracheotomy care techniques in hospitals with head and neck/ENT surgical departments. *Cancer Nursing*, 7(1), 23–32.

Harris, R. B. & Hyman, R. B. (1984). Clean vs. sterile tracheostomy care and level of pulmonary infection. *Nursing Research*, 33(2), 80–85.

Langrehr, E. A., Washburn, S. C. & Guthrie, M. P. (1981). Oxygen insufflation during endotracheal suctioning. *Heart and Lung*, 10(6), 1028–1036.

Larson, E. (1970). Bacterial colonization of tracheal tubes of patients in a surgical intensive care unit. *Nursing Research*, 19(2), 122–128.

Skelley, B. F. H., Deeren, S. M. & Powaser, M. M. (1980). The effectiveness of two preoxygenation methods to prevent endotracheal suction–induced hypoxemia. *Heart and Lung*, 9(2), 316–323.

Touch

Cannon, R. B. (1977). The development of maternal touch during early mother-infant interaction. *JOGN Nursing*, 6(2), 28–33.

Copstead, L. C. (1980). Effects of touch on self-appraisal and interaction appraisal for permanently institutionalized older adults. *Journal of Gerontological Nursing*, 6(12), 747–752.

Heidt, P. (1981). Effect of therapeutic touch on anxiety level of hospitalized patients. *Nursing Research*, 30(1), 32–37.

Jay, S. S. (1982). The effects of gentle human touch on mechanically ventilated very-short-gestation infants. *Maternal-Child Nursing Journal*, 11(4), 199–256.

Keller, E. & Bzdek, V. M. (1986). Effects of therapeutic touch on tension headache pain. *Nursing Research*, 35(2), 101–106.

Kramer, M., Chamorro, I., Green, D. & Knudtson, F. (1975). Extra tactile stimulation of the premature infant. *Nursing Research*, 24(5), 324–334.

Krieger, D. (1973). The relationship of touch, with intent to help or heal, to subjects' in-vivo hemoglobin values: a study in personalized interaction. *Proceedings of the Ninth American Nurses Association Nursing Research Conference*. American Nurses' Association Publication (Nu 00322-05), pp. 39–58.

Krieger, D. (1975). Therapeutic touch: the imprimatur of nursing. *American Journal of Nursing*, 75(5), 784–787.

Langland, R. M. & Panicucci, C. L. (1982). Effects of touch on communication with elderly confused clients. *Journal of Gerontological Nursing*, 8(3), 152–155.

McCorkle, R. (1974). Effects of touch on seriously ill patients. *Nursing Research*, 23(2), 125–132.

Mills, M. E., Thomas, S. A., Lynch, J. J. & Katcher, A. H. (1976). Effect of pulse palpation on cardiac arrhythmia in coronary care patients. *Nursing Research*, 25(5), 378–382.

Quinn, J. F. (1984). Therapeutic touch as energy exchange: testing the theory. *Advances in Nursing Science*, 6(2), 42–49.

Randolph, G. L. (1984). Therapeutic and physical touch: physiological response to stressful stimuli. *Nursing Research*, 33(1), 33–36.

Rowlands, D. (1984). Therapeutic touch: its effects on the depressed elderly. *Australian Nurses Journal*, 13(11), 45–46, 52.

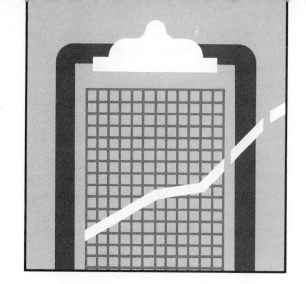

22

Future of Nursing Research

Great strides have been made in nursing research during the 1970s and 1980s. These strides are evident in the nursing literature, where an increasing number of complex, scholarly studies have been published by sophisticated nurse researchers. However, there are still many unresolved problems in nursing that require investigation. In addition, trends such as an increase in the elderly population, emphasis on health prevention and promotion, advancement of health care technology and emphasis on cost-effectiveness in the health care system hold many opportunities for nursing research. The need for nursing research in the 1990s and in the twenty-first century will be even greater than it is now, as nursing attempts to keep pace with the changing needs of society and the rapid advancement of technology. The research problems of the future will require an increasing number of sophisticated researchers conducting innovative, complex quantitative and qualitative studies.

The future goal of nursing research is to generate a relevant, organized body of knowledge that provides a basis for nursing practice and education in the twenty-first century. Through research, nursing knowledge can be refined to meet the changing health needs of consumers, to encompass the changing health care system and to promote the profession of nursing. This final chapter addresses future research priorities based on predicted changes in health care.

Some strategies are identified that could facilitate the growth of research in nursing, such as (1) the development of a scientific community, (2) the utilization of diverse and innovative methodological strategies and (3) the expansion of political and consumer awareness of nursing research.

Future Research Priorities

The broad focus of nursing research is to generate knowledge about the total person's (individual, family and community) response to health promotion, prevention of illness, illness, rehabilitation, habilitation and dying within their environment. Nursing research is also conducted to generate knowledge about the health care system, the educational preparation of nurses and the evolution of the nursing profession. Thus, identifying the future priorities for nursing research involves examining the projected health needs of consumers, the projected changes in the health care system and the predictions about the nursing profession. The Cabinet on Nursing Research of the American Nurses' Association (1985) developed a paper entitled "Directions for Nursing Re-

---

TABLE 22–1
Predictions About Consumers of Nursing Services

1. Persons over the age of 65 will make up nearly 15 per cent of the U.S. population. Eighty per cent of the elderly will live with one or more chronic illnesses.
2. Increased cultural diversity will characterize American society.
3. Health problems induced by lifestyle, chronic illness, and the environment will be responsible for a large proportion of illnesses, disabilities, and deaths.
4. Abuse of alcohol and drugs, including tobacco, will be responsible for significant health care expenses and limited productivity.
5. New mental health problems will be produced by rapid technological and social change, especially by the shift from a labor-oriented to an information-oriented society.
6. Poverty, violence, and traumatic injury will produce complex physical and mental health problems.
7. People who have survived catastrophic illnesses and children who are born prematurely or with congenital anomalies will experience prolonged life spans, and many will live with chronic disabilities.
8. People will survive previously fatal illnesses, living with organ transplants and mechanical substitutes for vital organs. Although these technologies will extend longevity, they will also generate new problems in adjustment to new technology and demands of self-care.
9. Cancer, heart disease, arthritis, chronic pulmonary diseases, diabetes, Alzheimer's disease, and other diseases more prevalent during the middle and late adult years will produce major needs for individual and family adaptation and will command a major proportion of health resources.
10. People will assume greater responsibility for their own health care because of their increased consciousness about health, economic necessity, and social pressure. Consumers will demand high-quality services and the right to self-determination from all health professionals.
11. Complex health care technology will become commonplace in the home, because persons with health problems previously requiring hospitalization will be discharged much earlier.
12. People will select health care providers and services from multiple options available to them, and they will exercise increased self-determination and discretion in use of the health care system.

(From American Nurses' Association, Cabinet on Nursing Research: *Directions for nursing research: toward the twenty-first century.* Kansas City, Missouri: American Nurses' Association, 1985, pp. 1–2; with permission.)

TABLE 22-2
Predictions About Health Care Systems

1. Improved quality of life as well as an extended life span and decreased morbidity will be the major goals of health care.
2. Cost-containment will remain a major focus of national health policy. Factors blocking consumers' access to necessary health services will remain a major concern of nursing.
3. Federal resources for health care will decrease, placing increased demands for support on individuals and the private sector.
4. Families will have increased responsibility for the care of their elderly and ill at a time when family size and family economic resources are decreasing.
5. People will have increased access to care because services will be provided in a variety of settings, including workplaces, schools, community health centers, community nursing centers, day-care settings, and homes. Services will focus on health promotion, illness prevention, and optimum adaptation to chronic illness.
6. The critically ill and injured will receive care in regional treatment centers staffed by highly skilled specialists capable of practicing in a technologically complex and rapidly changing treatment environment.

(From American Nurses' Association, Cabinet on Nursing Research: *Directions for nursing research: toward the twenty-first century.* Kansas City, Missouri: American Nurses' Association, 1985, p. 2; with permission.)

search: Toward the Twenty-First Century." Within this paper, the cabinet members made some predictions about the consumers of nursing service (Table 22–1), the health care systems (Table 22–2) and the nursing profession (Table 22–3) by the year 2000.

TABLE 22-3
Predictions About Nursing

1. Nurses will need a broad knowledge base in order to deliver comprehensive health promotion and preventive services to individuals and families in homes, schools, workplaces, and community nursing centers.
2. Nurses will need specialized knowledge in order to care for the critically ill, acutely ill, and chronically ill in technologically sophisticated treatment centers and in long-term care facilities.
3. Nurses will experience an accelerated rate of change in clinical therapeutics because of the rapid infusion of new scientific information.
4. Nurses will continue to target services to vulnerable populations, especially the very young and the very old, those from diverse cultures, and those whose access to health services is limited because of their economic status, health status, or age.
5. Nursing services will complement families' resources for caring for the chronically ill, disabled, elderly, and dying.
6. The complexity of health care problems and the need for knowledge from diverse areas will require increased collaboration among nurses and other health professionals.
7. Nurses will need undergraduate educational preparation that includes a broad knowledge base in the areas of human health, ethics, and nursing therapeutics.
8. Graduate education will be essential in order to prepare specialized practitioners for technologically complex care of the critically ill and to prepare advanced practitioners for health promotion and maintenance.
9. Research centers will exist in large university settings in which a cadre of nurse scientists will generate knowledge in areas designated by the pofession as important to its social mandate.
10. Nurses will continue to deliver high-quality health care in cost-effective modes.

(From American Nurses' Association, Cabinet on Nursing Research: *Directions for nursing research: toward the twenty-first century.* Kansas City, Missouri: American Nurses' Association, 1985, p. 2; with permission.)

TABLE 22–4
Priorities for Nursing Research

1. Promote health, well-being, and ability to care for oneself among all age, social, and cultural groups.
2. Minimize or prevent behaviorally and environmentally induced health problems that compromise the quality of life and reduce productivity.
3. Minimize the negative effects of new health technologies on the adaptive abilities of individuals and families experiencing acute or chronic health problems.
4. Ensure that the care needs of particularly vulnerable groups, such as the elderly, children with congenital health problems, individuals from diverse cultures, the mentally ill, and the poor, are met in effective and acceptable ways.
5. Classify nursing practice phenomena.
6. Ensure that principles of ethics guide nursing research.
7. Develop instruments to measure nursing outcomes.
8. Develop integrative methodologies for the holistic study of human beings as they relate to their families and lifestyles.
9. Design and evaluate alternative models for delivering health care and for administering health care systems so that nurses will be able to balance high quality and cost-effectiveness in meeting the nursing needs of identified populations.
10. Evaluate the effectiveness of alternative approaches to nursing education for the kind of practice that requires broad knowledge and a wide repertoire of skills and for the kind of practice that requires specialized knowledge and a focused set of skills.
11. Identify and analyze historical and comtemporary factors that influence the shaping of nursing professionals' involvement in national health policy development.

(From American Nurses' Association, Cabinet on Nursing Research: *Directions for nursing research: toward the twenty-first century.* Kansas City, Missouri: American Nurses' Association, 1985, pp. 2–3; with permission.)

Based on these predictions, the Cabinet on Nursing Research identified 11 priorities for nursing research (Table 22–4). Graduate students, practicing nurses and nurse scientists must be aware of these priorities when selecting an area for investigation. The focus of nursing research for the 1980s has been to generate and refine knowledge for clinical practice, and this is still a strong focus for the 1990s and the twenty-first century. Many of the current clinical research topics will be the focus of future research, but some new topics are also being identified for investigation. Based on the priorities identified by the cabinet members, we have identified a few research topics and related questions that might facilitate the development of future studies (Table 22–5).

Development of a Scientific Community

A scientific community is a cohesive group of scholars within a discipline. These scholars are supportive colleagues as well as competitors in conducting research (Fawcett, 1980). As a group, these scholars stimulate the creation of new research ideas and the development of innovative methodologies to conduct research (Hinshaw, 1983). They share their research endeavors, debate relevant issues and scrutinize each other's work. These activities frequently increase researcher commitment and productivity. A strong scientific community in nursing could provide an important source of social influence on nursing research. The community members could have an impact on the quality and quantity of the problems studied, the methodologies used, the studies published and the theories generated.

TABLE 22–5
Future Research Topics and Related Questions

Research Topic	Questions Requiring Investigation
Health care of the elderly	1. How do the health needs (physical, psychological, social and spiritual) of the elderly differ from those of other age groups? 2. How have the changing patterns of families influenced the health and health care of the elderly? 3. What productive roles can the elderly fulfill in society? 4. How can family members be assisted in coping with the health needs of their elderly members? 5. What settings (currently existing or proposed) can provide effective health care for the elderly? 6. What nursing interventions and implementation processes will effectively meet the health needs of the elderly? 7. What is the role of the elderly in promoting their own health and preventing illnesses? How can this role of health promotion and illness prevention be expanded? 8. How has lifestyle (such as poverty or positive and negative health habits) and environment (such as technological advances) affected the health of the elderly?
Physically challenged, chronic illness, chronic disability	1. What are the health needs (physical, psychological, social and spiritual) of individuals experiencing chronic illness and disability? 2. What is the impact of living with chronic illness and disability for multiple years on the individual and family? 3. What nursing services and interventions can be effective in promoting the adjustment of individuals and families to chronic illness? 4. How can technological advances (such as computerized mechanical devices) be used to promote self-care of the physically challenged (chronically disabled) person? 5. How can high-quality care be delivered in cost-effective ways to individuals with chronic disabilities? 6. What role can a physically challenged person perform in promoting his or her own health and the health of others with similar conditions? 7. What nursing interventions will be effective in helping individuals and families cope with new health technologies (such as organ transplants)?
Health promotion, illness prevention	1. What lifestyle and environmental factors increase the quantity and quality of life? 2. What is the impact of specific health promotions behaviors (such as not taking drugs, smoking or abusing alcohol) on the life of an individual and family? 3. What nursing interventions are effective in facilitating long-term lifestyle changes? 4. Which are the best settings and methods for providing health education? 5. What nursing interventions are effective in promoting health and preventing illness in persons of all age groups and levels of health? 6. How cost-effective is health promotion and illness prevention care? 7. How can environment be altered to promote health and prevent illness? 8. How can technological advancements be used to promote health and prevent illness among all age groups? 9. What historical factors have had an impact on the health care of individuals and groups? How have these factors affected the health needs of people and the health care system?

The development of a scientific community requires preparation of qualified researchers who are actively involved in conducting research. These expert researchers discuss with other nurses the utilization of research findings in practice, how to conduct research and the development of a theory base for nursing practice. They serve as mentors for novice researchers and collaborate with other researchers and clinicians in conducting studies. Academic preparation, mentorship and collaboration are activities that serve to increase the size and productivity of a scientific community.

PREPARATION OF RESEARCHERS

The discipline of nursing is in the process of developing a scientific community, and adequate preparation of researchers is an essential first step. The preparation of a researcher begins at the baccalaureate level and continues through postdoctorate work. In order to achieve the goals of the nursing profession, nurses must learn not only how to conduct research but also to value the process and be committed to furthering the impact of research on nursing practice. Recognizing the value of research and developing an inquiring attitude regarding nursing practice must be encouraged in the baccalaureate educational process (Levin, 1983). The baccalaureate-prepared nurse must actively read research, critique study findings and use the findings in practice. He or she can also be involved in research activities by identifying potential problems, participating as a subject and serving as a research assistant.

Master's level education needs to build upon the background of baccalaureate education, which fosters knowledge and utilization of research findings. Through master's educational preparation, the nurse must gain knowledge of the research process and receive support in conducting a study. Replication of previous studies is frequently undertaken by master's level nurses and is extremely important in the future to determine the extent to which the findings are reliable and generalizable (Reynolds & Haller, 1986). Master's-prepared nurses should collaborate with expert researchers and continue their involvement in conducting clinical research.

The complex knowledge and skills needed for unique, innovative research projects frequently require doctoral preparation. The development of instruments to measure nursing concepts (methodological research) requires doctoral preparation. Complex, funded research projects often require that the primary investigator have a minimum of doctoral preparation. Currently, many of the senior authors of published studies hold doctorate degrees (Brown, Tanner & Padrick, 1984). However, the number of doctoral-prepared nurses is still low. The Cabinet on Nursing Research (1985) indicated that the minimal per cent of the total nursing population with a doctorate by 1990 should be 0.5 per cent and by 1995, it should be 1 percent. In order to achieve these goals, financial support must be made more available for doctoral students in nursing.

The current question is whether doctoral preparation is adequate for the development of a scientific community. The complex research problems of the 1990s and the twenty-first century and the methodology required to investigate these problems will require even more sophistication. Future researchers will need postdoctoral preparation. Through postdoctoral work, researchers gain increased research knowledge and skills, develop a commitment to a research career and often identify an area for a lifetime of study. In the future, there will be an increased need for postdoctoral educational experiences and post-doctoral fellowships for students.

Adequate educational preparation is not enough. Researchers must be committed to conducting research, and frequently this commitment involves years, and sometimes a lifetime, of work to generate answers to clinical problems. Researchers must learn to designate the time and to generate the funds needed to conduct studies (Rittenmeyer, 1982). In addition, an environment must be developed in academic and clinical settings to foster and support research. Researchers must acquire and maintain access to subjects, equipment and personnel. Administrators can facilitate the conduct of research by promoting an environment that is supportive of research. Incentives and rewards can be built into the environment to increase researcher productivity. It is hoped that research will become a higher priority for nurses as knowledge of its benefits increases. Possibly by the 1990s or the twenty-first century, research will be an integral part of the nurse's normal workload in a variety of settings.

MENTOR RELATIONSHIP

A *mentor* serves as a role model in scientific endeavors and is someone the mentee or protege admires and seeks to emulate. Socialization in the research role is facilitated with a mentor. The mentee not only learns the process of conducting research but often acquires desirable personality traits, such as curiosity, persistence, dedication, competence, independence and self-confidence (Fagan & Fagan, 1983). A mentor relationship usually lasts for 2 or 3 years. Because of the time commitment, mentoring usually involves faculty and postdoctoral fellows, doctoral students and occasionally master's students (Mercer, 1984). However, mentor relationships could be effective in the practice setting to promote the conduct of research. Clinical agencies are now hiring nurse researchers who can serve as mentors to nurse clinicians who are interested in becoming researchers.

Frequently, mentor relationships are developed because the mentor and mentee have a mutual interest in a research topic or a specific research problem. Students might become involved in the research of a faculty member; this can stimulate a mentor relationship. The mentor provides support, guidance and criticism in the development and implementation of a study, grant proposal and/or article for publication. The mentee stimulates ideas in the mentor by raising questions and sharing current research findings. In addition, the mentee could assist with data collection and analysis and with the development of the research report.

Two issues that should be discussed in the early phase of a mentor relationship are authorship and ownership of ideas (Mercer, 1984). The publications from the research should be anticipated, and the authorship of these publications should be determined. The order of the authors' names on each publication should also be decided upon. When individuals work together, many ideas are generated, and sometimes taking another's ideas as one's own is as serious as taking another's written work. The ideas generated during the relationship should be recorded, and ownership should be identified. When the relationship is terminated, the future use of ideas should be determined to the satisfaction of both the mentor and the mentee.

The opportunities for mentorship in nursing have been very limited. The development of a scientific community can be facilitated by and can facilitate the mentoring process. The growing number of expert researchers must take responsibility for mentoring the novice researchers. Through mentor relationships, scientists can know that their research will continue. In some situations, mentor relationships turn into collegial relationships in which the individuals collaborate as peers in conducting research.

MODELS FOR RESEARCH

Academic-Based and Agency-Based Models

Traditionally, nurses have conducted research using an academic-based or an agency-based model. In an academic-based model, researchers identify their own area of interest and investigate problems that they believe are important. These researchers are often involved in conducting basic research that is critical to the scientific community but has no immediate application to practice. In the academic-based model, the research usually takes place in the university and involves academicians and their graduate students. The advantages of this model include the freedom to investigate a problem of choice in an environment where research is a desired activity and where there is easy access to resources such as computers, statisticians, laboratories and other researchers.

In the agency-based model, studies are conducted in sponsoring agencies, and the research problems are often identified by administrators or clinicians. Thus, an agency hires a researcher to generate answers to specific questions relevant to the agency (Engstrom, 1984). Werley (1972) established the first agency-based research department in the 1950s. Advantages to using this model are (1) the investigation of relevant clinical problems, (2) involvement of clinicians in research, (3) conduct of research in real settings and (4) establishment of relationships among researchers, administrators and clinicians.

There are problems with both models. The problems that have been identified with the academic-based research model include the relevance of the studies to clinical practice, the dissemination of research findings and the designation of faculty time for research. The problems associated with the agency-based model include the generalizability and dissemination of the results outside the sponsoring agency, the risk of investigator bias, the limited resources available within one agency and the generation of research that is usually oriented toward problem solving but not toward the expansion of fundamental knowledge (Engstrom, 1984).

Collaborative Research Model

The collaborative research model was developed to combine the advantages of the academic-based and agency-based models. Two common models for collaboration are the complementary and the supplementary models (Hagstrom, 1965). In the complementary model, researchers treat each other as equals and share equal responsibilities and rewards in conducting research. In this type of model, participants elect to collaborate with each other based on their interests and expertise. The collaborative relationship evolves over time with a testing of individual commitment and honesty in the relationship. Interdisciplinary and multidisciplinary collaboration frequently involve the complementary approach.

In the supplementary model, there is usually a division of labor, with one individual having the major responsibility for the study. The members usually have unequal levels of rank, prestige, responsibility and credit. The researcher with major responsibility usually selects the members for collaboration based on the specific expertise that each individual can contribute to the study (Speer, McLane, White, Whall, King, Buckwalter, Lasky & Lederman, 1985). In some studies, both complementary and supplementary models of collaboration are used.

The use of collaborative models in conducting research has advantages and disadvantages. The advantages of collaborative research include (1) increased access to facilities, (2) increased availability of subjects, (3) increased intellectual stimulation, (4) reduced social isolation, (5) increased availability of resources, (6) increased peer review and feedback, (7) possible increased dissemination and utilization of findings, (8) increased opportunities for replication and (9) greater possibility of conducting research relevant to nursing practice. The disadvantages of the collaborative process include (1) excessive competition, (2) delayed decision making, (3) frustration, (4) unfair distribution of awards, (5) rejection of certain members, (6) territoriality problems, (7) budgeting problems, (8) poor communication and (9) not completing the study (Engstrom, 1984; Speer et al., 1985).

The number of collaborative research projects in nursing is increasing. A recent review of the literature indicated that 7 per cent of the published studies were collaborative between 1952 and 1953 and that 40 per cent were collaborative in 1980 (Brown et al., 1984). Three common types of collaboration that have evolved in nursing are (1) interdisciplinary and multidisciplinary collaboration, (2) collaboration among expert nurse researchers and (3) collaboration among academic and clinical agencies.

Interdisciplinary and Multidisciplinary Collaboration □ Nurses work in settings with a variety of professionals. These environments provide many opportunities for interdisciplinary and multidisciplinary collaboration for conducting research. Interdisciplinary collaboration involves researchers from different disciplines working together on the same research problem. Multidisciplinary collaboration involves professionals from different disciplines working parallel to one another on similar research problems (Oberst, 1980). Advantages of these types of collaboration projects are that the researchers have different areas of expertise and resources to share that could improve the research methodology. Since these researchers work in different disciplines, they often have unique ideas about how to study a problem. Today, interdisciplinary and multidisciplinary collaboration projects are more likely to receive external funding than previously (Engstrom, 1984).

Collaboration Among Expert Researchers ☐ More and more researchers are collaborating in conducting an individual study or in conducting many related studies. Organizations such as the Western Council for Higher Education in Nursing (WCHEN) have encouraged the conduct of collaborative research projects among expert researchers. WCHEN sponsored workshops to facilitate collaboration among nurses of various clinical backgrounds and research expertise (Krueger, Nelson & Wolanin, 1978). Three types of collaborative projects were identified: (1) multiple settings–single study, (2) vertical building and (3) horizontal building. In the multiple setting–single study type of project, the researchers conduct the same study in multiple settings to gain an adequate sample size. The researchers usually have a common interest in a particular problem, and they design a study in which they can pool their data for analysis.

In the vertical building type of project, the researchers are involved with concurrent replications of a study in which different patients are used. For example, the same study might be conducted using patients experiencing heart disease, respiratory disease and renal disease. Clinical trials are an example of vertical building projects. In a clinical trial, a protocol is developed that synthesizes the research base related to a nursing intervention. The protocol indicates the design and the methodology to be used in the clinical trial (Firlit, Kemp & Walsh, 1986). The studies are concurrent or simultaneous replications that are conducted using the protocol with different patients in different settings.

The third type of collaborative project, horizontal building, involves using a single theoretical framework, and each researcher conducts a complementary piece of research to clarify a certain area of the framework. The researchers have a common problem area of interest, but they each select a different research purpose and often study different variables. They use a variety of research designs, measurement tools and data collection and analysis techniques. These horizontal building projects are referred to as *cluster studies*. For example, cluster studies were conducted by the Tube Feeding Group, which was formed from the WCHEN workshops. This group consisted of seven nurse researchers in four geographic locations. Their common area of interest was "nursing interventions in problems of tube feeding" (Bergstrom, Hansen, Grant, Hanson, Kubo, Padilla & Wong, 1984, p. 21). They developed descriptive and experimental studies using different research designs, variables and measurement tools to study nursing measures in the identified problem area.

Collaboration Among University-Based Researchers and Agency-Based Clinicians ☐ Collaborative research projects have been encouraged between members of academic agencies and clinical agencies. In fact, collaboration among expert researchers sometimes involves university-based researchers and agency-based clinicians. In these types of collaborative projects, the expertise of the researchers and the resources of the agencies can be combined to facilitate the conduct of research. The Conduct and Utilization of Research in Nursing (CURN) project was conducted to stimulate collaborative research between university-based researchers and agency-based clinicians (Horsley, Crane, Crabtree & Wood, 1983; Loomis, 1982). The CURN project provided partial funding for the research proposals developed by these teams.

One of us, Grove, has been part of a collaborative research project among university-based researchers and agency-based clinicians. Based on this collaborative experience, guidelines have been identified that might promote effective collaboration among researchers and clinicians. The following steps should be taken early in the formulation of a collaborative project:

1. A research topic and potential research purposes should be identified.
2. Members selected for or who request to be part of the collaborative project must have an interest in the project and an expertise to offer the group.
3. The role of each member should be openly discussed and clearly identified, including the leader or co-leaders of the project.
4. The decision-making process should be clearly outlined, with an indication of how conflicts will be resolved.
5. The specific scientific tasks to be performed should be identified.
6. The scientific tasks are designated to members of the group.
7. A budget should be developed for the project that indicates who or which agencies will be responsible for specific expenses. The group should also budget for hidden costs and indicate who will be responsible for handling unexpected expenses.
8. A mechanism for frequent, at least weekly, communication should be identified. If the group members are close geographically, communication is usually less of a problem.
9. Specific deadlines for completion of the project should be set. Plans should be developed to deal with the possibility of not meeting the deadlines.
10. Ownership of the data should be determined.
11. An extremely important step in planning is deciding who gets the credit. Those responsible for the development of the research report, presentation of that report and authorship of publications should be determined.

Future Conduct of Research in Nursing

DEVELOPING A RESEARCH TRADITION

Currently, there is a conflict among nurse scientists regarding the selection of a research tradition for nursing (Gorenberg, 1983). Research traditions indicate the conceptual boundaries for the domain of inquiry and provide prescriptive norms for how the domain is to be investigated (Laudan, 1981). This means that these traditions direct the conduct of research and the development of theory. Some nurse scientists support the scientific method that involves the conduct of quantitative research, whereas others support the conduct of qualitative research. However, the concern is really not which research tradition to follow but what questions need to be answered and how these questions can best be answered. A research tradition will evolve as nurse scientists determine the research approaches that generate solutions to the problems relevant to the discipline of nursing (Laudan, 1981). The effectiveness of a research tradition can be evaluated by addressing the following questions: "(1) Is it workable? (2) Does it simultaneously offer rational acceptance and scientific progress that can be linked in ways not explained by previous models? (3) Is it more widely applicable in the history of science than alternative models?" (Gorenberg, 1983, p. 348). In the future, it appears that both quantitative and qualitative approaches will be used in the generation of nursing knowledge. In fact, some investigators are incorporating both strategies in a particular study (Bargagliotti, 1983).

THEORY-BASED RESEARCH

Regardless of whether quantitative or qualitative research is conducted, the studies of the future must be theory based. Currently, many of the published studies do not have an explicitly stated framework. Brown et al.'s (1984) review of research articles published in 1980 indicated that 35 per cent of the studies had implied frameworks, and only 14 per cent of the studies had explicitly stated frameworks. Most of these frameworks were selected from the disciplines of physiology, psychology and sociology, not nursing. The studies of the future need to have explicitly stated frameworks that guide the generation and refinement of nursing theory. A study's theoretical or conceptual framework must clearly direct the design of the study and be linked to the study findings. Hopefully, in the future, more researchers will use nursing models as conceptual frameworks for their research (Flaskerud, 1984).

DEVELOPMENT OF INNOVATIVE METHODOLOGIES

A scientific community provides stimulation for the development and implementation of complex, innovative methodologies. Nurse researchers must pursue new designs, methods of measurements and data analysis techniques in generating the knowledge essential for nursing practice. Two recent reviews of the research literature are used to identify the methodological trends that have occurred over the last 30 years. Brown, Tanner and Padrick (1984) examined 137 studies from four nursing research journals (*Nursing Research, International Journal of Nursing Studies, Research in Nursing and Health* and *Western Journal of Nursing Research*) published in 1952–1953, 1960, 1970 and 1980. Jacobsen and Meininger (1985) examined 434 research articles in three nursing research journals (*Nursing Research, Research in Nursing and Health* and *Western Journal of Nursing Research*) published in 1956, 1961, 1966, 1971, 1976, 1981 and 1983. These methodological trends provide direction in making recommendations for the future.

Design

Brown *et al.* (1984) and Jacobsen and Meininger (1985) noted that the use of experimental designs was greatest at the end of the 1960s and the beginning of the 1970s. Through the 1970s and 1980s, the use of experimental designs has continued to decrease. Most of the studies examined by Brown *et al.* and Jacobsen and Meininger were observational with cross-sectional designs. The findings of Jacobsen and Meininger are presented in Table 22–6. Often the data were collected at one point in time; rarely (25 per cent) did the studies include observations at more than one point in time. In the studies designed to measure the impact of interventions, the data were frequently collected too soon after the implementation of the intervention to detect a difference (Brown *et al.*, 1984). Very few of the studies (24 per cent) over the last 30 years have been longitudinal (Jacobsen & Meininger, 1985).

In the future, research is needed to examine trends and processes that exist in clinical practice. For example, studies are needed to examine patterns of care that are provided to patients experiencing different illnesses. Longitudinal designs are needed to examine the trends, processes and patterns relevant to the practice and profession. Jacobsen and Meininger (1985) noted that the number of trend studies was increasing in the 1980s. In addition, innovative designs should be developed to address some of the complex problems confronting nursing. Designs for health promotion and prevention studies are needed to examine the impact of these behaviors on individuals' levels of health. Multivariate designs are needed to examine the many variables that have an impact on the health of the elderly and those experiencing chronic illnesses. More meta-analysis designs are needed to develop an understanding of the findings from many studies. Repeated measures designs are needed to examine the impact of nursing interventions, and the designs of these studies must provide sufficient time for the intervention to make an impact.

TABLE 22–6
Relative Frequency of Principle Designs Used in Nursing
Research Articles by Year

				Year				All
Design	**1956**	**1961**	**1966**	**1971**	**1976**	**1981**	**1983**	**Years**
Experimental								
True	11%	9%	10%	14%	4%	11%	9%	9%
Quasi-	0%	9%	31%	18%	32%	12%	11%	18%
Observational								
Cross-sectional	56%	52%	36%	46%	52%	47%	56%	49%
Longitudinal	33%	30%	24%	22%	12%	30%	24%	24%
N	9	23	42	50	50	66	75	315

(From Jacobsen, B. S. & Meininger, J. C.: The designs and methods of published nursing research: 1956–1983. *Nursing Research,* 34, 307, 1985; with permission.)

Methods of Measurement

During the last 30 years, the most common method of measurement used was the questionnaire. Frequently, the questionnaires were developed for a specific study without documentation of their validity and reliability. As recently as the published studies of the 1980s, researchers were still not documenting the reliability and validity of their instruments (Brown *et al.*, 1984). Instruments were frequently borrowed from other disciplines without determining the usefulness of these instruments in measuring nursing concepts. The studies of the future must incorporate a variety of measurement tools. Extensive methodological research is needed to generate instruments that validly measure the concepts relevant to nursing. Valid and reliable methods of measurements must be used in all studies, and the reliability and validity of the measurement tools must be included in the publication of the study findings.

Subjects and Settings

Many of the studies in the 1950s were conducted using students and health care providers as subjects. However, the use of patients as subjects has greatly increased, from 17 per cent in 1956 to 66 per cent in 1983 (Table 22–7). It is necessary for the trend of using patients as subjects to continue in the future. In addition, families, groups such as professional and self-help organizations, and health care agencies should be studied. Researchers should strive for larger samples using probability sampling techniques. In order to study a variety of populations, studies must be conducted in unique settings such as clinics, workplaces, homes, nursing homes and nurse-managed centers.

Data Analysis

The researchers of the future will need a stronger statistical background. The complex designs involving measurement of many variables will require complex analysis techniques. With greater frequency, researchers will employ complex techniques such as factor analyses, discriminant function analyses, multiple regression analyses and analyses of variance. Researchers will also need to be more sophisticated in qualitative data analysis. In the future, some nurses will

TABLE 22–7
Type of Subjects in Nursing Research Articles by Year

Type of Subject	Year							All Years
	1956	1961	1966	1971	1976	1981	1983	
Patient/client oriented	17%	24%	42%	39%	39%	50%	66%	46%
Health care provider oriented	83%	62%	56%	61%	61%	47%	33%	52%
Other	—	15%	2%	—	—	3%	1%	2%
N	12	34	52	61	64	88	84	395

(From Jacobsen, B. S. & Meininger, J. C.: The designs and methods of published nursing research: 1956–1983. *Nursing Research,* <u>34</u>, 307, 1985; with permission.)

probably be developing their own analysis techniques to examine certain types of data.

Awareness of Nursing Research

There is a need for nurses, politicians and consumers to be aware of the research conducted in nursing. Many mechanisms are being developed, and many more are needed to communicate nursing research findings. Werley and Fitzpatrick (1983, 1984 & 1985) have devised a strategy for summarizing and communicating research findings. Since 1983, they have been publishing a volume entitled *Annual Review of Nursing Research*. These publications include selected research topics and summaries of the research (current scientific knowledge) related to these topics. The areas covered in these volumes include research on nursing practice, nursing care delivery, nursing education, the profession of nursing and other research. The research on nursing practice includes topics such as infants and young children; school-age children and adolescents; adulthood; death, dying and terminal illness; family research; anxiety and conflict in pregnancy; experience of being a parent; health promotion and illness prevention; coping with elective surgery; school nursing; teenage pregnancy; and cross-cultural nursing research. The research on nursing care delivery includes topics such as nursing staff turnover; interorganizational relations; assessment of quality of nursing care; public health nursing evaluation, education and professional issues; nurse practitioners and primary care; and nursing diagnosis. The research on nursing education includes topics such as teaching-learning process, nursing students, curriculum, continuing education and doctoral education of nurses. The research on the profession of nursing includes such topics as socialization and roles, information processing in nursing practice, ethical inquiry and cost-effectiveness analysis. These publications are potentially effective mechanisms for increasing nurses' awareness of nursing research.

A central, computerized information system is needed in nursing. This system can be used to store and rapidly retrieve published and unpublished research. A nursing information system can also be used to disseminate research findings to university-based researchers, clinicians and other members of society. With the rapid advancement of technology, a national information system that will increase the awareness of nursing research might soon be a reality. The next step will be the development of an international information system. Currently, researchers are communicating findings at international nursing research conferences, such as the conference entitled "New Frontiers in Nursing Research" in Canada in May, 1986.

POLITICIAN AWARENESS OF NURSING RESEARCH

Additional strategies are needed to increase politicians' awareness of the research that has been conducted and the future research that is needed in nursing. Publications and media presentations must be developed to communicate research findings to health policy makers (American Nurses Association, 1985). These publications and presentations must demonstrate the research expertise of nurses. In addition, nurse scientists must actively pursue federal funding for research. In the past, most of the research funds have been designated for studies involving the diagnosis and cure of disease. Nursing research has focused on prevention of illness and quality care for the chronically ill (Larson, 1984); therefore, nursing has been receiving a very small percentage of the federal research and development (R & D) funds. As indicated in Figure 22–1, nurses are receiving only 0.8 per cent of these funds (Larson, 1984). The American Nurses Association (1985) indicated that funding for nursing research must be at least $50 million by 1990 and $75 million by 1995. In addition, they indicated that $5 million was needed for major equipment by 1990 and $10 million by 1995.

Center for Nursing Research

Only recently has the need for nursing research been brought to the attention of the scientific community and the politicians. The 1983 Institute of Medicine report entitled "Nursing and nursing education: public policies and private actions" strongly supported a federally sponsored center for nursing research:

> A substantial share of the health care dollar is expended on direct nursing care, yet the professionals who deliver this care work without the benefit of a strong organizational base to stimulate and support scientific investigation in their field. The committee believes that a center of nursing research is needed at a high level in the federal government to be a focal point for promoting the growth of quality nursing research (p. 216).

In 1985, the American Nurses Association accomplished a major political victory for nursing research with the creation of a National Center for Nursing Research. This center for nursing research was created after 2 years of work and two presidential vetoes (Bauknecht, 1986). The purpose of the center is "the conduct, support and dissemination of information regarding basic and clinical nursing research, training and other programs in patient care research" (Bauknecht, 1985, p. 2). Having a center for nursing research complies with

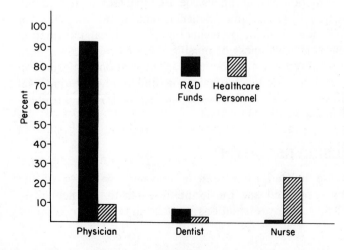

FIGURE 22–1. Percent of total health care personnel and percent of federal R & D funds for three professional groups.*

*Group includes physicians, dentists, and registered nurses (excludes administrative, construction, and training allocations). (From Larson, E.: Health policy and NIH: implications for nursing research. *Nursing Research*, 33, 352, 1984, with permission.)

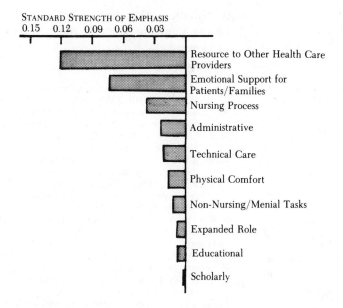

FIGURE 22–2. Nursing activities on television: 1950 through 1979.

(From Kalisch, P. A., Kalisch, B. J. & Clinton, J.: The world of nursing on prime time television: 1950–1980. *Nursing Research,* 31, 358, 1982; with permission.)

the recommendation of the Institute of Medicine (IOM), which was to establish an organizational entity within the federal structure to place nursing research in the mainstream of scientific inquiry and accountability (Aiken, 1983). An advisory council for the center will be appointed by the Secretary of Health and Human Services and will make recommendations to the Secretary regarding the Center's activities. The National Center for Nursing Research will be established under the National Institutes of Health (NIH), which will provide greater visibility for nursing research at the federal level. The Center for Nursing Research will probably make it possible to expand the number of experienced nurse researchers and to increase nurse researchers' interactions with researchers in other health research disciplines (Bauknecht, 1985). It is hoped that this is only one of many steps that can be taken to further the visibility of nursing research.

CONSUMER AWARENESS OF NURSING RESEARCH

There is a need to increase consumers' awareness of the scientific endeavors of nurses. Most consumers do not view nurses as researchers and scholars. Kalisch, Kalisch and Clinton (1982) noted that a scholarly image of nurses has not been projected on television during the last 20 years. The nursing activities that have been portrayed on television from 1950 to 1979 are presented in Figure 22–2. Most of the nurse characters (82 per cent) worked in a hospital and served as resources to other health care providers.

The professional organization needs to conduct a mass media campaign to promote the image of the nurse as a scholar, a theorist and a researcher (Hinshaw, 1983). This campaign should involve communication by a variety of media, including newspaper, radio and television. Consumers should know the contributions that nurses are making to the body of scientific knowledge. Through nursing research, the quality of the health care provided to consumers will improve.

References

Aiken, L. H. (1983). Nursing's future: public policies, private actions. *American Journal of Nursing*, 83(10), 1440–1444.

American Nurses Association, Cabinet on Nursing Research (1985). *Directions for nursing research: toward the twenty-first century*. Kansas City, Missouri: American Nurses Association.

Andreoli, K. G. & Musser, L. A. (1985). Trends that may affect nursing's future. *Nursing and Health Care*, 6(1), 46–51.

Bargagliotti, L. A. (1983). Researchmanship: the scientific method and phenomenology: toward their peaceful coexistence in nursing. *Western Journal of Nursing Research*, 5(4), 409–411.

Barnard, K. E. (1982). Proceedings of the 1982 Conference of the Western Society for Research in Nursing. The research cycle: nursing, the profession, the discipline. *Western Journal of Nursing Research*, 4(3), 1–12.

Bauknecht, V. L. (1985). Capital commentary: NIH bill passes, includes nursing research center. *American Nurse*, 17(10), 2.

Bauknecht, V. L. (1986). Congress overrides veto, nursing gets center for research. *American Nurse*, 18(1), 1, 24.

Bergstrom, N., Hansen, B. C., Grant, M., Hanson, R., Kubo, W., Padilla, G. & Wong, H. L. (1984). Collaborative nursing research: anatomy of a successful consortium. *Nursing Research*, 33(1), 20–25.

Brogan, D. R. (1982). Professional socialization to a research role: interest in research among graduate students in nursing. *Research in Nursing and Health*, 5(3), 113–122.

Brown, J. S., Tanner, C. A. & Padrick, K. P. (1984). Nursing's search for scientific knowledge. *Nursing Research*, 33(1), 26–32.

Engstrom, J. L. (1984). University, agency, and collaborative models for nursing research: an overview. *Image: The Journal of Nursing Scholarship*, 16(3), 76–80.

Evans, L. K., Dienemann, J. & Dahlen, R. (1986). University-based nursing research centers: a strategic investment. *Nursing Economics*, 4(1), 23–30.

Fagan, M. M. & Fagan, P. D. (1983). Mentoring among nurses. *Nursing and Health Care*, 13(2), 77–82.

Fawcett, J. (1980). Editorial: on development of a scientific community in nursing. *Image*, 12(3), 51–52.

Firlit, S. L., Kemp, M. G. & Walsh, M. (1986). Strategies for teaching nursing research: preparing master's students to develop clinical trials. *Western Journal of Nursing Research*, 8(1), 106–109.

Flaskerud, J. H. (1984). Nursing models as conceptual frameworks for research. *Western Journal of Nursing Research*, 6(2), 153–155.

Gorenberg, B. (1983). The research tradition of nursing: an emerging issue. *Nursing Research*, 32(6), 347–349.

Gortner, S. R. (1980). Nursing research: out of the past and into the future. *Nursing Research*, 29(4), 204–207.

Hagerty, B. (1986). A second look at mentors. *Nursing Outlook*, 341, 16–19.

Hagstrom, W. O. (1965). *Scientific community*. New York: Basic Books.

Hinshaw, A. S. (1983). Proceedings of the 1983 Conference of the Western Society for Research in Nursing. The image of nursing research: issues and strategies. *Western Journal of Nursing Research*, 5(3), 1–13.

Hinshaw, A. S. (1984). Theoretical model testing: full utilization of data. *Western Journal of Nursing Research*, 6(1), 5–9.

Horsley, J. A., Crane, J., Crabtree, M. K. & Wood, D. J. (1983). *Using research to improve nursing practice: a guide, CURN Project*. New York: Grune & Stratton, Inc.

Institute of Medicine. (1983). *Nursing and nursing education: public policies and private actions*. Washington, DC: National Academy Press.

Jacobsen, B. S. & Meininger, J. C. (1985). The designs and methods of published nursing research: 1956–1983. *Nursing Research*, 34(5), 306–312.

Jacox, A. K. (1980). Strategies to promote nursing research. *Nursing Research*, 29(4), 213–217.

Jacox, A. K. (1985). Science and politics: the background and the issues surrounding the controversial proposal for a national institute of nursing. *Nursing Outlook*, 33(2), 78–84.

Kalisch, B. (1975). Creativity and nursing research. *Nursing Outlook*, 23(5), 314–319.

Kalisch, P. A., Kalisch, B. J. & Clinton, J. (1982). The world of nursing on prime time television, 1950 to 1980. *Nursing Research*, 31(6), 358–363.

Krueger, J. C., Nelson, A. H. & Wolanin, M. O. (1978). *Nursing research: development, collaboration, and utilization*. Rockville, Maryland: Aspen Systems Corporation.

Lancaster, J. (1985). The perils and joys of collaborative research: what to look for—and what to avoid—when putting together a research team. *Nursing Outlook*, 33(5), 231–232.

Larson, E. (1984). Health policy and NIH: implications for nursing research. *Nursing Research*, 33(6), 352–356.

Larson, E. (1986). Guidelines for collaborative research with industry. *Nursing Economics*, 4(3), 131–133.

Laudan, L. (1981). A problem-solving approach to scientific progress. In I. Hacking (Ed.), *Scientific revolutions* (pp. 144-155). Oxford, England: Oxford University Press.

Levin, R. F. (1983). Research for the undergraduate: too much, too soon. *Nursing Outlook*, 31(5), 258–259.

Loomis, M. E. (1982). Resources for collaborative research. *Western Journal of Nursing Research*, 4(1), 65–74.

Loomis, M. E. (1985). Emerging content in nursing: an analysis of dissertation abstracts and titles: 1976-1982. *Nursing Research*, 34(2), 113–119.

Meisenhelder, J. B. (1982). Networking and nursing. *Image*, 14(3), 77–80.

Mercer, R. T. (1984). Student involvement in faculty research: a mentor's view. *Western Journal of Nursing Research*, 6(4), 433–437.

Mitsunaga, B. K. (1981). The use of knowledge and health policy planning: forms and functions of the relationships. *Western Journal of Nursing Research*, 3(3), 1–8.

Murphy, S. O. (1985). Contexts for scientific creativity: applications to nursing. *Image*, 17(4), 103–107.

Newman, M. A. (1982). What differentiates clinical research? *Image*, 14(3), 86–88.

Oberst, M. T. (1980). Nursing research: new definitions, collegial approaches. *Cancer Nursing*, 3(6), 459.

Paletta, J. L. (1980). Nursing research: an integral part of professional nursing. *Image*, 12(1), 3–6.

Reynolds, M. A. & Haller, K. B. (1986). Using research in practice: a case for replication in nursing—part I. *Western Journal of Nursing Research*, 8(1), 113–116.

Rittenmeyer, P. A. (1982). The evolution of nursing research. *Western Journal of Nursing Research*, 4(2), 223–225.

Speer, J., McLane, A., White, M. A., Whall, A., King, J. M., Buckwalter, K. C., Lasky, P. & Lederman, R. (1985). Symposium: development of a research group. Collaboration and the research process. *Western Journal of Nursing Research*, 7(1), 32–39.

Stanford, E. D. (1980). Directions for research in nursing. *Nursing Research*, 29(4), 203.

Stinson, S. M., Kerr, J. C., Giovannetti, P., Field, P. & MacPhail, J. (Eds.) (1986). *New frontiers in nursing research*. Proceedings of the International Nursing Research Conference. Edmonton, Alberta, Canada.

Werley, H. H. (1972). This I believe about clinical nursing research. *Nursing Outlook*, 20(11), 718–722.

Werley, H. H. & Fitzpatrick, J. J. (1983). *Annual review of nursing research* (Vol. 1). New York: Springer Publishing Company.

Werley, H. H. & Fitzpatrick, J. J. (1984). *Annual review of nursing research* (Vol. 2). New York: Springer Publishing Company.

Werley, H. H. & Fitzpatrick, J. J. (1985). *Annual review of nursing research* (Vol. 3). New York: Springer Publishing Company.

White, D. L. & Hamel, P. K. (1986). National center for nursing research: how it came to be. *Nursing Economics*, 4(1), 19–22.

Appendices

APPENDIX K
Table of Probabilities Associated With Values as Large as Observed Values of *H* in the *Kruskal-Wallis* One-Way Analysis of Variance by Ranks

APPENDIX L
Table of Probabilities Associated With Values as Large as Observed Values of χ_r^2 in the Friedman Two-Way Analysis of Variance by Ranks

APPENDIX M
Statistical Power Tables

APPENDIX A
Table of Random Numbers

71510	68311	48214	99929	64650	13229
36921	58733	13459	93488	21949	30920
23288	89515	58503	46185	00368	82604
02668	37444	50640	54968	11409	36148
82091	87298	41397	71112	00076	60029
47837	76717	09653	54466	87988	82363
17934	52793	17641	19502	31735	36901
92296	19293	57583	86043	69502	12601
00535	82698	04174	32342	66533	07875
54446	08795	63563	42296	74647	73120
96981	68729	21154	56182	71840	66135
52397	89724	96436	17871	21823	04027
76403	04655	87277	32593	17097	06913
05136	05115	25922	07123	31485	52166
07645	85123	20945	06370	70255	22806
32530	98883	19105	01769	20276	59402
60427	03316	41439	22012	00159	08461
51811	14651	45119	97921	08063	70820
01832	53295	66575	21384	75357	55888
83430	96917	73978	87884	13249	28870
00995	28829	15048	49573	65278	61493
44032	88720	73058	66010	55115	79227
27929	23392	06432	50201	39055	15529
53484	33973	10614	25190	52647	62580
51184	31339	60009	66595	64358	14985
31359	77470	58126	59192	23371	25190
37842	44387	92421	42965	09736	51873
94596	61368	82091	63835	86859	10678
58210	59820	24710	23225	45788	21426
63354	29875	51058	29958	61221	61200
79958	67599	74103	49824	39306	15069
56328	26905	34454	53965	66617	22137
72806	64421	58711	68436	60301	28620
91920	96081	01413	27281	19397	36231
05010	42003	99866	20924	76152	54090
88239	80732	20778	45726	41481	48277
45705	96458	13918	52375	57457	87884
64274	26236	61096	01309	48632	00431
63731	18917	21614	06412	71008	20255
39891	75337	89452	88092	61012	38072
26466	03735	39891	26362	86817	48193
33492	70485	77323	01016	97315	03944
04509	46144	88909	55261	73434	62538
63187	57352	91208	33555	75943	41669
64651	38741	86190	38197	99113	59694
46792	78975	01999	78892	16177	95747
78076	75002	51309	18791	34162	32258
05345	79268	75608	29916	37005	09213
10991	50452	02376	40372	45077	73706

APPENDIX B
Cumulative Normal Distribution (Z)

Z	X	Area	Z	X	Area
−3.25	$\mu - 3.25\sigma$	.0006	−1.00	$\mu - 1.00\sigma$	.1587
−3.20	$\mu - 3.20\sigma$	.0007	− .95	$\mu - .95\sigma$	.1711
−3.15	$\mu - 3.15\sigma$	.0008	− .90	$\mu - .90\sigma$	.1841
−3.10	$\mu - 3.10\sigma$	.0010	− .85	$\mu - .85\sigma$	.1977
−3.05	$\mu - 3.05\sigma$	.0011	− .80	$\mu - .80\sigma$	.2119
−3.00	$\mu - 3.00\sigma$	.0013	− .75	$\mu - .75\sigma$	.2266
−2.95	$\mu - 2.95\sigma$	.0016	− .70	$\mu - .70\sigma$	.2420
−2.90	$\mu - 2.90\sigma$	.0019	− .65	$\mu - .65\sigma$	.2578
−2.85	$\mu - 2.85\sigma$	.0022	− .60	$\mu - .60\sigma$	.2743
−2.80	$\mu - 2.80\sigma$	.0026	− .55	$\mu - .55\sigma$	.2912
−2.75	$\mu - 2.75\sigma$	.0030	− .50	$\mu - .50\sigma$	.3085
−2.70	$\mu - 2.70\sigma$	.0035	− .45	$\mu - .45\sigma$	.3264
−2.65	$\mu - 2.65\sigma$	.0040	− .40	$\mu - .40\sigma$	.3446
−2.60	$\mu - 2.60\sigma$	.0047	− .35	$\mu - .35\sigma$	.3632
−2.55	$\mu - 2.55\sigma$	.0054	− .30	$\mu - .30\sigma$	.3821
−2.50	$\mu - 2.50\sigma$	.0062	− .25	$\mu - .25\sigma$	.4013
−2.45	$\mu - 2.45\sigma$	.0071	− .20	$\mu - .20\sigma$	.4207
−2.40	$\mu - 2.40\sigma$	.0082	− .15	$\mu - .15\sigma$	.4404
−2.35	$\mu - 2.35\sigma$	.0094	− .10	$\mu - .10\sigma$	.4602
−2.30	$\mu - 2.30\sigma$	.0107	− .05	$\mu - .05\sigma$	.4801
−2.25	$\mu - 2.25\sigma$	.0122			
−2.20	$\mu - 2.20\sigma$	.0139			
−2.15	$\mu - 2.15\sigma$	.0158	.00	μ	.5000
−2.10	$\mu - 2.10\sigma$	.0179			
−2.05	$\mu - 2.05\sigma$	.0202			
−2.00	$\mu - 2.00\sigma$	.0228	.05	$\mu + .05\sigma$	.5199
−1.95	$\mu - 1.95\sigma$	.0256	.10	$\mu + .10\sigma$	.5398
−1.90	$\mu - 1.90\sigma$	.0287	.15	$\mu + .15\sigma$	.5596
−1.85	$\mu - 1.85\sigma$	.0322	.20	$\mu + .20\sigma$	.5793
−1.80	$\mu - 1.80\sigma$	.0359	.25	$\mu + .25\sigma$	.5987
−1.75	$\mu - 1.75\sigma$	.0401	.30	$\mu + .30\sigma$	.6179
−1.70	$\mu - 1.70\sigma$	.0446	.35	$\mu + .35\sigma$	.6368
−1.65	$\mu - 1.65\sigma$	.0495	.40	$\mu + .40\sigma$	.6554
−1.60	$\mu - 1.60\sigma$	.0548	.45	$\mu + .45\sigma$	.6736
−1.55	$\mu - 1.55\sigma$	.0606	.50	$\mu + .50\sigma$	.6915
−1.50	$\mu - 1.50\sigma$	.0668	.55	$\mu + .55\sigma$	.7088
−1.45	$\mu - 1.45\sigma$	.0735	.60	$\mu + .60\sigma$	.7257
−1.40	$\mu - 1.40\sigma$	.0808	.65	$\mu + .65\sigma$	.7422
−1.35	$\mu - 1.35\sigma$	.0885	.70	$\mu + .70\sigma$	.7580
−1.30	$\mu - 1.30\sigma$	.0968	.75	$\mu + .75\sigma$	.7734
−1.25	$\mu - 1.25\sigma$	.1056	.80	$\mu + .80\sigma$	.7881
−1.20	$\mu - 1.20\sigma$	.1151	.85	$\mu + .85\sigma$	.8023
−1.15	$\mu - 1.15\sigma$	.1251	.90	$\mu + .90\sigma$	.8159
−1.10	$\mu - 1.10\sigma$	.1357	.95	$\mu + .95\sigma$	.8289
−1.05	$\mu - 1.05\sigma$	.1469	1.00	$\mu + 1.00\sigma$	.8413

Table continued on opposite page

APPENDIX B (*continued*)

Z	X	Area	Z	X	Area
1.05	$\mu + 1.05\sigma$	.8531	−4.265	$\mu - 4.265\sigma$	.00001
1.10	$\mu + 1.10\sigma$	.8643	−3.719	$\mu - 3.719\sigma$	.0001
1.15	$\mu + 1.15\sigma$	.8749	−3.090	$\mu - 3.090\sigma$	.001
1.20	$\mu + 1.20\sigma$	.8849	−2.576	$\mu - 2.576\sigma$	.005
1.25	$\mu + 1.25\sigma$	.8944	−2.326	$\mu - 2.326\sigma$	.01
1.30	$\mu + 1.30\sigma$	.9032	−2.054	$\mu - 2.054\sigma$	.02
1.35	$\mu + 1.35\sigma$	.9115	−1.960	$\mu - 1.960\sigma$	.025
1.40	$\mu + 1.40\sigma$	.9192	−1.881	$\mu - 1.881\sigma$	.03
1.45	$\mu + 1.45\sigma$	.9265	−1.751	$\mu - 1.751\sigma$	.04
1.50	$\mu + 1.50\sigma$	.9332	−1.645	$\mu - 1.645\sigma$	.05
1.55	$\mu + 1.55\sigma$	.9394	−1.555	$\mu - 1.555\sigma$	.06
1.60	$\mu + 1.60\sigma$	.9452	−1.476	$\mu - 1.476\sigma$	.07
1.65	$\mu + 1.65\sigma$	.9505	−1.405	$\mu - 1.405\sigma$	.08
1.70	$\mu + 1.70\sigma$	.9554	−1.341	$\mu - 1.341\sigma$	.09
1.75	$\mu + 1.75\sigma$	.9599	−1.282	$\mu - 1.282\sigma$	.10
1.80	$\mu + 1.80\sigma$	.9641	−1.036	$\mu - 1.036\sigma$	.15
1.85	$\mu + 1.85\sigma$	.9678	−.842	$\mu - .842\sigma$	.20
1.90	$\mu + 1.90\sigma$	.9713	−.674	$\mu - .674\sigma$	.25
1.95	$\mu + 1.95\sigma$	.9744	−.524	$\mu - .524\sigma$	.30
2.00	$\mu + 2.00\sigma$	.9772	−.385	$\mu - .385\sigma$	.35
2.05	$\mu + 2.05\sigma$	.9798	−.253	$\mu - .253\sigma$	.40
2.10	$\mu + 2.10\sigma$	.9821	−.126	$\mu - .126\sigma$	.45
2.15	$\mu + 2.15\sigma$	.9842	0	μ	.50
2.20	$\mu + 2.20\sigma$	.9861	.126	$\mu + .126\sigma$	.55
2.25	$\mu + 2.25\sigma$	.9878	.253	$\mu + .253\sigma$	.60
2.30	$\mu + 2.30\sigma$	.9893	.385	$\mu + .385\sigma$	.65
2.35	$\mu + 2.35\sigma$	.9906	.524	$\mu + .524\sigma$	.70
2.40	$\mu + 2.40\sigma$	.9918	.674	$\mu + .674\sigma$	.75
2.45	$\mu + 2.45\sigma$	.9929	.842	$\mu + .842\sigma$	.80
2.50	$\mu + 2.50\sigma$	.9938	1.036	$\mu + 1.036\sigma$	.85
2.55	$\mu + 2.55\sigma$	.9946	1.282	$\mu + 1.282\sigma$	.90
2.60	$\mu + 2.60\sigma$	.9953	1.341	$\mu + 1.341\sigma$	.91
2.65	$\mu + 2.65\sigma$	.9960	1.405	$\mu + 1.405\sigma$	.92
2.70	$\mu + 2.70\sigma$	.9965	1.476	$\mu + 1.476\sigma$	.93
2.75	$\mu + 2.75\sigma$	.9970	1.555	$\mu + 1.555\sigma$	.94
2.80	$\mu + 2.80\sigma$	.9974	1.645	$\mu + 1.645\sigma$	.95
2.85	$\mu + 2.85\sigma$	.9978	1.751	$\mu + 1.751\sigma$	.96
2.90	$\mu + 2.90\sigma$	.9981	1.881	$\mu + 1.881\sigma$	.97
2.95	$\mu + 2.95\sigma$	.9984	1.960	$\mu + 1.960\sigma$	.975
3.00	$\mu + 3.00\sigma$	.9987	2.054	$\mu + 2.054\sigma$	.98
3.05	$\mu + 3.05\sigma$	.9989	2.326	$\mu + 2.326\sigma$	.99
3.10	$\mu + 3.10\sigma$	.9990	2.576	$\mu + 2.576\sigma$	.995
3.15	$\mu + 3.15\sigma$	.9992	3.090	$\mu + 3.090\sigma$	.999
3.20	$\mu + 3.20\sigma$	.9993	3.719	$\mu + 3.719\sigma$	.9999
3.25	$\mu + 3.25\sigma$	.9994	4.265	$\mu + 4.265\sigma$	.99999

(From Dixon, W. J. and Massey, F. J. Jr.: *Introduction to statistical analysis* (3rd ed). New York: McGraw-Hill Book Company, 1969; with permission.)

Percentage Points of Student's t Distribution

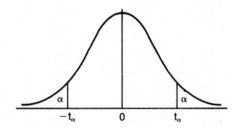

APPENDIX C (*continued*)

df	α .25 2α .50	.20 .40	.15 .30	.10 .20	.05 .10	.025 .05	.01 .02	.005 .01	.0005 .001
1	1.000	1.376	1.963	3.078	6.314	12.706	31.821	63.657	636.619
2	.816	1.061	1.386	1.886	2.920	4.303	6.965	9.925	31.598
3	.765	.978	1.250	1.638	2.353	3.182	4.541	5.841	12.924
4	.741	.941	1.190	1.533	2.132	2.776	3.747	4.604	8.610
5	.727	.920	1.156	1.476	2.015	2.571	3.365	4.032	6.869
6	.718	.906	1.134	1.440	1.943	2.447	3.143	3.707	5.959
7	.711	.896	1.119	1.415	1.895	2.365	2.998	3.499	5.408
8	.706	.889	1.108	1.397	1.860	2.306	2.896	3.355	5.041
9	.703	.883	1.100	1.383	1.833	2.262	2.821	3.250	4.781
10	.700	.879	1.093	1.372	1.812	2.228	2.764	3.169	4.587
11	.697	.876	1.088	1.363	1.796	2.201	2.718	3.106	4.437
12	.695	.873	1.083	1.356	1.782	2.179	2.681	3.055	4.318
13	.694	.870	1.079	1.350	1.771	2.160	2.650	3.012	4.221
14	.692	.868	1.076	1.345	1.761	2.145	2.624	2.977	4.140
15	.691	.866	1.074	1.341	1.753	2.131	2.602	2.947	4.073
16	.690	.865	1.071	1.337	1.746	2.120	2.583	2.921	4.015
17	.689	.863	1.069	1.333	1.740	2.110	2.567	2.898	3.965
18	.688	.862	1.067	1.330	1.734	2.101	2.552	2.878	3.922
19	.688	.861	1.066	1.328	1.729	2.093	2.539	2.861	3.883
20	.687	.860	1.064	1.325	1.725	2.086	2.528	2.845	3.850
21	.686	.859	1.063	1.323	1.721	2.080	2.518	2.831	3.819
22	.686	.858	1.061	1.321	1.717	2.074	2.508	2.819	3.792
23	.685	.858	1.060	1.319	1.714	2.069	2.500	2.807	3.767
24	.685	.857	1.059	1.318	1.711	2.064	2.492	2.797	3.745
25	.684	.856	1.058	1.316	1.708	2.060	2.485	2.787	3.725
26	.684	.856	1.058	1.315	1.706	2.056	2.479	2.779	3.707
27	.684	.855	1.057	1.314	1.703	2.052	2.473	2.771	3.690
28	.683	.855	1.056	1.313	1.701	2.048	2.467	2.763	3.674
29	.683	.854	1.055	1.311	1.699	2.045	2.462	2.756	3.659
30	.683	.854	1.055	1.310	1.697	2.042	2.457	2.750	3.646
40	.681	.851	1.050	1.303	1.684	2.021	2.423	2.704	3.551
60	.679	.848	1.046	1.296	1.671	2.000	2.390	2.660	3.460
120	.677	.845	1.041	1.289	1.658	1.980	2.358	2.617	3.373
∞	.674	.842	1.036	1.282	1.645	1.960	2.326	2.576	3.291

(From Fisher, R. A. and Yates, F.: *Statistical tables for biological, agricultural, and medical research* (6th ed.). London: Longman Group Ltd., 1978. [Previously published by Oliver & Boyd Ltd. Edinburgh]; and by permission of the authors and publishers.)

APPENDIX D
Percentage Points of the F Distribution

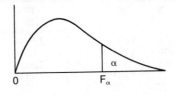

$\alpha = .05$

Degrees of Freedom

v_1

v_2	1	2	3	4	5	6	7	8	9
1	161.4	199.5	215.7	224.6	230.2	234.0	236.8	238.9	240.5
2	18.51	19.00	19.16	19.25	19.30	19.33	19.35	19.37	19.38
3	10.13	9.55	9.28	9.12	9.01	8.94	8.89	8.85	8.81
4	7.71	6.94	6.59	6.39	6.26	6.16	6.09	6.04	6.00
5	6.61	5.79	5.41	5.19	5.05	4.95	4.88	4.82	4.77
6	5.99	5.14	4.76	4.53	4.39	4.28	4.21	4.15	4.10
7	5.59	4.74	4.35	4.12	3.97	3.87	3.79	3.73	3.68
8	5.32	4.46	4.07	3.84	3.69	3.58	3.50	3.44	3.39
9	5.12	4.26	3.86	3.63	3.48	3.37	3.29	3.23	3.18
10	4.96	4.10	3.71	3.48	3.33	3.22	3.14	3.07	3.02
11	4.84	3.98	3.59	3.36	3.20	3.09	3.01	2.95	2.90
12	4.75	3.89	3.49	3.26	3.11	3.00	2.91	2.85	2.80
13	4.67	3.81	3.41	3.18	3.03	2.92	2.83	2.77	2.71
14	4.60	3.74	3.34	3.11	2.96	2.85	2.76	2.70	2.65
15	4.54	3.68	3.29	3.06	2.90	2.79	2.71	2.64	2.59
16	4.49	3.63	3.24	3.01	2.85	2.74	2.66	2.59	2.54
17	4.45	3.59	3.20	2.96	2.81	2.70	2.61	2.55	2.49
18	4.41	3.55	3.16	2.93	2.77	2.66	2.58	2.51	2.46
19	4.38	3.52	3.13	2.90	2.74	2.63	2.54	2.48	2.42
20	4.35	3.49	3.10	2.87	2.71	2.60	2.51	2.45	2.39
21	4.32	3.47	3.07	2.84	2.68	2.57	2.49	2.42	2.37
22	4.30	3.44	3.05	2.82	2.66	2.55	2.46	2.40	2.34
23	4.28	3.42	3.03	2.80	2.64	2.53	2.44	2.37	2.32
24	4.26	3.40	3.01	2.78	2.62	2.51	2.42	2.36	2.30
25	4.24	3.39	2.99	2.76	2.60	2.49	2.40	2.34	2.28
26	4.23	3.37	2.98	2.74	2.59	2.47	2.39	2.32	2.27
27	4.21	3.35	2.96	2.73	2.57	2.46	2.37	2.31	2.25
28	4.20	3.34	2.95	2.71	2.56	2.45	2.36	2.29	2.24
29	4.18	3.33	2.93	2.70	2.55	2.43	2.35	2.28	2.22
30	4.17	3.32	2.92	2.69	2.53	2.42	2.33	2.27	2.21
40	4.08	3.23	2.84	2.61	2.45	2.34	2.25	2.18	2.12
60	4.00	3.15	2.76	2.53	2.37	2.25	2.17	2.10	2.04
120	3.92	3.07	2.68	2.45	2.29	2.17	2.09	2.02	1.96
∞	3.84	3.00	2.60	2.37	2.21	2.10	2.01	1.94	1.88

Table continued on opposite page

APPENDIX D (*continued*)

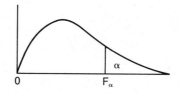

$$\alpha = .01$$

v_1

10	12	15	20	24	30	40	60	120	∞	v_2
241.9	243.9	245.9	248.0	249.1	250.1	251.1	252.2	253.3	254.3	1
19.40	19.41	19.43	19.45	19.45	19.46	19.47	19.48	19.49	19.50	2
8.79	8.74	8.70	8.66	8.64	8.62	8.59	8.57	8.55	8.53	3
5.96	5.91	5.86	5.80	5.77	5.75	5.72	5.69	5.66	5.63	4
4.74	4.68	4.62	4.56	4.53	4.50	4.46	4.43	4.40	4.36	5
4.06	4.00	3.94	3.87	3.84	3.81	3.77	3.74	3.70	3.67	6
3.64	3.57	3.51	3.44	3.41	3.38	3.34	3.30	3.27	3.23	7
3.35	3.28	3.22	3.15	3.12	3.08	3.04	3.01	2.97	2.93	8
3.14	3.07	3.01	2.94	2.90	2.86	2.83	2.79	2.75	2.71	9
2.98	2.91	2.85	2.77	2.74	2.70	2.66	2.62	2.58	2.54	10
2.85	2.79	2.72	2.65	2.61	2.57	2.53	2.49	2.45	2.40	11
2.75	2.69	2.62	2.54	2.51	2.47	2.43	2.38	2.34	2.30	12
2.67	2.60	2.53	2.46	2.42	2.38	2.34	2.30	2.25	2.21	13
2.60	2.53	2.46	2.39	2.35	2.31	2.27	2.22	2.18	2.13	14
2.54	2.48	2.40	2.33	2.29	2.25	2.20	2.16	2.11	2.07	15
2.49	2.42	2.35	2.28	2.24	2.19	2.15	2.11	2.06	2.01	16
2.45	2.38	2.31	2.23	2.19	2.15	2.10	2.06	2.01	1.96	17
2.41	2.34	2.27	2.19	2.15	2.11	2.06	2.02	1.97	1.92	18
2.38	2.31	2.23	2.16	2.11	2.07	2.03	1.98	1.93	1.88	19
2.35	2.28	2.20	2.12	2.08	2.04	1.99	1.95	1.90	1.84	20
2.32	2.25	2.18	2.10	2.05	2.01	1.96	1.92	1.87	1.81	21
2.30	2.23	2.15	2.07	2.03	1.98	1.94	1.89	1.84	1.78	22
2.27	2.20	2.13	2.05	2.01	1.96	1.91	1.86	1.81	1.76	23
2.25	2.18	2.11	2.03	1.98	1.94	1.89	1.84	1.79	1.73	24
2.24	2.16	2.09	2.01	1.96	1.92	1.87	1.82	1.77	1.71	25
2.22	2.15	2.07	1.99	1.95	1.90	1.85	1.80	1.75	1.69	26
2.20	2.13	2.06	1.97	1.93	1.88	1.84	1.79	1.73	1.67	27
2.19	2.12	2.04	1.96	1.91	1.87	1.82	1.77	1.71	1.65	28
2.18	2.10	2.03	1.94	1.90	1.85	1.81	1.75	1.70	1.64	29
2.16	2.09	2.01	1.93	1.89	1.84	1.79	1.74	1.68	1.62	30
2.08	2.00	1.92	1.84	1.79	1.74	1.69	1.64	1.58	1.51	40
1.99	1.92	1.84	1.75	1.70	1.65	1.59	1.53	1.47	1.39	60
1.91	1.83	1.75	1.66	1.61	1.55	1.50	1.43	1.35	1.25	120
1.83	1.75	1.67	1.57	1.52	1.46	1.39	1.32	1.22	1.00	∞

Table continued on following page

APPENDIX D (*continued*)

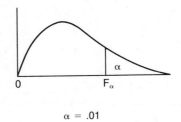

$$\alpha = .01$$

Degrees of Freedom

$$v_1$$

v_2	1	2	3	4	5	6	7	8	9
1	4052	4999.5	5403	5625	5764	5859	5928	5982	6022
2	98.50	99.00	99.17	99.25	99.30	99.33	99.36	99.37	99.39
3	34.12	30.82	29.46	28.71	28.24	27.91	27.67	27.49	27.35
4	21.20	18.00	16.69	15.98	15.52	15.21	14.98	14.80	14.66
5	16.26	13.27	12.06	11.39	10.97	10.67	10.46	10.29	10.16
6	13.75	10.92	9.78	9.15	8.75	8.47	8.26	8.10	7.98
7	12.25	9.55	8.45	7.85	7.46	7.19	6.99	6.84	6.72
8	11.26	8.65	7.59	7.01	6.63	6.37	6.18	6.03	5.91
9	10.56	8.02	6.99	6.42	6.06	5.80	5.61	5.47	5.35
10	10.04	7.56	6.55	5.99	5.64	5.39	5.20	5.06	4.94
11	9.65	7.21	6.22	5.67	5.32	5.07	4.89	4.74	4.63
12	9.33	6.93	5.95	5.41	5.06	4.82	4.64	4.50	4.39
13	9.07	6.70	5.74	5.21	4.86	4.62	4.44	4.30	4.19
14	8.86	6.51	5.56	5.04	4.69	4.46	4.28	4.14	4.03
15	8.68	6.36	5.42	4.89	4.56	4.32	4.14	4.00	3.89
16	8.53	6.23	5.29	4.77	4.44	4.20	4.03	3.89	3.78
17	8.40	6.11	5.18	4.67	4.34	4.10	3.93	3.79	3.68
18	8.29	6.01	5.09	4.58	4.25	4.01	3.84	3.71	3.60
19	8.18	5.93	5.01	4.50	4.17	3.94	3.77	3.63	3.52
20	8.10	5.85	4.94	4.43	4.10	3.87	3.70	3.56	3.46
21	8.02	5.78	4.87	4.37	4.04	3.81	3.64	3.51	3.40
22	7.95	5.72	4.82	4.31	3.99	3.76	3.59	3.45	3.35
23	7.88	5.66	4.76	4.26	3.94	3.71	3.54	3.41	3.30
24	7.82	5.61	4.72	4.22	3.90	3.67	3.50	3.36	3.26
25	7.77	5.57	4.68	4.18	3.85	3.63	3.46	3.32	3.22
26	7.72	5.53	4.64	4.14	3.82	3.59	3.42	3.29	3.18
27	7.68	5.49	4.60	4.11	3.78	3.56	3.39	3.26	3.15
28	7.64	5.45	4.57	4.07	3.75	3.53	3.36	3.23	3.12
29	7.60	5.42	4.54	4.04	3.73	3.50	3.33	3.20	3.09
30	7.56	5.39	4.51	4.02	3.70	3.47	3.30	3.17	3.07
40	7.31	5.18	4.31	3.83	3.51	3.29	3.12	2.99	2.89
60	7.08	4.98	4.13	3.65	3.34	3.12	2.95	2.82	2.72
120	6.85	4.79	3.95	3.48	3.17	2.96	2.79	2.66	2.56
∞	6.63	4.61	3.78	3.32	3.02	2.80	2.64	2.51	2.41

Table continued on opposite page

APPENDIX D (*continued*)

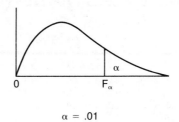

$\alpha = .01$

					v_1					
10	12	15	20	24	30	40	60	120	∞	
										v_2
6056	6106	6157	6209	6235	6261	6287	6313	6339	6366	1
99.40	99.42	99.43	99.45	99.46	99.47	99.47	99.48	99.49	99.50	2
27.23	27.05	26.87	26.69	26.60	26.50	26.41	26.32	26.22	26.13	3
14.55	14.37	14.20	14.02	13.93	13.84	13.75	13.65	13.56	13.46	4
10.05	9.89	9.72	9.55	9.47	9.38	9.29	9.20	9.11	9.02	5
7.87	7.72	7.56	7.40	7.31	7.23	7.14	7.06	6.97	6.88	6
6.62	6.47	6.31	6.16	6.07	5.99	5.91	5.82	5.74	5.65	7
5.81	5.67	5.52	5.36	5.28	5.20	5.12	5.03	4.95	4.86	8
5.26	5.11	4.96	4.81	4.73	4.65	4.57	4.48	4.40	4.31	9
4.85	4.71	4.56	4.41	4.33	4.25	4.17	4.08	4.00	3.91	10
4.54	4.40	4.25	4.10	4.02	3.94	3.86	3.78	3.69	3.60	11
4.30	4.16	4.01	3.86	3.78	3.70	3.62	3.54	3.45	3.36	12
4.10	3.96	3.82	3.66	3.59	3.51	3.43	3.34	3.25	3.17	13
3.94	3.80	3.66	3.51	3.43	3.35	3.27	3.18	3.09	3.00	14
3.80	3.67	3.52	3.37	3.29	3.21	3.13	3.05	2.96	2.87	15
3.69	3.55	3.41	3.26	3.18	3.10	3.02	2.93	2.84	2.75	16
3.59	3.46	3.31	3.16	3.08	3.00	2.92	2.83	2.75	2.65	17
3.51	3.37	3.23	3.08	3.00	2.92	2.84	2.75	2.66	2.57	18
3.43	3.30	3.15	3.00	2.92	2.84	2.76	2.67	2.58	2.49	19
3.37	3.23	3.09	2.94	2.86	2.78	2.69	2.61	2.52	2.42	20
3.31	3.17	3.03	2.88	2.80	2.72	2.64	2.55	2.46	2.36	21
3.26	3.12	2.98	2.83	2.75	2.67	2.58	2.50	2.40	2.31	22
3.21	3.07	2.93	2.78	2.70	2.62	2.54	2.45	2.35	2.26	23
3.17	3.03	2.89	2.74	2.66	2.58	2.49	2.40	2.31	2.21	24
3.13	2.99	2.85	2.70	2.62	2.54	2.45	2.36	2.27	2.17	25
3.09	2.96	2.81	2.66	2.58	2.50	2.42	2.33	2.23	2.13	26
3.06	2.93	2.78	2.63	2.55	2.47	2.38	2.29	2.20	2.10	27
3.03	2.90	2.75	2.60	2.52	2.44	2.35	2.26	2.17	2.06	28
3.00	2.87	2.73	2.57	2.49	2.41	2.33	2.23	2.14	2.03	29
2.98	2.84	2.70	2.55	2.47	2.39	2.30	2.21	2.11	2.01	30
2.80	2.66	2.52	2.37	2.29	2.20	2.11	2.02	1.92	1.80	40
2.63	2.50	2.35	2.20	2.12	2.03	1.94	1.84	1.73	1.60	60
2.47	2.34	2.19	2.03	1.95	1.86	1.76	1.66	1.53	1.38	120
2.32	2.18	2.04	1.88	1.79	1.70	1.59	1.47	1.32	1.00	∞

(From Merrington, M. and Thompson, C. M.: Biometrika, *33*:73–78, 1943; with permission.)

Critical Values of the χ^2 Distribution

df	$P_{0.5}$	P_{01}	$P_{02.5}$	P_{05}	P_{10}	P_{90}	P_{95}	$P_{97.5}$	P_{99}	$P_{99.5}$
1	.000039	.00016	.00098	.0039	.0158	2.71	3.84	5.02	6.63	7.88
2	.0100	.0201	.0506	.1026	.2107	4.61	5.99	7.38	9.21	10.60
3	.0717	.115	.216	.352	.584	6.25	7.81	9.35	11.34	12.84
4	.207	.297	.484	.711	1.064	7.78	9.49	11.14	13.28	14.86
5	.412	.554	.831	1.15	1.61	9.24	11.07	12.83	15.09	16.75
6	.676	.872	1.24	1.64	2.20	10.64	12.59	14.45	16.81	18.55
7	.989	1.24	1.69	2.17	2.83	12.02	14.07	16.01	18.48	20.28
8	1.34	1.65	2.18	2.73	3.49	13.36	15.51	17.53	20.09	21.96
9	1.73	2.09	2.70	3.33	4.17	14.68	16.92	19.02	21.67	23.59
10	2.16	2.56	3.25	3.94	4.87	15.99	18.31	20.48	23.21	25.19
11	2.60	3.05	3.82	4.57	5.58	17.28	19.68	21.92	24.73	26.76
12	3.07	3.57	4.40	5.23	6.30	18.55	21.03	23.34	26.22	28.30
13	3.57	4.11	5.01	5.89	7.04	19.81	22.36	24.74	27.69	29.82
14	4.07	4.66	5.63	6.57	7.79	21.06	23.68	26.12	29.14	31.32
15	4.60	5.23	6.26	7.26	8.55	22.31	25.00	27.49	30.58	32.80
16	5.14	5.81	6.91	7.96	9.31	23.54	26.30	28.85	32.00	34.27
18	6.26	7.01	8.23	9.39	10.86	25.99	28.87	31.53	34.81	37.16
20	7.43	8.26	9.59	10.85	12.44	28.41	31.41	34.17	37.57	40.00
24	9.89	10.86	12.40	13.85	15.66	33.20	36.42	39.36	42.98	45.56
30	13.79	14.95	16.79	18.49	20.60	40.26	43.77	46.98	50.98	53.67
40	20.71	22.16	24.43	26.51	29.05	51.81	55.76	59.34	63.69	66.77
60	35.53	37.48	40.48	43.19	46.46	74.40	79.08	83.30	88.38	91.95
120	83.85	86.92	91.58	95.70	100.62	140.23	146.57	152.21	158.95	163.64

(From Dixon, W. J. and Massey, F. J. Jr.: *Introduction to statistical analysis* (3rd ed.). New York: McGraw-Hill Book Company, 1969; with permission.)

Table of Probabilities Associated with Values as Small as Observed Values of U in the Mann-Whitney Test

$n_2 = 3$			
U \ n_1	1	2	3
0	.250	.100	.050
1	.500	.200	.100
2	.750	.400	.200
3		.600	.350
4			.500
5			.650

$n_2 = 4$				
U \ n_1	1	2	3	4
0	.200	.067	.028	.014
1	.400	.133	.057	.029
2	.600	.267	.114	.057
3		.400	.200	.100
4		.600	.314	.171
5			.429	.243
6			.571	.343
7				.443
8				.557

$n_2 = 5$					
U \ n_1	1	2	3	4	5
0	.167	.047	.018	.008	.004
1	.333	.095	.036	.016	.008
2	.500	.190	.071	.032	.016
3	.667	.286	.125	.056	.028
4		.429	.196	.095	.048
5		.571	.286	.143	.075
6			.393	.206	.111
7			.500	.278	.155
8			.607	.365	.210
9				.452	.274
10				.548	.345
11					.421
12					.500
13					.579

$n_2 = 6$						
U \ n_1	1	2	3	4	5	6
0	.143	.036	.012	.005	.002	.001
1	.286	.071	.024	.010	.004	.002
2	.428	.143	.048	.019	.009	.004
3	.571	.214	.083	.033	.015	.008
4		.321	.131	.057	.026	.013
5		.429	.190	.086	.041	.021
6		.571	.274	.129	.063	.032
7			.357	.176	.089	.047
8			.452	.238	.123	.066
9			.548	.305	.165	.090
10				.381	.214	.120
11				.457	.268	.155
12				.545	.331	.197
13					.396	.242
14					.465	.294
15					.535	.350
16						.409
17						.469
18						.531

APPENDIX F (*continued*)

	n_1 1	2	3	4	5	6	7
U							
0	.125	.028	.008	.003	.001	.001	.000
1	.250	.056	.017	.006	.003	.001	.001
2	.375	.111	.033	.012	.005	.002	.001
3	.500	.167	.058	.021	.009	.004	.002
4	.625	.250	.092	.036	.015	.007	.003
5		.333	.133	.055	.024	.011	.006
6		.444	.192	.082	.037	.017	.009
7		.556	.258	.115	.053	.026	.013
8			.333	.158	.074	.037	.019
9			.417	.206	.101	.051	.027
10			.500	.264	.134	.069	.036
11			.583	.324	.172	.090	.049
12				.394	.216	.117	.064
13				.464	.265	.147	.082
14				.538	.319	.183	.104
15					.378	.223	.130
16					.438	.267	.159
17					.500	.314	.191
18					.562	.365	.228
19						.418	.267
20						.473	.310
21						.527	.355
22							.402
23							.451
24							.500
25							.549

Table header: $n_2 = 7$

APPENDIX F (*continued*)

					$n_2 = 8$						
n_1 / U	1	2	3	4	5	6	7	8	t	Normal
0	.111	.022	.006	.002	.001	.000	.000	.000	3.308	.001
1	.222	.044	.012	.004	.002	.001	.000	.000	3.203	.001
2	.333	.089	.024	.008	.003	.001	.001	.000	3.098	.001
3	.444	.133	.042	.014	.005	.002	.001	.001	2.993	.001
4	.556	.200	.067	.024	.009	.004	.002	.001	2.888	.002
5		.267	.097	.036	.015	.006	.003	.001	2.783	.003
6		.356	.139	.055	.023	.010	.005	.002	2.678	.004
7		.444	.188	.077	.033	.015	.007	.003	2.573	.005
8		.556	.248	.107	.047	.021	.010	.005	2.468	.007
9			.315	.141	.064	.030	.014	.007	2.363	.009
10			.387	.184	.085	.041	.020	.010	2.258	.012
11			.461	.230	.111	.054	.027	.014	2.153	.016
12			.539	.285	.142	.071	.036	.019	2.048	.020
13				.341	.177	.091	.047	.025	1.943	.026
14				.404	.217	.114	.060	.032	1.838	.033
15				.467	.262	.141	.076	.041	1.733	.041
16				.533	.311	.172	.095	.052	1.628	.052
17					.362	.207	.116	.065	1.523	.064
18					.416	.245	.140	.080	1.418	.078
19					.472	.286	.168	.097	1.313	.094
20					.528	.331	.198	.117	1.208	.113
21						.377	.232	.139	1.102	.135
22						.426	.268	.164	.998	.159
23						.475	.306	.191	.893	.185
24						.525	.347	.221	.788	.215
25							.389	.253	.683	.247
26							.433	.287	.578	.282
27							.478	.323	.473	.318
28							.522	.360	.368	.356
29								.399	.263	.396
30								.439	.158	.437
31								.480	.052	.481
32								.520		

(From Mann, H. B. and Whitney, D. R.: Ann. Math. Statist., *18*:52–54, 1947; with permission.)

APPENDIX G

Table of Critical Values of U in the Mann-Whitney Test

TABLE G–1
Critical Values of U for a One-Tailed Test at $\alpha = .001$ or for a Two-Tailed Test at $\alpha = .002$

n_1 \ n_2	9	10	11	12	13	14	15	16	17	18	19	20
1												
2												
3									0	0	0	0
4		0	0	0	1	1	1	2	2	3	3	3
5	1	1	2	2	3	3	4	5	5	6	7	7
6	2	3	4	4	5	6	7	8	9	10	11	12
7	3	5	6	7	8	9	10	11	13	14	15	16
8	5	6	8	9	11	12	14	15	17	18	20	21
9	7	8	10	12	14	15	17	19	21	23	25	26
10	8	10	12	14	17	19	21	23	25	27	29	32
11	10	12	15	17	20	22	24	27	29	32	34	37
12	12	14	17	20	23	25	28	31	34	37	40	42
13	14	17	20	23	26	29	32	35	38	42	45	48
14	15	19	22	25	29	32	36	39	43	46	50	54
15	17	21	24	28	32	36	40	43	47	51	55	59
16	19	23	27	31	35	39	43	48	52	56	60	65
17	21	25	29	34	38	43	47	52	57	61	66	70
18	23	27	32	37	42	46	51	56	61	66	71	76
19	25	29	34	40	45	50	55	60	66	71	77	82
20	26	32	37	42	48	54	59	65	70	76	82	88

APPENDIX G (*continued*)

TABLE G–2
Critical Values of U for a One-Tailed Test at α = .01 or for a Two-Tailed Test at α = .02

n_1 \ n_2	9	10	11	12	13	14	15	16	17	18	19	20
1												
2					0	0	0	0	0	0	1	1
3	1	1	1	2	2	2	3	3	4	4	4	5
4	3	3	4	5	5	6	7	7	8	9	9	10
5	5	6	7	8	9	10	11	12	13	14	15	16
6	7	8	9	11	12	13	15	16	18	19	20	22
7	9	11	12	14	16	17	19	21	23	24	26	28
8	11	13	15	17	20	22	24	26	28	30	32	34
9	14	16	18	21	23	26	28	31	33	36	38	40
10	16	19	22	24	27	30	33	36	38	41	44	47
11	18	22	25	28	31	34	37	41	44	47	50	53
12	21	24	28	31	35	38	42	46	49	53	56	60
13	23	27	31	35	39	43	47	51	55	59	63	67
14	26	30	34	38	43	47	51	56	60	65	69	73
15	28	33	37	42	47	51	56	61	66	70	75	80
16	31	36	41	46	51	56	61	66	71	76	82	87
17	33	38	44	49	55	60	66	71	77	82	88	93
18	36	41	47	53	59	65	70	76	82	88	94	100
19	38	44	50	56	63	69	75	82	88	94	101	107
20	40	47	53	60	67	73	80	87	93	100	107	114

APPENDIX G (*continued*)

TABLE G–3
Critical Values of U for a One-Tailed Test at $\alpha = .025$ or for a Two-Tailed Test at $\alpha = .05$

n_1 \ n_2	9	10	11	12	13	14	15	16	17	18	19	20
1												
2	0	0	0	1	1	1	1	1	2	2	2	2
3	2	3	3	4	4	5	5	6	6	7	7	8
4	4	5	6	7	8	9	10	11	11	12	13	13
5	7	8	9	11	12	13	14	15	17	18	19	20
6	10	11	13	14	16	17	19	21	22	24	25	27
7	12	14	16	18	20	22	24	26	28	30	32	34
8	15	17	19	22	24	26	29	31	34	36	38	41
9	17	20	23	26	28	31	34	37	39	42	45	48
10	20	23	26	29	33	36	39	42	45	48	52	55
11	23	26	30	33	37	40	44	47	51	55	58	62
12	26	29	33	37	41	45	49	53	57	61	65	69
13	28	33	37	41	45	50	54	59	63	67	72	76
14	31	36	40	45	50	55	59	64	67	74	78	83
15	34	39	44	49	54	59	64	70	75	80	85	90
16	37	42	47	53	59	64	70	75	81	86	92	98
17	39	45	51	57	63	67	75	81	87	93	99	105
18	42	48	55	61	67	74	80	86	93	99	106	112
19	45	52	58	65	72	78	85	92	99	106	113	119
20	48	55	62	69	76	83	90	98	105	112	119	127

APPENDIX G (*continued*)

TABLE G–4
Critical Values of *U* for a One-Tailed Test at α = .05 or for a Two-Tailed Test at
α = .10

n_1 \ n_2	9	10	11	12	13	14	15	16	17	18	19	20
1											0	0
2	1	1	1	2	2	2	3	3	3	4	4	4
3	3	4	5	5	6	7	7	8	9	9	10	11
4	6	7	8	9	10	11	12	14	15	16	17	18
5	9	11	12	13	15	16	18	19	20	22	23	25
6	12	14	16	17	19	21	23	25	26	28	30	32
7	15	17	19	21	24	26	28	30	33	35	37	39
8	18	20	23	26	28	31	33	36	39	41	44	47
9	21	24	27	30	33	36	39	42	45	48	51	54
10	24	27	31	34	37	41	44	48	51	55	58	62
11	27	31	34	38	42	46	50	54	57	61	65	69
12	30	34	38	42	47	51	55	60	64	68	72	77
13	33	37	42	47	51	56	61	65	70	75	80	84
14	36	41	46	51	56	61	66	71	77	82	87	92
15	39	44	50	55	61	66	72	77	83	88	94	100
16	42	48	54	60	65	71	77	83	89	95	101	107
17	45	51	57	64	70	77	83	89	96	102	109	115
18	48	55	61	68	75	82	88	95	102	109	116	123
19	51	58	65	72	80	87	94	101	109	116	123	130
20	54	62	69	77	84	92	100	107	115	123	130	138

(From Siegel, S.: *Nonparametric statistics for the behavioral sciences.* New York: McGraw-Hill Book Company, 1956, as adapted from Auble, D.: Bulletin of Institute of Educational Research at Indiana University, Vol. 1, No. 2, 1953; with permission.)

APPENDIX H
Percentiles of the Kolmogorov–Smirnov Test Statistic

		One-Sided Test: α =				
		.90	.95	.975	.99	.995
		Two-Sided Test: α =				
		.80	.90	.95	.98	.99
n_1	n_2					
3	3	.667	.667			
3	4	.750	.750			
3	5	.667	.800	.800		
3	6	.667	.667	.833		
3	7	.667	.714	.857	.857	
3	8	.625	.750	.750	.875	
3	9	.667	.667	.778	.889	.889
3	10	.600	.700	.800	.900	.900
3	12	.583	.667	.750	.833	.917
4	4	.750	.750	.750		
4	5	.600	.750	.800	.800	
4	6	.583	.667	.750	.833	.833
4	7	.607	.714	.750	.857	.857
4	8	.625	.625	.750	.875	.875
4	9	.556	.667	.750	.778	.889
4	10	.550	.650	.700	.800	.800
4	12	.583	.667	.667	.750	.833
4	16	.563	.625	.688	.750	.812
5	5	.600	.600	.800	.800	.800
5	6	.600	.667	.667	.833	.833
5	7	.571	.657	.714	.829	.857
5	8	.550	.625	.675	.800	.800
5	9	.556	.600	.689	.778	.800
5	10	.500	.600	.700	.700	.800
5	15	.533	.600	.667	.733	.733
5	20	.500	.550	.600	.700	.750
6	6	.500	.667	.667	.833	.833
6	7	.548	.571	.690	.714	.833
6	8	.500	.583	.667	.750	.750
6	9	.500	.556	.667	.722	.778
6	10	.500	.567	.633	.700	.733
6	12	.500	.583	.583	.667	.750
6	18	.444	.556	.611	.667	.722
6	24	.458	.500	.583	.625	.667
7	7	.571	.571	.714	.714	.714
7	8	.482	.589	.625	.732	.750
7	9	.492	.556	.635	.714	.746
7	10	.471	.557	.614	.700	.714
7	14	.429	.500	.571	.643	.714
7	28	.429	.464	.536	.607	.643
8	8	.500	.500	.625	.625	.750
8	9	.444	.542	.625	.667	.750
8	10	.475	.525	.575	.675	.700
8	12	.458	.500	.583	.625	.667

Table continued on opposite page

APPENDIX H (*continued*)

n_1	n_2					
8	16	.438	.500	.563	.625	.625
8	32	.406	.438	.500	.563	.594
9	9	.444	.556	.556	.667	.667
9	10	.467	.500	.578	.667	.689
9	12	.444	.500	.556	.611	.667
9	15	.422	.489	.533	.600	.644
9	18	.389	.444	.500	.556	.611
9	36	.361	.417	.472	.528	.556
10	10	.400	.500	.600	.600	.700
10	15	.400	.467	.500	.567	.633
10	20	.400	.450	.500	.550	.600
10	40	.350	.400	.450	.500	.576
11	11	.454	.454	.545	.636	.636
12	12	.417	.417	.500	.583	.583
12	15	.383	.450	.500	.550	.583
12	16	.375	.438	.479	.542	.583
12	18	.361	.417	.472	.528	.556
12	20	.367	.417	.467	.517	.567
13	13	.385	.462	.462	.538	.615
14	14	.357	.429	.500	.500	.571
15	15	.333	.400	.467	.467	.533
16	16	.375	.375	.438	.500	.563
17	17	.353	.412	.412	.471	.529
18	18	.333	.389	.444	.500	.500
19	19	.316	.368	.421	.473	.473
20	20	.300	.350	.400	.450	.500
21	21	.286	.333	.381	.429	.476
22	22	.318	.364	.364	.454	.454
23	23	.304	.348	.391	.435	.435
24	24	.292	.333	.375	.417	.458
25	25	.280	.320	.360	.400	.440

For other sample sizes, let $C = \sqrt{\dfrac{n_1 + n_2}{n_1 n_2}}$, and use as an approximation:

		1.07C	1.22 C	1.36 C	1.52 C	1.63 C

(From Marascuilo, L. A. and McSweeney, M.: *Nonparametric and distribution-free methods for the social sciences*. Monterey, California: Brooks/Cole Publishing Company, as adapted from Massey, F. J. Jr: Ann. Math. Statist., *23*:435–441, 1952; with permission.)

Table of Critical Values of *r* in the Runs Test

Given in the bodies of Table I-1 and Table I-2 are various critical values of *r* for various values of n_1 and n_2. For the one-sample runs test, any value of *r* which is equal to or smaller than that shown in Table I-1 or equal to or larger than that shown in Table I-2 is significant at the .05 level. For the Wald-Wolfowitz two-sample runs test, any value of *r* which is equal to or smaller than that shown in Table I-1 is significant at the .05 level.

TABLE I-1

n_2 \ n_1	2	3	4	5	6	7	8	9	10	11	12	13	14	15	16	17	18	19	20
2											2	2	2	2	2	2	2	2	2
3				2	2	2	2	2	2	2	2	2	3	3	3	3	3	3
4			2	2	2	3	3	3	3	3	3	3	3	4	4	4	4	4
5		2	2	3	3	3	3	3	4	4	4	4	4	4	4	5	5	5
6	2	2	3	3	3	3	4	4	4	4	5	5	5	5	5	5	6	6
7	2	2	3	3	3	4	4	5	5	5	5	5	6	6	6	6	6	6
8	2	3	3	3	4	4	5	5	5	6	6	6	6	6	7	7	7	7
9	2	3	3	4	4	5	5	5	6	6	6	7	7	7	7	8	8	8
10	2	3	3	4	5	5	5	6	6	7	7	7	7	8	8	8	8	9
11	2	3	4	4	5	5	6	6	7	7	7	8	8	8	9	9	9	9
12	2	2	3	4	4	5	6	6	7	7	7	8	8	8	9	9	9	10	10
13	2	2	3	4	5	5	6	6	7	7	8	8	9	9	9	10	10	10	10
14	2	2	3	4	5	5	6	7	7	8	8	9	9	9	10	10	10	11	11
15	2	3	3	4	5	6	6	7	7	8	8	9	9	10	10	11	11	11	12
16	2	3	4	4	5	6	6	7	8	8	9	9	10	10	11	11	11	12	12
17	2	3	4	4	5	6	7	7	8	9	9	10	10	11	11	11	12	12	13
18	2	3	4	5	5	6	7	8	8	9	9	10	10	11	11	12	12	13	13
19	2	3	4	5	6	6	7	8	8	9	10	10	11	11	12	12	13	13	13
20	2	3	4	5	6	6	7	8	9	9	10	10	11	12	12	13	13	13	14

APPENDIX I (*continued*)

TABLE I-2

n_2 \ n_1	2	3	4	5	6	7	8	9	10	11	12	13	14	15	16	17	18	19	20
2																			
3																			
4				9	9														
5			9	10	10	11	11												
6			9	10	11	12	12	13	13	13	13								
7				11	12	13	13	14	14	14	14	15	15	15					
8				11	12	13	14	14	15	15	16	16	16	16	17	17	17	17	17
9					13	14	14	15	16	16	16	17	17	18	18	18	18	18	18
10					13	14	15	16	16	17	17	18	18	18	19	19	19	20	20
11					13	14	15	16	17	17	18	19	19	19	20	20	20	21	21
12					13	14	16	16	17	18	19	19	20	20	21	21	21	22	22
13						15	16	17	18	19	19	20	20	21	21	22	22	23	23
14						15	16	17	18	19	20	20	21	22	22	23	23	23	24
15						15	16	18	18	19	20	21	22	22	23	23	24	24	25
16							17	18	19	20	21	22	23	23	24	25	25	25	25
17							17	18	19	20	21	22	23	23	24	25	25	26	26
18							17	18	19	20	21	22	23	24	25	25	26	26	27
19							17	18	20	21	22	23	23	24	25	26	26	27	27
20							17	18	20	21	22	23	24	25	25	26	27	27	28

(From Siegel, S.: *Nonparametric statistics for the behavioral sciences.* New York: McGraw-Hill Book Company, 1956, as adapted from Swed, F. S. and Eisenhart, C.: Ann. Math. Statist., *14*:83–86, 1943; with permission.)

APPENDIX J
Critical Values for the Wilcoxon Signed Rank Test

$(N = 5(1)50)$

One-sided	Two-sided	N=5	N=6	N=7	N=8	N=9	N=10	N=11	N=12	N=13	N=14	N=15	N=16
P=.05	P=.10	1	2	4	6	8	11	14	17	21	26	30	36
P=.025	P=.05		1	2	4	6	8	11	14	17	21	25	30
P=.01	P=.02			0	2	3	5	7	10	13	16	20	24
P=.005	P=.01				0	2	3	5	7	10	13	16	19

One-sided	Two-sided	N=17	N=18	N=19	N=20	N=21	N=22	N=23	N=24	N=25	N=26	N=27	N=28
P=.05	P=.10	41	47	54	60	68	75	83	92	101	110	120	130
P=.025	P=.05	35	40	46	52	59	66	73	81	90	98	107	117
P=.01	P=.02	28	33	38	43	49	56	62	69	77	85	93	102
P=.005	P=.01	23	28	32	37	43	49	55	61	68	76	84	92

One-sided	Two-sided	N=29	N=30	N=31	N=32	N=33	N=34	N=35	N=36	N=37	N=38	N=39
P=.05	P=.10	141	152	163	175	188	201	214	228	242	256	271
P=.025	P=.05	127	137	148	159	171	183	195	208	222	235	250
P=.01	P=.02	111	120	130	141	151	162	174	186	198	211	224
P=.005	P=.01	100	109	118	128	138	149	160	171	183	195	208

One-sided	Two-sided	N=40	N=41	N=42	N=43	N=44	N=45	N=46	N=47	N=48	N=49	N=50
P=.05	P=.10	287	303	319	336	353	371	389	408	427	446	466
P=.025	P=.05	264	279	295	311	327	344	361	379	397	415	434
P=.01	P=.02	238	252	267	281	297	313	329	345	362	380	398
P=.005	P=.01	221	234	248	262	277	292	307	323	339	356	373

(From Wilcoxon, F. and Wilcox, R. A.: Some rapid approximate statistical procedures (revised edition). Pearl River, New York: Lederle Laboratories, 1964; with permission.)

Table of Probabilities Associated with Values as Large as Observed Values of *H* in the *Kruskal-Wallis* One-Way Analysis of Variance by Ranks

Sample Sizes					Sample Sizes				
n_1	n_2	n_3	*H*	*p*	n_1	n_2	n_3	*H*	*p*
2	1	1	2.7000	.500	4	3	2	6.4444	.008
								6.3000	.011
2	2	1	3.6000	.200				5.4444	.046
								5.4000	.051
2	2	2	4.5714	.067				4.5111	.098
			3.7143	.200				4.4444	.102
3	1	1	3.2000	.300	4	3	3	6.7455	.010
3	2	1	4.2857	.100				6.7091	.013
			3.8571	.133				5.7909	.046
								5.7273	.050
3	2	2	5.3572	.029				4.7091	.092
			4.7143	.048				4.7000	.101
			4.5000	.067					
			4.4643	.105	4	4	1	6.6667	.010
								6.1667	.022
3	3	1	5.1429	.043				4.9667	.048
			4.5714	.100				4.8667	.054
			4.0000	.129				4.1667	.082
								4.0667	.102
3	3	2	6.2500	.011					
			5.3611	.032	4	4	2	7.0364	.006
			5.1389	.061				6.8727	.011
			4.5556	.100				5.4545	.046
			4.2500	.121				5.2364	.052
								4.5545	.098
3	3	3	7.2000	004				4.4455	.103
			6.4889	.011					
			5.6889	.029					
			5.6000	.050	4	4	3	7.1439	.010
			5.0667	.086				7.1364	.011
			4.6222	.100				5.5985	.049
								5.5758	.051

Table continued on following page

APPENDIX K (*continued*)

Sample Sizes			H	p	Sample Sizes			H	p
n_1	n_2	n_3			n_1	n_2	n_3		
4	1	1	3.5714	.200				4.5455	.099
								4.4773	.102
4	2	1	4.8214	.057					
			4.5000	.076	4	4	4	7.6538	.008
			4.0179	.114				7.5385	.011
								5.6923	.049
4	2	2	6.0000	.014				5.6538	.054
			5.3333	.033				4.6539	.097
			5.1250	.052				4.5001	.104
			4.4583	.100					
			4.1667	.105	5	1	1	3.8571	.143
4	3	1	5.8333	.021	5	2	1	5.2500	.036
			5.2083	.050				5.0000	.048
			5.0000	.057				4.4500	.071
			4.0556	.093				4.2000	.095
			3.8889	.129				4.0500	.119
								5.6308	.050
5	2	2	6.5333	.008				4.5487	.099
			6.1333	.013				4.5231	.103
			6.1600	.034					
			5.0400	.056	5	4	4	7.7604	.009
			4.3733	.090				7.7440	.011
			4.2933	.122				5.6571	.049
								5.6176	.050
5	3	1	6.4000	.012				4.6187	.100
			4.9600	.048				4.5527	.102
			4.8711	.052					
			4.0178	.095	5	5	1	7.3091	.009
			3.8400	.123				6.8364	.011
								5.1273	.046
5	3	2	6.9091	.009				4.9091	.053
			6.8218	.010				4.1091	.086
			5.2509	.049				4.0364	.105
			5.1055	.052					
			4.6509	.091	5	5	2	7.3385	.010
			4.4945	.101				7.2692	.010
								5.3385	.047

Table continued on opposite page

APPENDIX K (*continued*)

Sample Sizes			H	p	Sample Sizes			H	p
n_1	n_2	n_3			n_1	n_2	n_3		
5	3	3	7.0788	.009				5.2462	.051
			6.9818	.011				4.6231	.097
			5.6485	.049				4.5077	.100
			5.5152	.051					
			4.5333	.097	5	5	3	7.5780	.010
			4.4121	.109				7.5429	.010
								5.7055	.046
5	4	1	6.9545	.008				5.6264	.051
			6.8400	.011				4.5451	.100
			4.9855	.044				4.5363	.102
			4.8600	.056					
			3.9873	.098	5	5	4	7.8229	.010
			3.9600	.102				7.7914	.010
								5.6657	.049
5	4	2	7.2045	.009				5.6429	.050
			7.1182	.010				4.5229	.099
			5.2727	.049				4.5200	.101
			5.2682	.050					
			4.5409	.098	5	5	5	8.0000	.009
			4.5182	.101				7.9800	.010
								5.7800	.049
5	4	3	7.4449	.010				5.6600	.051
			7.3949	.011				4.5600	.100
			5.6564	.049				4.5000	.102

(From Siegel, S.: *Nonparametric statistics for the behavioral sciences.* New York: McGraw-Hill Book Company, 1956, as adapted from Kruskal, W. H. and Wallis, W. A.: J. Am. Statist. Assoc., *47*:614–617, 1952; with permission.)

Table of Probabilities Associated with Values as Large as Observed Values of χ_r^2 in the Friedman Two-Way Analysis of Variance by Ranks

TABLE L = 1. $k = 3$

$N = 2$		$N = 3$		$N = 4$		$N = 5$	
χ_r^2	p	χ_r^2	p	χ_r^2	p	χ_r^2	p
0	1.000	.000	1.000	.0	1.000	.0	1.00
1	.833	.667	.944	.5	.931	.4	.954
3	.500	2.000	.528	1.5	.653	1.2	.691
4	.167	2.667	.361	2.0	.431	1.6	.522
		4.667	.194	3.5	.273	2.8	.367
		6.000	˙.028	4.5	.125	3.6	.182
				6.0	.069	4.8	.124
				6.5	.042	5.2	.093
				8.0	.0046	6.4	.039
						7.6	.024
						8.4	.0085
						10.0	.00077

Table continued on opposite page

APPENDIX L (*continued*)

χ_r^2	p	χ_r^2	p	χ_r^2	p	χ_r^2	p

N = 6		N = 7		N = 8		N = 9	
χ_r^2	p	χ_r^2	p	χ_r^2	p	χ_r^2	p
.00	1.000	.000	1.000	.00	1.000	.000	1.000
.33	.956	.286	.964	.25	.967	.222	.971
1.00	.740	.857	.768	.75	.794	.667	.814
1.33	.570	1.143	.620	1.00	.654	.889	.865
2.33	.430	2.000	.486	1.75	.531	1.556	.569
3.00	.252	2.571	.305	2.25	.355	2.000	.398
4.00	.184	3.429	.237	3.00	.285	2.667	.328
4.33	.142	3.714	.192	3.25	.236	2.889	.278
5.33	.072	4.571	.112	4.00	.149	3.556	.187
6.33	.052	5.429	.085	4.75	.120	4.222	.154
7.00	.029	6.000	.052	5.25	.079	4.667	.107
8.33	.012	7.143	.027	6.25	.047	5.556	.069
9.00	.0081	7.714	.021	6.75	.038	6.000	.057
9.33	.0055	8.000	.016	7.00	.030	6.222	.048
10.33	.0017	8.857	.0084	7.75	.018	6.889	.031
12.00	.00013	10.286	.0036	9.00	.0099	8.000	.019
		10.571	.0027	9.25	.0080	8.222	.016
		11.143	.0012	9.75	.0048	8.667	.010
		12.286	.00032	10.75	.0024	9.556	.0060
		14.000	.000021	12.00	.0011	10.667	.0035
				12.25	.00086	10.889	.0029
				13.00	.00026	11.556	.0013
				14.25	.000061	12.667	.00066
				16.00	.0000036	13.556	.00035
						14.000	.00020
						14.222	.000097
						14.889	.000054
						16.222	.000011
						18.000	.0000006

APPENDIX L (*continued*)

TABLE L = 2. $k = 4$

χ_r^2	p	χ_r^2	p	χ_r^2	p	χ_r^2	p
N = 2		**N = 3**		**N = 4**			
.0	1.000	.2	1.000	.0	1.000	5.7	.141
.6	.958	.6	.958	.3	.992	6.0	.105
1.2	.834	1.0	.910	.6	.928	6.3	.094
1.8	.792	1.8	.727	.9	.900	6.6	.077
2.4	.625	2.2	.608	1.2	.800	6.9	.068
3.0	.542	2.6	.524	1.5	.754	7.2	.054
3.6	.458	3.4	.446	1.8	.677	7.5	.052
4.2	.375	3.8	.342	2.1	.649	7.8	.036
4.8	.208	4.2	.300	2.4	.524	8.1	.033
5.4	.167	5.0	.207	2.7	.508	8.4	.019
6.0	.042	5.4	.175	3.0	.432	8.7	.014
		5.8	.148	3.3	.389	9.3	.012
		6.6	.075	3.6	.355	9.6	.0069
		7.0	.054	3.9	.324	9.9	.0062
		7.4	.033	4.5	.242	10.2	.0027
		8.2	.017	4.8	.200	10.8	.0016
		9.0	.0017	5.1	.190	11.1	.00094
				5.4	.158	12.0	.000072

(From Siegel, S.: *Nonparametric statistics for the behavioral sciences.* New York: McGraw-Hill Book Company, 1956, as adapted from Friedman, M.: J. Am. Statist. Assoc., *32*:688–689, 1937; with permission.)

APPENDIX M
Statistical Power Tables

TABLE M-1
Power of t Test of $m_1 = m_2$ at $a_1 = .01$

n	d_c											
		.10	**.20**	**.30**	**.40**	**.50**	**.60**	**.70**	**.80**	**1.00**	**1.20**	**1.40**
8	1.31	02	03	04	05	08	12	14	19	30	43	57
9	1.22	02	03	04	06	09	13	16	22	35	49	63
10	1.14	02	03	04	07	10	14	18	25	40	55	70
11	1.08	02	03	05	07	11	15	21	28	45	61	76
12	1.02	02	03	05	08	12	17	23	31	49	66	81
13	.98	02	03	05	08	13	19	26	34	53	71	85
14	.94	02	03	06	09	14	20	28	38	57	75	88
15	.90	02	04	06	10	15	22	31	41	61	79	90
16	.87	02	04	06	10	16	24	34	44	64	82	92
17	.84	02	04	07	11	18	26	36	47	68	85	94
18	.81	02	04	07	12	19	27	38	49	71	87	95
19	.79	02	04	07	13	20	29	40	51	74	89	96
20	.77	02	04	08	13	21	30	42	54	76	91	97
21	.75	02	05	08	14	22	32	44	56	79	93	98
22	.73	02	05	08	15	23	34	46	59	81	94	98
23	.71	02	05	09	15	24	36	48	61	83	95	99
24	.70	02	05	09	16	25	37	50	64	85	95	99
25	.68	02	05	10	17	27	39	53	66	87	96	99
26	.67	02	05	10	17	28	41	55	68	89	97	99
27	.65	02	05	10	18	29	42	57	70	90	97	*
28	.64	02	05	11	19	30	44	59	72	91	98	
29	.63	02	06	11	19	31	46	60	74	92	98	
30	.62	03	06	11	20	32	48	62	75	93	99	
31	.61	03	06	12	21	34	50	64	77	94	99	
32	.60	03	06	12	22	35	51	66	79	94	99	
33	.59	03	06	13	22	36	52	67	80	95	99	
34	.58	03	06	13	23	37	53	69	81	95	99	
35	.57	03	07	13	24	38	55	70	83	96	*	
36	.56	03	07	14	25	40	56	72	84	96		
37	.55	03	07	14	26	41	58	73	85	97		
38	.55	03	07	15	26	42	60	75	86	97		
39	.54	03	07	15	27	43	61	76	87	98		
40	.53	03	07	15	28	45	62	78	88	98		
42	.52	03	08	16	30	47	64	80	90	98		
44	.51	03	08	17	31	49	67	82	91	99		
46	.49	03	08	18	33	51	69	83	93	99		
48	.48	03	08	19	34	53	71	85	94	99		

Table continued on following page

APPENDIX M (*continued*)

TABLE M-1 *continued*

n	d_c	.10	.20	.30	.40	.50	.60	.70	.80	1.00	1.20	1.40
							d					
50	.47	03	09	20	36	55	73	87	95	99	*	*
52	.46	03	09	21	37	57	75	88	95	*		
54	.45	04	10	21	39	59	77	90	96			
56	.45	05	10	22	40	61	79	91	97			
58	.44	05	10	23	41	62	81	92	97			
60	.43	05	11	24	43	64	82	93	98			
64	.42	05	11	26	46	68	85	94	98			
68	.40	05	12	27	49	71	87	96	99			
72	.39	05	12	29	52	74	89	97	99			
76	.38	05	13	31	55	76	91	97	99			
80	.37	05	14	33	57	78	92	98	*			
84	.36	06	15	34	60	81	94	99				
88	.35	06	16	36	62	83	95	99				
92	.35	06	16	38	64	85	96	99				
96	.34	06	17	39	66	86	96	99				
100	.33	06	18	41	69	88	97	*				
120	.30	07	21	49	77	93	99					
140	.28	07	25	57	84	96	*					
160	.26	07	29	63	89	98						
180	.25	08	33	69	93	99						
200	.23	09	37	75	95	*						
250	.21	11	46	84	98							
300	.19	13	55	91	99							
350	.18	16	61	95	*							
400	.16	18	69	97								
450	.16	20	75	98								
500	.15	22	80	99								
600.	.13	27	87	*								
700	.12	32	92									
800	.12	37	95									
900	.11	42	97									
1000	.10	46	98									

APPENDIX M (*continued*)

TABLE M-2
Power of t Test of $m_1 = m_2$ at $a_1 = .05$

n	d_c	.10	.20	.30	.40	.50	.60	.70	.80	1.00	1.20	1.40
8	.88	07	10	13	19	25	31	38	46	61	74	85
9	.82	07	11	15	20	27	34	41	50	66	79	88
10	.78	08	11	16	22	29	36	45	53	70	83	91
11	.74	08	12	17	23	31	39	48	57	74	86	94
12	.70	08	12	18	25	33	41	51	60	77	89	96
13	.67	08	13	18	26	34	44	54	63	80	91	97
14	.64	08	13	19	27	36	46	57	66	83	93	98
15	.62	08	13	20	28	38	48	59	69	85	94	98
16	.60	09	14	21	30	40	51	62	72	87	95	99
17	.58	09	14	22	31	42	53	64	74	89	96	99
18	.56	09	15	22	32	43	55	66	76	90	97	99
19	.55	09	15	23	33	45	57	68	78	92	98	*
20	.53	09	15	24	34	46	59	70	80	93	98	
21	.52	09	16	25	36	48	60	72	82	94	99	
22	.51	09	16	26	37	50	62	74	83	95	99	
23	.50	10	16	26	38	51	64	76	85	96	99	
24	.48	10	17	27	39	53	66	77	86	96	99	
25	.47	10	17	28	40	54	67	79	88	97	99	
26	.46	10	18	28	41	55	69	80	89	97	*	
27	.46	10	18	29	42	57	70	82	90	98		
28	.45	10	18	30	43	58	72	83	90	98		
29	.44	10	19	30	44	59	73	84	91	98		
30	.43	10	19	31	46	61	74	85	92	99		
31	.42	10	19	32	47	62	76	86	93	99		
32	.42	11	20	33	48	63	77	87	93	99		
33	.41	11	20	33	49	64	78	88	94	99		
34	.40	11	20	34	50	66	79	89	95	99		
35	.40	11	21	34	50	67	80	89	95	99		
36	.39	11	21	35	51	68	81	90	96	99		
37	.39	11	21	36	52	69	82	91	96	*		
38	.38	11	22	36	53	70	83	91	96			
39	.38	11	22	37	54	71	84	92	97			
40	.37	11	22	38	55	72	84	93	97			
42	.36	12	23	39	57	74	86	94	98			
44	.35	12	24	40	59	75	87	95	98			
46	.35	12	24	41	60	77	89	95	99			
48	.34	12	25	43	62	79	90	96	99			

Table continued on following page

APPENDIX M (*continued*)

TABLE M-2 *continued*

N	d_c	.10	.20	.30	.40	.50	.60	.70	.80	1.00	1.20	1.40
							d					
50	.33	12	26	44	63	80	91	97	99	*	*	*
52	.33	13	26	45	65	81	92	97	99			
54	.32	13	27	46	66	83	93	98	99			
56	.31	13	28	47	68	84	93	98	99			
58	.31	13	28	49	69	85	94	98	*			
60	.30	13	29	50	70	86	95	98				
64	.29	14	30	52	73	88	96	99				
68	.28	14	31	54	75	90	97	99				
72	.28	15	33	56	77	91	97	99				
76	.27	15	34	58	79	92	98	*				
80	.26	15	35	60	81	93	98					
84	.26	16	36	61	82	94	99					
88	.25	16	37	63	84	95	99					
92	.24	17	38	65	85	96	99					
96	.24	17	40	66	87	96	99					
100	.23	17	41	68	88	97	*					
120	.21	19	46	75	93	99						
140	.20	21	51	80	95	99						
160	.18	23	56	85	97	*						
180	.17	24	60	88	98							
200	.16	26	64	91	99							
250	.15	30	72	96	*							
300	.13	34	79	98								
350	.12	37	84	99								
400	.12	41	88	*								
450	.11	44	91									
500	.10	47	93									
600	.10	53	97									
700	.09	59	98									
800	.08	64	99									
900	.08	68	*									
1000	.07	72										

APPENDIX M (*continued*)

TABLE M-3
Power of t Test of $m_1 = m_2$ at $a_1 = .10$

n	d_c	.10	.20	.30	.40	.50	.60	.70	.80	1.00	1.20	1.40
8	.67	13	18	24	30	37	44	53	60	74	85	92
9	.63	14	19	25	32	39	47	56	64	78	88	94
10	.59	14	19	26	34	42	50	59	67	81	91	96
11	.57	14	20	27	35	44	53	62	70	84	93	97
12	.54	15	21	28	37	46	56	65	73	87	94	98
13	.52	15	21	29	38	48	58	68	76	89	96	99
14	.50	15	22	30	40	50	61	70	79	90	97	99
15	.48	15	23	31	42	52	63	72	81	92	97	99
16	.46	16	23	32	43	54	65	75	83	93	98	*
17	.45	16	24	33	44	56	67	76	84	94	98	
18	.44	16	24	34	46	58	69	78	86	95	99	
19	.42	16	25	35	47	59	70	80	87	96	99	
20	.41	16	25	36	48	61	72	82	89	97	99	
21	.40	17	26	37	50	62	74	83	90	97	99	
22	.39	17	26	38	51	64	75	84	91	98	*	
23	.38	17	27	39	52	65	77	86	92	98		
24	.38	17	27	40	53	67	78	87	93	98		
25	.37	17	28	41	55	68	79	88	94	99		
26	.36	18	28	41	56	69	80	89	94	99		
27	.35	18	29	42	57	70	82	90	95	99		
28	.35	18	29	43	58	72	83	91	95	99		
29	.34	18	30	44	59	73	84	91	96	99		
30	.33	18	30	45	60	74	85	92	96	95		
31	.33	19	31	45	61	75	86	93	97	*		
32	.32	19	31	46	62	76	86	93	97			
33	.32	19	32	47	63	77	87	94	97			
34	.31	19	32	48	64	78	88	94	98			
35	.31	19	33	48	65	79	89	95	98			
36	.30	19	33	49	66	80	89	95	98			
37	.30	20	33	50	66	80	90	96	98			
38	.30	20	34	51	67	81	91	96	99			
39	.29	20	34	51	68	82	91	96	99			
40	.29	20	35	52	69	83	92	97	99			
42	.28	20	35	53	70	84	93	97	99			
44	.28	21	36	55	72	85	94	98	99			
46	.27	21	37	56	73	86	94	98	99			
48	.26	21	38	57	75	88	95	98	*			

Table continued on following page

APPENDIX M (*continued*)

TABLE M-3 *continued*

n	d_c	.10	.20	.30	.40	.50	.60	.70	.80	1.00	1.20	1.40
							d					
50	.26	22	39	58	76	89	96	99	*	*	*	*
52	.25	22	39	59	77	90	96	99				
54	.25	22	40	61	78	90	97	99				
56	.24	22	41	62	80	91	97	99				
58	.24	23	42	63	81	92	97	99				
60	.24	23	42	64	82	93	98	99				
64	.23	24	44	66	83	94	98	*				
68	.22	24	45	68	85	95	99					
72	.21	25	47	70	87	96	99					
76	.21	25	48	71	88	96	99					
80	.20	26	49	73	89	97	99					
84	.20	26	51	74	90	97	*					
88	.19	27	52	76	91	98						
92	.19	27	53	77	92	98						
96	.19	28	54	79	93	99						
100	.18	29	55	80	94	99						
120	.17	31	60	85	96	*						
140	.15	33	65	89	98							
160	.14	35	69	92	99							
180	.14	37	73	94	99							
200	.13	39	76	96	*							
250	.11	44	83	98								
300	.10	48	88	99								
350	.10	52	91	*								
400	.09	55	94									
450	.09	59	96									
500	.08	62	97									
600	.07	67	99									
700	.07	72	99									
800	.06	76	*									
900	.06	80										
1000	.06	83										

APPENDIX M (*continued*)

TABLE M-4
Power of t Test of $m_1 = m_2$ at $a_2 = .01$

n	d_c	.10	.20	.30	.40	.50	.60	.70	.80	1.00	1.20	1.40
8	1.49	01	02	02	03	05	07	09	12	21	33	46
9	1.38	01	02	02	04	05	08	11	15	25	39	54
10	1.28	01	02	03	04	06	09	12	17	29	45	61
11	1.21	01	02	03	04	07	10	14	20	33	50	67
12	1.15	01	02	03	05	07	11	16	22	38	55	72
13	1.10	01	02	03	05	08	12	18	25	42	61	77
14	1.05	01	02	03	06	09	14	20	27	46	65	81
15	1.01	01	02	04	06	10	15	22	30	50	70	85
16	.97	01	02	04	07	11	16	24	33	54	73	88
17	.94	01	02	04	07	12	18	26	35	57	77	90
18	.91	01	02	04	08	12	19	28	38	61	80	92
19	.88	01	02	05	08	13	21	30	41	64	83	94
20	.86	01	02	05	09	14	22	32	44	67	85	95
21	.83	01	03	05	09	15	24	34	46	70	87	96
22	.81	01	03	05	10	16	25	36	49	73	89	97
23	.79	01	03	06	10	17	27	38	51	75	91	98
24	.78	01	03	06	11	18	28	40	54	78	92	98
25	.76	01	03	06	11	19	30	42	56	80	93	99
26	.74	01	03	06	12	20	31	44	58	82	95	99
27	.73	01	03	07	12	21	33	46	60	84	95	99
28	.71	02	03	07	13	22	34	48	63	85	96	99
29	.70	02	03	07	14	23	36	50	65	87	97	*
30	.69	02	03	07	14	24	37	52	66	88	97	
31	.68	02	04	08	15	25	39	54	68	89	98	
32	.66	02	04	08	15	26	40	56	70	91	98	
33	.65	02	04	08	16	27	42	57	72	92	98	
34	.64	02	04	08	17	28	43	59	74	92	99	
35	.63	02	04	09	17	30	45	61	75	93	99	
36	.62	02	04	09	18	31	46	62	77	94	99	
37	.62	02	04	09	18	32	48	64	78	95	99	
38	.61	02	04	10	19	33	49	66	80	95	99	
39	.60	02	04	10	20	34	50	67	81	96	*	
40	.59	02	04	10	20	35	52	68	82	96		
42	.58	02	05	11	22	37	55	71	84	97		
44	.56	02	05	12	23	39	57	74	86	98		
46	.55	02	05	12	24	41	60	76	88	98		
48	.54	02	05	13	26	43	62	78	90	99		

Table continued on following page

APPENDIX M (*continued*)

TABLE M-4 *continued*

n	d_c	.10	.20	.30	.40	.50	.60	.70	.80	1.00	1.20	1.40
							d					
50	.53	02	06	14	27	45	64	81	91	99	*	*
52	.51	02	06	14	28	47	67	82	92	99		
54	.50	02	06	15	30	49	69	84	93	99		
56	.50	02	06	16	31	51	71	86	94	*		
58	.49	02	06	16	32	53	73	87	95			
60	.48	02	07	17	34	55	75	88	96			
64	.46	02	07	18	36	58	78	91	97			
68	.45	02	08	20	39	62	81	93	98			
72	.44	02	08	21	42	65	84	94	98			
76	.42	03	09	23	44	68	86	95	99			
80	.41	03	09	24	47	71	88	96	99			
84	.40	03	10	26	50	74	90	97	99			
88	.39	03	10	27	52	76	91	98	*			
92	.38	03	11	29	54	78	93	98				
96	.38	03	11	30	57	80	94	99				
100	.37	03	12	32	59	82	95	99				
120	.34	04	15	39	69	90	98	*				
140	.31	04	18	47	77	94	99					
160	.29	05	21	54	84	97	*					
180	.27	05	25	60	88	98						
200	.26	06	29	66	92	99						
250	.23	07	36	78	97	*						
300	.21	09	45	86	99							
350	.20	10	53	92	*							
400	.18	12	60	95								
450	.17	14	66	97								
500	.16	16	72	98								
600	.15	20	81	*								
700	.14	24	88									
800	.13	28	92									
900	.12	33	95									
1000	.12	37	97									

APPENDIX M (*continued*)

TABLE M-5
Power of t Test of $m_1 = m_2$ at $a_2 = .05$

n	d_c	.10	.20	.30	.40	.50	.60	.70	.80	.100	.120	1.40
8	1.07	05	07	09	11	15	20	25	31	46	60	73
9	1.00	05	07	09	12	16	22	28	35	51	65	79
10	.94	06	07	10	13	18	24	31	39	56	71	84
11	.89	06	07	10	14	20	26	34	43	61	76	87
12	.85	06	08	11	15	21	28	37	46	65	80	90
13	.81	06	08	11	16	23	31	40	50	69	83	93
14	.78	06	08	12	17	25	33	43	53	72	86	94
15	.75	06	08	12	18	26	35	45	56	75	88	96
16	.72	06	08	13	19	28	37	48	59	78	90	97
17	.70	06	09	13	20	29	39	51	62	80	92	98
18	.68	06	09	14	21	31	41	53	64	83	94	98
19	.66	06	09	15	22	32	43	55	67	85	95	99
20	.64	06	09	15	23	33	45	58	69	87	96	99
21	.62	06	10	16	24	35	47	60	71	88	97	99
22	.61	06	10	16	25	36	49	62	73	90	97	99
23	.59	06	10	17	26	38	51	64	75	91	98	*
24	.58	06	10	17	27	39	53	66	77	92	98	
25	.57	06	11	18	28	41	55	68	79	93	99	
26	.56	06	11	19	29	42	56	69	80	94	99	
27	.55	06	11	19	30	43	58	71	82	95	99	
28	.54	07	11	20	31	45	59	73	83	96	99	
29	.53	07	12	20	32	46	61	74	85	96	99	
30	.52	07	12	21	33	47	63	76	86	97	*	
31	.51	07	12	21	34	49	64	77	87	97		
32	.50	07	12	22	35	50	65	78	88	98		
33	.49	07	13	22	36	51	67	80	89	98		
34	.48	07	13	23	37	53	68	81	90	98		
35	.48	07	13	23	38	54	70	82	91	98		
36	.47	07	13	24	39	55	71	83	92	99		
37	.46	07	14	25	39	56	72	84	92	99		
38	.46	07	14	25	40	57	73	85	93	99		
39	.45	07	14	26	41	58	74	86	94	99		
40	.45	07	14	26	42	60	75	87	94	99		
42	.43	07	15	27	44	62	77	89	95	99		
44	.42	07	15	28	46	64	79	90	96	*		
46	.41	08	16	30	48	66	81	91	97			
48	.41	08	16	31	49	68	83	92	97			

Table continued on following page

APPENDIX M (*continued*)

TABLE M-5 *continued*

n	d_c	d										
		.10	.20	.30	.40	.50	.60	.70	.80	1.00	1.20	1.40
50	.40	08	17	32	50	70	84	93	98	*	*	*
52	.39	08	17	34	51	71	86	94	98			
54	.38	08	18	34	53	73	87	95	98			
56	.37	08	18	35	55	74	88	96	99			
58	.37	08	19	36	57	76	89	96	99			
60	.36	08	19	37	58	77	90	97	99			
64	.35	09	20	39	61	80	92	98	99			
68	.34	09	21	41	64	82	93	98	*			
72	.33	09	22	43	66	85	94	99				
76	.32	09	23	45	69	86	95	99				
80	.31	10	24	47	71	88	96	99				
84	.30	10	25	49	73	90	97	99				
88	.30	10	26	51	75	91	98	*				
92	.29	10	27	52	77	92	98					
96	.29	11	28	54	79	93	99					
100	.28	11	29	56	80	94	99					
120	.26	12	34	64	87	97	*					
140	.24	13	38	71	92	99						
160	.22	14	43	76	95	99						
180	.21	16	47	81	97	*						
200	.20	17	51	85	98							
250	.18	20	61	92	99							
300	.16	23	69	96	*							
350	.15	26	75	98								
400	.14	29	81	99								
450	.13	32	85	99								
500	.12	35	88	*								
600	.11	41	93									
700	.10	46	96									
800	.10	52	98									
900	.09	56	99									
1000	.09	61	99									

APPENDIX M (*continued*)

Table M-6
Power of t Test of $m_1 = m_2$ at $a_2 = .10$

n	d_c	.10	.20	.30	.40	.50	.60	.70	.80	1.00	1.20	1.40
8	.88	11	12	15	20	25	31	38	46	61	74	85
9	.82	11	13	16	21	27	34	42	50	66	79	89
10	.78	11	13	17	22	29	37	45	53	70	83	92
11	.74	11	13	18	24	31	39	48	57	74	86	94
12	.70	11	14	19	25	33	42	51	60	77	89	96
13	.67	11	14	19	26	34	44	54	63	80	91	97
14	.64	11	14	20	27	36	46	57	66	83	93	98
15	.62	11	15	21	29	38	49	59	69	85	94	98
16	.60	11	15	21	30	40	51	62	72	87	95	99
17	.58	11	15	22	31	42	53	64	74	89	96	99
18	.56	11	16	23	32	43	55	66	76	90	97	99
19	.55	11	16	24	33	45	57	68	78	92	98	*
20	.53	12	16	24	35	47	59	70	80	93	98	
21	.52	12	17	25	36	48	61	72	82	94	99	
22	.51	12	17	26	37	50	62	74	83	95	99	
23	.50	12	17	26	38	51	64	76	85	96	99	
24	.48	12	18	27	39	53	66	77	86	96	99	
25	.47	12	18	28	40	54	67	79	88	97	99	
26	.46	12	18	29	41	55	69	80	89	97	*	
27	.46	12	19	29	42	57	70	82	90	98		
28	.45	12	19	30	44	58	72	83	90	98		
29	.44	12	19	31	45	59	73	84	91	98		
30	.43	12	20	31	46	61	74	85	92	99		
31	.42	13	20	32	47	62	76	86	93	99		
32	.42	13	20	33	48	63	77	87	93	99		
33	.41	13	21	33	49	64	78	88	94	99		
34	.40	13	21	34	50	66	79	89	95	99		
35	.40	13	21	35	51	67	80	89	95	99		
36	.39	13	22	35	52	68	81	90	96	99		
37	.39	13	22	36	52	69	82	91	96	*		
38	.38	13	22	37	53	70	83	91	96			
39	.38	13	23	37	54	71	84	92	97			
40	.37	13	23	38	55	72	84	93	97			
42	.36	13	24	39	57	74	86	94	98			
44	.35	14	24	40	58	75	87	95	98			
46	.35	14	25	41	60	77	89	95	99			
48	.34	14	25	43	62	79	90	96	99			

Table continued on following page

APPENDIX M (*continued*)

Table M-6 *continued*

n	d_c	.10	.20	.30	.40	.50	.60	.70	.80	1.00	1.20	1.40
							d					
50	.33	14	26	44	63	80	91	97	99	*	*	*
52	.33	14	27	45	65	81	92	97	99			
54	.32	14	27	46	66	83	93	98	99			
56	.31	15	28	47	68	84	93	98	99			
58	.31	15	29	49	69	85	94	98	*			
60	.30	15	29	50	70	86	95	98				
64	.29	15	30	52	73	88	96	99				
68	.28	16	32	54	75	90	97	99				
72	.28	16	33	56	77	91	97	99				
76	.27	16	34	58	79	92	98	*				
80	.26	17	35	60	81	93	98					
84	.26	17	36	61	82	94	98					
88	.25	17	37	63	84	95	99					
92	.24	18	39	65	85	96	99					
96	.24	18	40	66	87	96	99					
100	.23	18	41	68	88	97	99					
120	.21	20	46	75	93	99	*					
140	.20	22	51	80	95	99						
160	.18	23	56	85	97	*						
180	.17	25	60	88	98							
200	.16	26	64	91	99							
250	.15	30	72	96	*							
300	.13	34	79	98								
350	.12	37	84	99								
400	.12	41	88	*								
450	.11	44	91									
500	.10	47	93									
600	.10	53	97									
700	.09	59	98									
800	.08	64	99									
900	.08	68	*									
1000	.07	72										

APPENDIX M (*continued*)

Table M-7
Power of F Test at a = .01, u = 1

n	F_c	.05	.10	.15	.20	.25	.30	.35	.40	.50	.60	.70	.80
2	98.503	01	01	01	01	02	02	03	04	04	05	06	08
3	21.198	01	01	01	02	02	02	03	04	05	07	09	11
4	13.745	01	01	01	02	02	03	04	05	07	10	14	19
5	11.259	01	01	02	02	03	03	05	06	10	15	21	29
6	10.044	01	01	02	02	03	04	06	08	13	20	29	40
7	9.330	01	01	02	03	04	05	07	10	17	26	38	50
8	8.861	01	01	02	03	04	06	09	12	21	32	46	60
9	8.531	01	02	02	03	05	07	10	14	25	39	54	68
10	8.285	01	02	02	04	06	08	12	17	29	45	61	75
11	8.096	01	02	03	04	06	09	14	19	34	51	67	81
12	7.946	01	02	03	05	07	11	16	22	38	56	73	86
13	7.823	01	02	03	05	08	12	18	25	42	61	78	89
14	7.721	01	02	03	05	08	13	20	28	46	66	82	92
15	7.636	01	02	03	06	09	15	22	30	50	70	85	94
16	7.562	01	02	04	06	10	16	24	33	54	74	88	96
17	7.499	01	02	04	07	11	17	26	36	58	78	91	97
18	7.444	01	02	04	07	12	19	28	39	62	81	92	98
19	7.396	01	02	04	08	13	20	30	41	65	83	94	98
20	7.353	01	02	04	08	14	22	32	44	68	86	95	99
21	7.314	01	02	05	08	15	24	34	47	71	88	96	99
22	7.280	01	03	05	09	16	25	37	49	73	90	97	99
23	7.248	01	03	05	09	17	27	39	52	76	91	98	*
24	7.220	01	03	05	10	18	28	41	54	78	93	98	
25	7.194	01	03	06	10	19	30	43	57	80	94	99	
26	7.171	01	03	06	11	20	31	45	59	82	95	99	
27	7.149	01	03	06	12	21	33	47	61	84	96	99	
28	7.129	01	03	06	12	22	35	49	63	86	96	99	
29	7.110	01	03	07	13	23	36	50	65	87	97	*	
30	7.093	01	03	07	13	24	38	53	67	89	97		
31	7.077	02	03	07	14	25	39	55	69	90	98		
32	7.062	02	03	07	15	26	41	56	71	91	98		
33	7.048	02	04	08	15	27	42	58	73	92	99		
34	7.035	02	04	08	16	28	44	60	75	93	99		
35	7.023	02	04	08	17	30	45	62	76	94	99		
36	7.011	02	04	08	17	31	47	63	78	94	99		
37	7.001	02	04	09	18	32	48	65	79	95	99		
38	6.990	02	04	09	19	33	50	66	80	96	99		
39	6.981	02	04	09	19	34	51	68	82	96	*		

Table continued on following page

APPENDIX M (*continued*)

Table M-7 *continued*

n	F_c	.05	.10	.15	.20	.25	.30	.35	.40	.50	.60	.70	.80
40	6.971	02	04	10	20	35	53	69	83	97	*	*	*
42	6.954	02	04	10	21	37	55	72	85	97			
44	6.939	02	05	11	23	39	58	75	87	98			
46	6.925	02	05	11	24	41	60	77	89	98			
48	6.912	02	05	12	25	44	63	79	90	99			
50	6.901	02	05	13	27	46	65	81	92	99			
52	6.890	02	05	13	28	48	67	83	93	99			
54	6.880	02	06	14	30	50	70	85	94	99			
56	6.871	02	06	15	31	52	72	86	95	*			
58	6.862	02	06	16	33	54	73	88	95				
60	6.854	02	06	16	34	56	75	89	96				
64	6.840	02	07	18	37	59	79	91	97				
68	6.828	02	07	19	40	63	82	93	98				
72	6.817	02	08	21	42	66	84	95	99				
76	6.807	02	08	22	45	69	87	96	99				
80	6.798	02	09	24	48	72	89	97	99				
84	6.790	03	09	25	50	74	90	97	*				
88	6.783	03	10	27	53	77	92	98					
92	6.776	03	10	29	55	79	93	98					
96	6.770	03	11	30	57	81	94	99					
100	6.764	03	11	32	60	83	95	99					
120	6.742	03	14	40	70	90	98	*					
140	6.727	04	17	47	78	95	99						
160	6.715	04	21	54	84	97	*						
180	6.706	04	24	61	89	99							
200	6.699	05	28	67	92	99							
250	6.686	07	37	79	97	*							
300	6.677	08	45	87	99								
350	6.671	10	53	92	*								
400	6.667	11	60	95									
450	6.663	13	67	97									
500	6.661	15	73	99									
600	6.656	19	82	*									
700	6.653	24	88										
800	6.651	28	93										
900	6.649	32	95										
1000	6.648	37	97										

APPENDIX M (*continued*)

Table M-8
Power of F Test at a = .01, u = 2

n	F_c	.05	.10	.15	.20	.25	.30	.35	.40	.50	.60	.70	.80
								f					
2	30.817	01	01	01	01	02	02	03	03	03	04	06	07
3	10.925	01	01	01	02	02	02	03	04	05	07	10	13
4	8.022	01	01	01	02	02	03	04	05	08	12	17	24
5	6.927	01	01	02	02	03	04	05	07	11	18	27	38
6	6.359	01	01	02	02	03	05	07	09	16	26	38	51
7	6.013	01	01	02	03	04	06	08	11	21	33	48	63
8	5.780	01	01	02	03	05	07	10	14	26	41	58	73
9	5.614	01	02	02	04	05	08	12	17	31	49	67	81
10	5.488	01	02	03	04	06	10	14	21	37	56	74	87
11	5.390	01	02	03	04	07	11	17	24	42	63	80	91
12	5.313	01	02	03	05	08	13	19	27	48	69	85	94
13	5.249	01	02	03	05	09	14	22	31	53	74	89	96
14	5.195	01	02	03	06	10	16	24	34	58	79	92	98
15	5.150	01	02	04	06	11	18	27	38	62	82	94	99
16	5.111	01	02	04	07	12	20	30	41	67	86	96	99
17	5.078	01	02	04	07	13	21	32	45	70	89	97	99
18	5.048	01	02	04	08	14	23	35	48	74	91	98	*
19	5.022	01	02	05	09	15	25	38	52	77	93	98	
20	4.999	01	02	05	09	17	27	40	55	80	94	99	
21	4.977	01	03	05	10	18	29	43	58	83	95	99	
22	4.959	01	03	05	10	19	31	46	61	85	96	*	
23	4.943	01	03	06	11	20	33	48	64	87	97		
24	4.928	01	03	06	12	22	35	51	65	89	98		
25	4.914	01	03	06	12	23	37	53	69	91	98		
26	4.901	01	03	07	13	24	39	56	71	92	99		
27	4.889	01	03	07	14	26	41	58	74	93	99		
28	4.878	01	03	07	15	27	43	60	76	94	99		
29	4.868	01	03	07	15	28	45	62	78	95	99		
30	4.859	02	03	08	16	30	47	65	80	96	*		
31	4.850	02	04	08	17	31	49	67	81	96			
32	4.842	02	04	08	18	33	51	69	83	97			
33	4.834	02	04	09	19	34	53	70	84	98			
34	4.827	02	04	09	19	35	54	72	86	98			
35	4.820	02	04	09	20	37	56	74	87	98			
36	4.814	02	04	10	21	38	58	76	88	99			
37	4.808	02	04	10	22	40	59	77	89	99			
38	4.802	02	04	10	23	41	61	79	90	99			
39	4.797	02	04	11	24	42	63	80	91	99			

Table continued on following page

APPENDIX M (*continued*)

Table M-8 *continued*

n	F_c	.05	.10	.15	.20	.25	.30	.35	.40	.50	.60	.70	.80
40	4.791	02	05	11	25	44	64	81	92	99	*	*	*
42	4.782	02	05	12	26	46	67	84	94	*			
44	4.774	02	05	13	28	49	70	86	95				
46	4.766	02	05	14	30	51	73	88	96				
48	4.760	02	05	14	32	54	75	90	97				
50	4.753	02	06	15	33	56	77	91	97				
52	4.747	02	06	16	35	59	79	92	98				
54	4.742	02	06	17	37	61	81	93	98				
56	4.737	02	06	18	39	63	83	94	99				
58	4.732	02	07	19	40	65	85	95	99				
60	4.728	02	07	20	42	67	86	96	99				
64	4.720	02	08	22	46	71	89	97	99				
68	4.713	02	08	24	49	75	91	98	*				
72	4.707	02	09	26	52	78	93	99					
76	4.702	02	09	28	55	81	95	99					
80	4.697	03	10	30	58	83	96	99					
84	4.693	03	10	32	61	85	97	*					
88	4.689	03	11	34	64	88	97						
92	4.685	03	12	36	67	89	98						
96	4.682	03	13	38	69	91	98						
100	4.678	03	13	40	72	92	99						
120	4.666	04	17	49	82	97	*						
140	4.657	04	21	58	89	99							
160	4.651	05	26	66	93	99							
180	4.646	05	30	73	96	*							
200	4.642	06	34	79	98								
250	4.634	07	45	89	99								
300	4.629	09	56	95	*								
350	4.626	11	65	97									
400	4.623	13	72	99									
450	4.621	16	79	*									
500	4.620	18	84										
600	4.617	24	91										
700	4.616	29	95										
800	4.614	35	98										
900	4.613	40	99										
1000	4.612	46	99										

APPENDIX M (*continued*)

Table M-9
Power of F test at a = .01, u = 3

n	F_c	.05	.10	.15	.20	.25	.30	.35	.40	.50	.60	.70	.80
						f							
2	16.694	01	01	01	01	02	02	02	03	04	05	06	07
3	7.591	01	01	01	02	02	03	03	04	06	08	12	16
4	5.953	01	01	01	02	02	03	04	06	09	15	22	31
5	5.292	01	01	02	02	03	04	06	08	14	23	34	48
6	4.938	01	01	02	03	04	05	08	11	20	32	47	63
7	4.718	01	01	02	03	04	06	10	14	26	42	59	75
8	4.568	01	02	02	03	05	08	12	17	32	51	69	84
9	4.460	01	02	02	04	06	10	15	21	39	59	78	90
10	4.378	01	02	03	04	07	11	17	25	45	67	84	94
11	4.313	01	02	03	05	08	13	20	29	52	74	89	97
12	4.262	01	02	03	05	09	15	23	34	58	79	92	98
13	4.219	01	02	03	06	10	17	27	38	63	84	95	99
14	4.183	01	02	04	07	12	19	30	42	68	88	97	99
15	4.153	01	02	04	07	13	22	33	46	73	91	98	*
16	4.126	01	02	04	08	14	24	36	50	77	93	99	
17	4.104	01	02	04	09	16	26	40	54	81	95	99	
18	4.084	01	02	05	09	17	29	43	58	84	96	99	
19	4.067	01	02	05	10	19	31	46	62	86	97	*	
20	4.051	01	03	05	11	20	33	49	65	89	98		
21	4.038	01	03	06	11	22	36	52	68	91	99		
22	4.025	01	03	06	12	23	38	55	71	92	99		
23	4.013	01	03	06	13	25	40	58	74	94	99		
24	4.003	01	03	07	14	26	43	61	77	95	99		
25	3.993	01	03	07	15	28	45	63	79	96	*		
26	3.984	01	03	07	16	30	48	66	81	97			
27	3.976	01	03	08	17	31	50	68	83	97			
28	3.969	02	03	08	18	33	52	71	85	98			
29	3.962	02	04	08	19	35	54	73	87	98			
30	3.955	02	04	09	20	36	56	75	88	99			
31	3.949	02	04	09	21	38	58	77	90	99			
32	3.944	02	04	10	22	40	60	79	91	99			
33	3.939	02	04	10	23	41	62	80	92	99			
34	3.934	02	04	10	24	43	64	82	93	99			
35	3.929	02	04	11	25	45	66	83	94	*			
36	3.925	02	04	11	26	46	68	85	94				
37	3.921	02	05	12	27	48	70	86	95				
38	3.917	02	05	12	28	49	71	87	96				
39	3.914	02	05	13	29	51	73	88	96				

Table continued on following page

APPENDIX M (*continued*)

Table M-9 *continued*

n	F_c	.05	.10	.15	.20	.25	.30	.35	.40	.50	.60	.70	.80
							f						
40	3.910	02	05	13	30	53	74	89	97	*	*	*	*
42	3.904	02	05	14	32	56	77	91	98				
44	3.898	02	06	15	34	58	80	93	98				
46	3.893	02	06	16	36	61	82	94	99				
48	3.889	02	06	17	38	64	84	95	99				
50	3.884	02	06	18	41	66	86	96	99				
52	3.880	02	07	19	43	69	88	97	99				
54	3.876	02	07	21	45	71	90	97	*				
56	3.873	02	07	22	47	73	91	98					
58	3.870	02	08	23	49	75	92	98					
60	3.867	02	08	24	51	77	93	99					
64	3.862	02	09	26	55	81	95	99					
68	3.857	02	09	29	59	84	96	99					
72	3.853	03	10	31	62	87	97	*					
76	3.849	03	11	34	65	89	98						
80	3.845	03	11	36	69	91	99						
84	3.842	03	12	38	72	93	99						
88	3.839	03	13	41	74	94	99						
92	3.837	03	14	43	77	95	99						
96	3.834	03	15	45	79	96	*						
100	3.832	03	16	48	81	97							
120	3.824	04	21	59	90	99							
140	3.818	04	26	68	95	*							
160	3.813	05	31	76	97								
180	3.810	06	36	82	99								
200	3.807	07	42	87	99								
250	3.802	09	54	95	*								
300	3.798	11	66	98									
350	3.796	13	75	99									
400	3.794	16	82	*									
450	3.793	19	87										
500	3.792	22	91										
600	3.790	29	96										
700	3.789	35	98										
800	3.788	42	99										
900	3.787	49	*										
1000	3.787	55											

APPENDIX M (*continued*)

Table M-10
Power of F Test at a = .01, u = 4

n	F_c	.05	.10	.15	.20	.25	.30	.35	.40	.50	.60	.70	.80
								f					
2	11.392	01	01	01	01	02	02	02	03	04	05	06	08
3	5.994	01	01	01	02	02	02	03	04	06	10	14	20
4	4.893	01	01	01	02	03	03	04	06	11	18	27	39
5	4.431	01	01	02	02	03	05	06	09	17	28	42	57
6	4.177	01	01	02	03	04	06	09	12	23	39	56	73
7	4.018	01	01	02	03	05	08	11	16	31	50	69	84
8	3.910	01	02	02	04	06	09	14	21	39	60	78	91
9	3.828	01	02	03	04	07	11	17	25	46	69	86	95
10	3.769	01	02	03	05	08	13	21	30	54	76	91	97
11	3.721	01	02	03	05	09	15	24	35	60	82	94	99
12	3.682	01	02	03	06	11	18	28	40	67	87	96	99
13	3.649	01	02	04	07	12	20	32	45	72	90	98	*
14	3.623	01	02	04	07	13	23	35	50	77	93	99	
15	3.601	01	02	04	08	15	26	39	54	81	95	99	
16	3.581	01	02	05	09	17	28	43	59	85	97	*	
17	3.564	01	02	05	10	18	31	47	63	88	98		
18	3.549	01	03	05	11	20	34	50	67	90	98		
19	3.536	01	03	06	11	22	37	54	70	92	99		
20	3.524	01	03	06	12	24	39	57	74	94	99		
21	3.514	01	03	06	13	26	42	60	77	95	*		
22	3.504	01	03	07	14	27	45	64	80	96			
23	3.495	01	03	07	15	29	48	67	82	97			
24	3.487	01	03	07	16	31	50	69	84	98			
25	3.480	01	03	08	17	33	53	72	86	98			
26	3.473	01	03	08	19	35	55	74	88	99			
27	3.467	02	04	09	20	37	58	77	90	99			
28	3.462	02	04	09	21	39	60	79	91	99			
29	3.457	02	04	10	22	41	63	81	92	99			
30	3.452	02	04	10	23	43	65	83	93	*			
31	3.448	02	04	11	24	45	67	84	94				
32	3.443	02	04	11	25	47	69	86	95				
33	3.439	02	04	12	27	49	71	87	96				
34	3.436	02	05	12	28	50	73	89	97				
35	3.432	02	05	13	29	52	75	90	97				
36	3.429	02	05	13	30	54	76	91	98				
37	3.426	02	05	14	32	56	78	92	98				
38	3.423	02	05	14	33	57	79	93	98				
39	3.420	02	05	15	34	59	81	94	99				

Table continued on following page

APPENDIX M (*continued*)

Table M-10 *continued*

n	F_c	.05	.10	.15	.20	.25	.30	.35	.40	.50	.60	.70	.80
40	3.418	02	05	15	35	61	82	94	99	*	*	*	*
42	3.413	02	06	17	38	64	85	96	99				
44	3.409	02	06	18	40	67	87	97	99				
46	3.405	02	06	19	43	70	89	97	*				
48	3.401	02	07	20	45	72	91	98					
50	3.398	02	07	22	48	75	92	98					
52	3.395	02	07	23	50	77	93	99					
54	3.392	02	08	24	52	79	94	99					
56	3.389	02	08	26	55	81	95	99					
58	3.386	02	09	27	57	83	96	99					
60	3.384	02	09	28	59	85	97	*					
64	3.380	02	10	31	63	88	98						
68	3.376	03	11	34	67	90	98						
72	3.373	03	11	37	71	92	99						
76	3.371	03	12	39	74	94	99						
80	3.368	03	13	42	77	95	*						
84	3.366	03	14	45	80	96							
88	3.364	03	15	48	82	97							
92	3.361	03	16	50	84	98							
96	3.360	03	17	53	86	98							
100	3.358	03	19	55	88	99							
120	3.352	04	24	67	94	*							
140	3.347	05	30	76	98								
160	3.344	06	37	84	99								
180	3.341	06	43	89	*								
200	3.339	07	49	93									
250	3.335	10	63	98									
300	3.332	12	74	99									
350	3.330	15	82	*									
400	3.329	19	89										
450	3.328	22	93										
500	3.327	26	96										
600	3.326	34	98										
700	3.325	42	*										
800	3.324	49											
900	3.323	56											
1000	3.323	63											

APPENDIX M (*continued*)

Table M-11
Power of F Test at a = .01, u = 5

n	F_c	.05	.10	.15	.20	.25	.30	.35	.40	.50	.60	.70	.80
2	8.746	01	01	01	01	02	02	02	03	04	05	07	09
3	5.064	01	01	01	02	02	03	03	04	07	11	17	24
4	4.248	01	01	02	02	03	04	05	07	12	21	32	46
5	3.895	01	01	02	02	03	05	07	10	19	33	49	66
6	3.699	01	01	02	03	04	07	10	14	28	45	64	80
7	3.576	01	01	02	03	05	08	13	19	36	57	76	90
8	3.489	01	02	02	04	07	10	16	24	45	67	85	95
9	3.426	01	02	03	05	08	13	20	30	53	76	91	98
10	3.388	01	02	03	05	09	15	24	35	61	83	95	99
11	3.339	01	02	03	06	10	18	28	41	68	88	97	*
12	3.309	01	02	04	07	12	21	32	46	74	92	98	
13	3.284	01	02	04	07	14	24	37	52	79	95	99	
14	3.263	01	02	04	08	15	27	41	57	84	97	*	
15	3.244	01	02	05	09	17	30	45	62	87	98		
16	3.229	01	02	05	10	19	33	49	66	90	99		
17	3.215	01	03	05	11	21	36	53	70	92	99		
18	3.203	01	03	06	12	23	39	57	74	94	99		
19	3.192	01	03	06	13	25	42	61	77	96	*		
20	3.182	01	03	07	14	27	45	64	81	97			
21	3.174	01	03	07	15	30	48	68	83	98			
22	3.166	01	03	07	16	32	51	71	86	98			
23	3.159	01	03	08	18	34	54	74	88	99			
24	3.153	01	03	08	19	36	57	76	90	99			
25	3.147	01	04	09	20	38	60	79	91	99			
26	3.142	02	04	09	21	40	63	81	93	*			
27	3.137	02	04	10	23	43	65	83	94				
28	3.133	02	04	10	24	45	67	85	95				
29	3.129	02	04	11	25	47	70	87	96				
30	3.125	02	04	11	27	49	72	88	97				
31	3.121	02	04	12	28	51	74	90	97				
32	3.118	02	05	12	29	53	76	91	98				
33	3.115	02	05	13	31	55	78	92	98				
34	3.112	02	05	14	32	57	80	93	98				
35	3.109	02	05	14	34	59	81	94	99				
36	3.107	02	05	15	35	61	83	95	99				
37	3.104	02	05	16	36	63	84	95	99				
38	3.102	02	06	16	38	64	86	96	99				
39	3.100	02	06	17	39	66	87	97	99				

Table continued on following page

APPENDIX M (*continued*)

Table M-11 *continued*

n	F_c	.05	.10	.15	.20	.25	.30	.35	.40	.50	.60	.70	.80
40	3.097	02	06	18	41	68	88	97	*	*	*	*	*
42	3.093	02	06	19	43	71	90	98					
44	3.090	02	07	20	46	74	92	98					
46	3.087	02	07	22	49	77	93	99					
48	3.084	02	07	23	52	79	94	99					
50	3.081	02	08	25	54	81	96	99					
52	3.079	02	08	26	57	84	96	*					
54	3.076	02	09	28	59	85	97						
56	3.074	02	09	30	61	87	98						
58	3.072	02	10	31	64	89	98						
60	3.070	02	10	33	66	90	99						
64	3.067	03	11	36	70	92	99						
68	3.064	03	12	39	74	94	99						
72	3.061	03	13	42	77	96	*						
76	3.059	03	14	45	80	97							
80	3.057	03	15	48	83	98							
84	3.055	03	16	51	86	98							
88	3.053	03	18	54	88	99							
92	3.052	03	19	57	90	99							
96	3.050	04	20	60	91	99							
100	3.049	04	21	62	93	*							
120	3.044	04	28	74	97								
140	3.040	05	35	83	99								
160	3.037	06	42	89	*								
180	3.035	07	49	93									
200	3.033	08	55	96									
250	3.030	11	70	99									
300	3.028	14	80	*									
350	3.026	18	88										
400	3.025	22	93										
450	3.024	26	96										
500	3.023	30	98										
600	3.022	39	99										
700	3.022	47	*										
800	3.021	56											
900	3.021	63											
1000	3.020	70											

*Power values below this point are greater than .995.

(From Cohen, J.: *Statistical power analysis for the behavioral sciences* (rev. ed.). New York: Academic Press, 1977; with permission.)

Glossary

Abstract Thinking. Thinking that is oriented toward the development of an idea without application to, or association with, a particular instance. This type of thinking is independent of time and space.

Accessible Population. The portion of the target population to which the researcher has reasonable access.

Accidental Sampling. The subjects are included in the study because they happened to be in the right place at the right time; also known as convenience or incidental sampling.

Analysis of Covariance (ANCOVA). A statistical procedure designed to reduce the error term (or variance within groups) by partialing out the variance due to a confounding variable by performing regression analysis prior to performing ANOVA.

Analysis of Variance (ANOVA). A statistical test used to examine differences among two or more groups by comparing the variability between the groups with the variability within the groups.

Analysis Step of a Critique. Involves examining the logic links connecting one study element with another.

Anonymity. Protection of the subjects so that their identity cannot be linked with their individual responses, even by the researcher.

Applied Research. Scientific investigation conducted to answer a clinical question or solve a practice-related problem.

Assumptions. Statements that are taken for granted or are considered true, even though they have not been scientifically tested.

Attribute Variables. Characteristics or elements of the subject that are collected to describe the sample.

Authority. A person with expertise and power who is able to influence opinion and behavior.

Autonomous Agents. Prospective subjects must be informed about a proposed study and allowed to voluntarily choose to participate or not participate.

Basic Research. Scientific investigation that involves the generation of "knowledge for knowledge's sake" or for the pleasure of learning and finding truth.

Benefit-Risk Ratio. Researchers and reviewers of research balance the potential benefits and risks in a study to promote the conduct of research ethically.

741

Bias. Any influence or action in a study that distorts the findings.

Bivariate Analysis. Statistical procedures that involve the comparison of summary values from two groups on the same variable or of two variables within a group.

Body of Knowledge. Information, facts, principles and theories that are organized by the beliefs accepted in a discipline at a given time.

Borrowing. The appropriation and use of knowledge from other fields or disciplines to guide nursing practice.

Bracketing. Suspending or laying aside what is known about an experience being studied; a technique used in qualitative research.

Breach of Confidentiality. When a researcher by accident or direct action allows an unauthorized person to have access to raw data of a study.

Case Study Design. An intensive exploration of a single unit of study—a person, family, group, community or institution—or a very small number of subjects who are examined intensively.

Causal Relationship. The relationship between two variables where one variable (independent variable) is thought to cause or determine the presence of the other variable (dependent variable).

Cell. The intersection between the row and column in a table where a specific numerical value is inserted.

Central Processing Unit (CPU). The device that controls the computer operations and includes the internal memory, the control unit and the arithmetic and logic unit.

Chi-Square (χ^2) Test. A statistical procedure for determining significant differences between observed frequencies within the data and frequencies that were expected. This test can be used with nominal level data.

Cluster Sampling. A sampling frame is developed that includes a list of all the states, cities, institutions or organizations (clusters) that could be used in a study. A randomized sample of these states, cities, institutions or organizations would then be used in the study.

Codebook. Documents the location or the column(s) that represent each variable and other information entered in a computer file.

Coding. The process of transforming qualitative data into numerical symbols that can be computerized.

Coercion. An overt threat of harm or excessive reward is presented by one person to another in order to obtain compliance, such as coercing subjects to participate in research.

Co-Investigators. In a research grant, professionals whose salaries are being paid partially or in full by the grant funding.

Communication of Findings. Involves the development of a research report that is disseminated effectively and efficiently to selected audiences.

Comparative Descriptive Designs. Designs to examine and describe differences in variables in two or more groups that occur naturally in a setting.

Comparison Step of a Critique. Involves examining the extent to which the researcher followed the "rules" for an ideal study; the ideal is compared to the real.

Comprehension Step of a Critique. Involves identifying and understanding the meaning of the explicit and implicit elements of the study.

Complex Hypothesis. An hypothesis that predicts the relationship between two (or more) independent and/or two (or more) dependent variables.

Computer Hardware. The machinery or physical equipment of the computer, which includes the input device, central processing unit (CPU), output device and external storage device.

Computerized Database. A structured compilation of information that can be scanned and retrieved by computer, enabling this data to be used in research.

Computer Software. The instructions or programs that direct the operations of the computer hardware.

Concept. A word or idea to which abstract meaning is attached.

Concept Analysis. A strategy that involves examining the attributes or characteristics of a concept.

Conceptual Clustering Step of a Critique. Current knowledge in a specific area of study is carefully analyzed, relationships are examined and the knowledge is organized theoretically. Conceptual clustering maximizes the meaning attached to research findings, highlights gaps in knowledge and generates new research questions.

Conceptual Definition. Defines the personal knowledge or connotative meaning of a word. These meanings are often difficult to express; the meaning is "known" but not easily put into words.

Conceptual Framework. An organization or matrix of concepts that provides a focus for inquiry.

Conclusions. Derived from the study findings, constituting a synthesis of the findings.

Concrete Thinking. Thinking that is oriented toward and limited by tangible things or events that are observed and/or experienced in reality. The focus of concrete thinking is immediate events that are limited by time and space.

Confidence Interval. A range within which the value of the population parameter is estimated to be.

Confidentiality. The management of private data in research so that subjects' identities are not linked with their responses.

Consent Form. A written, tape-recorded or videotaped form used to document a subject's agreement to participate in a study.

Construct Validity. The degree to which the instrument measures the construct being investigated. Thus, it examines the fit between the conceptual definitions and operational definitions.

Consultants. Individuals hired for a specific task during the study period.

Content Analysis. The technique that provides a systematic means of measuring the frequency, order or intensity of occurrence of words, phrases or sentences.

Content Validity. Verifies that the method of measurement actually measures the expected content. A subtype of content validity is face validity.

Control. The imposing of "rules" by the researcher to decrease the possibility of error and thus increase the probability that the study's findings are an accurate reflection of reality.

Control Group. The group of subjects that is not exposed to the experimental treatment; the response of the control group is compared with the experimental group(s).

Correlational Analysis. Statistical procedures conducted to determine the direction of a relationship (positive or negative) between two variables and the magnitude (or strength) of the relationship.

Correlational Coefficient. Indicates the degree of relationship between two variables; the coefficients range in value from +1.00 (perfect positive relationship) to 0.00 (no relationship) to −1.00 (perfect negative or inverse relationship).

Correlational Research. The systematic investigation of relationships between (among) two or more variables. The primary aim is to explain the nature of relationships in the real world and not to examine cause and effect.

Criterion-Referenced Testing. The comparison of a subject's score with a criterion of achievement that includes the definition of target behaviors. When these behaviors are mastered, the subject is considered proficient in the behavior.

Critical Analysis of Nursing Studies. The carefully thought out examination of a nursing study, in which the merits and faults and the meaning and significance of the study are examined. The critique process involves five steps: comprehension, comparison, analysis, evaluation and conceptual clustering.

Cross-Sectional Designs. Designs used to examine groups of subjects in various stages of development simultaneously with the intent of inferring trends over time.

Cultural Immersion. A technique used in ethnographic research for gaining increased familiarity with such things as language, sociocultural norms, traditions and other social dimensions in a culture.

Data. Pieces of information that are collected during a study.

Data Analysis. A mechanism for reducing and organizing data to produce findings that require interpretation by the researcher.

Data Coding Sheet. A sheet for organizing and recording data for rapid entry into the computer.

Data Collection. The precise, systematic gathering of information relevant to the research subproblems.

Debriefing. After the study is completed, subjects are informed of the actual purpose of the study and the results that were obtained.

Deception. The actual misinforming of subjects for research purposes.

Deductive Reasoning. Reasoning from a general premise to a particular situation or conclusion.

Degrees of Freedom (df). The freedom of a score's value to vary given the other existing scores' values and the established sum of these scores. Degrees of freedom equal the sample size minus 1 ($df = N - 1$).

Delphi Technique. A method of measuring the judgments of a group of experts, assessing priorities or making forecasts.

Dependent Variable. The response, behavior or outcome that the researcher wishes to predict or explain. Changes in the dependent variable are presumed to be caused by the independent variable.

Descriptive Research. Provides an accurate portrayal or account of characteristics of a particular individual, situation or group. These studies are a means of discovering new meaning, describing what exists, determining the frequency with which something occurs and/or categorizing information.

Design. Directs the researcher in planning and implementing the study in a way that is most likely to achieve the intended goal. It is a blueprint for the conduct of a study.

Developmental Grant Proposals. Proposals written to obtain funding for the development of a new program in nursing.

Diary. A record of events kept by a subject over time that is collected and analyzed by researchers.

Diffusion. In research, this is the process by which research findings are communicated through certain channels over time among the members of the discipline.

Diminished Autonomy. Subjects who have a decreased ability to voluntarily give informed consent because of legal or mental incompetence, terminal illness or confinement to an institution.

Directional Hypothesis. An hypothesis that states the specific nature of the relationship between two or more variables.

Empirical Generalization. The research findings that have been verified through multiple studies and gradually become a part of a discipline's scientific body of knowledge.

Ethical Principles. Principles relevant to the conduct of research involving human subjects: principle of respect for persons, principle of beneficence and principle of justice.

Ethnographic Research. The investigation of cultures through an in-depth study of the members of the culture. The ethnographic research process is the systematic collection, description and analysis of data to develop a theory of cultural behavior.

Evaluation Step of a Critique. This step involves examining the meaning and significance of the study according to set criteria. The present study is compared with previous studies conducted in the field of interest.

Experimental Designs. Designs that provide the greatest amount of control possible in order to more closely examine causality. Types of experimental designs include pretest-post-test control group design, post-test only control group design, Solomon four-group design, randomized block design, factorial designs, nested designs, multivariate designs, repeated measures designs with counterbalancing and randomized clinical trials.

Experimental Group. The subjects who are exposed to the experimental treatment.

Experimental Research. Objective, systematic, controlled investigation for the purpose of predicting and controlling phenomena. The purpose of this type of research is to examine probability and causality among selected variables.

Exploratory Research. Formative studies to gain new insights, discover new ideas and/or increase knowledge of a phenomenon.

External Criticism. A method of determining the validity of source materials in historical research. It involves knowing where, when, why and by whom a document was written.

External Storage Device or Secondary Memory. A mechanism for permanently storing data and programs.

External Validity. The extent to which study findings can be generalized beyond the sample used in the study.

Extraneous Variables. Variables that exist in all studies and that can affect the measurement of the study variables and the examination of the relationships within a study.

Fair Treatment, Right to. In research, the fair selection and treatment of subjects during the course of a study.

Findings. The translated and interpreted results from a study.

Frame of Reference or Framework. An abstract conceptualization that places the study within a context of meaning. A structure that links components of the study together and links the study findings to nursing's body of knowledge.

Framework. See Frame of Reference.

Frequency Distribution. A statistical procedure that involves listing all possible measures of a variable and tallying each datum on the listing.

Generalization. Extends the implications of the findings from the sample that was studied to the larger population.

Gestalt. Organization of knowledge about a particular phenomenon into a cluster of linked ideas. The clustering and interrelatedness enhance the meaning of the ideas.

Grounded-Theory Research. A type of research approach used in discovering what problems exist in a social scene and how the persons involved handle them. The research process involves formulation, testing and redevelopment of propositions until a theory is developed.

Hawthorne Effect. A psychological response in which the research subjects change their behavior simply because they are subjects in a study, not because of the research treatment.

Highly Controlled Settings. Artificially constructed environments that are developed for the sole purpose of conducting research, such as laboratories and research centers.

Historical Research. A narrative description or analysis of events that occurred in the remote or recent past.

History. An event that is not related to the planned study but occurs during the time of the study. History could influence the responses of subjects to the treatment.

Hypothesis. Formal statement of the expected relationships between two or more variables.

Implications. The meanings that the research conclusions have for the body of knowledge.

Incomplete Disclosure. Subjects are not totally informed about the purpose of a study because that knowledge might alter the subjects' actions. Following the study, the subjects must be debriefed.

Independent Variable. The treatment or experimental variable that is manipulated or varied by the researcher to create an effect on the dependent variable.

Indirect Measurement. Used with abstract concepts, when the concepts are not measured directly but, rather, indicators or attributes of the concepts are used to represent the abstraction.

Inductive Reasoning. Reasoning from particular instances to a general premise or conclusion.

Inferential Statistics. Statistics designed to allow inference from a sample statistic to a population parameter; commonly used to test hypotheses of similarities and differences in subsets of the sample under study.

Informed Consent. The prospective subject's agreement to voluntarily participate in a study, which is reached after assimilation of essential information.

Input Device. Enables the user to enter data and instructions into the computer system.

Institutional Review. A process in which a study is examined for ethical concerns by a committee of peers.

Instrumentation. The application of specific rules to develop a measurement device or instrument.

Internal Criticism. Involves examination of the reliability of historical documents.

Internal Validity. The extent to which the effects detected in the study are a true reflection of reality, rather than being due to the effects of extraneous variables.

Interpretation of Findings. The evidence from data analysis is carefully examined, organized and given meaning. The conclusions drawn from the findings provide the basis for making recommendations for further study.

Interrater Reliability. The degree of consistency between two raters who are independently assigning ratings to a variable being investigated.

Interrupted Time Series Designs. These designs are similar to descriptive time designs except that a treatment is applied at some point in the observations.

Interval Level Measurement. Interval scales have equal numerical distances between intervals of the scale in addition to following the rules of mutually exclusive categories, exhaustive categories and rank ordering. Temperature is an example of an interval scale.

Interviews. Structured or unstructured verbal communication between the researcher and the subject in which information is provided to the researcher.

Introspection. A process of turning your attention inward toward your own thoughts that is used in qualitative research.

Intuiting. Process of actually "looking at" the phenomenon; the individual focuses all awareness and energy on the subject of interest. A technique used in qualitative research.

Intuition. An awareness or knowing that seems to come unbidden. A feeling or sense that usually cannot be logically explained, "gut feeling" or "hunch."

Invasion of Privacy. When private information is shared without an individual's knowledge or against his or her will.

Kurtosis. The degree of peakedness of the curve shape that is related to the spread of variance of scores.

Landmark Studies. Major studies that generate knowledge that influences a discipline and sometimes society in general.

Level of Significance. The cut-off point used to determine whether the samples being tested are members of the same population or of different populations. The common levels of significance are 0.05 and 0.01.

Likert Scales. A scale designed to determine the opinion or attitude of a subject; it contains a number of declarative statements with a scale after each statement.

Limitations. Restrictions in the study that may decrease the generalizability of the findings. There are conceptual and methodological limitations.

Logic. A science that involves valid ways of relating ideas to promote human understanding.

Longitudinal Designs. Designs used to examine changes in the same subjects over an extended period of time.

Magnitude Estimation. A strategy to estimate the degree of difference between groups.

Magnitude Scale. A scale that is a line 100 mm in length. The extremes of stimuli are placed at each end of the line, and the subject is asked to place a mark through the line to indicate the intensity of the stimuli.

Maturation. The unplanned and unrecognized changes experienced during a study, such as growing older, wiser, stronger, hungrier or more tired, that can influence the findings of a study.

Mean. The value obtained by summing all the scores and dividing that total by the number of scores being summed.

Measurement. The process of assigning numbers to objects, events or situations in accord with some rule.

Measurement Error. The difference between what exists in reality and what is measured by a research tool.

Measures of Central Tendency. Statistical procedures for determining the center of a distribution of scores; mode, median and mean.

Measures of Dispersion. Statistical procedures for examining how scores vary or are dispersed around the mean. Measures of dispersion include range, difference scores, sum of squares, variance and standard deviation.

Median. The score at the exact center of the ungrouped frequency distribution.

Mentor. Someone who serves as a role model in scientific endeavors.

Meta-Analysis Design. A design that involves the merging of findings from many studies that have examined the same phenomenon.

Methodological Design. A design used to develop the validity and reliability of instruments to measure constructs used as variables in research.

Minimal Risk. The risks of harm anticipated in the proposed research are not greater, considering probability and magnitude, than those ordinarily encountered in daily life or during the performance of routine physical or psychological examinations or tests.

Mode. The numerical value or score that occurs with the greatest frequency in a distribution.

Model. A pictorial demonstration, using illustrations or mathematical formulas, that helps clarify the relationships being explained.

Mortality. Subjects drop out of a study before completion, which creates a threat to the internal validity.

Multivariate Analyses. Statistical techniques used to concurrently examine more than two variables; such techniques include multiple correlation, partial correlation, multiple regression, factor analysis, analysis of covariance and meta-analysis.

Natural Settings. Uncontrolled, real-life situations that are sometimes referred to as field settings.

Negative Relationship. The scores being correlated vary inversely (in opposite directions). Thus, when one score is high, the other score is low.

Networking. A process of developing channels of communication between people with common interests in many parts of the country.

Network Sampling. A sampling technique that takes advantage of social networks and the fact that friends tend to hold characteristics in common. When the researcher has found a few subjects with the needed criteria, they are asked for their assistance in getting in touch with others with similar characteristics.

Nominal Level Measurement. Lowest level of measurement that is used when data can be organized into categories that are exclusive and exhaustive, but the categories cannot be compared (for example, gender, race, marital status and nursing diagnoses).

Nondirectional Hypothesis. An hypothesis which states that a relationship exists but does not predict the exact nature of the relationship.

Nonequivalent Control Group Designs. Designs in which the control group is not selected by random means. Types of these designs include the one-group post-test only design, post-test only design with nonequivalent groups and one-group pretest-post-test design.

Nonparametric Statistics. Statistical techniques used when the assumptions of parametric statistics are not met.

Nonprobability Sampling. Not every element of the population has an opportunity for selection in the sample; examples include accidental sampling, quota sampling, purposive sampling and network sampling,.

Norm-Referenced Testing. The use of standardized tests that have been carefully developed over years and have extensive reliability and validity data available.

Normal Curve. A curve that is symmetrical and unimodal and has continuous values; also called a bell-shaped curve.

Null Hypothesis. An hypothesis that states that there is no relationship between the variables being studied.

Nursing Research. A scientific process that validates old knowledge and generates new knowledge that directly and indirectly influences clinical nursing practice.

Objectives, Research. Clear, concise declarative statements that direct research. Objectives state what characteristics of a variable are to be identified and/ or described.

Observational Measurement. The use of structured and unstructured observation to measure study variables.

Obtained Score. The actual score or value assigned to a subject on a measurement tool.

One-Tailed Test of Significance. An analysis used with directional hypotheses where extreme statistical values of interest are thought to occur on a single tail of the curve.

Open Context. Requires deconstruction of the sedimented view, which allows one to see the depth and complexity within the phenomenon being examined; used in qualitative research.

Operational Definition. A way of defining variables that makes them measurable in the real world.

Ordinal Level Measurement. Level of measurement in which data can be assigned to categories of an attribute that can be ranked. However, it cannot be demonstrated that the intervals between the ranked categories are equal, for example, levels of education, degrees of coping and levels of mobility.

Output Devices. Devices used to display, print or store the information generated from a computer.

Parameter. A characteristic of a population.

Parametric Statistics. Statistical techniques used when three assumptions are met: (1) the sample was drawn from a normal distribution, (2) random sampling techniques were used and (3) the data were measured at least at the interval level.

Partial Correlation Design. A design developed to eliminate the influence of a third variable and to determine the magnitude of the relationship between the two remaining variables.

Partially Controlled Setting. An environment that is manipulated or modified in some way by the researcher.

Path Analysis Design. Design developed to determine the accuracy of a theoretical model.

Personal Experience. Gaining knowledge by being personally involved in an event, situation or circumstance; used in qualitative research.

Phenomenological Research. An inductive, descriptive research approach, developed from phenomenological philosophy. The aim of phenomenological research is to describe an experience as it is lived by the person.

Physiological Measurement. Techniques used to measure physiological variables either directly or indirectly, for example, techniques to measure variables such as heart rate, mean arterial pressure and total lung capacity.

Pilot Study. Smaller version of a proposed study conducted to refine the methodology. It should be as similar to the proposed study as possible, using similar subjects, the same setting and the same data collection and analysis techniques.

"Pink Sheet." A letter indicating the rejection of a research grant proposal and a critique by the scientific committee that reviewed the proposal.

Population. All elements (for example, individuals, objects, events) that meet certain criteria for inclusion in a given universe.

Positive Relationship. The scores being correlated vary together (in the same direction). Thus, both the scores will be either high or low.

Power. The probability that a statistical test will detect a significant difference that exists; power analysis is conducted to determine the power of a study.

Predictive Validity or Criterion Validity. Determines the effectiveness of the instrument as a predictor of a future event.

Preproposal. A short document of four to five pages plus appendix that is written to explore the funding possibilities for a research project.

Primary Source. A source that is written by the person who originated or is responsible for generating the ideas published.

Principal Investigator (PI). In a research grant, the individual who will have primary responsibility for administering the grant and will interact with the funding agency during the period of the grant.

Privacy. The freedom an individual has to determine the time, extent and general circumstances under which private information will be shared with or withheld from others.

Probability Sampling. Sampling techniques in which every member (element) of the population has a probability higher than zero of being selected for the sample; also referred to as random sampling. Examples of probability sampling include simple random sampling, stratified random sampling, cluster sampling, systematic sampling and random assignment.

Problem-Solving Process. Systematic identification of a problem, determination of goals related to the problem, identification of possible solutions to achieve those goals, implementation of selected solutions and evaluation of goal achievement.

Process. Includes a purpose, a series of actions and a goal.

Projective Techniques. A method of measuring responses of individuals to unstructured or ambiguous situations as a means of describing attitudes, desires, personality characteristics and motives of the individuals. One such test is the Rorschach Inkblot Test.

Proposition. An abstract statement that further clarifies the relationship between two concepts.

Purposive Sampling. Judgmental sampling that involves the conscious selection by the researcher of certain subjects or elements to include in a study.

Q Sort. A technique of comparative rating where a subject sorts cards with statements on them into piles (usually 7 to 10 piles). The rating is from best to worst or from most useful to least useful.

Qualitative Research. A systematic, subjective approach used to describe life experiences and give them meaning.

Quantitative Research. A formal, objective, systematic process for obtaining information about the world. This research method is used to describe, test relationships and examine cause and effect relationships.

Quasi-Experimental Research. A type of research conducted to explain relationships and/or clarify why certain events happen. These studies are also a means of examining causality.

Query Letter. A letter sent to an editor of a journal to determine interest in publishing an article, or a letter sent to a funding agency to determine interest in funding a particular study.

Questionnaire. A printed self-report form designed to elicit information that can be obtained through written responses of the subject.

Question, Research. An interrogative statement that focuses on what variables are to be described and what relationships might exist among the variables.

Quota Sampling. An accidental sampling technique with an added feature—a strategy to ensure the inclusion of subject types that are likely to be underrepresented in the accidental sample.

Random Assignment. A process whereby each subject has an equal opportunity for being assigned to one group or another.

Random Error. An error that causes individuals' observed scores to vary haphazardly around their true score.

Random Sampling or Probability Sampling. A process whereby every member (element) of the population has a probability higher than zero of being selected for the sample.

Random Variation. The expected difference that occurs when one examines different subjects from the same population.

Range. The simplest measure of dispersion obtained by subtracting the lowest score from the highest score.

Ratio Level Measurement. Ratio level is the highest form of measure and meets all the rules of other forms of measure: mutually exclusive categories, exhaustive categories, rank ordering, equal spacing between intervals and a continuum of values. In addition, ratio level of measurement has an absolute zero, such as weight.

Reasoning. Processing and organizing knowledge for application to selected situations in order to reach conclusions.

Referencing. Comparing a subject's score against a standard. Two types of testing that involve referencing are norm-referenced testing and criterion-referenced testing.

Relevant Literature. Sources that are pertinent or highly important in providing the in-depth knowledge needed to study a selected problem.

Reliability. The degree of consistency that a measurement technique has in measuring the concept of interest.

Reliability Testing. A measure of the amount of random error in the measurement technique.

Replication. Repeating the work of other investigators.

Research. Diligent, systematic inquiry or investigation to validate old knowledge and generate new knowledge.

Research Grant Proposal. Proposal developed to obtain funding specifically to conduct a study.

Research Problem. A question or statement that clarifies the problem area to be investigated.

Research Proposal. A written plan that identifies the major elements of the study, such as the research problem, purpose, subproblems and frame of reference, and outlines the methods and procedures to be used in studying the subproblems.

Research Purpose. A clear, concise statement of "why" the study is being conducted or the goal of the study. The purpose is generated from the problem statement and focuses on the development of the study.

Research Subproblems. Research objectives, questions or hypotheses.

Research Topics. Broad problem areas that provide the basis for generating research problems.

Research Tradition. Indicates the conceptual boundaries for the domain of inquiry and provides prescriptive norms for how the domain is to be investigated.

Results. The outcomes from data analysis that are generated for each research subproblem.

Review of Relevant Literature. Conducted to determine the knowledge that currently exists concerning a selected research problem.

Rigor. The striving for excellence in research. Associated with discipline, scrupulous adherence and strict accuracy.

Robust. The analysis will yield accurate results even if some of the assumptions are violated by the data used for the analysis.

Role-Modeling. Learning by imitating the role and behaviors of an exemplar.

Sample. A subset of the population that is selected for a particular investigation.

Sampling. The process of selecting a group of people, events, behaviors or other elements that are representative of the population being studied.

Sampling Error. The difference between a sample statistic and a population parameter.

Scale. A self-report form of measurement that is composed of several items that are thought to measure the construct being studied. A scale requires the subject to rate a construct on a continuum; scales are often developed to measure psychosocial variables.

Science. A coherent, organized body of research findings and tested theories related to a specific field of knowledge. Science is both a product and a process.

Scientific Community. A cohesive group of scholars within a discipline who stimulate the creation of new research ideas and the development of innovative methodologies to conduct research.

Secondary Source. A source that summarizes and/or quotes content from primary sources.

Sedimented View. Seeing things within a specific frame of reference, world view or theory. This gives a sense of reality, certainty, security and, seemingly, control.

Seeking Approval for the Conduct and/or Funding of a Study. A process that involves submission of a research proposal to a selected group for review and, in many situations, verbally defending that proposal.

Semantic Differential. A scale that consists of two opposite adjectives with a seven-point scale between them. The subject is to select one point on the scale that best describes his or her view of the concept being examined.

Serendipity. The accidental discovery of something valuable during the conduct of a study.

Simple Hypothesis. An hypothesis that states a relationship between two variables.

Skewness. A curve that is not symmetrical that is developed from an asymmetrical distribution of scores.

Split-Half Reliability. The instrument items are split in half, and a correlational procedure is performed between the two halves. This strategy is a way of getting at test-retest reliability without administering the test twice.

Standard Deviation. A measure of dispersion that is calculated by taking the square root of the variance.

Standard Scores. Express deviations from the mean (difference scores) in terms of standard deviation units. Standard scores are called Z scores, where the mean is zero and the standard deviation is 1.

Statistic. A numerical value obtained from a sample used to estimate the parameters of a population.

Statistical Conclusion Validity. The concern with whether the conclusions about relationships drawn from statistical analysis are an accurate reflection of the real world.

Stratified Random Sampling. Sampling that is used in situations in which the researcher knows some of the variables in the population that are critical to achieving representativeness.

Subjects. Members of a sample who participate in a study.

Summary or Descriptive Statistics. Statistics that allow the researcher to organize the data in ways that give meaning and facilitate insight. Summary statistics include frequency distributions and measures of central tendency.

Survey Design. A design in which data are collected with questionnaires or through personal interviews about an identified population.

Systematic Sampling. Type of sampling conducted when an ordered list of all members of the population is available. The process involves selecting every kth individual on the list, using a starting point that is selected randomly.

Systematic Variance or Systematic Bias. A consequence of selecting subjects whose scores are different in some way from the population at large.

Target Population. The population from which the sample is chosen and to which study findings are generalized.

Testable Hypothesis. One that contains variables that are observable or measurable in the real world.

Test-Retest Reliability. Determination of the stability or consistency of a measurement technique by correlating the scores obtained from repeated measures.

Theoretical Framework. A general, abstract explanation of the interrelationships of the concepts to be investigated in a study; an expression of an existing theory.

Theory. A way of explaining some segment of the empirical world; an expression of a perception of a part of the empirical world.

Time Dimensional Designs. Designs used to examine sequence and patterns of change, growth or trends across time.

Time-Lag. The span of time between the generation of new knowledge through research and the use of this knowledge in practice.

Tradition. "Truths" or beliefs that are based on customs and past trends.

Trend Designs. Designs used to examine changes in the general population in relation to a particular phenomenon.

Trial and Error. Using an approach with an unknown outcome in a situation of uncertainty, where other sources of knowledge are unavailable.

t-test. A parametric test used to examine the difference between two means.

Two-Tailed Test of Significance. The analysis used for a nondirectional hypothesis where the researcher assumes that an extreme score can occur in either tail.

Type I Error. An error that occurs when the researcher concludes that the samples tested are from different populations (there is a significant difference between groups) when, in fact, the samples are from the same population (there is no significant difference between groups).

Type II Error. An error that occurs when the researcher concludes that there is no significant difference between the samples examined when, in fact, a difference exists.

Use of Researcher's Personality. In qualitative research, the researcher must use his or her personality to become closely involved with the subject's experience in order to interpret it. The researcher must remain open to the perceptions of the subject.

Utilization of Research Findings. The use of knowledge generated through research to guide nursing practice.

Validity. The determination of the extent to which the instrument actually reflects the abstract construct being examined.

Variable. Attributes, properties and/or characteristics of persons, events or objects that are examined in a study.

Variance. A measure of dispersion that is calculated by determining the mean of the sum of squares.

Author Index

Pages in *italics* refer to illustrations.

Subject Index

Note: Page numbers in italics refer to illustrations. Page numbers followed by t refer to tables.